Clinical Orthopedics for the Physical Therapist Assistant

Steven G. Lesh, MPA, PT, SCS, ATC

Assistant Professor of Physical Therapy
Arkansas State University
Jonesboro, Arkansas

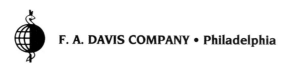

F. A. DAVIS COMPANY • Philadelphia

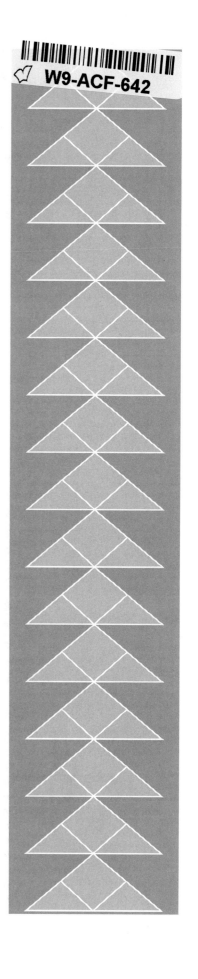

F. A. Davis Company
1915 Arch Street
Philadelphia, PA 19103

Printed in the United States of America

Last digit indicates print number: 10 9 8 7 6 5 4 3 2 1

Publisher: Jean-François Vilain
Developmental Editor: Sharon Lee
Cover Designer: Louis J. Forgione

As new scientific information becomes available through basic and clinical research, recommended treatments and drug therapies undergo changes. The author(s) and publisher have done everything possible to make this book accurate, up to date, and in accord with accepted standards at the time of publication. The authors, editors, and publisher are not responsible for errors or omissions or for consequences from application of the book, and make no warranty, expressed or implied, in regard to the contents of the book. Any practice described in this book should be applied by the reader in accordance with the professional standards of care used in regard to the unique circumstances that may apply in each situation. The reader is advised always to check product information (package inserts) for changes and new information regarding dose and contraindications before administering any drug. Caution is especially urged when using new or infrequently ordered drugs.

Library of Congress Cataloging-in-Publication Data

Lesh, Steven G.
    Clinical orthopedics for the physical therapist assistant / Steven G. Lesh.
      p. ; cm.
    Includes bibliographical references and index.
    ISBN 0-8036-0449-1
    1. Physical therapy.   2. Physical therapy assistants.   3. Orthopedics.   4. Orthopedics—Case studies. I. Title.
    [DNLM: 1. Musculoskeletal Diseases—therapy.   2. Orthopedic Procedures.
    3. Physical Therapy. WE 140 L629c 2000]
    RM701 .L47 2000
    616.7—dc21
                                     99-045181

DEDICATION

"To Diana, my wife, who helps me to see the world through the eyes of the PTA,
and to McKenzie and Reaghan, my daughters, who help me to see the world through the eyes of a child.
Thank you for granting me the strength and ability to complete this project."

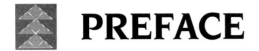

PREFACE

As we enter the twenty-first century, we in the physical therapy profession are under great pressure to graduate professionals from our academic programs to fill the demand of the private sector. Health-care reform, the aging population, and trends toward wellness in the United States have elevated physical therapy to one of the most sought-after occupations. The physical therapist assistant (PTA) has grown in popularity both within the profession and in the academic ranks. Community colleges have found the two-year PTA degree to be an attractive offering and have seen tremendous growth in enrollment.

This book was written especially to address the educational needs of the physical therapist assistant. Traditionally, PTA curricula used parts of or watered down versions of physical therapist textbooks, leaving a significant knowledge gap between what is presented to the PTA student and what is written. Most, if not all, texts were geared toward the prerequisite level of the PT, not the PTA student. With that deficit in mind, this text was created to provide PTA students with the knowledge and skills they need to become successful clinicians.

Because the PTA is moving from an exclusive role of modality technician to an integral part of the delivery of physical therapy services, the physical therapy profession must continue to improve the knowledge base of PTAs, if the PTA is expected to succeed in this expanded role. *Clinical Orthopedics for the Physical Therapist Assistant* is just such a textbook. It is designed to provide clinically relevant material to the PTA concerning the implementation of directed treatment plans. The text covers three broad sections, which present a general foundation of orthopedic principles, specific orthopedic conditions, and interactive case studies that allow the PTA student the opportunity to practice the newly acquired orthopedic concepts and develop critical inquiry skills.

The first section covers general orthopedic principles, including the role of the PTA in the implementation of physical therapy services, exercise principles, range of motion, mechanical properties of the human body, tissue response to healing, normal aging, and mobilization concepts. These are broad wide-ranging concepts that in their own right could constitute an entire textbook, but I feel it is beneficial to address these topics in the compact format of the PTA curriculum to give the PTA student a broad-based foundation related to orthopedic management.

The second section differs from most orthopedic textbooks in two ways. First, it follows the life-span development approach in covering orthopedic conditions rather than the traditional presentation by anatomically involved joints. Some practicing professionals find this difficult to follow. However, I argue that most physical therapy professionals treat their clients as individuals and not according to the anatomical joint that is involved. Therefore, it should be logical to study the client and then the condition, rather than the condition systematically applied to the client. I find it difficult to talk about total knee replacements and anterior cruciate ligament reconstructions in the same lecture even though both conditions involve the knee joint anatomically. These two conditions of the knee present different aspects of an individual's growth and development with different concerns and rehabilitation approaches. Second, this textbook has integrated the goals and preferred practice patterns found in the *Guide to Physical Therapy Practice* to help promote consistency and enhance delivery of physical therapy services provided by the PTA.

The final section of the text is an interactive case study approach to implementation of clinical orthopedics. This section, designed to work in conjunction with the lab instructor and lab instructor's guide, will expand the scenarios as clinical decisions are made or will alter the delivery of scenarios as unexpected conditions arise. Presented in the case studies are some of the clinical aspects related to orthopedic physical therapy that are covered in this textbook. The student will be asked to make clinical decisions within the scope of practice of the PTA, participate in academic investigations, and promote lifelong learning. This text should not be considered a complete reference book for all orthopedic cases that the PTA may encounter. Professional literature and other related texts should be used to develop a comprehensive inquiry into the orthopedic management of the physical therapy client. Also presented in this section are brief practice scenarios that give the student ample opportunity to simulate clinical experiences in orthopedic management.

I would like to thank the people at F. A. Davis who have made this an enjoyable experience, especially Jean-François Vilain, who took this chance on me to produce a textbook. My peer reviewers were a critical part of the final presentation of this text, and without them I could not have finished the project. A special thanks goes to the College of Nursing and Health Professions at Arkansas State University, which put up with me trying to meet my deadlines. Thanks to the ASU Radiologic Sciences Program and to the ASU Athletic Department for helping me to acquire figures for this text. To the wonderful people at One on One Gymnastics in Jonesboro, thanks for letting me take some pictures. Thanks to Kent Watkins for developing my pictures and helping me achieve my first professional goal of becoming a published photojournalist. I would like to thank all of my previous students who kept me on my toes and challenged me to promote greater learning. Lastly, a special thanks to all of my clients who taught me something new each day and gave me such pride to be a member of the physical therapy profession.

Steven G. Lesh, MPA, PT, SCS, ATC

REVIEWERS

Joyce Marie Peters, PT
Chair, PTA Program
Endicott College
Beverly, Massachusetts

Carol A. Maritz, MS, PT
Assistant Professor of PT
Assistant Director of PTA Program
Allegheny University of Health Science
Philadelphia, Pennsylvania

Jacqueline J. Shakar, MS, PT, AT
Program Director PTA
Mount Wachusett Community College
Worcester, Massachusetts

Alice F. Cain, PT
Associate Professor
Program Director PTA
Stark State College of Technology
Canton, Ohio

Christine Kowalski, M. Ad.Ed., PTA
Program Director PTA
Elgin Community College
Burlington, Wisconsin

Phillip H. Warren, MPH, MPT, OCS
Instructor
Fayetteville Technical Community College
Newton Grove, North Carolina

Julie Muertz, M.Ed., PT
PTA Program
Belleville Area College
Belleville, Illinois

CONTENTS

part I

GENERAL ORTHOPEDIC PRINCIPLES

chapter 1

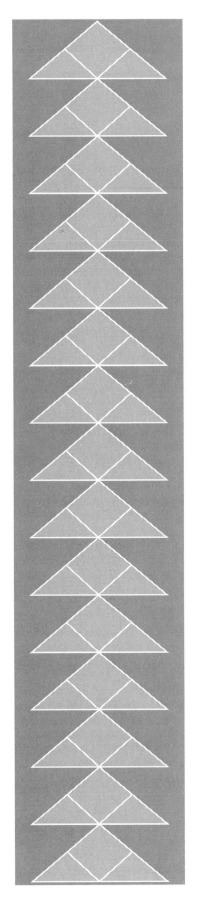

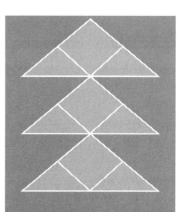

Role of the Physical Therapist Assistant in Orthopedics

OBJECTIVES

After reading this chapter, the PTA student will be able to:
1. Discuss the team concept of physical therapy as it relates to the orthopedic client, including the roles of each team member.
2. Discuss the role of the supervising physical therapist, including the appropriate level of supervision level for the PTA.
3. Discuss when the PTA can and cannot modify a treatment plan.
4. Identify the need for client education in physical therapy.
5. Discuss client compliance issues relevant to physical therapy intervention.

 # THE PHYSICAL THERAPIST ASSISTANT IN THE ORTHOPEDIC JOB MARKET

The profession of physical therapy has experienced a growth through the 1980s and 1990s unlike any other profession during the same period. Educational institutions have responded by increasingly graduating qualified clinicians to fill the significant job demand presented by the health-care industry. Physical therapist (PT) and physical therapist assistant (PTA) graduates have seen a steady supply of jobs available to them, with markets increasing in the fields of home health, long-term care, outpatient orthopedics, sports medicine, inpatient rehabilitation, pediatrics, and acute care. The PTA continues to grow in both supply and demand in all of these physical therapy fields, finding ample practice opportunities.

The role of the PTA in orthopedics continues to evolve as more graduates progressively enter the workplace and as legal reform changes the face of service delivery for the practice of physical therapy. PTA educational programs in the United States are graduating clinicians skilled in the uses of therapeutic exercise, modalities, and health education. In the orthopedic environment, the PTA is able to implement the orthopedic plan of treatment established by the supervising therapist to guide the client along the path of recovery after disability. Clients that may benefit from the therapeutic skills possessed by a PTA include those with joint replacements, muscular injuries, skeletal injuries, sports injuries, repetitive use injuries, traumatic injuries, and pediatric orthopedic injuries. This chapter identifies current issues relative to the legal, ethical, and practical roles of the PTA in the delivery of orthopedic physical therapy services.

PERCEPTION OF THE PHYSICAL THERAPIST ASSISTANT ROLE

Published studies relative to the perceived role of the PTA in delivering physical therapy services have stirred debate among professionals concerning the true role of the assistant. Schunk et al,[1] found in a survey of Oregon PTAs, that physical therapists often underuse the PTA in the delivery of physical therapy services. Robinson et al,[2] supported the same notion as late as 1992 when 51.6% of the respondent physical therapists reported not receiving information about the clinical roles of the PTA when they were in physical therapy school. Robinson concluded that there existed "evidence that therapist perceptions on selected activities are incongruent with guidelines outlining PTA function [which may suggest] the potential for inefficient or inappropriate utilization of the PTA." As the clinical roles of the PTA continue to mature, partial burden to educate health professionals on the proper use of the assistant may be placed on the shoulders of the PTA.

 TEAM APPROACH

THE CLIENT

The **team approach** constitutes the interacting of involved team members to achieve a common goal. The most important and significant team member for the profession of physical therapy is the client. The **client** is the person seeking skilled treatment for the alleviation of pain, restoration of lost function, or education on a medical condition. The client should be an active participant in the treatment program from beginning to end. Often in the medical community, the client is put into a passive participation role, having procedures done to him or her, having tests without understandable explanations, or receiving treatments lying passively in a room. When implementing a treatment program, the PTA should remember that the role of the client should be an active process. The assistant should work to educate and empower the clients to help themselves (Box 1–1).

THE PHYSICIAN

The traditional point of entry into the medical system has been the **physician**. The physician is the medical professional who diagnoses a condition for the client and prescribes appropriate medical intervention. This medical professional could potentially cover a wide referral base, including the medical doctor (MD), orthopedic surgeon, chiropractor (DC), osteopathic physician (DO), podiatrist

Team Approach
An approach that constitutes the interacting of involved team members to achieve a common goal.

Client
The person seeking skilled treatment for the alleviation of pain, restoration of lost function, or education on a medical condition.

Physician
The medical professional who diagnoses a condition for the client and prescribes appropriate medical intervention.

__ Box 1–1 _____

ACTIVE VERSUS PASSIVE PARTICIPATION OF THE CLIENT

Active Participation

- Asking the client to state his or her goals.
- Having the client demonstrate a home program for you.
- Finding ways for the client to alleviate his or her own pain.
- Allowing the client to express his or her concerns.
- Educating the client regarding the medical process.

Passive Participation

- Telling the client the goals of therapy.
- Giving the client a sheet and telling him or her to "do these at home."
- "Stating I [therapist] will make you [client] feel better."
- Telling the client what is typical for his or her condition.
- Funneling the client through the system.

(DPM), and dentist (DDS). The physician may identify a specific treatment protocol with duration and frequency or issue a general "evaluation and treat appropriately" order to the physical therapist.

The traditional role of the physician as the medical entry point is being challenged by recent legislative trends granting direct access to the physical therapy profession. **Direct access** allows the physical therapist to evaluate and treat a client without a medical referral. This recent trend in physical therapy continues to evolve and currently has different interpretations from state to state. Some states still require a medical referral for physical therapy, whereas others allow only a limited physical therapy evaluation. Still other states permit full physical therapy services without the client ever seeing a physician. A medical referral from a physician is typically required by most insurance companies to grant payment of physical therapy services rendered. This small but relevant issue is currently limiting the effectiveness of most physical therapy direct access legislation.

Direct Access
A form of health-care access that allows the PT to evaluate and treat a client without a medical referral.

THE THIRD-PARTY PAYER

Third-Party Payer
The party responsible for reimbursement of medical services provided by a medical professional.

The **third-party payer** is responsible for reimbursement for medical services provided by a medical professional. This team member is often overlooked in the delivery of health-care services, but if actively involved from the initial onset of the client's medical condition, can be a significantly helpful player. Prompt and accurate reimbursement of medical services provided to a client is critical to help cover the medical provider's expenses. If the third-party payer is involved early, ensuring that appropriate procedures are followed and benefits are confirmed, reimbursement may be received earlier than if the appropriate procedures were not followed. The reimbursement from the third-party payer can take several forms (Table 1–1) and can often dictate the extent or degree of services delivered.

Private Insurance Companies

The private insurance company has been the traditional form of coverage for the individual client receiving physical therapy services. Benefits are usually paid directly to the provider of the services for qualified conditions and treatments. In some cases, the benefits are paid to the individual, who then is responsible for paying the extent of the bill accrued from the provider.

Medicare

Medicare is the insurance program funded by the federal government that covers elderly and disabled persons (after a qualifying waiting period). This payer has been very influential in shaping the delivery of physical therapy services in the United States since its inception in 1965. Medicare currently has limitation caps on services available by the physical therapy profession, thus greatly limiting the amount of physical therapy that can be provided to Medicare recipients. A significant aspect to the degree in which physical therapy services are reimbursed by Medicare revolves around demonstrating an improvement in the functional status of the client.

___ *Table 1–1* ___

FORMS OF THIRD-PARTY PAYER REIMBURSEMENT	
Fee for Service	Paid to provider after qualified service, *or*
	Paid to individual after qualified service.
	Noncovered services are not reimbursable.
Capitation	Predetermined reimbursement rates per medical condition.
	Noncovered services are not reimbursable.
	Health maintenance organizations (HMOs).
	Qualified services are covered under plan, except benefits are
	not paid to the provider because the provider is employed
	directly by the HMO.
Self-Pay	Client pays out of own pocket.

Managed Care

Managed care is the aspect of third-party reimbursement that seeks to dictate coverage of medical services by medical providers. *Taber's*[3] defines managed care as "a variety of methods of financing and organizing the delivery of health care in which costs are contained by controlling the provisions of services." This aspect of reimbursement has been a proactive stance by the insurance companies to use statistical and fiscal management to define medical treatment and regulate perceived uncontrolled health-care spending. Through a series of contractual agreements and negotiated services, the insurance company develops a network of approved medical providers (hospitals, physicians, therapists). The managed care client may then seek medical attention from that established list of medical professionals. Typically, before physical therapy services can be rendered, the proposed plan of treatment or possibly even an evaluation must be approved by the managed care company. After the submission of necessary documentation, the managed care company will approve (or deny) reimbursement for an allotted number of treatment sessions. The therapy team must effectively manage the allowed number of treatment sessions to promote the functional return of the orthopedic client. As of the writing of this text, managed care has become heavily entrenched in the urban sectors of the United States and is gradually increasing its influence in the rural sectors. Managed care as a form of medical reimbursement will play a significant role in the shaping of physical therapy services over the next few years.

Health maintenance organizations (HMOs) are a specialized form of managed care. The client purchases a health-care program from a comprehensive medical provider with an emphasis on preventative medicine. All medical services must be preapproved and provided by the HMO, which typically owns and operates the medical facilities and employs the medical personnel. The option of seeking medical services outside of the HMO is generally discouraged, and the clients who do are usually not reimbursed.

Managed Care
A variety of methods of financing and organizing the delivery of health care in which costs are contained by controlling the provisions of services.

Case Managers

Case managers, when involved, are a vital aspect of the team approach in rehabilitation efforts and are frequently used in workers' compensation claims.

Case Manager
The team member responsible for coordinating health-care benefits for the involved client and monitoring effectiveness of the medical treatment.

The **case manager** is responsible for coordinating health-care benefits for the involved client and monitoring the effectiveness of the prescribed medical treatment. Periodically, the case manager may attend treatment sessions or physicians' appointments with the client. The team must communicate effectively with the case manager to ensure that the benefits for the client will be maximized.

PHYSICAL THERAPIST

Physical Therapist (PT)
The team member who evaluates the client's medical condition, establishes the physical therapy diagnosis, determines the plan of treatment, delegates appropriate services, periodically re-evaluates the client, supervises the PTA, and may or may not implement treatment.

The **physical therapist** (PT) is the team member who evaluates the client's medical condition (either on referral from a physician or via direct access), determines a physical therapy diagnosis, establishes the plan of treatment complete with appropriate therapeutic goals, delegates appropriate services, and periodically re-evaluates the client. The PT also supervises the PTA, the athletic trainer (in some clinical settings), and support personnel. Implementation of the prescribed treatment may or may not be an active role of the PT. In some settings, such as rehabilitation hospitals or outpatient clinics, the PT may evaluate and treat his or her own clients without significant use of the assistant. In other settings, such as long-term care facilities and acute care facilities, the PT may evaluate and delegate the treatment program to the assistant serving in the supervisory role.

The use of the assistant by the PT in the various settings may depend on several factors. First, the physical therapist may have an organizational system within the facility that either dictates or prohibits the use of assistants for some or all medical conditions. Second, the use of the assistant by the PT may revolve around a comfort level or bias by the supervising therapist. Some PTs may or may not feel comfortable using the PTA. Third, legal issues may dictate to what extent an assistant can be used. Some states prohibit the assistant from delivering physical therapy services when the supervising therapist is not readily available. Lastly, reimbursement issues may dictate the use or nonuse of the assistant. Some insurance companies may limit reimbursement for different levels of professional intervention.

ATHLETIC TRAINER

Athletic Trainer (AT)
The team member who provides for the care and prevention of athletic injuries in traditional or clinical settings.

A special member of the orthopedic team is the **athletic trainer** (AT). Traditionally, the AT works with a sports team at the professional, collegiate, or secondary level providing for the care and prevention of athletic injuries. In recent years, however, ATs are increasingly being found in outpatient clinics working with private-pay clients or in community outreach programs. Licensure laws for the AT vary tremendously from state to state in terms of granting or prohibiting certain actions and interventions in a nontraditional athletic training environment.

PHYSICAL THERAPIST ASSISTANT

Physical Therapist Assistant (PTA)
The team member who implements the plan of treatment, monitors the effectiveness of services, and ensures the safety of the client.

The role of the **physical therapist assistant** (PTA) on the orthopedic team is to implement the plan of treatment established by the PT, monitor the effectiveness of delivered services by interim assessments, modify delivery of services according to established standards, and ensure the safety of the client. The PTA must communicate effectively with all appropriate team members to report the progression or regression of the client during the implemented physical therapy services.

PHYSICAL THERAPY AIDE OR TECHNICIAN

In states where it is allowed by law, facilities may choose to use nonlicensed personnel to aid in the delivery of physical therapy services. The physical therapy aide or physical therapy technician typically possesses on-the-job training with a few facilities having a certification process for their employees. The roles for the aide or technician are to prepare the area and to clean up the facilities used by the PT or the PTA. The operative aspect of this team member is that he or she is nonlicensed and should not be placed in a position to monitor the safety of the client or to determine the effectiveness of the treatment protocol.

SUPERVISION OF THE PHYSICAL THERAPIST ASSISTANT

AMERICAN PHYSICAL THERAPY ASSOCIATION GUIDE FOR CONDUCT

The American Physical Therapy Association (APTA) House of Delegates adopted (1982) and later amended (1991) the "Standards of Ethical Conduct for the Physical Therapist Assistant," providing an ethical framework for the practice affiliate (PTA) members.[4] Standard 1 of the document states that "physical therapist assistants provide service under the supervision of a physical therapist," and Standard 4 states that "physical therapist assistants provide services within the limits of the law." The interpreting standards by the APTA regarding PTA supervision are listed in Box (1–2).

Legal Issues

Many states have adopted specific practice acts defining the role of the PTA in clinical practice. Some states identify specific time frames between evaluation by the PT and subsequent re-evaluations, whereas other states define direct supervision and general supervision. Many states use national guidelines set by the APTA for designing practice acts, but the end result after the political process is that the rules for each state vary. Liability issues for the PTA revolve around the accepted practice for the PTA in his or her state or jurisdictional region. The PTA should investigate the applicable laws of his or her particular state pertaining to the practice as a PTA, because the statues may not be identical to the guidelines suggested by the national associations.

MODIFICATIONS OF THE TREATMENT PLAN

The PTA is generally not permitted to modify the treatment plan. Exceptions present for allowable modifications by the PTA in response to changes in the client's acute physiological status. Some debate exists and varies among state practice acts as to whether the PTA can make incremental changes within the scope of the treatment plan to progress the client toward meeting established goals. See Box 1–3 for a further discussion of appropriate and inappropriate changes in treatment plans by the PTA.

For the PTA to deliver safe and effective treatment, the assistant must have a working knowledge of all appropriate indications, precautions, and contraindications for the client's medical condition, as well as a strong background in the

Box 1–2

GUIDE FOR CONDUCT OF THE AFFILIATE MEMBER

Standard 1: Physical therapist assistants provide services under the supervision of a physical therapist.

1.1 *Supervisory Relationship*

- Physical therapist assistants shall work under the supervision and direction of a physical therapist who is properly credentialed in the jurisdiction in which the physical therapist assistant practices.

1.2 *Performance of Services*

a. Physical therapist assistants may not initiate or alter a treatment program without prior evaluation by and approval of the supervising physical therapist.
b. Physical therapist assistants may modify a specific treatment procedure in accordance with changes in patient status.
c. Physical therapist assistants may not interpret data beyond the scope of their physical therapist assistant education.
d. Physical therapist assistants may respond to inquiries regarding patient status to appropriate parties within the protocol established by a supervising physical therapist.
e. Physical therapist assistants shall refer inquiries regarding patent prognosis to a supervising physical therapist.

(From APTA, 111 N. Fairfax St., Alexandria, VA 22314-1488, with permission.)

Box 1–3

MODIFICATIONS IN THE PLAN OF TREATMENT BY THE PHYSICAL THERAPIST ASSISTANT

Three scenarios are presented describing situations in such away that the PTA has the opportunity to modify in the plan of treatment (POT). One is clearly appropriate, one falls into a gray area of appropriateness, and the third is clearly inappropriate.

Scenario A: Appropriate Modification of an Established Plan of Treatment

The PTA is working in an acute care hospital with a client who recently underwent a total knee replacement. The POT calls for (1) continuous passive motion for 3 hours two times per day, (2) gait training with a standard walker over level surfaces, (3) therapeutic exercises including heel slides, quad sets, ankle pumps, and straight-leg raises.

   The PTA upon arriving at the morning treatment session listens to complaints from the client about how bad the back of her knee and calf hurt last night. Upon examination of the client's surgical knee, the PTA observes

(Continued)

Box 1–3

MODIFICATIONS IN THE PLAN OF TREATMENT BY THE PHYSICAL THERAPIST ASSISTANT (Continued)

warmth and redness over the posterior aspect of the knee and calf. Upon squeezing the posterior calf and simultaneously dorsiflexing the ankle (Homans' sign), the client reports pain.

The PTA decides to change the POT for the morning session, halting all therapies and activity, and consults the supervising PT immediately. In this scenario, the PTA suspects a possible deep venous thrombosis and appropriately changes the POT to ensure the safety of the client.

Scenario B: Gray Area Modification of an Established Plan of Treatment

The PTA is working in an acute care hospital with a client who recently underwent a total hip replacement. The POT calls for (1) therapeutic exercises of gluteal sets, straight-leg raises, heel slides, and ankle pumps; (2) gait training over level surfaces with a standard walker; and (3) transfer training. One of the long term goals includes client to be independent with gait skills using appropriate assistive device over level surfaces short functional distances.

After working extensively with the client on gait skills using a standard walker, an uncomplicated progression of the client moves toward independent use of the walker. The PTA chooses to progress the assistive device from a walker to a straight cane.

In this scenario, this presents a gray area of whether it is or is not appropriate to modify the plan of treatment. Clearly, the POT calls for a standard walker, but the goals suggest progressing to the most functional and appropriate assistive device. An appropriate way for the PTA to practice safely is to discuss the progression with the supervising therapist before acting.

Scenario C: Inappropriate Modification of an Established Plan of Treatment

The PTA is working in an outpatient clinic with a client with a diagnosis of rotator cuff strain. The established POT calls for (1) moist heat, (2) ultrasound, and (3) passive range of motion (PROM) to the involved shoulder.

After working with the client for 1 week with no improvement, the PTA decides to change treatment modalities from ultrasound to interferential current and from PROM to active range of motion.

In this scenario, this modification of treatment is clearly inappropriate and outside the scope of practice of the PTA. If this situation had actually occurred, the PTA would be performing an act of commission exposing himself or herself to possible liability claims and possible job dismissal.

rationale for the therapeutic interventions. The physical therapy services are being delegated by the supervising therapist to the PTA for the safe and effective delivery to the client.

Client Safety

Client safety during the delivery of treatment procedures must be the foremost consideration of the assistant. During the treatment interaction with the client, the assistant should be continually observing the client's responses both physiologically and psychologically. In relation to physiological concerns, the assistant should understand normal bodily parameters and be able to respond accordingly to changes in heart rate, blood pressure, respiratory rate, pain, and level of consciousness. Psychologically, the assistant should be aware of motivational concerns and compliance issues. The PTA should be able to discuss the positive and negative aspects of the treatment program with the supervising PT to ensure the most effective delivery of physical therapy services. Other areas related to client safety include (1) ensuring that the equipment is in a safe and working order, (2) practicing within the boundaries of educational background, and (3) using proper body mechanics and guarding techniques.

 ## CLIENT EDUCATION

Client Education
A planned learning experience using a combination of methods such as teaching, counseling, and behavior modification techniques that influence patients' knowledge and health behavior.

Client education as defined by Bartlett[5] is "a planned learning experience using a combination of methods such as teaching, counseling and behavior modification techniques which influence patients' knowledge and health behavior." Gahimer and Domholdt[6] concluded that client education in physical therapy is regularly provided covering information about the medical condition and home program instruction. In the profession of physical therapy, striving to restore lost function is one of the critical motivators. By educating the client and related parties, physical therapy professionals can enhance the therapeutic benefits of their services. Education can take the forms:

> Verbal Instruction
> Active Demonstration by the Clinician
> Handwritten Instructions
> Preprinted Exercise Programs
> Educational Handouts Regarding Medical Condition, Wellness, and Stress
>   Relief
> Videos on Medical Condition
> Support Groups
> Community Resources
> Internet Resources on Medical Condition
> Educational Classes (e.g., Back School)

Repetition is usually critical for most people to become familiar with a task or behavior. To ensure that the education message was received by the client, the PTA can (1) repeat instructions, (2) have the client verbally repeat the instructions, or (3) have the client demonstrate the activity. The PTA as part of the orthopedic team must be able to participate actively in the education of clients, their families, and other health-care providers to promote positive outcomes in the field of physical therapy.

COMPLIANCE

Compliance is the willingness of the client to regularly perform an exercise program or implement the suggested therapeutic intervention. The issue of compliance with home exercise programs in physical therapy is of great concern, not only from the standpoint of improving a client's medical condition, but also from that of judging the effectiveness of the prescribed treatment. Home exercise programs, suggestions by the therapist, or lifestyle changes may or may not be effective for a specific client. Effectiveness of a treatment program can only be judged when the client has been compliant with the physical therapy instructions. When a client is compliant with the program recommendations, improvements may be observed. However, if no improvements are noted, then changes in the program may be implemented.[7] Sluijs et al.[8] have identified three factors that strongly correlate to the noncompliance of clients performing recommended exercise programs. These include (1) perceived barriers by the client, (2) lack of positive feedback, and (3) perceived helplessness by the client (Box 1–4).

During the implementation of the physical therapy plan of treatment, the PTA plays a critical role in ensuring compliance of the client. Methods to improve compliance that the PTA can use include (1) identifying reasons for noncompliance, (2) involving the client in constructing a solution, (3) making home programs fit the client's schedule and needs, (4) giving positive feedback, (5) empowering the client to help himself or herself, and (6) educating the client on the need for exercise.

 ## SUMMARY

The team approach to health care is the interaction of the involved team members to achieve a common goal. The most important member of the team is the client who is seeking skilled medical treatment and should be empowered to be an active participant. The team also consists of the physician, who diagnoses and prescribes appropriate medical treatment; the third-party payer, who is responsible for the payment of approved medical services; the case manager, who coordinates and monitors medical services; the PT, who evaluates, re-evaluates, delegates, and supervises physical therapy services; the AT, who provides for the prevention and care of athletic injuries; and the PTA, who implements the plan of

Compliance
The willingness of the client to regularly perform an exercise program or implement the suggested therapeutic intervention.

Box 1–4

COMMON COMPLAINTS FROM CLIENTS LEADING TO NONCOMPLIANCE

- "Exercising takes too much of my time."
- "I don't like to exercise."
- "These exercises weren't adjusted to my needs."
- "There are not enough hours in the day to exercise."
- "I forgot to exercise."
- "It hurts to exercise."

treatment and ensures client safety. The PTA practices under the supervision of a properly credentialed PT and adjusts the plan of treatment only in response to changes in client status to ensure client safety. Client education is the learning process by which health-care professionals attempt to influence the attitudes and behaviors of clients to promote positive successes of prescribed treatments. Compliance is the willingness of the client to regularly perform or accept the suggested therapeutic intervention. Changes to a therapeutic program or evaluation of successes (or failures) can be made only if a client has been compliant. The PTA plays a critical role in helping the client to be compliant with the prescribed program. Complete Case Study 1 (p. 469) for a review of the concepts in this chapter.

 # REFERENCES

1. Schunk, C, et al: PTA practice: In reality. Clinical Management 12(6):88, 1992.
2. Robinson, AJ, et al: Physical therapists' perception of the roles of the physical therapist assistant. Phys Ther 74:571, 1994.
3. Taber's Cyclopedic Medical Dictionary, ed 18th. FA Davis, Philadelphia. p 1159.
4. Guide for Conduct of the Affiliate Member: APTA Core Documents. PT Magazine of Physical Therapy 6(1):81, 1998.
5. Bartlett, EE: At last, a definition (editorial). Patient Education and Counseling 7:323, 1985.
6. Gahimer, JE, and Domholdt, E: Amount of patient education in physical therapy practice and perceived effects. Phys Ther 76:1089, 1996.
7. Sluijs, EM, and Knibbe, JJ: Patient compliance with exercises: Different theoretical approaches to short-term and long-term compliance: Patient Education and Counseling. 17:191, 1991.
8. Sluijs, EM, et al: Correlates of exercise compliance in physical therapy. Phys Ther 73:771, 1993.

 # BIBLIOGRAPHY

Bartlett, EE: At last, a definition (editorial). Patient Education and Counseling 7:323, 1985.

Gahimer, JE, and Domholdt, E: Amount of patient education in physical therapy practice and perceived effects. Phys Ther 76:1089, 1996.

Guide for Conduct of the Affiliate Member: APTA Core Documents. PT Magazine of Physical Therapy. 6(1):81, 1998.

Robinson, AJ, et al: Physical therapists' perception of the roles of the physical therapist assistant. Phys Ther 74:571, 1994.

Schunk, C, et al: PTA practice: In reality. Clinical Management 12(6):88, 1992.

Sluijs, EM, et al: Correlates of exercise compliance in physical therapy. Phys Ther 73:771, 1993.

Sluijs, EM, and Knibbe, JJ: Patient compliance with exercises: Different theoretical approaches to short-term and long-term compliance: Patient Education and Counseling 17:191, 1991.

Taber's Cyclopedic Medical Dictionary, ed 18. FA Davis, Philadelphia. p 1159.

chapter 2

Exercise Principles

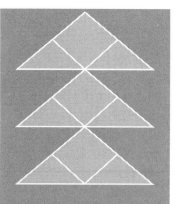

Skeletal Muscle
The organ system responsible for producing active motion at joints and maintaining upright posture by generating force through a series of contracting, lengthening, or holding. The two methods by which strength gains can be realized are the hypertrophy of muscle fibers and the increased recruitment of motor units.

OBJECTIVES

After completing this chapter, the PTA student will be able to:
1. Identify the structural components of human skeletal muscle.
2. Discuss the importance of the all-or-none law in orthopedic rehabilitation.
3. Discuss the overload principle of muscle strengthening.
4. Relate physiological limitations to strengthening.
5. Discuss the clinical significance of the terms *muscular strength, muscular endurance*, and *muscular power*.
6. Differentiate types of exercise, giving positive and negative effects related to orthopedic rehabilitation.
7. Identify the elements of the exercise prescription.
8. Identify various types of exercise equipment used in orthopedic rehabilitation.

 ## STRUCTURE OF THE MUSCLE

Skeletal muscle is the organ system responsible for producing active motion at joints and maintaining upright posture by generating force through a series of shortening, lengthening, or holding events. The size and shape of a muscle are related to the functional demands of the muscle, but despite the great functional differences of many of the skeletal muscles, the cellular structure remains about the same.[1-3] As stated by Binder-Macleod[4] in his introduction to the special skeletal muscle series published in P*hysical Therapy*, "Understanding the structure and function of skeletal muscle is central to the practice of physical therapy." This chapter provides the PTA student with an overview of the anatomic and histological structure of human skeletal muscle, followed by a discussion of the exercise principles and applications used in physical therapy relative to the functioning of muscle tissue.

Skeletal muscle is typically referred to as voluntary or striated muscle. The term *voluntary* is used because the muscle can be controlled consciously. The muscle is considered *striated* because of the microscopic appearance of the fibers. The striated appearance is the representation of the **sarcomere**, which is the functional contractile unit of the muscle containing the actin and myosin protein cross-bridges. See Figure 2–1 for a breakdown of the components within the sarcomere. The sarcomere is encased in a cell membrane called the sarcolemma, which houses the transverse tubules (T-tubules) that transmit the action potential to the interior of the muscle, resulting in a muscle contraction.[5] Functionally, the muscle is divided into contractile elements, which are responsible for force generation; and noncontractile elements, which join the muscle to the bone. Many sarcomeres, cylindrical in shape, form a myofibril; in turn, many myofibrils form a muscle fiber. Many muscle fibers are joined to form a fascicle, and many fascicles form a muscle (Fig. 2–2).

A continuous network of connective tissue envelops the contractile elements found within skeletal muscle. This network allows for the transfer of forces from the contracting muscle to the bony structure to produce movement. The noncontractile elements or connective tissue surrounding the muscle fiber is referred to as

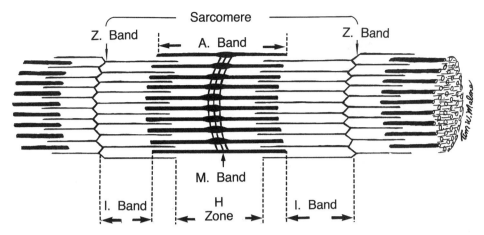

FIG. 2–1

The sarcomere. The portion of the myofibril located between the Z bands is the sarcomere. The A band represents the overlap of the actin and myosin filaments. The H zone contains only myosin and the I band contains only actin. (From Norkin & Levangie, p 95, with permission.)

endomysium. Surrounding the fascicle is the connective tissue called perimysium, and the epimysium surrounds the muscle in its entirety (see Fig. 2–3). The outer sheath of the muscle continues into the tendon and is attached to bones by Sharpey's fibers that become continuous with the periosteum of the bone. The noncontractile component of skeletal muscle is a frequent site of injury in orthopedic conditions.[1,3]

Neurologically, the muscle fibers are stimulated to contract from a single anterior horn cell found in the spinal cord. The connection is made via a single alpha motor neuron carried within a peripheral nerve (axon) to the muscle (motor end plate), where it divides into a few or many branches. The muscle fiber is innervated only from one anterior horn cell, but an anterior horn cell may innervate several muscle fibers. The alpha motor neuron and all of the muscle fibers that it innervates is referred to as a **motor unit** (Fig. 2–4A).[3,6] If a motor unit innervates many muscle fibers, then that particular motor unit will tend to be used in gross motor activities. Examples include the muscles used for knee extension or ankle plantar flexion. Conversely, if a motor unit has only a few muscle fibers under its control, then that motor unit will tend to be more oriented towards fine motor skills, such as finger flexion (Fig 2–4B).[1,3]

For a motor unit to be activated, an adequate (or threshold) stimulus from the anterior horn cell must be transmitted. If the threshold is reached, then a contraction of the muscle fibers associated with the motor unit is realized. Different motor units have different levels of threshold activation. Some are very sensitive, needing only a relatively small threshold to be reached before activation. Others require a greater amount of stimulus before the threshold is reached and a muscular contraction is produced. As the muscle fibers contract, tension is developed within the body of the muscle to perform the desired activity. The varying thresholds of motor unit activation allow for a graded or progressive contraction of the entire muscle. For motor tasks requiring only a small amount of muscular force, the lower threshold motor units are stimulated. However, for task requiring greater amounts of force, a larger stimulus is produced, activating all of the motor units equal to or less than the threshold level

Sarcomere
The functional contractile unit of the muscle containing actin and myosin cross-bridges.

Motor Unit
The alpha motor neuron and all of the muscle fibers it innervates.

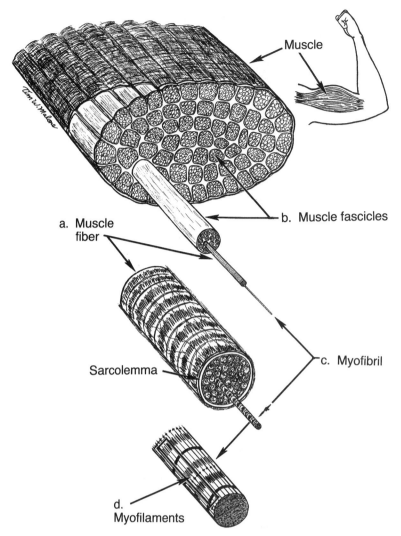

FIG. 2–2
Composition of skeletal muscle. (A) The muscle fiber is enclosed in a cell membrane called the **sarcolemma.** (B) Groups of muscle fibers form bundles called **fasciculi.** (C) The muscle fiber contains myofibrillar structures called **myofibrils.** (D) The myofibril is composed of thick myosin and thin actin myofilaments. (From Norkin & Levangie, p 94, with permission.)

transmitted. The threshold concept is demonstrated by activating enough motor units to hold an egg between the thumb and index finger without damaging the egg. If a greater stimulus is transmitted, then more motor units with greater thresholds will be activated, causing the thumb and index finger to break the egg.

All-or-None Law
Law referring to the fact that each muscle fiber contracts maximally or not at all.

The **all-or-none law** refers to the fact that each muscle fiber contracts maximally or not at all after the threshold stimulus has been reached. The understanding of this principle is critical when applying the exercise principles that are discussed later in this chapter. When a motor unit is adequately stimulated, all of the muscle fibers of that particular motor unit will contract fully or not at all. This, however, does not mean that the entire muscle is fully contracted every time a motor unit is stimulated. As discussed previously, a muscle may have few or many motor units

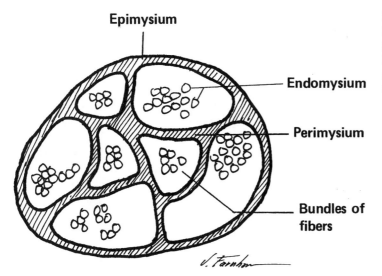

Epimysium

Endomysium

Perimysium

Bundles of fibers

FIG. 2–3
Muscular connective tissue. A schematic cross-sectional view of the connective tissue in a muscle. Notice that the inner layers of the perimysium are continuous with the outer layers of the epimysium (From Norkin & Levangie, p 103, with permission.)

in its entirety. The process of fully contracting the muscle is achieved by the repeated firing of motor units asynchronously or at differing times. The force of the muscular contraction also is varied by the number of motor units activated or by the frequency of the motor units activated.[3] See Box 2–1 for a discussion of synchronous versus asynchronous contraction of skeletal muscle.

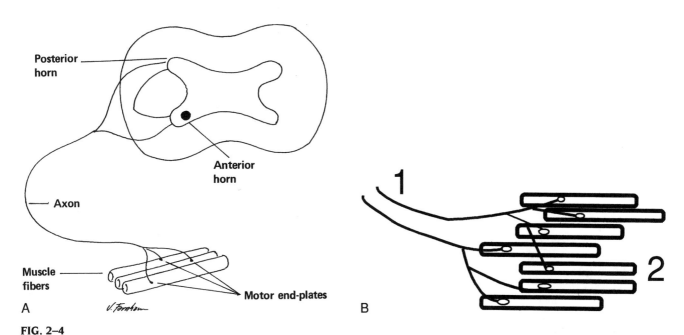

Posterior horn

Anterior horn

Axon

Muscle fibers

Motor end-plates

A

B

FIG. 2–4
(A) Motor unit (From Norkin & Levangie, p 98, with permission.) **(B) Motor unit.** The motor axon (1) innervates many or few muscle fibers (2) making a motor unit. The size of the motor unit can range from several thousand muscle fibers per motor axon to as few as three muscle fibers per motor axon. The muscle fibers need not be adjacent to receive stimulation from the motor axon.

_ Box 2–1 _

SYNCHRONOUS VERSUS ASYNCHRONOUS MUSCULAR CONTRACTION

The human body demonstrates a wide spectrum of muscle contraction (tension development) ability, from fine-skilled motor movement to gross powerful motor movement. This amazing ability can be demonstrated in almost every muscle in the body and is realized by the ability of the central nervous system to identify exactly how many motor units are needed for a particular task, how often the motor units need to be activated, and in what order the motor units are to be activated. Some constants (assuming the absence of pathology) exist in the motor unit contraction system, and those include (1) the speed at which the impulse travels from the anterior horn cell to the motor end plate, and (2) that every muscle fiber innervated in that particular motor unit will contract fully or not at all (all-or-none law).

For a slow-skill movement, the central nervous system tends to recruit the smaller-sized motor units first and tends to properly time the activation of those units to complete the task. If a fast, powerful movement is needed, then the central nervous system will again activate from smaller to larger motor units in a rapid fashion to produce enough tension within the muscle to complete the task. If a sustained contraction is needed, the nervous system will fire selected motor units repeatedly and asynchronously to sustain a smooth contraction before fatiguing. A tetanic contraction is when the muscle contracts fully firing every motor unit in a synchronous fashion. This is seen in pathological conditions such as tetany or seizure disorders and can result in fatigue and damage of the muscular elements. Clinically, physical therapy professionals can produce a synchronous tetanic muscle contraction through the use of functional electrical stimulation or neuromuscular stimulation. I have often thought the term "functional" electrical stimulation was an oxymoron because the muscle contraction that is produced via the electrical stimulation is not how the muscle functionally contracts in the human body. The electrical stimulation that excites the motor units tends to recruit larger motor units first without any benefit of asynchronous timing of the central nervous system. I am a big believer in the use of electrical stimulation in muscular rehabilitation, but the PTA must realize the benefits and limitations of this modality and allow adequate rest time to prevent fatigue as well as to encourage the client to participate actively in the muscle contraction, trying to restore normal asynchronous timing of the impaired muscle.

Overload Principle
Principle that states that to produce a strength change in skeletal muscle, the muscle must be progressively overloaded past the metabolic and physiological capacity of the selected muscle.

 RESISTIVE AND OVERLOAD PRINCIPLE

In beginning the discussion of the principles behind the therapeutic exercises prescribed in physical therapy, how skeletal muscles respond to exercise and stress is presented. The **overload principle** is related to the concept that in order to produce an adaptive strength change in skeletal muscle, the muscle must be progressively overloaded past the metabolic and physiological capacity of the selected muscle.[7–9] The **specificity of exercise principle** demonstrates that gains and adaptations of the trained muscle will only be realized in the patterns in which the muscle is exercised. For example, training the triceps brachii muscle by performing elbow extension against a resistance will strengthen the triceps performing that motion. It will not, however, make the triceps muscle more efficient at throwing a football. To make the entire arm more efficient at throwing a football, a client must eventually throw a football. The **reversibility principle** is simply stated in the old saying, "If you don't use it, then you'll lose it." Adaptive changes that are gained in a muscle after training will begin to reverse in as little as 3 days if the program of exercise is halted.[9–11] Clinically, these principles are significantly relevant to the programs of rehabilitation that are designed and implemented. If weak muscles are not stressed enough to produce an adaptive physiological change, then none will occur. If you focus on quadriceps femoris strengthening only by performing quad sets (isometric), then the muscle may not be ready for the eccentric demands of functional gait activities. If the continuation of a successful rehabilitation program is not pursued, then the client may lose the strength gains and positive benefits that were achieved.

Specificity of Exercise Principle
Principle that states that gains and adaptations of the trained muscle will be realized only in the patterns in which they are exercised

Reversibility Principle
Principle that states that adaptive changes realized in a muscle will reverse if program of exercise is halted.

PHYSIOLOGICAL LIMITATIONS

Each of the previously mentioned principles will have limiting factors depending on the size, shape, and characteristics of skeletal muscle. The type of fibers found within the muscle, the ability to generate force within a muscle, and the method by which fuel is produced for the working muscle will also limit the abilities of the clinician to strengthen or train the muscle.

FIBER TYPES

For the purpose of discussion in this text, two general types of fibers found in skeletal muscle are discussed: (1) slow twitch and (2) fast twitch. There are in fact several subcategories identified in skeletal muscle fibers as well as an extensive, complex body of knowledge that examines the utilization of fiber types (Table 2–1).[12–15] Slow-twitch fibers (type I fibers) are generally fatigue resistant and tend to contract slowly. The function of slow-twitch fibers is to perform long-duration tasks. Fast-twitch fibers (type II fibers) tend to fatigue significantly faster than slow-twitch ones, but are capable of generating forceful contractions at a faster rate than slow-twitch fibers. Type II fibers are geared toward functional use in anaerobic or short-duration activities requiring high intensity. Each skeletal muscle constitutes a blend of these two fiber types giving a tendency of the entire muscle (depending on which fiber type is dominant) to function either aerobically or anaerobically. In the human body, as a generality, postural muscles tend to be oriented toward slow-twitch type I fibers, whereas the power muscles of the extremities designed for locomotion have a combination of type I and type II fibers.[8]

Despite the inherent blending of muscle fiber types, a client should be trained for function. Hopp[10] stated, in her review of the effects of age and resistance training on skeletal muscle, that "it is difficult . . . to draw conclusions about a muscle's contractile properties [function] based solely on its metabolic properties [fiber type] or about a muscle's metabolic properties based solely on its

--- **Table 2-1** ---

COMPEXITY OF SKELETAL MUSCLE FIBER COMPOSITION

The following table represents the many differing methods to classify skeletal muscle fibers. Clamann[12] strongly recommended against trying to make a table of equivalencies among muscle fiber types, as the methods of establishing criteria differ significantly. The purpose of this table is to illustrate the complexity of identifying skeletal muscle fiber types, not to identify definitively every histochemical aspect of skeletal muscle fibers. Please refer to the referenced article by Clamann for a more comprehensive review.

Color	Metabolism	Speed of Contraction	Fiber Type (Pette et al.[21])	Fiber Type (Henneman et al.[22])	Oxidative Capacity (Peter et al.[20])
Red fibers	Aerobic	Slow twitch	Type I	B	Slow oxidative
White fibers	Anaerobic	Fast twitch	Type IIb	A	Fast glycolytic
	Both	Fast twitch	Type IIa	C	Fast oxidative glycolytic
			Type IIc		

contractile properties." Under normal daily activities, high-velocity, high-intensity actions are not required. These normal activities fall within the physiological firing range of motor units dominated by slow-twitch fibers. Unless great demand activities are placed on the skeletal system, fast-twitch fibers typically will not be recruited. Most clients treated in the physical therapy profession will recruit slow-twitch fibers primarily. The functional aspect of the activity must be identified to properly rehabilitate a client. If high-intensity, high-speed actions are needed (fast-twitch fibers), then tasks designed to train fast-twitch fibers (high intensity) should be incorporated into the treatment program. Fast-twitch fibers will not have improved performance if these training guidelines are not reached. Memorization of the exact fiber-type composition of skeletal muscle is not essential for the PTA student. However, it is important to focus on the skeletal muscle's function and on the rehabilitation efforts to exercise the muscle as it was designed to operate.

FORCE OF CONTRACTION

There are two methods by which the PTA can promote functional strength gains in a client and increase the force of contraction of a muscle. The first method is known as **hypertrophy** of muscle fibers, or growth in cross-sectional size of the fiber itself. Strength is directly related to the size of a muscle and thus the larger the diameter of the muscle, the greater its ability to generate force.[9] As stated in the overload principle, with resistance training an adaptive response (increase strength) is produced by increasing the size of the muscle fiber over a period of time. A common misconception related to the strengthening of muscles is that the number of muscle fibers actually increase with training. There has been no researched evidence in human subjects to support this theory. The reduction of the size of the muscle fiber is referred to as **atrophy**, and this is a common complication seen in physical therapy after surgical procedures, prolonged bedrest, or simply disuse.

The second method by which an assistant can promote strengthening of orthopedic clients is by the **recruitment of motor units.** Clamann[12] showed that by adding progressively more motor units to form a muscular contraction, the greatest range of forces are produced. This process is responsible for the more rapid "strength" gains that are seen day to day in therapy as the efficiency of the

Hypertrophy
The growth in cross-sectional size of a muscle fiber in response to training.

Atrophy
Reduction of the size of a muscle fiber.

Recruitment of Motor Units
The neurological sequencing process by which progressively larger motor units are activated to generate sufficient force to perform a task.

neuromuscular system improves with repetitive training. Manifestations of the orderly recruitment of motor units include proportional control and smooth movement. When lifting a glass, the sequencing of activating motor units progresses from the very small units to the larger units until sufficient force is generated to support the glass without breaking it. As an orthopedic client learns through repetition the exercise demands placed on a muscle, the neuromuscular timing of when and how to turn on motor units is improved resulting in functional strength gains. This can readily be seen postsurgically when a client almost immediately loses muscular strength, but regains the strength relatively quickly over the next few days. There indeed may be some adaptive hypertrophy of muscle fibers occurring, but most of the immediate strength gains can be attributed to the recruitment of motor units.

AEROBIC VERSUS ANAEROBIC EXERCISE

There are three distinct energy systems that can be used by the body when a demand is placed upon skeletal muscle: (1) the adenosine triphosphate–phosphocreatine (ATP-PC) energy system, (2) the anaerobic glycolytic energy system, and (3) the aerobic energy system. Each system has unique features and characteristics producing energy to be used by muscles in response to specific demands. Each system obeys the specificity of exercise principle in that using an individual system will only improve muscular function when that system is activated.

Clinically, when an assistant trains a client to perform straight-leg raises after a total knee replacement to strengthen the quadriceps femoris muscle, sufficient strength and endurance to perform that specific exercise does not necessarily make the muscle performance sufficiently enhanced for stair climbing. By only strengthening the quadriceps femoris muscle in a supine position for short periods, the client does not use the different energy systems needed to produce functional gains. This issue should not be confused with overall body conditioning and strength improvement postsurgery, but in order to functionally improve climbing steps, a client must eventually climb steps.

The **adenosine triphosphate–phosphocreatine** (ATP-PC) energy system is very brief in nature (lasting less than 30 seconds of exercise), uses energy stores (ATP-PC) found directly in the muscle, and can produce a great amount of power. The system is designed for short-duration, high-intensity activities and is replenished when the muscle is at rest.[16] This system is highly responsive to the nutrition of a client because it is based off of energy stores found directly in the muscle. If your client is in a state of general malnutrition, there may not be an adequate store of energy in the muscle to perform brief, intense activities such as going from sit to stand or climbing one flight of stairs. These seem to be relatively easy tasks for the healthy individual, but to some of the clients treated in physical therapy, these tasks can be paramount to climbing to the top of a skyscraper (Fig. 2–5).

The **anaerobic glycolytic energy system** uses glucose (glycogen) as fuel, producing ATP (energy source) directly in the muscle with lactic acid as a by-product. This system is short in duration, lasting from the 30 to 90 seconds of activity, and does not produce as much energy as the first system, but it is the chief source of energy during the first 2 minutes of activity after the ATP-PC system is depleted. This system will allow for only moderate intensity over a short period. Comparative examples of energy system utilization include the difference between a sprint race of 100 m (typically only 10 to 15 seconds in duration) where the ATP-PC system supplies fuel for working muscles and the 800-m race (typically

Adenosine Triphosphate–Phosphocreatine (ATP-PC) Energy System
The energy system used for quick burst of energy using energy stores found directly in the muscle. It is able to generate a significant amount of force over a very short period.

Anaerobic Glycolytic Energy System
The energy system used to produce energy for the muscle during the first 2 minutes of activity after the ATP-PC system has been exhausted by burning glucose (glycogen) as a fuel to synthesize ATP.

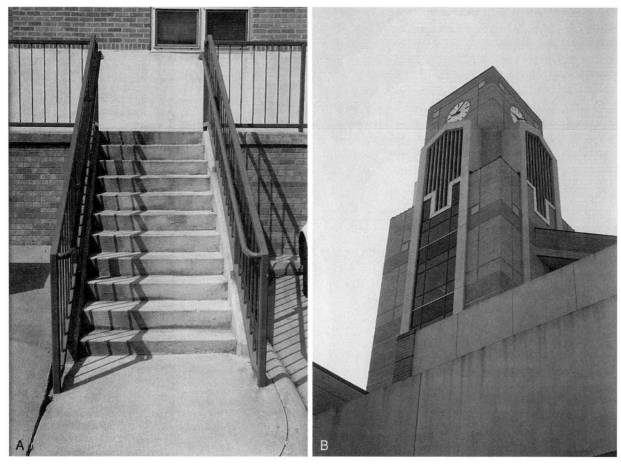

FIG. 2–5
ATP-PC Energy System. This energy system is designed for quick bursts of energy to perform activities lasting less than 30 seconds. Climbing a flight of steps (A) to a healthy individual may utilize only the ATP-PC system, but to the debilitated or malnutritioned individual those same steps may be paramount to climbing to the top of a bell tower (B).

Aerobic Energy System
The energy system that produces a significant amount of energy by metabolizing oxygen with a fuel (glucose, fat, or proteins), resulting in ATP production. It is predominantly used after 2 minutes of sustained activities when large muscle groups are involved.

2 to 2.5 minutes in duration) that exhausts first the ATP-PC and then the anaerobic glycolytic system.[16]

The **aerobic energy system** is the almost endless supply of energy within the human body and is used predominantly after the second minute of activity. The uniqueness of this system is the utilization of oxygen to build ATP within the mitochondria (engines of the muscle cell) using glycogen, fats, and proteins (in that order) as fuel. These components are "burned" to produce the necessary energy for the muscle to operate. The capacity to produce energy is almost 90 times greater than that with the two previous energy systems. This system is highly dependant on the ability of the body to transport oxygen to the muscle to be utilized in the aerobic system. The energy transport system consists of many elements including (1) the ability of the heart to adequately pump blood, (2) the ability of the lungs to exchange oxygen into the blood and remove waste products, (3) the ability of the blood to carry oxygen (hemoglobin), (4) the ability to exchange oxygen from the capillary beds to the muscle needing the oxygen, and (5) the ability to adequately remove waste products from the working muscle. A physical therapy client may be successful ambulating within the home where short distances and frequent rests can be taken, but may have difficulty performing community ambulation if the aerobic energy system is not adequate.[16]

Clinically, the assistant must understand the principles of energy source utilization by their clients to ensure successful treatment application. It must be understood that the discussed energy systems are not absolute, and there exists overlap in the body's use of each source of ATP production, but a certainty may be implied that when a client is in a poor state of health, the ability of his or her body to sufficiently produce energy may be impaired. For quick bursts of energy, ATP is supplied by the ATP-PC system. For short-duration (1 to 2 minutes), intense activities, ATP is supplied by the ATP- PC and anaerobic glycolytic system and can be recharged and ready to produce for another similar activity after resting for 2 to 4 minutes. Activities that are of moderate intensity using large muscle groups and last for less than 5 minutes may see all three energy systems used. This is often a frequent scenario in the field of physical therapy. Lastly, activities that last 20 to 30 minutes at less than maximal intensity are producing ATP from the aerobic system.[16]

 ## TYPES OF EXERCISE

In the physical therapy profession, there are many differing opinions, styles, and approaches to the rehabilitation of orthopedic clients. The underlying premise for all physical therapy rehabilitation practices lies in the ability to skillfully apply exercise principles to enhance the functional abilities of the client. This section discusses the types of muscular contractions and types of exercises that are commonly used for physical therapy rehabilitation.

MUSCULAR STRENGTH

The ability of the muscle to develop force against some resistance is known as **muscular strength.** To observe an increase in strength, the muscular contraction must be progressively overloaded, as stated by the overload principle. Clinically, the development of muscular strength is highly visible as clients are asked to lift progressively heavier weights. To promote the increased strength of a client, the assistant can encourage lifting of heavier objects in a controlled manner over relatively few repetitions.[8,9]

Muscular Strength
The ability of the muscle to develop force against some resistance.

MUSCULAR ENDURANCE

The ability of the muscle to perform repeated contractions over time is referred to as **muscular endurance.** Clinically, muscular endurance plays a significant role. The client may effectively possess adequate strength to move a load, but may not possess adequate endurance to move the load over a safe and functional distance. Most activities of daily living have an endurance element, not exclusively a strength element. However, most exercise programs designed to improve muscular strength will also produce endurance gains as well.[17] The assistant can promote muscular endurance gains by having the client perform repeated tasks with relatively low resistance over a longer period (many repetitions). The patterns used to improve muscular endurance can be performed in anatomic planes (repeated shoulder flexion) or in a functional manner (lifting a plate into a cabinet). In physical therapy treatments where clients often have painful, dysfunctional pathologies, the low-resistance and high-repetition approach may be more comfortable and produce less irritation as compared with exercises of higher resistance.[8,9]

Muscular Endurance
The ability of the muscle to perform repeated contractions over time.

MUSCULAR POWER

Muscular Power
The ability of the muscle to develop force quickly (strength × velocity).

The ability of the muscle to develop force quickly is termed **muscular power.** This muscular event is a coordinated effort joining muscular strength and velocity of movement. The activities required during athletic competition (throwing a baseball, a gymnastics tumbling run) are often described as power movements. The athlete must be able to generate tremendous amounts of strength but must also possess the ability to develop that strength quickly. Exercises designed to enhance power incorporate not only the development of strength, but the added element of speed moving the load quickly, efficiently, and in a controlled manner. Clinically, the athlete can perform functional exercises at greater intensity and then progressively lessen the time needed to complete the activity. Examples include box jumps, resisted leaping machines, medicine ball tosses, and the category of exercises referred to as plyometrics (to be discussed later in this chapter). Unless the assistant has an athletic client population, the clinical utilization of these power exercises will be minimal.[8,9]

MUSCULAR CONTRACTIONS

Isometric Contraction
A type of contraction produced when the muscle develops force internally but produces no external movement. The load is equal to the force.

Isotonic Contraction
A type of contraction produced when the muscle is activated, force develops, and movement is seen about the skeletal joint.

Concentric Contraction
A type of isotonic contraction in which the muscle shortens. The force is greater than the load.

Eccentric Contraction
A type of isotonic contraction in which the muscle lengthens. The load is greater than the force.

When skeletal muscle is stimulated and force is produced inside the muscle with no apparent change in the angle of the joint, an **isometric** contraction is demonstrated. On a kinesiological basis, the load or resistance is equal to the force developed and a balance is realized. An **isotonic** contraction is produced when the muscle is activated, force develops, and movement is seen about the skeletal joint. Kinesiologically, when the force developed by the muscle is greater than the resistance, a shortening of the muscle is produced and is referred to as a **concentric** contraction. Conversely, **eccentric** contractions occur when the load is greater than the force developed resulting in a controlled lengthening of the muscle. Figure 2–6 demonstrates the differences between skeletal muscle contractions. Each form of skeletal muscle contraction adheres to the specificity of exercise principle described earlier in this chapter. The PTA must secure the knowledge of how a muscle functions in a given situation to properly exercise and promote functional return.[8]

 EXERCISE APPLICATIONS

ISOMETRIC

Isometric exercise programs are those designed to be static or nonmoving in nature. Significant force and tension are generated within the muscle, despite the fact that no actual work is done (work is measured as force × distance: with no movement, the work result is zero). Adaptive strength changes can occur with isometric exercise programs if performed in a progressive fashion. These exercises are frequently prescribed in the early stages of rehabilitation because the static nature of the exercise may avoid irritation to a painful joint.[8,9,18–20] Historically, isometric exercises were believed to develop strength adaptations only in the specific position that the exercise was performed (specificity of exercise). Gardner[19] reported in 1963 that significant strength gains were realized only at the isometric training angle, and this conclusion was later supported by other published studies.[21,22] However, more recent studies have disputed this conclusion, now showing that isometric exercises will produce measurable strength gains

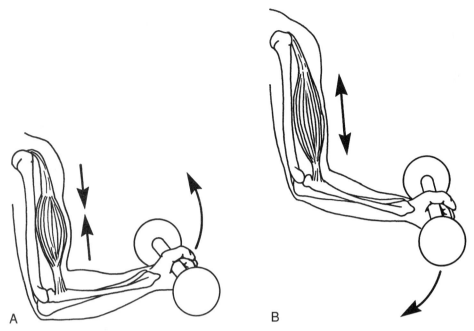

FIG. 2–6
Differences between skeletal muscle contractions. (A) demonstrates a concentric contraction as the muscle actively shortens lifting the weight against the forces of gravity, while (B) demonstrates an eccentric contraction as the muscle actively lengthens controlling the weight as it is lowered with gravity. (From Minor MA and Lippert LS: Kinesiology Laboratory Manual for the Physical Therapist Assistant, FA Davis, Philadelphia, 1998, p 9, with permission.)

at other points in the range of motion.[23] Bandy and Hanten[18] demonstrated in a 1993 study involving isometric strengthening of the quadriceps femoris muscle that strength gains were realized at angles in which exercising did not occur and that the greatest gains were seen when the isometric exercise was performed when the muscle was in a lengthened state.

Clinical Applications

Clinically, isometric exercises can be used (1) to retard muscle atrophy, (2) to strengthen a muscle when motion of the joint is contraindicated or painful, (3) to assist with circulation of blood, (4) to promote relaxation or reduce spasm of a muscle, and (5) when the client is unable to perform more advanced exercises. Types of isometric exercises include (1) muscle setting, (2) resistive isometrics, and (3) stabilization exercises.

Muscle Setting. The muscle-setting protocol is often a beginning exercise to warm the muscle or is used greatly for deconditioned individuals when other forms of exercise may be too strenuous. When performed properly, the muscle set is a low-intensity exercise performed against no resistance. The client tightens the muscle, shortening the muscle belly without moving the adjacent joints for a range of 6 to 10 seconds before relaxing. The exercise is repeated 10 to 15 times. "Quad sets" and "glut sets" are two well-used setting exercises (Fig. 2–7).[8,9]

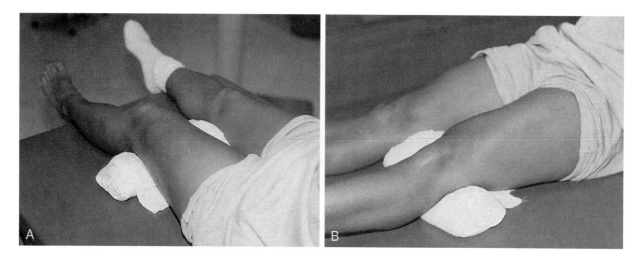

FIG. 2–7
Quad sets. (A) The knee is extended with a supportive bolster or towel roll under the knee and the client contracts the quadriceps maximally without producing movement and holds for a count of 6–10 before relaxing. (B) The exercise is then repeated 10–15 times.

Resistive Isometrics. Resistive isometric exercises are of a higher intensity than muscle setting and usually performed against either a manual or mechanical resistance. These exercises are used when the client is unable to perform active movement for a medical reason (pain, recent surgery), but it is desired to increase strength. As the study by Bandy and Hanten suggested, the muscle should be placed in a lengthened position before the resistive isometric exercise is performed to produce general strength gains throughout the range of motion (ROM); however, the traditional approach of applying resistance at various points in the ROM is still practiced.[8,9]

Stabilization Exercises. Stabilization exercises is a relatively new concept in orthopedic rehabilitation applied to a basic function of muscles that support skeletal structures. When a muscle cocontracts with an opposing muscle group, then a state of stability is reached about that joint. This cocontraction is necessary for postural control as well as for stabilizing proximal structures (shoulder girdle) to allow for distal movement (the arm). Exercises designed in an environment where the stability of a dynamic joint is challenged strengthen muscles in an isometric fashion. These concepts are used frequently in proprioceptive neuromuscular facilitation (PNF) techniques as well as in dynamic lumbar stabilization exercises for the spine.[8,24]

Contraindications. Contraindications for the performance of isometric exercises include (1) any time that contraction of the muscle would prevent healing, or (2) clients with prior history of cardiovascular disease or cerebrovascular accident. Isometric exercise can produce an increase in blood pressure if performed against a substantial resistance. This may be undesirable in clients with a history of blood pressure–related pathologies. The Valsalva maneuver occurs when a client tightens the abdomen forcing air up against a closed glottis (appearance of holding one's breath), resulting in increased intrathoracic pressure, decreased return of blood to the heart, and increased blood pressure.[25] This maneuver is frequently performed when clients are doing resistive exercises because it gives the "feeling" of increased power and strength or maybe even the feeling of increased effort. However, no real benefits are found from physical therapy clients performing the Valsalva maneuver, and as mentioned previously, it can be potentially harmful. A smooth coordination of exhaling on the exertion of force should be encouraged while performing any type of resistive movement or exercise.

ISOTONIC

Isotonic exercises are designed to develop tension in the muscle and produce a shortening (concentric) or lengthening (eccentric) of the muscle length. This classic form of exercise may be performed by placing resistance to the movement either by manual or by mechanical means. The term *isotonic* means "same tension"; however, that term is not quite descriptive of the tension being developed within the muscle, because indeed a significant amount of change is occurring throughout the ROM. As the contraction occurs and a shortening of the muscle is produced, a peak tension will be reached at some point but will not remain constant through the entire motion.[26] The maximum amount of resistance that can be successfully moved will be equal to the weakest point in the ROM. This is analogous to the "weakest" link in the chain because the chain will only support as much tension as the weakest aspect.

Clinical Applications

Concentric. Isotonic exercises can take the form of concentric exercises, eccentric exercises, or a combination of both. Concentric exercises shorten the muscle by moving a load against the forces of gravity or in a gravity-lessened environment with the load being mechanical or manual in nature. Examples of concentric exercises include lifting free weights, raising ankle weights, pulling on resistive tubing, using weight machines, performing water exercises, or providing manual resistance as a person actively shortens a muscle. Eccentric exercises are those exercises performed by lowering the resistance with gravity to a resting point. The same machines or equipment used for concentric exercises are also used during eccentric exercises with the exception of water therapy. In a water environment, the effects of gravity are significantly lessened. During water programs, alternating concentric contractions are performed by the client instead of the combination of concentric followed by an eccentric contraction. The full benefits of water programs will be discussed in the second part of this text.

Eccentric. Eccentric exercises have played an increasingly important role in the rehabilitation of physical therapy clients. The functional roles of most lower-extremity muscles during gait and activities of daily living (ADLs) are eccentric in nature. Shock absorption is one role of lower-extremity muscles that is a type of eccentric activity. Eccentric contractions have been termed the "negative" contraction, with concentric being the "positive." Weight lifters place great emphasis on performing negative contractions to build strength, power, and definition. It has been shown in several studies that maximal eccentric contractions develop greater muscle tension than either concentric or isometric contractions.[8,26,27] The added tension development is produced from the elastic properties of the noncontractile elements (tendons, connective tissue sheath) found in the muscle. The added assistance of the noncontractile elements in controlling an eccentric load allows the eccentric contraction to be neurologically more efficient than concentric contractions. The eccentric contraction recruits fewer motor units than a concentric contraction to perform an equal amount of work.[28] This can be very beneficial during rehabilitation when a muscle is significantly weak because the involved client may be able to perform eccentric exercises more easily as compared with concentric exercises. Dean[28] suggested that eccentric exercises "may allow patients to improve their work capacity and use energy more efficiently, and thus, to do more work with reduced energy expenditure and subjective fatigue."

Precautions. Eccentric exercises should be performed within the abilities (or disabilities) of the client. First, the Valsalva maneuver (as with isometric exercises) should be avoided because of the possibility of increasing blood pressure and decreasing blood flow to the heart. The PTA should ensure that the client is breathing regularly during exercise, and caution must be used when eccentrically exercising clients with cardiovascular or hypertensive disease. Second, microtrauma to the skeletal muscle tissue tends to occur more readily with slow-velocity, high-intensity eccentric exercises as compared with concentric exercises. This can lead to delayed-onset muscle soreness (DOMS). This condition is characterized by muscular stiffness, tenderness, and pain with active movement that usually arises 24 to 48 hours after eccentric loading the muscle.[29] DOMS may be undesired in the physical therapy client because producing new, painful symptoms may (1) delay healing of the involved structures, (2) discourage the client, or even (3) potentially anger the referring physician. Fitzgerald et al.[30] suggested that clients who are weak in nature or prone to muscular dysfunction (e.g., polio, postpolio syndrome, Guillain-Barré syndrome) may need to avoid strenuous eccentric activities. Also, because of the increased tension development of the noncontractile elements in the eccentric contraction over concentric exercises, clients who have had surgery involving musculotendinous components (tendon or muscle repairs) may have eccentric exercises introduced later in the rehabilitation program, thus allowing sufficient healing time of the noncontractile elements to occur.

Speed of Contraction.

The speed of contraction is considered important when performing isotonic exercises for two reasons: (1) safety and (2) force generation to produce an adaptive change. When performing an exercise against resistance, the faster the exercise is performed, then the greater the possibility of the client's losing control of that motion. If the load is out of control, possible injury to the client may result. For the safety of the client, ensure that all exercises are done slowly and under control to prevent injury. Secondly, as momentum increases during the exercise performance, the less the muscle being trained has to work, and thus strengthening benefits are not being appreciated to produce an adaptive change. Griffin[26] demonstrated that greater forces are generated during eccentric and concentric contractions at slower velocities.

Resistance: Mechanical versus Manual.

As mentioned previously, the load or resistance for isotonic exercises may take two forms: either mechanical or manual. Figures 2–8 through 2–17 contain photographs and descriptions of tools to accomplish mechanical resistive exercise programs. Failure to discuss manual resistance as a mode of exercise would be to neglect one of the greatest tools (hands) that the assistant has at his or her disposal (another tool being the mind!). Manual resistive isotonic exercises can be applied in either a concentric or an eccentric fashion as well as isometrically, as mentioned earlier in the chapter. The resistance can be applied (1) following anatomical planes of motion, (2) in combinations of motion, or (3) in functional patterns.

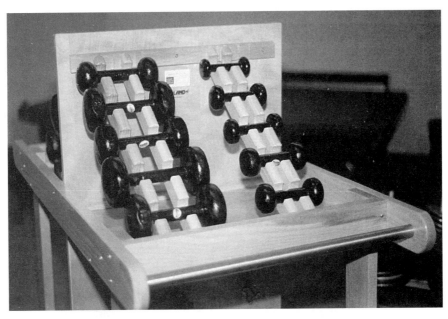

FIG. 2–8
Hand weights. Small hand weights are commonly used for resistive strengthening exercises involving the upper extremity.

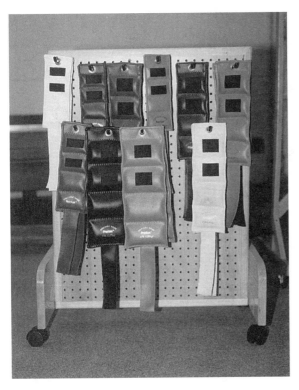

FIG. 2–9
Ankle weights. These types of weights are easily secured to either the upper or lower extremity to provide resistance during exercise.

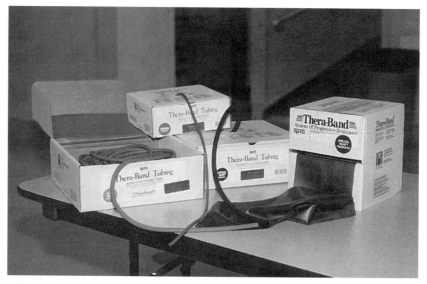

FIG. 2–10
Resistive tubing and bands. This form of resistive exercise equipment is easily portable and can be adapted to almost any joint in the body.

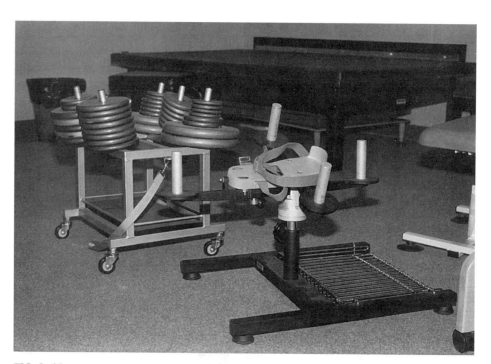

FIG. 2–11
Ankle mechanical resistance machine. The ankle can be strengthened by placing resistance (plates) in the sagittal or frontal planes.

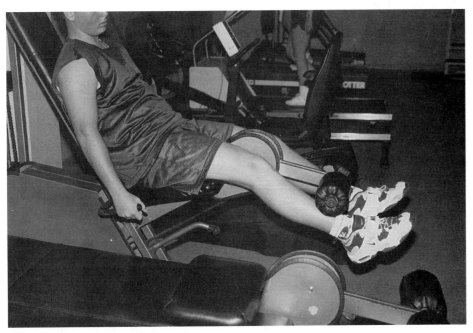

FIG. 2–12
Knee extension mechanical resistance. Through the use of a pulley system, this free standing resistance machine places progressive resistance on the knee extensor muscles.

Clinical Applications. Clinically, the assistant should use manual resistance (1) when the client is significantly weak and the use of mechanical resistance may be harmful, (2) when careful, controlled movements are required postsurgically, (3) when the muscle throughout the ROM needs to be challenged by increasing or decreasing resistance according to the length-strength relationship, and (4) as a reeducation tool to provide manual feedback to the client to ensure proper use of weakened muscles. The assistant should (1) explain the procedure to the client; (2) place the client in a comfortable position; (3) move limb passively through ROM demonstrating the desired motion, being confident with your hand placement, and ensuring client trust; (4) instruct client to produce pain-free maximal effort; and 5) ensure proper breathing patterns.

Verbal commands given by the therapist to the client should suggest exactly what the client is to perform. The term "hold" works well for producing an isometric contraction; however, the statement "Don't let me move you" often turns into a tug-of-war. "Push" or "pull" works well if the desired exercise is concentric in nature with "Slowly control the motion," or "Let me slowly push or pull" if eccentric exercises are the goal. Make sure that the commands are appropriate to the client's learning and listening ability; at no time should it turn into an arm-wrestling contest. If the client is not producing the desired action, the assistant is in control of the resistance and can easily stop a procedure to prevent possible injury to the client or to ensure proper use of the exercise techniques.

Factors Influencing Resistance. In a relevant kinesiology text,[3,31] the assistant should learn the different types of lever systems. The application of the different types of lever systems in the human body can greatly affect the amount of force generated. In a lever system, the components include the lever, the force, the resistance (load) and the fulcrum (axis). Depending on the alignment of the system

FIG. 2–13
Shoulder horizontal flexion mechanical resistance. This type of machine has affectionately been named the "pect deck" for the resistance training provided to the horizontal flexor muscles of the shoulder.

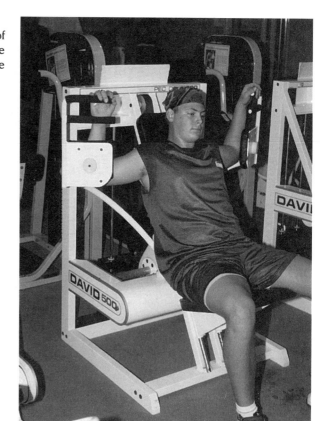

(first, second, or third class) and the distances of the force (force arm) and resistance (resistance arm) from the fulcrum, movement is produced to overcome the resistance. If no movement is produced, then a greater force may be applied or the application of the force may be moved farther from the fulcrum. This has great clinical implications because the assistant can modulate the amount of force being generated internally by the client in two fashions: (1) increasing the amount of force applied by the assistant, and (2) moving hand placement proximally (to decrease) or distally (to increase).

The amount of resistance applied by the assistant presents a significant drawback to the use of manual resistance—the documentation aspect. In physical therapy, we do not have a significantly easy way to quantify manual resistance. The terms used in documentation related to manual resistance are "minimal," "moderate," and "maximal." These terms do not, however, relate to a specific, easily quantified amount and may vary among clinicians applying the force and clients performing the exercise. The mechanical resistance environment provides a more consistent means of documentation. It is clear and relatively accurate to document the difference between a 2-lb ankle weight and a 3-lb weight when used during exercise.

Clinical Techniques. Through experience, the assistant will be able to appropriately use the terms minimal, moderate, and maximal resistance applied manually. Regardless of the technical amount of force applied by the assistant, the force applied should be proportionate to the tolerance and abilities of the client

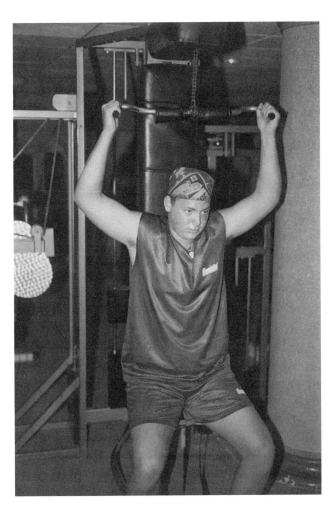

FIG. 2-14
Shoulder extension mechanical resistance. By pulling down on the overhead bar, resistance is applied through a system of pulleys to the shoulder extensor muscles as well as the elbow flexor muscles.

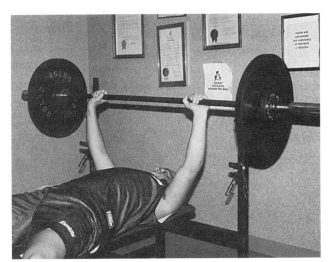

FIG. 2-15
Shoulder and elbow mechanical resistance. The bench press, using free weights, has been a classic resistance exercise to strengthen the elbow extensor muscles and the horizontal flexor muscles of the shoulder.

FIG. 2–16
Wall pulley. Pulley systems are used to change the direction of resistance and can be applied to a variety of exercises and body joints.

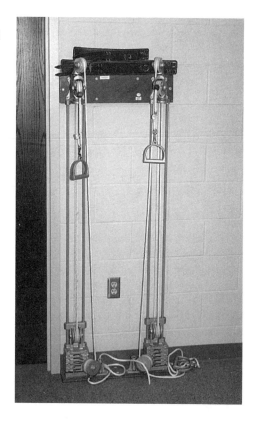

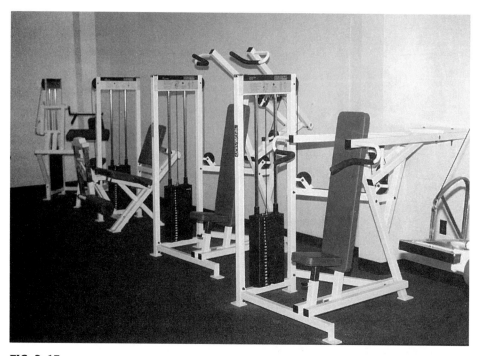

FIG. 2–17
Free-standing weight machines. These large machines use levers and pulley systems to apply resistance in a variety of positions and movements.

without producing pain or harm. Gradient pressure, or gently applying progressively greater resistance, is much more desirable than sudden, abrupt changes. By changing hand placement either proximally or distally through which the force is applied, the assistant can also cause changes in internal force production. Generally, the force is applied just distally to the joint being exercised, but it may be moved farther distally encompassing a second joint, if and only if the second joint is stable and free of pathology. Be keenly aware that by moving force application distally, the amount of torque is significantly increased and physical damage to the client can be done with relatively little force application. Clients with a history of osteoporosis, steroid therapy, and rheumatoid arthritis are prone to fracture; thus, the assistant must apply force judiciously.

During the application of manual resistance, the assistant should ensure that the client is properly stabilized and no substitutions or unwanted motion is occurring. Usually, stabilization occurs near or at the origin (proximal attachment) of the muscle being exercised. A number of repetitions should be followed for documentation and progression purposes ranging from 5 to 20 times performing the exercise. If the client develops pain or tremors or is unable to continue because of fatigue, the exercise should be halted. Figures 2–18 through 2–30 demonstrate application of manual resistance techniques to selected body parts.

Applying resistance in functional movement patterns was introduced by Knott and Voss[32] through the treatment concept of PNF. The treatment approach of PNF

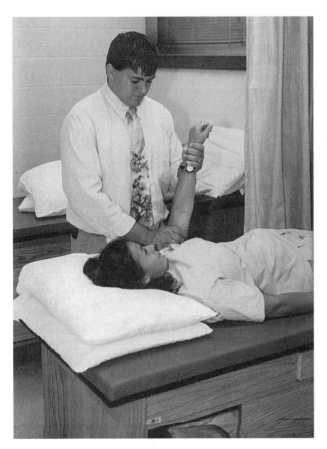

FIG. 2–18
Manual resistance. Shoulder flexion—resistance is applied by the examiner on the anterior portion of the upper arm, resisting the concentric contraction of shoulder flexion. Stabilization of the scapula and the trunk comes from the plinth. Distal pressure on the forearm is applied only if the elbow is stable and pain free. Always remember that the farther you place your hand from the joint in motion, the greater the amount of force that is generated by the client. As the arm is returned to the table from a fully flexed position, resistance may be given to the extensors concentrically or to the flexors eccentrically. If the arm is nonmoving as force is being generated by the client, then the contraction is isometric in nature.

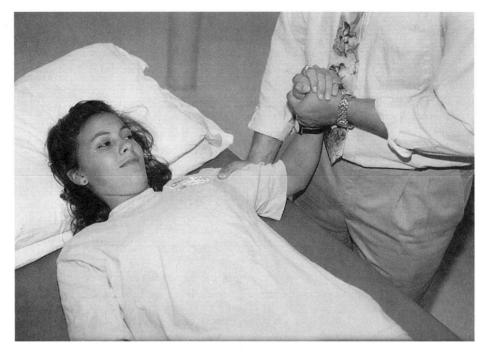

FIG. 2–19

Manual resistance. Shoulder abduction—The assistant applies resistance to the lateral aspect of the upper arm as the client concentrically abducts the arm. If necessary, stabilization superiorly on the scapula may be needed to limit scapular elevation. As the client adducts the upper extremity from an abducted position, the assistant may apply concentric resistance to the adductors by placing a hand on the medial upper arm or eccentrically resisting the abductors by keeping the original hand placement as concentric abduction and by stating "slowly let your arm down; don't work against me."

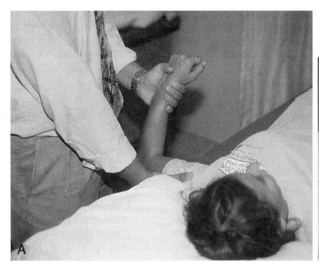
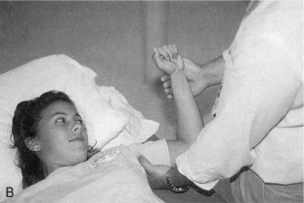

FIG. 2–20

Manual resistance. Shoulder internal and external rotation—With the arm positioned at 90° of elbow flexion and shoulder abduction, resistance is applied to the anterior surface of the forearm for concentric internal rotation (A), or the posterior surface of the forearm for concentric external rotation (B). During the return motion to the starting position, resistance can be applied either eccentrically or concentrically as desired. Stabilization is applied on the upper extremity. The same resistive exercise may be performed with the elbow at the side of the client if the abducted position causes discomfort.

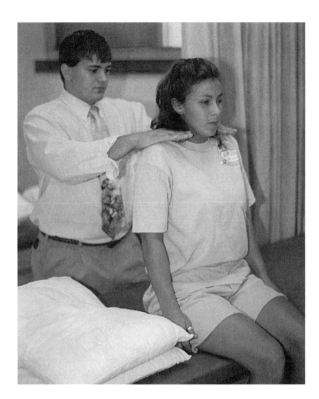

FIG. 2–21
Manual resistance. Scapular elevation—This is performed either sitting (pictured) or supine by resisting the movement of scapular elevation concentrically. From this position, the assistant easily can eccentrically resist scapular elevation as well.

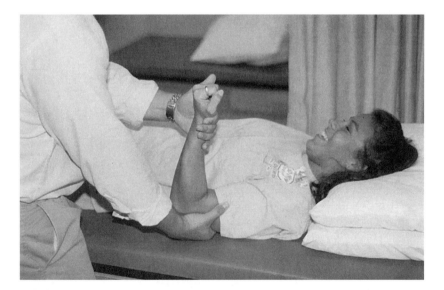

FIG. 2–22
Manual resistance. Elbow flexion—By positioning the patient supine, the trunk is easily stabilized, allowing resistance to be placed on the anterior surface of the forearm concentrically resisting elbow flexion. Eccentric resistance to the elbow flexors can be applied by asking the client to slowly control the motion as you gently resist on the anterior surface of the forearm allowing the elbow to extend. The forearm may be in either a neutral (brachioradialis), supinated (biceps brachii) or pronated (brachialis) position, emphasizing different muscular elements of elbow flexion.

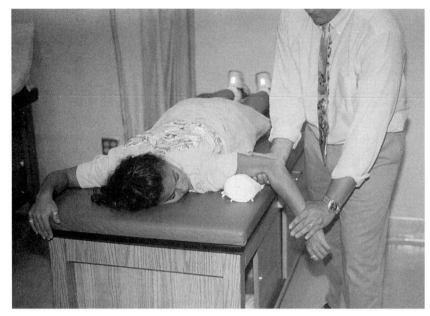

FIG. 2–23
Manual resistance. Elbow extension—The prone position works well for stabilizing the trunk and upper arm. Place a towel roll under the upper extremity and apply resistance on the lateral aspect of the distal forearm as the client extends the elbow concentrically. Eccentric resistance may be applied with the same hand positioning as the elbow slowly flexes.

FIG. 2–24
Manual resistance. Hip flexion and knee flexion—In the supine position, resist simultaneously at the anterior thigh (hip flexion) and posterior lower leg (knee flexion) to perform this combination concentric motion. Stabilization of the pelvis is provided by the table and adequate abdominal strength, however, if the client is having difficulty maintaining pelvic positioning against the resisted hip flexion (possible excessive anterior rotation), have the client place the opposite foot on the table by flexing the hip and knee. By shifting the lower hand placement under the heel and the upper hand placement under the thigh during the return motion, concentric hip and knee extension can be manually resisted.

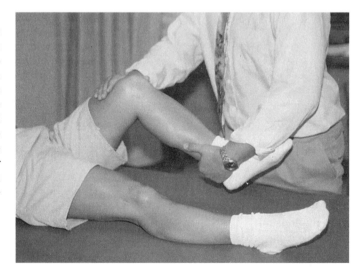

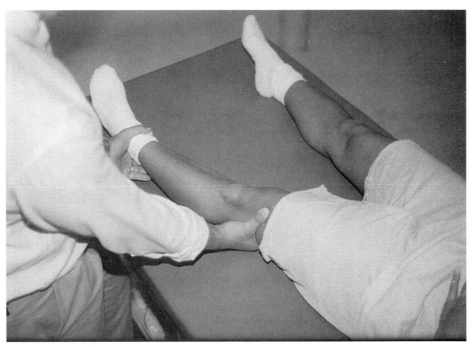

FIG. 2–25
Manual resistance. Hip abduction and adduction—Supine positioning with stabilization from the plinth allows the ability to apply resistance to the lateral aspect of the thigh or the lateral aspect of the lower leg (or combination or both) to concentrically train the hip abductors. Resisted adduction is performed concentrically by moving the hand placement to the medial aspects of the thigh and/or lower leg. Ensure that the toes keep pointing toward the ceiling (neutral position of hip) because rotation of the hip will allow a substitution by the hip flexors.

has been adopted by many orthopedic therapists using certain elements and techniques. It is out of the scope of this text to cover the entire spectrum of PNF, but Chapter 3 presents a discussion of PNF techniques applied to the orthopedic environment.

ISOKINETIC EXERCISES

Isokinetic exercises are those in which the muscle is actively shortening or lengthening against a fixed speed or velocity. Another means of describing isokinetic exercise is "accommodative resistance." This type of contraction does not occur naturally in the body, but it was theorized that by providing a constant speed of contraction for the muscle, the maximum resistance is provided throughout the ROM. A special machine is needed to perform this type of exercise and is used frequently either as an assessment tool or as a conditioning tool (Fig. 2–31). The amount of resistance that is produced depends directly on the effort of the client through the ROM. The popularity of isokinetic exercise use grew to a peak in the late 1980s, largely because of the objective data and documentation that were produced. Other advantages of isokinetic training include (1) the ability to accommodate the resistance through the ROM, (2) the safety of the client during exercise as the resistance is in response to the client's effort, (3) accurateness of equipment and testing procedures, and (4) the ability to adjust to pain and

Isokinetic Exercises
Exercises in which the muscle is actively shortening or lengthening, contracting against a fixed speed or velocity. A special machine is needed to perform this type of exercise because it does not occur naturally in the human body.

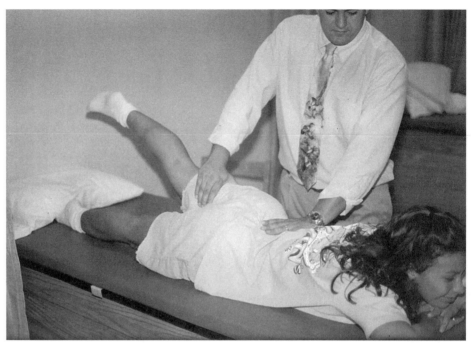

FIG. 2–26
Manual resistance. Hip extension—As mentioned in Figure 2–24, the hip extensors can be concentrically resisted from the supine position or as pictured here in the prone position. Ensure proper stabilization of the pelvis by placing hand or forearm across the posterior aspect of pelvis and then applying resistance to posterior thigh as the client concentrically extends the hip. Eccentric hip extension can be resisted easily from the same hand placement. This exercise can easily produce hamstring cramping if the knee is in a flexed position due to the two-joint nature of the muscle. Avoid extremes in hip extension motion; this may cause an anterior rotation of the pelvis and hyperextension of the lumbar spine.

FIG. 2–27
Manual resistance. Knee flexion—As mentioned in Figure 2–24, knee flexion may be manually resisted in the supine position or as pictured here. In the prone position, resistance can be applied to the posterior lower leg and stabilized at the posterior hip joint as the client concentrically contracts the hamstrings. Eccentric resistance can be applied from the same hand positioning. Ensure that there is adequate room anteriorly for the patella to slide in the femoral groove and that compression is not occurring because this may elicit pain.

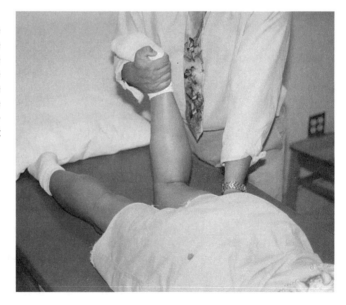

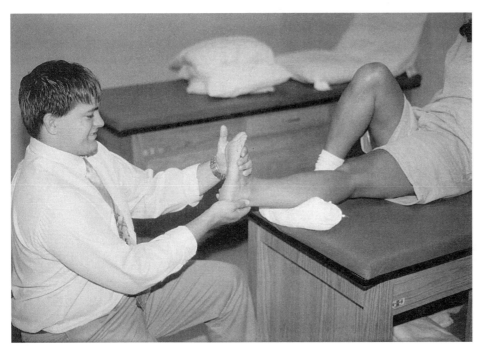

FIG. 2–28
Manual resistance. Ankle dorsiflexion—By applying resistance to the dorsum of the foot, dorsiflexion can be resisted concentrically or eccentrically.

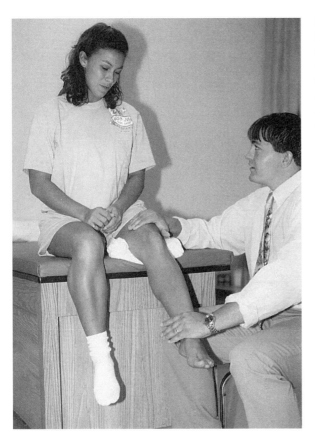

FIG. 2–29
Manual resistance. Knee extension—Sitting is typically utilized when applying manual resistance to the knee extensor muscles. The assistant can apply resistance distally over the anterior aspect of the tibia when the client concentrically performs knee extension as well as during eccentric lengthening of the quadriceps. This open chain activity should be avoided if the client has poor trunk and pelvis stability or if the compressive forces at the patella elicit pain.

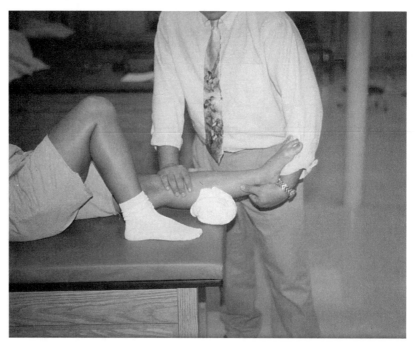

FIG. 2–30
Manual resistance. Ankle plantarflexion—In the supine long sit position, the assistant can grasp the posterior aspect of the client's calcaneus, resting the metatarsal heads of the client against the forearm of the assistant. This position allows for resisted plantar flexion either concentrically or eccentrically. Stabilize proximally on the tibia without compressing the patella.

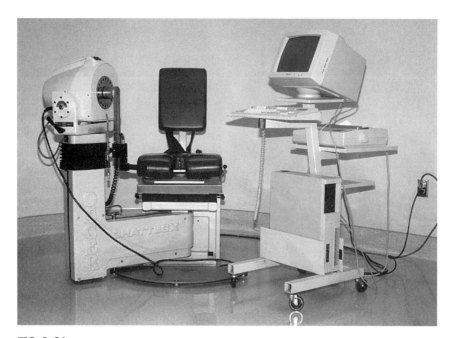

FIG. 2–31
Isokinetic equipment. Isokinetic exercises are performed on a special machine that provides a constant speed of contraction in either an eccentric or concentric fashion resulting in accommodating maximal resistance throughout the entire ROM.

fatigue. However, the extreme cost of equipment (machines can be in excess of $50,000), the complexity of routine setup, the availability of appropriate equipment, and the nonfunctional nature of isokinetic training (positioning in non–weight-bearing postures) has reduced the demand in orthopedic rehabilitation. Box 2–2 presents a comparison of isometric, isotonic, and isokinetic exercises.[9,33]

OPEN KINEMATIC CHAIN EXERCISES

Open kinematic chain (OKC) exercises are those in which the distal end segment of the extremity, being either the hand or the foot, is moving free in space. Exercise characteristics include (1) the use of individual muscle groups, (2) single axis and plane movement, and (3) non–weight-bearing positions. The OKC principle will not predict what will occur at adjacent joints: A limb may move in an open-chain environment either independently or in unison with the surrounding joints. The upper extremity typically functions in open-chain patterns such, as bending of the elbow in performing a biceps curl. Traditional exercises in physical therapy have been mostly open chain in nature regardless of whether the exercises were applied to the upper or lower extremity.[3,34]

Open Kinematic Chain
Exercises in which the distal end of the extremity, being either the hand or the foot, is free in space.

CLOSED KINEMATIC CHAIN EXERCISES

Closed kinematic chain (CKC) exercises are those in which the distal end segment of the extremity, being either the hand or the foot, is in contact with the ground. The closed system incorporates muscles and joints acting in a predictable manner, blending weight-bearing forces and eccentric muscle control during movement of the limb. The lower extremity typically functions in closed-chain patterns, such as sitting down into a chair. For this activity to successfully occur, flexion of the knee and hip along with ankle dorsiflexion must work in concert. A recent trend in physical rehabilitation has moved the traditional exercise spectrum from OKC toward the biomechanical principles of CKC. Figure 2–32A demonstrates the different aspects of closed and open kinematic chain activities.[3,34]

Closed Kinematic Chain
Exercises in which the distal end of the extremity, being either the hand or the foot, is contacted with the ground.

Clinical Implications

To understand the basis of open and closed kinematic chain exercises, visualize the effects of doing activities when the foot is on the ground as compared with when the foot is not on the ground. Most, if not all, functional activities for the lower extremity occur when the foot is on the ground in some fashion or another. Remembering the specificity of exercise principle would demand the assistant to exercise the muscle or muscle group in the fashion to which the muscle or muscle group will be asked to perform functionally. By placing the foot in a weight-bearing position to perform a selected exercise, the muscles of the entire lower extremity become involved by providing stabilization or controlling the effects of gravity. Another benefit of closed-chain performance is promoting the natural joint compressive forces when the force from the ground is transmitted up from the foot, through the ankle and to the knee and hip. Intermittent compressive forces encourage joint nourishment from the synovial fluid and promote stability of a joint. Conversely, open-chain exercise produces a shearing force in which one part of the articular surface slides across the other, which can be damaging to the joint surfaces and soft-tissue structures. Figure 2–32B demonstrates the differing forces that are created at the knee joint. A third benefit of closed-chain exercises is the

Box 2-2

ADVANTAGES AND DISADVANTAGES OF ISOMETRIC, ISOTONIC, AND ISOKINETIC EXERCISES[8,9,34]

Advantages of Isometric Exercise

It promotes strength gains.
It can be used early in rehabilitation with low risk of joint irritation.
It can slow the muscle atrophy process.
Muscle pumping action helps reduce swelling and promotes circulation.
It begins the muscule reeducation process (learning to use muscle again after surgery).
Minimal to no equipment is needed.
There may be a carryover effect strengthening other parts of the ROM than just angle of exercise.
It is an excellent tool if client is unable to perform more advanced exercises.

Advantages of Isotonic Exercise

It is easy to progress client.
The cost of equipment (ankle weights, elastic tubing) is relatively low.
It possesses both an eccentric and concentric component.
It can improve muscular strength and endurance.
It promotes muscule reeducation.

Advantages of Isokinetic Exercise

Variable resistance is safe for client.
Variable resistance promotes maximal load through entire ROM.
It allows good documentation through computer charts and graphs.
The testing procedure is easily reproducible.
It can improve muscular strength, endurance, and power.
High-speed motions tend to have less joint compression forces.

Disadvantages of Isometric Exercise

No work (force × distance) is performed.
Strengthening may be limited to position of exercise.
It may be difficult to get best effort from client (motivation).
It does not significantly improve muscular endurance or power.
There is no eccentric component.

Disadvantages of Isotonic Exercise

Weakest link in chain: only able to load that is equal to the weakest part of the ROM.
Momentum may not produce strength gains.
It may be unsafe to client if he or she has poor strength, control, or coordination.
Its benefit is limited to improving muscular power.
Eccentric component may promote muscular soreness (DOMS).

(Continued)

— **Box 2–2** ————————————————

ADVANTAGES AND DISADVANTAGES OF ISOMETRIC, ISOTONIC, AND ISOKINETIC EXERCISES[8,9,34] **(Continued)**

Disadvantages of Isokinetic Exercise

Cost of equipment is high, and availability is limited.
Expert knowledge and skill are needed to set up equipment.
A lot of time is involved to perform session.
It may be difficult to get best effort from client (motivation).
Eccentric component may promote muscular soreness (DOMS).
Non–weight-bearing positioning may not be functional in nature for the client.

neural timing and proprioceptive benefits that are promoted. The client, by performing activities when the foot is on the ground, relearns the balance and timing needed to perform functional activities. Table 2–2 presents an overall comparison of the different kinematic chain exercises. Examples of kinematic chain exercises are also presented in Figures 2–33 and 2–34.[8,9,35]

Closed-chain exercises have limitations as well and are not applicable in every situation. The client must have at least a partial to full weight-bearing status and

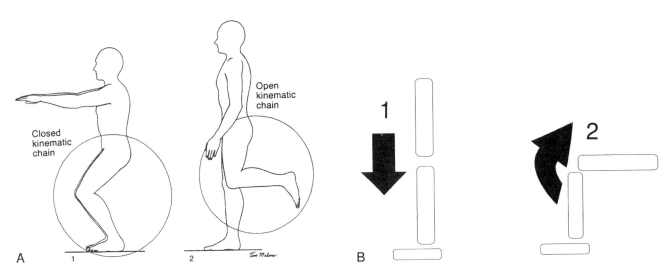

FIG. 2–32

(A) Open and closed kinematic chains. (1) In a closed kinematic chain, knee flexion is accompanied by hip flexion and ankle dorsiflexion. (2) Knee motion in an open kinematic chain may occur with or without motion at the hip and ankle. (From Norkin & Levangie, p 69, with permission.) **(B) Compressive and shearing forces at the knee.** In a weight-bearing posture (1—closed chain) the forces at the knee typically are compressive in nature approximating the joint surfaces, while in a non–weight-bearing (2—open chain) the forces are shearing in nature as the tibia slides anteriorly on the femoral condyles. Compressive forces are more beneficial to the nourishment of the joint surfaces while shearing forces can be damaging.

___ **Table 2–2** ___

COMPARISON OF OPEN AND CLOSED KINEMATIC CHAIN EXERCISES (OKC VS. CKC)[3,8,9,35]

Parameter	OKC	CKC
Definition	Distal end segment is free	Distal end segment fixed
Axis of motion	Single	Multiple
Planes of movement	Cardinal planes	Triplanar
Stabilization	External (straps, belts)	Internal (postural, cocontraction)
Movement	Isolated	Coordinated and functional
Resistance	Artificial external load	Body weight
Purpose of movement	Proactive (moving load)	Reactive (to body weight)
Neural motor unit recruitment	Isolated	Functional recruitment
Neural feedback (proprioception)	Inaccurate, nonfunctional	Appropriate timing
Exercise fatigue detected	Momentary motor failure	Substitution patterns
Joint stability	Long axis distraction	Joint compression
Variability of exercises	Limited by design	Unlimited potential
Mechanical effects on joint surface	Shear	Compression
Advantages	Improve muscular strength	Parallels actual muscle function
	Simple movement patterns	Promotes joint nourishment
		Promotes stability of a joint
		Appropriate neural timing
Disadvantages	Increased shearing forces	Must be PWB to Full WB
	Limited function	Must have good balance
	Limited proprioception	Must support body weight

PWB = partial weight bearing; WB = weight bearing.

good balance in order to participate. Pool therapy can provide an environment in which closed-chain exercises can be performed while the effects of gravity are significantly lessened protecting a weight-bearing status; however, as previously discussed, pool therapy tends to limit eccentric contractions. The client must also possess adequate lower-extremity strength to support the weight of the body and prevent the possibility of falls. Open-chain exercises can be used to begin the rehabilitation process, increasing the strength of the antigravity muscles. When the client has demonstrated adequate strength, closed-chain exercises may gradually be introduced. By using an appropriate combination of the two approaches of kinematic chain exercises, the assistant should find ample variety of which the client can be exercised to promote the return of function.[3,8]

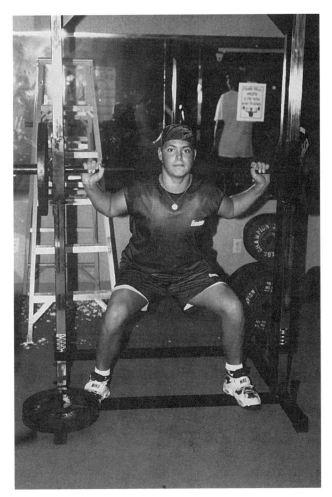

FIG. 2–33
Closed chain exercise: Standing squat. The knee and hip extensor muscles are worked in an eccentric fashion as the weight is lowered, moving the knee and hip into a position of flexion. The same muscles then work concentrically to return the athlete to a standing position. Compare this activity to performing hip and knee flexion resistively in an open chain environment.

PLYOMETRIC EXERCISES

The concept of **plyometric exercises** uses the neurophysiological principle of applying a quick stretch to an eccentrically loaded muscle followed by a forceful concentric contraction. This type of exercise attempts to merge speed of movement with strength (power) and is typically incorporated into the later stages of the rehabilitation of athletes. Plyometric exercise tends to simulate the body's functioning during high-stress running, jumping and bounding. Typically, large muscle groups of the trunk and lower and upper extremities are incorporated in functional patterns. The following are some guidelines for when to use plyometrics: (1) exercises are specific to the functional goals of the client, (2) exercise quality is desired over exercise quantity, (3) the client should be able to participate with maximal effort, (4) adequate recovery time should be incorporated into the program, and (5) exercises should be progressive.

In designing an exercise program that uses plyometrics, the therapist must examine the amount of force developed (intensity) in concert with the speed of the activity. Categories of plyometric exercise include: (1) jumping in place, (2) standing jumps, (3) multiple-response jumps and hops, (4) in-depth jumping and box drills, (5) bounding, and (6) high-stress, sport-specific drills.[36] This

Plyometric Exercises
Exercises that use the neurophysiological principle of applying a quick stretch to an eccentrically loaded muscle followed by a forceful concentric contraction.

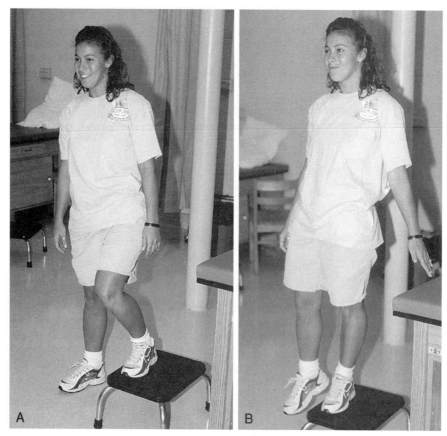

FIG. 2–34
Closed chain exercise: Lateral step up. Compare the functioning of the ankle muscles (A) raising the weight of the body up on to the step, then (B) lowering the body to the ground. By exercising the lower extremity in a position of function, the assistant encourages proper eccentric/concentric utilization of muscle, encourages balance and proprioceptive feedback, and joint compression.

concept of exercise is used almost exclusively in the sports rehabilitation arena just prior to the release of the athlete in order to facilitate the return to competition. Because the explosive type of exercises demanded in a plyometric program place tremendous stress on the skeletal system and requires great timing, balance, and strength to prevent injury to the client, these exercises should be used judiciously.[9]

AEROBIC EXERCISES

Aerobics
Prolonged, low-intensity exercises designed to stress and strengthen the cardiovascular system.

Exercises that are designed to stress and strengthen the cardiovascular system are referred to as **aerobics** or aerobic exercises. To produce an aerobic exercise, the client must use large muscle groups in a repeated fashion over some time. Walking, running, swimming, riding a stationary bike, or exercising on a treadmill or upper extremity ergometer are all common means of aerobic exercise (Figs. 2–35 through 2–38). Endurance is a measure of fitness that refers to the ability of the muscle or the cardiovascular system to perform work over a long period. Adaptation to greater levels of performance of the cardiovascular or muscular system will occur if the exercise regimem is of sufficient intensity, duration, and frequency and is also dependent on the client's original state of health.[16] When considering the state of health of an individual, generally, a person who trains aerobically will need to increase the intensity of exercises if further adaptation is desired. However, a person in a deconditioned state of health may only need to begin aerobic exercises to see an adaptation. This varies dramatically depending on the presence or absence of pathology in the client.

To determine what level of aerobic exercise a client should begin, often a cardiac stress test is performed. This process is used for high-risk clients (e.g., post–myocardial infarction) in cardiac rehabilitation environments to develop safe guidelines of exercise tolerance. A stress test consists of measuring heart rate and oxygen consumption while increasing the amount of work performed during the aerobic activity (Fig. 2–39). Parameters of safe exercise are developed for the client from the stress test incorporating the intensity (how hard the client is

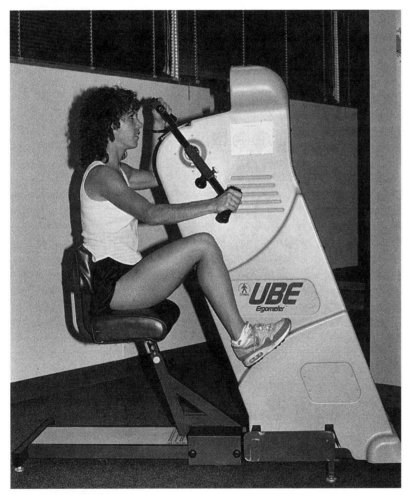

FIG. 2–35
Aerobic exercise. UBE—Utilizing the major muscle groups of the upper extremity can produce an aerobic exercise. This is of great benefit to those with lower extremity pathologies who can not effectively sustain endurance-related activities (From Kisner & Colby, p. 106, with permission.)

FIG. 2–36
Aerobic exercise. Treadmill—Common aerobic conditioning tool.

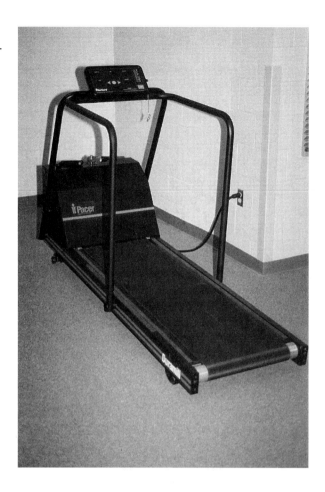

FIG. 2–37
Aerobic exercise. Stationary bike—Common aerobic conditioning tool. Participation by the client may be limited by orthopedic limitations or functional ROM deficits in the lower extremities.

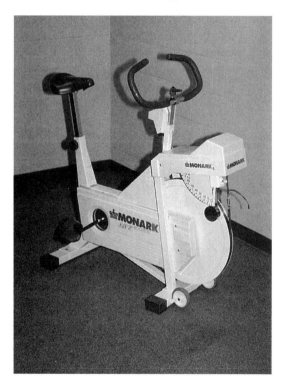

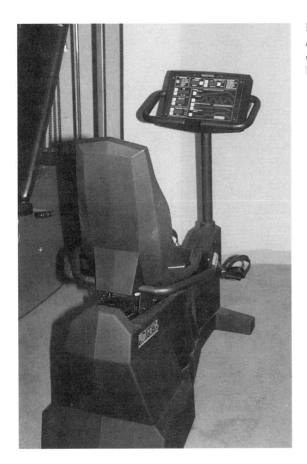

FIG. 2–38
Aerobic exercise. Recumbent bike—Often utilized for the more comfortable seated position, as compared to the upright stationary bike.

exercising), the duration (how long each session), and the frequency (how often). The assistant may then use the established parameters to implement an aerobic conditioning program.[16]

The intensity is typically measured in terms of a percentage of the maximum heart rate of the client. In healthy, young individuals, using the simple formula of 220 minus the age of the client can determine the maximum heart rate (MaxHR = 220 – age). To produce a conditioning response the intensity must be 60% to 85% of the MaxHR and can be targeted by multiplying the desired percentage by the MaxHR. When aerobically exercising clients with pathologies, a second method to establish a target HR is more reliable. Karvonen's formula is used with 0.6 as the intensity factor:

$$\text{Target HR} = [0.6 \, (\text{peak HR} - \text{resting HR})] + \text{resting HR}$$

After the target HR is established, exercising of the client can be monitored by taking the client's pulse.[16,37]

Duration of aerobic exercise is typically measured in minutes. There has been some debate to what is the most appropriate and effective duration needed for aerobic exercise. Historically, guidelines have been 20 minutes of aerobic exercise at an intensity of 70% MaxHR. General guidelines to produce an adaptive change in the client's aerobic system include: (1) more intense aerobic exercising needs shorter durations, and (2) less intense aerobic exercising needs longer durations to produce the same results. These general guidelines are dependent on the

FIG. 2–39
Cardiac stress test. Using elaborate measuring equipment, a client's maximal oxygen consumption during exercise can be determined, as well as heart rate and rhythm. Exercise base lines can be determined from the data collected (From Kisner & Colby, p 121, with permission.)

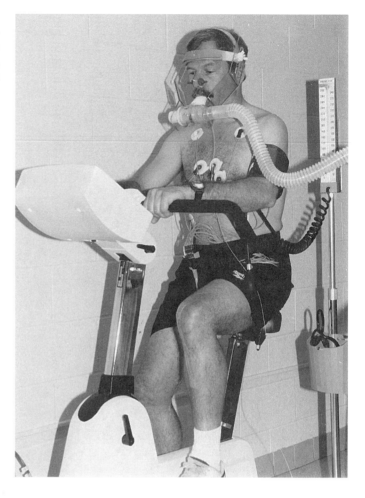

inherent abilities and disabilities of the client. For a deconditioned client, aerobic activities as little as 5 minutes daily may be sufficient to begin the adaptive change process; however, for the peak athlete, a more intense duration of 30 minutes may be needed. Clinically, the assistant must understand that exercise periods greater than 45 minutes may put the client at risk for injury to the musculoskeletal system.[16]

The frequency of aerobic exercise is measured in how many days per week and varies depending on the health state of the client. Aerobic exercise as little as twice per week may benefit some clients by giving adequate time for recovery and preventing overuse injuries, whereas the peak athlete may demand some form of aerobic exercise at least daily. Historically, the 3 to 4 times per week has been accepted as the proper frequency, but the assistant must ensure that an aerobic program is customized to fit the client's needs and abilities.[16]

 EXERCISE PRESCRIPTION

The exercise prescription is the basis of the plan of treatment in which the supervising physical therapist identifies what type of activity will be performed by the client, how often the activity will be performed, and how the activity should be progressed. The presentation of the exercise prescription may take several forms, ranging from general terms in the plan of a Subjective findings, Objective findings, Assessment, and Plan (SOAP) note to carefully identified exercise protocols that are in a preprinted format. Many companies now produce interchangeable home exercise cards, allowing the therapist to easily custom-tailor an exercise prescription to the individual client's specific needs. Figure 2–40 represents such an interchangeable system that is published by Therapy Skills Builders of San Antonio, Texas. Exercise prescriptions should be well designed to meet the client's needs and should be easy for the client to follow. The student PTA may be exposed to a wide variety of styles and protocols; however, the exercise prescription possesses many subcomponents in common. These common elements make the therapeutic plan of action easy to follow for both the client and the assistant.

COMPONENTS OF THE PRESCRIPTION

The term **frequency** refers to how often a client will perform the exercise prescription and is usually measured in times per day or times per week. **Duration** refers to how long each exercise session will last and can be measured in minutes or the number of times an exercise was performed. The number of **repetitions** refers to how many times an exercise is performed during that particular session and is grouped into how many **sets** that particular exercise was performed for that many repetitions. **Intensity** is how hard the client is exercising and can take several different forms of measurement, including a percentage of a targeted heart rate or how much weight is being used. The **mode** is what type of exercise the client is performing. For examples of exercise prescriptions, see Table 2–3.

WHEN TO ADVANCE THE CLIENT

Progression of exercise is critical for the continued success of an exercise program. As exercise produces strength gains in the client, progressive overloading must occur for strength gains to be continued. There exists many differing opinions regarding when and how to progress a client, but the underlying premise must be to progress as tolerated by the client. Kisner and Colby[8] stated in their text on therapeutic exercise that "it is difficult to make comparisons or determine which [exercise] protocol is best." Generally, the assistant will be working with clients with significant impairment and, thus, must tailor the progression to the response of each client. A concept of exercise progression was termed by Delorme and Watkins[38] in 1948 as **progressive resistive exercise (PRE)**. It is a frequently used term and concept in the physical therapy profession, even if the actual described principles are not exactly followed. See Table 2–4 for a discussion of the procedure for PRE.

When progressing a client clinically, the PTA must take three factors into consideration. First, as mentioned previously, the ability of the client to progress must be determined. The assistant can easily vary at each session the exercise determinants in the number of repetitions, sets, and/or load performed by the client and document accordingly the degree of success or lack of success. Adequate documentation for a client is necessary to show progression of tolerance or lack of tolerance, and this forms the basis on which judgements are made in future treatment sessions. The second consideration includes the physician and the specific orders or protocols given for the client. Depending on the physician and the condition of the client, a wide variety of exercise protocols may be given

Frequency
Frequency means how often.

Duration
Duration means how long.

Repetition
Repetition means how many.

Sets
Sets means how many groups of repetitions.

Intensity
Intensity means how hard.

Mode
Mode means what type of exercise.

Progressive Resistive Exercise (PRE)
Term coined by Delorme in 1948 for a method of progressively overloading the muscle to produce an adaptive strength change. The principles are still used today in physical therapy.

Elbow Extension — Active

_____ arm above head, elbow pointing to ceiling. Straighten elbow.

Hold ____ counts.

Repeat ____ times.

Progress to ____ lbs. at wrist/hand.

Knee Extension — Active

Stand with back against wall. Slide bottom down until knees are bent halfway.

Hold ____ counts.

Repeat ____ times.

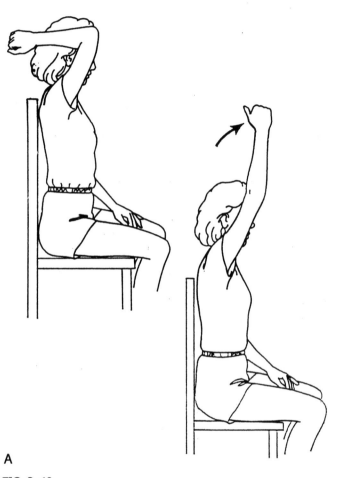

A

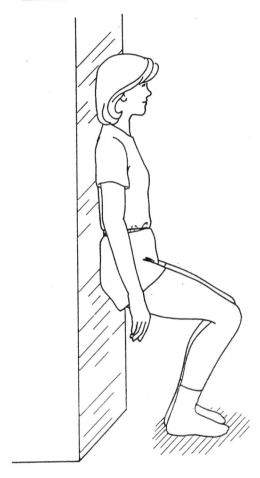

B

FIG. 2–40

Preprinted home exercise programs. "Progressive Individualized Exercises (PIE)," written by Joelle Schneider and Joan Cecil Passanisi, is an example of a complete set of premade exercise cards covering the head, neck, trunk, and upper and lower extremities that gives the clinician the opportunity to easily custom make an exercise program for clients. The original cards are simply photocopied and then the exercise parameters are filled in by the clinician. (A) is an example of the card for active elbow extension and (B) is an example of a closed chain active knee extension card. (From *Progressive Individualized Exercises.* Copyright © 1989 by Therapy Skills Builders, a division of The Psychological Corporation, 555 Academic Court, San Antonio, TX 78204-2498 [http://www.hbtpc.com]. Reproduced by permission. All rights reserved.)

___ *Table 2–3* _____

EXERCISE PRESCRIPTION	
Example A	**Frequency:** 3x/wk **Duration:** 20 min **Intensity:** 65% of maxHR **Repetitions:** NA **Mode:** Stationary bike
Example B	**P:** The client will perform SLR with 3# bid 3 sets of 20 reps.

NA = not applicable; SLR = straight-leg raising.

___ *Table 2–4* _____

DELORME'S TECHNIQUE OF EXERCISE PROGRESSION (PROGRESSIVE RESISTIVE EXERCISE)[38]

1. First, determine the maximum amount of resistance a client can successfully lift for 10 repetitions (this is referred to as the 10 rep max or 10 RM).
2. Perform exercise progression as follows:
   a. 10 reps @ ½ 10 RM
   b. 10 reps @ ¾ 10 RM
   c. 10 reps @ full 10 RM
3. Have client take a brief period of rest between each set of reps.
4. Increase resistance weekly as strength increases.

as directives. Some physicians expect their clients to do as much resistance as possible as fast as possible. The assistant must carefully administer this approach without causing harm to their clients. Conversely, some physicians, believe that no resistance should ever be used on their clients and the only means available to increase strength would be increasing the number of repetitions performed by the client. Lastly, the assistant must communicate effectively with the supervising therapist to follow the intentions of the exercise prescription. As described earlier, an exercise prescription established by the supervising therapist may be very detailed in nature or relatively generalized. Depending on the specifics of individual state practice acts and the working relationship between the supervising PT and the PTA, progression of exercise parameters may or may not be built into the original plan. The supervising therapist may intend for the assistant to discuss plans of client progression before actual implementation. In other instances, the progression of exercise is included in the established protocols and discussion between the supervising PT and the assistant is not necessary. In performing the role of the PTA, it is wise not to assume any issues related to client progression and discuss suggestions with the supervising therapist.

 ## SUMMARY

Skeletal muscle is the organ system responsible for producing movement and maintaining upright posture in the body. The contractile structure of the voluntary skeletal or striated muscle from smallest to largest component consists of the sarcomere, myofibril, muscle fiber, fascicle, and muscle. The sarcomere is the functional contractile element of the muscle housing the actin and myosin cross-bridges. The muscle is attached to the bone through a series of continuous connective tissue allowing for the transfer of force from the muscle to the bone. A motor unit is the alpha motor neuron and all of the muscle fibers it innervates and follows the all-or-none law, which states that a muscle fiber will contract fully or not at all. Muscle contractions vary in amount of tension produced and speed of contraction by altering the number of and the timing of motor units activated. The overload principle, the specificity of exercise principle, and reversibility principle play critical roles in the development of rehabilitation programs for the physical therapy client. Physiological limitations to strengthening exist depending on the fiber type composition and function of a muscle. Type I muscle fibers are designed generally for postural functions, whereas type II muscle fibers are designed for powerful motions. Energy production systems in muscle will also limit the ability of a muscle to perform work and are described in three overlapping processes, including the ATP-PC system, the anaerobic system, and the aerobic system. The ability of the body to use an energy system properly is dependent on the individual's state of health. Muscular strength is the ability of the muscle to develop force against some resistance. Muscular endurance is the ability of the muscle to perform repeated contractions over a period of time. Muscular power is the ability of the muscle to develop force quickly (strength × velocity). Forms of muscle contractions can be either isometric or isotonic in nature and may be exercised by providing either manual resistance or mechanical resistance. Concentric contractions of the muscle occur when the muscle produces tension and actively shortens; eccentric contractions of the muscle occur when tension develops and the muscle lengthens. Isokinetic contractions do not naturally occur in the human body and are produced through the assistance a special machine in which the muscle contracts or lengthens against a fixed speed or velocity. Plyometrics are an explosive form of exercise designed to produce speed and strength and are used in the end stages of athletic rehabilitation. Aerobic exercises are designed to promote endurance and strength of the cardiovascular system. The exercise prescription is a tool by which the therapist communicates to the assistant and the client what activity is to be performed during the rehabilitation program. Exercise programs may follow different formats, but they should possess common components of frequency, duration, repetitions, sets, intensity, and mode. An exercise prescription should be tailored to the individual client and easy to follow. Progression of the exercise program is relevant to the outlined plan of the supervising therapist, the orders of the physician, and most important, the ability of the client to progress. Complete case studies for Chapter 2 (see p. 470–474) to review the concepts presented in this chapter.

 REFERENCES

1. Salter, RB: Textbook of Disorders and Injuries of the Musculoskeletal System: Williams & Wilkins, Baltimore, 1983.
2. Lieber, RL, and Bodine-Fowler, SC: Skeletal muscle mechanics: Implications for rehabilitation. Phys Ther 73:844, 1993.
3. Norkin, CC, and Levangie, PK: Joint Structure & Function: A Comprehensive Analysis, ed 2. FA Davis, Philadelphia, 1992.

4. Binder-Macleod, SA: Introduction: Skeletal muscle. Phys Ther 73:829, 1993.

5. Taber's Cyclopedic Medical Dictionary, ed 18. FA Davis, Philadelphia, 1996.

6. Moore, KL: Clinically Oriented Anatomy, ed 2. Williams & Wilkins, Baltimore, 1985.

7. Atha, J: Strengthening muscle. Exerc Sports Sci Rev 9:1, 1981.

8. Kisner, C, and Colby, LA: Therapeutic Exercise: Foundations and Techniques. 3rd ed. FA Davis, Philadelphia, 1996.

9. Prentice, WE: Rehabilitation Techniques in Sports Medicine, ed 2. Mosby, St. Louis, MO, 1994.

10. Hopp, JF: Effects of age and resistance training on skeletal muscle: a review. Phys Ther 73:361, 1993.

11. Weiss, LW, et al: Effects of heavy-resistance triceps surae muscle training on strength and muscularity of men and women. Phys Ther 68:208, 1988.

12. Clamann, HP: Motor unit recruitment and the gradation of muscle force. Phys Ther 73:830, 1993.

13. Peter, JB, et al: Metabolic profiles of the three fiber types of skeletal muscle in guinea pigs and rabbits. Biochemistry 11:2627, 1972.

14. Pette, D, and Vrbova, G: Neural control of phenotypic expression in mammalian muscle fibers. Muscle Nerve 8:676, 1985.

15. Henneman, E, and Olson, CB: Relations between structure and function in the design of skeletal muscle. J Neurophysiol 28:581, 1965.

16. Burnett, CN, and Glenn, TM: Principles of aerobic exercise. In Kisner, C, and Colby, LA (eds): Therapeutic Exercise: Foundations and Techniques, ed 3. FA Davis, Philadelphia, 1996.

17. Bandy, WD, et al: Adaptations of skeletal muscle to resistance training. J Orthop Sports Phys Ther 12:248, 1990.

18. Bandy, WD, and Hanten, WP: Changes in torque and electromyographic activity of the quadriceps femoris muscles following isometric training. Phys Ther 73:455, 1993.

19. Gardner, G: Specificity of strength changes of the exercised and nonexercised limb following isometric training. Research Quarterly 34:98, 1963.

20. Meyers, CR: Effects of two isometric routines on strength size and endurance in exercised and nonexercised arms. Research Quarterly 38:430, 1967.

21. Lindh, M: Increase of muscle strength from isometric quadriceps exercises at different knee angles. Scand J Rehabil Med 11:33, 1979.

22. Belka, D: Comparison of dynamic, static and combination training on dominant wrist flexor muscles. Research Quarterly 39:241, 1968.

23. Thepaut-Mathieu, C, et al: Myoelectrical and mechanical changes linked to length specificity during isometric training. J Appl Physiol 64:1500, 1988.

24. Sullivan PE, et al: An integrated approach to therapeutic exercise: Theory & clinical application. Reston Publishing, Reston, VA, 1982.

25. Taber's Cyclopedic Medical Dictionary, ed 18. FA Davis, Philadelphia. p 2059, 1996.

26. Griffin, JW: Differences in elbow flexion torque measured concentrically, eccentrically, and isometrically. Phys Ther 67:1205, 1987.

27. Singh, M, and Karpovich, PV: Isotonic and isometric forces of forearm flexors and extensors. J Appl Physiol 21:1435, 1966.

28. Dean, E: Physiology and therapeutic implications of negative work: a review. Phys Ther 68:233, 1988.

29. Yackzan, L, Adams, C, Francis, KT: The effects of ice massage on delayed muscle soreness. Am J Sports Med 12:159, 1984.

30. Fitzgerald, GK, Rothstein, JM, Mayhew, TP, and Lamb, RL: Exercise-induced muscle soreness after concentric and eccentric isokinetic contractions. Phys Ther 71:505, 1991.

31. Lippert, L: Clinical Kinesiology for the Physical Therapist Assistant, ed 2. FA Davis, Philadelphia, 1994.

32. Knott, M, and Voss, DM: Proprioceptive Neuromuscular Facilitation, ed 2. Harper & Row, New York. 1968.

33. Davies, GJ, et al: Assessment of strength. In Malone, TR, et al (eds): Orthopedic and Sports Physical Therapy, ed 3. Mosby, St. Louis, MO, 1997.

34. Sanders, B: Exercise and rehabilitation concepts. In Malone, TR, et al (eds): Orthopedic and Sports Physical Therapy, ed 3, Mosby, St. Louis, MO, 1997.

35. Greenfield, BH, and Tovin, BJ: The application of open and closed kinematic chain exercises in rehabilitation of the lower extremity. Journal of Back Musculoskeletal Rehabilitation 2:38, 1992.

36. Chu, D: Plyometric exercise. NSCA J 6:56, 1984.

37. Hilling, L, and Smith, J: Pulmonary rehabilitation. In Irwin, S, and Tecklin, JS (eds): Cardiopulmonary Physical Therapy, ed 3. Mosby, St. Louis, MO, 1995.

38. Delorme, T, and Watkins, A: Technics of progressive resistive exercise. Arch Phys Med Rehabil 29:263, 1948.

BIBLIOGRAPHY

Atha, J: Strengthening muscle. Exerc Sports Sci Rev 9:1, 1981.

Bandy, WD, and Hanten, WP: Changes in torque and electromyographic activity of the quadriceps femoris muscles following isometric training. Phys Ther 73:455, 1993.

Bandy, WD, et al.: Adaptations of skeletal muscle to resistance training. J Orthop Sports Phys Ther 12:248, 1990.

Belka, D: Comparison of dynamic, static and combination training on dominant wrist flexor muscles. Research Quarterly 39:241, 1968.

Binder-Macleod, SA: Introduction: Skeletal muscle. Phys Ther 73:829, 1993.

Burnett, CN, and Glenn, TM: Principles of aerobic exercise. In Kisner, C, and Colby, LA: Therapeutic Exercise: Foundations and Techniques, ed 3. FA Davis, Philadelphia, 1996.

Chu, D: Plyometric exercise. NSCA J 6:56, 1984.

Clamann, HP: Motor unit recruitment and the gradation of muscle force. Phys Ther 73:830, 1993.

Davies, GJ, et al: Assessment of strength. In Malone, TR, et al (eds): Orthopedic and Sports Physical Therapy, ed 3. Mosby, St. Louis, MO, 1997.

Dean, E: Physiology and therapeutic implications of negative work: A review. Phys Ther 68:233, 1988.

Delorme, T, and Watkins, A: Technics of progressive resistive exercise. Arch Phys Med Rehabil 29:263, 1948.

Fitzgerald, GK, et al: Exercise-induced muscle soreness after concentric and eccentric isokinetic contractions. Phys Ther 71:505, 1991.

Gardner, G: Specificity of strength changes of the exercised and nonexercised limb following isometric training. Research Quarterly 34:98, 1963.

Greenfield, BH, and Tovin, BJ: The application of open and closed kinematic chain exercises in the rehabilitation of the lower extremity. Journal of Back Musculoskeletal Rehabilitation 2:38, 1992.

Griffin, JW: Differences in elbow flexion torque measured concentrically, eccentrically, and isometrically. Phys Ther 67:1205, 1987.

Henneman, E, and Olson, CB: Relations between structure and function in the design of skeletal muscle. J Neurophysiol 28:581, 1965.

Hilling, L, and Smith, J: Pulmonary rehabilitation. In Irwin, S, and Tecklin, JS: Cardiopulmonary Physical Therapy, ed 3. Mosby, St. Louis, MO, 1995.

Hopp, JF: Effects of age and resistance training on skeletal muscle: A review. Phys Ther 73:361, 1993.

Kisner, C, and Colby, LA: Therapeutic Exercise: Foundations and Techniques, ed 3. FA Davis, Philadelphia, 1996.

Knott, M, and Voss, DM: Proprioceptive Neuromuscular Facilitation, ed 2. Harper & Row, New York. 1968.

Lieber, RL and Bodine-Fowler, SC: Skeletal muscle mechanics: Implications for rehabilitation. Phys Ther 73:844, 1993.

Lindh, M: Increase of muscle strength from isometric quadriceps exercises at different knee angles. Scand J Rehabil Med 11:33, 1979.

Lippert, L: Clinical Kinesiology for the Physical Therapist Assistant, ed 2. FA Davis, Philadelphia. 1994.

Meyers, CR: Effects of two isometric routines on strength size and endurance in exercised and nonexercised arms. Research Quarterly 38:430, 1967.

Moore, KL: Clinically Oriented Anatomy, ed 2. Williams & Wilkins, Baltimore, 1985.

Norkin, CC, and Levangie, PK: Joint Structure & Function: A Comprehensive Analysis, ed 2. FA Davis, Philadelphia, 1992.

Peter, JB, et al: Metabolic profiles of the three fiber types of skeletal muscle in guinea pigs and rabbits. Biochemistry 11:2627, 1972.

Pette, D, and Vrbova, G: Neural control of phenotypic expression in mammalian muscle fibers. Muscle Nerve 8:676, 1985.

Prentice, WE: Muscular strength and endurance. In Prentice, WE: Rehabilitation Techniques in Sports Medicine, ed 2. Mosby, St. Louis, MO, 1994.

Salter, RB: Textbook of Disorders and Injuries of the Musculoskeletal System, ed 2. Williams & Wilkins, Baltimore, 1983.

Sanders, B: Exercise and rehabilitation concepts. In Malone, TR, et al (eds): Orthopedic and Sports Physical Therapy, ed 3. Mosby, MO, St. Louis, 1997.

Singh, M, and Karpovich, PV: Isotonic and isometric forces of forearm flexors and extensors. J Appl Physiol 21:1435, 1966.

Sullivan PE, et al: An Integrated Approach to Therapeutic Exercise: Theory & Clinical Application. Reston Publishing, Reston, VA, 1982.

Taber's Cyclopedic Medical Dictionary, ed 18. FA Davis, Philadelphia, 1996.

Thepaut-Mathieu, C, et al: Myoelectrical and mechanical changes linked to length specificity during isometric training. J Appl Physiol 64:1500, 1988.

Weiss, LW, et al: Effects of heavy-resistance triceps surae muscle training on strength and muscularity of men and women. Phys Ther 68:208, 1988.

Yackzan, L, et al: The effects of ice massage on delayed muscle soreness. Am J Sports Med 12:159, 1984.

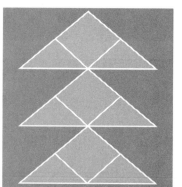

chapter 3

Range of Motion

Outline

After completing this chapter, the PTA student will be able to:
1. Define *range of motion* and describe the factors that influence range of motion.
2. Differentiate between passive, active, and active-assistive range of motion.
3. Identify the indications and contraindications of range of motion exercises.
4. Understand how to apply range of motion techniques.
5. Describe the neurophysiology related to flexibility in the human body.
6. Differentiate between mechanical and manual range of motion techniques.
7. Understand how to apply appropriate stretching methods to increase flexibility.

Key Words

active insufficiency
active assistive range of motion
active range of motion
agonistic muscle
antagonistic muscle
autogenic inhibition
ballistic stretching
facilitation
flexibility
golgi tendon organ
inhibition
intertester reliability
intratester reliability
mechanical elongation techniques
muscle spindle
passive insufficiency
passive range of motion
proprioceptive neuromuscular facilitation
range of motion
reciprocal inhibition
reliability
static stretching
validity

Range of Motion (ROM)
Range of motion is the fullest motion available about a joint.

RANGE OF MOTION

The fullest motion available about a joint is referred to as **range of motion** (ROM). Each joint in the human body has various amounts of available motion depending upon the soft-tissue structures that cross the joint, the shape of the joint surfaces, the age of the individual, the gender of the individual, and the type of motion occurring.[1,2]

FACTORS AFFECTING RANGE OF MOTION

Range of motion is affected by the structures that cross the joint, including ligaments, muscles, nerves, fascia, joint capsules, and blood vessels. The relative tension, or the ability of these structures to allow or prohibit motion at a joint, is critical in determining to what degree a joint will move. To demonstrate this principle, push the index finger of your right hand against the index finger of your left hand hyperextending the left index finger. During this investigation, be sure to keep both interphalangeal joints of the left hand fully extended. How far will the left index finger hyperextend? What are the limiting structures preventing this finger from touching the dorsum of the hand? Is it the same for all of your classmates? This investigation should produce a variety of results among your classmates. In general, the long finger flexor tendons of the left hand will limit the available ROM of the left index finger. Some individuals will have greater (or lesser) ROM depending on the flexibility of the tendons crossing the joints of the left index finger. Other soft-tissue structures (e.g., blood vessels, fascia, or joint capsule) may play an equally limiting role in the available motion of a joint.

Joint Structure

The shape of the joint surfaces can also dictate how far a joint will move. Comparing the elbow (humeroulnar) joint and the knee (femorotibial) joint will effectively demonstrate this concept. Full extension of the elbow joint is limited when the olecranon process fills the olecranon fossae, resulting in a stoppage of the extension motion. The elbow joint will not move into a greater ROM because of the bony limitation. Conversely, the knee joint has freedom to move into extension without significant bony limitation. In fact, soft-tissue structures (ligament and capsule) are major limiting factors in knee extension.

Age

The age of the individual will also play a role in the ability of a joint to move through the greatest amount of motion possible. Comparing the motion of a joint in a newborn infant to the same joint in a 79-year-old man will confirm different ranges of joint motion. Boone and Azen[3] demonstrated that a significant difference in average ROM measurements exists between children under 2 years and established adult average ROM measurements. Other authors[4,5] have concluded that a loss of joint motion exists as aging occurs, but they are inconclusive on absolute predictions that can be generalized to the entire adult population. Roach and Miles[6] found that published textbook ranges for normal motion values were not representative of the entire population of the United States and set out to identify normal ROM at the hip and knee. They concluded that until the age 74, losses in ROM should be considered abnormal (i.e., not a normal consequence of aging).

Gender

Some studies have addressed gender differences in establishing normal ROM measurements with the theory that gender will affect the ROM of a joint. For example, women (ages 21 to 69) tend to have less hip extension compared with their male counterparts, yet the same age group of women tend to demonstrate greater hip flexion.[7] Limitations noted in normal ROM when comparing gender tend to be specific to the joint involved, the type of motion, and the age of the client. Norkin and White[2] claimed that making judgements about joint limitations due to gender is difficult because gender-related norms have not been well established for all age groups.

Types of Motion

The type of motion that is occurring about a joint will also play a role in the availability of joint motion. Differences in ROM can be noted when the same joint is moved actively as compared with passively. This principle is demonstrated by lying prone and actively bending your knee. How far were you able to actively move your knee through the ROM? Now have someone push your heel closer to your buttock. Did the knee move through a further ROM? The hamstring muscle group is able to actively flex the knee in the prone position to an angle approaching 120° from the horizontal surface. At this point, the hamstring muscles are not able to physically contract further to produce motion about the joint. **Active insufficiency** occurs when a muscle can no longer actively shorten to move a joint through the ROM. The concept of active insufficiency is applied to the muscle that is performing the movement of the joint, or the **agonistic muscle.** The physical distance or the ability of the muscle to move a joint through the ROM is different for each muscle in the body and varies dramatically if the muscle functions at only one joint (one-joint muscles, such as the brachialis muscle) or at a combination of joints (multijoint muscles, such as the biceps brachii muscle). Figure 3–1A provides a visualization of the principle of active insufficiency.[1,8]

Active Insufficiency
Active insufficiency occurs when an agonistic muscle can no longer actively shorten to move a joint through the available ROM.

Agonistic Muscle
Agonistic muscle is the muscle about a moving joint that produces the desired motion.

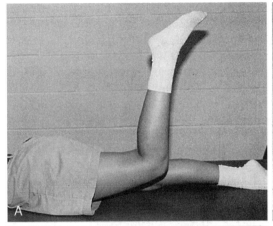

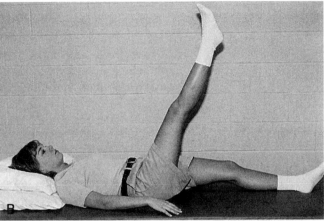

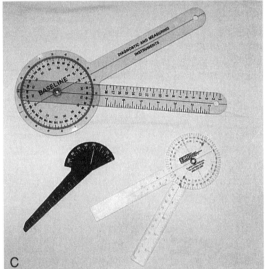

FIG. 3–1

(A) Active insufficiency. By performing prone hip extension and knee flexion simultaneously, the hamstring muscle becomes actively insufficient because it can no longer physically shorten to flex the knee or extend the hip. **(B) Passive insufficiency.** By performing supine hip flexion while keeping the knee extended and the pelvis stabilized, the hamstring muscle becomes passively insufficient because it can not physically lengthen to allow greater hip flexion. **(C) Standard goniometer.** This basic tool of the physical therapy profession is simply a protractor measuring incremental degrees with one moving and one stationary arm. Pictured here are a long-armed, short-armed, and finger goniometer. Norkin & White *Measurement in Joint Motion*: A *Guide to Goniometry* (FA Davis, 1995) covers the procedures and positioning for measuring the ROM of a joint.

Motion limitations can also be created by passive elements in the body. When performing the experiment in the previous paragraph, on reaching the contracting limits of the hamstring muscle to produce knee flexion, a partner can passively flex the knee to a greater distance. However, a tight or painful feeling may be felt in the anterior thigh as the quadriceps femoris muscle group reaches a passive limitation to full knee flexion. **Passive insufficiency** occurs when a muscle cannot passively lengthen further to allow complete ROM about a joint without producing internal damage to the muscular elements. For full knee flexion to occur, the **antagonistic muscle** (quadriceps femoris) must be able to relax passively and not oppose the motion of the agonist. Figure 3–1B provides a visualization of the principle of passive insufficiency.[1,8]

The assistant should be able to determine the nature of joint limitation due to contractile elements. The agonist may limit motion due to active insufficiency and the physical inability to contract any greater distance. The antagonist may limit ROM due to passive insufficiency and the physical inability to lengthen any greater distance permitting greater motion to occur. Joint motion may also be affected by a combination of both principles simultaneously. The hamstring muscles may not actively flex the knee through any greater ROM concurrent with the failure of the quadriceps muscles to passively lengthen adequately, allowing greater motion

Passive Insufficiency
Passive insufficiency occurs when an antagonistic muscle cannot passively lengthen further to allow complete ROM about a joint without producing internal damage to the muscular elements.

Antagonistic Muscle
Antagonistic muscle is the muscle opposite the agonist capable of opposing the desired motion.

into knee flexion. Lippert[8] reported that generally the agonist will reach a state of active insufficiency before the antagonist will become passively insufficient. Active and passive insufficiency are normal mechanical principles for each joint in the human body with normal or average ranges of motion produced; however, pathological conditions to the agonist (muscle or tendon damage) or the antagonist (muscle tightness) may further limit normal ROM.

BENEFITS OF RANGE OF MOTION

Range-of-motion exercises have been often associated with rehabilitation techniques and the profession of physical therapy, but their actual benefits are often misunderstood by the medical profession and the public. In general, ROM exercises are able to:

1. Promote the integrity of joint and soft-tissue structures
2. Lessen the potential of joint contractures
3. Use the mechanical properties of elasticity in the muscle
4. Assist in circulation and vascular drainage
5. Assist the movement of synovial fluid in the joint, which in turn provides nutrients to the articular cartilage
6. Promote a reduction in pain
7. Promote a positive environment for healing
8. Promote kinesthetic awareness (i.e., the client's awareness of movement)

The specific indications and contraindications for specific types of ROM exercises are discussed late in this chapter.[1]

MEASURING RANGE OF MOTION

There are many different tools used to measure the extent to which a joint is moving, but the most commonly accepted tool in the physical therapy profession is the standard goniometer (Fig. 3–1C). A goniometer is a version of the protractor used by children for drawing pictures and by architects to create exact angles. This device can help the examiner easily measure the available ROM about a moving or stationary joint. Alternative means to measure ROM include (1) fluid-based goniometers that work on the principle of a carpenter's level with an air bubble in a fluid-filled circular chamber, (2) tape measures, (3) visual estimates, (4) gravity-dependent inclinometers, and (5) electronic goniometers. For a more comprehensive description of alternative methods for assessing joint ROM, please refer to the text written by Norkin and White.[2]

Reliability

Reliability
The consistency of a measurement.

Reliability of a measurement is defined by Miller[9] as the consistency of the measurement. A highly reliable measurement is one that can generate a great deal of confidence, resulting in the measurement's being used for clinical decision making. A measurement of poor reliability should not be used for clinical decision making. The assistant may increase the reliability of a measurement by being consistent in the choice of the client position used during measurement, the device placement, the motion being analyzed, the device being used, and the examiner performing the measurement.[2]

When performing repeated measurements on a joint, consistency in the test position is critical. Measuring knee flexion supine during one assessment and prone in the next limits the reliability of the measurement. The position of the rectus femoris muscle has changed, being shortened at the hip in the first method and lengthened in the second. The routine use of established bony landmarks in goniometric alignment assists the reliability of the measurement. The inexperienced examiner must work to improve palpation skills of bony landmarks and knowledge of the appropriate test positions.

Reliability of the ROM measurement can also be decreased if the assistant in one treatment session measures the motion of the shoulder actively, and in the following treatment session passively. The assistant must document both the type of motion occurring and the position of the client during the measurement, in order for the measurement to be successfully reproduced. Consistency of the motion being analyzed is a critical factor in determining appropriate clinical decisions regarding the successes (or failures) of treatment programs.

When choosing a device for measuring ROM, the assistant can influence the reliability of an assessment. The use of different goniometers to measure the same joint will decrease reliability. Rheault et al.[10] examined the reliability between standard goniometers and fluid-based goniometers and found that although measurement results were similar, the two measuring devices cannot be used interchangeably in the clinic. The assistant should ensure that the documented results are produced with the same goniometer from session to session. A second consideration in making a choice of goniometer is using a long-armed versus a short-armed goniometer. Norkin and White[2] suggested that "examiners will find it easier and more accurate to use a large universal goniometer when measuring joints with large body segments, and a small goniometer when measuring joints with small body segments." Robson[11] in 1966 determined that long-armed goniometers are more accurate in the measurements of angles as compared with short-armed goniometers. However, more recent research by Rothstein et al.[12] and Riddle et al.[13] have suggested that there exists no difference in the reliability among short-armed and long-armed goniometers.

Intertester reliability and intratester reliability have often been the subjects of researched projects and professional literature. **Intertester reliability** addresses the consistency between two different clinicians performing the assessment. **Intratester reliability** addresses the consistency between the same clinician performing the assessment over different sessions or trials. Intratester reliability is generally more reliable using a standard goniometer than intertester reliability.[14] However, studies by Mitchell et al.[15] and Rheault et al.[10] found that intertester reliability can be equal to that of intratester reliability if both clinicians use standardized assessment procedures.

An area of little documented research is the reliability of visual estimates even though "estimations" of joint motion are frequently used in clinical practice. A study by Watkins et al.[14] addressed the reliability of clinical visual estimates. The authors reported that the visual estimates were slightly less reliable than goniometric measurements. In the conclusion section of the research, the authors stated: "the additional error associated with visual estimates could affect the usefulness of the measurements if a therapist is attempting to detect small changes in a patient's ROM." They also concluded that "[a] therapist can minimize error by using a goniometer and by standardizing patient position."

Validity

Compared with reliability, the concept of validity in ROM measurements is not as widely researched and documented in the professional literature. The **validity** of a measurement refers to the exactness or accuracy in which the measurement represents the actual ROM of the joint being measured. Stated simply: Does it

Intertester Reliability
The consistency between two different clinicians performing the assessment.

Intratester Reliability
The consistency between the same clinician performing the assessment over different sessions or trials.

Validity
The exactness of the measurement or how well the measurement represents the actual nature of the joint being measured.

measure what it is supposed to? In the physical therapy profession, it has been generally assumed that the validity of a goniometer measuring joint ROM is correct and that degree changes in the goniometer truly represent changes in the joint being measured.[16] The assistant is generally not concerned with the interpretation of the validity of standard goniometers in the everyday practice of his or her profession. The assistant will have a greater influence on the reliability of the instrument, as mentioned previously.

TYPES OF RANGE OF MOTION

Range of motion activities are a foundation of the therapeutic exercise that physical therapy clinicians use in developing intervention programs for their clients. Types of ROM activities will fall into four categories, depending on the involvement by the client performing the motion or exercise: active, active-assistive, passive, or resistive. To make sound clinical judgements, the clinician at all times should be aware of the safety and ability of the client to perform prescribed tasks or techniques and fully understand when to use (indications) and when not to use (contraindications) ROM activities.

Active Range of Motion

Active Range of Motion (AROM)
Exercises in which the client is actively moving the body part through the available motion with no assistance from the clinician.

Active range of motion (AROM) exercises are those in which the client is actively moving the body part through the available motion with no assistance from the clinician. An example of AROM would be demonstrated by having a client lift his or her arms overhead and then lower the arms to the side of the body. The motion produced moves the glenohumeral joint through the maximum amount of shoulder ROM followed by a return movement to the starting point at the side of the body (Fig. 3–2).

Active range of motion exercises are indicated in the following cases:

1. When the client is able to move the body part independently (assuming no medical contraindications to movement have been ordered by the physician)
2. To promote use of the contractile elements of the muscle
3. To provide neurological feedback from contracting muscles
4. To promote bone and soft-tissue integrity
5. To promote circulation and prevent deep venous thrombosis (DVT) formation
6. To enhance coordination and motor skills
7. To promote cardiovascular endurance[1]

Limitations of AROM include the fact that strength gains for an already strong muscle will not be produced by performing AROM. To strengthen an already strong muscle, progressive techniques must be implemented (see Chapter 2). Also, AROM will improve skill and coordination only in the exercise patterns that have been used (specificity of exercise principle).[1]

The assistant must also make appropriate clinical decisions regarding when the use of AROM activities may be harmful or not of benefit to the client. Absolute contraindications for AROM activities are situations in which motion will:

1. Disrupt the healing process
2. Cause undue harm to the client.

An example of motion disrupting to the healing process would be a healing fracture. An example of motion causing undue harm to the client would be the presence of a DVT in the lower extremity. Relative contraindications or precautions include the consideration of the effects of immobilization. There are instances in

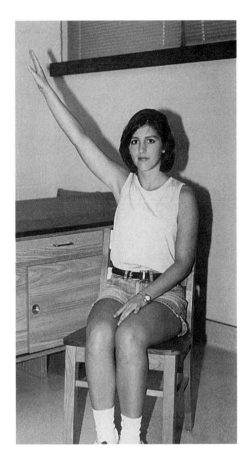

FIG. 3–2
AROM. The client lifts the arm overhead through an abduction motion without any assistance from the clinician.

which immobilization is more harmful than controlled motion activities. Researched evidence by Salter[17,18,19] has identified the positive effects of controlled motion early in rehabilitation efforts as compared with immobilization for most soft-tissue and synovial joint injuries. This research suggests that the clinical application of ROM activities within the pain-free ROM are beneficial to the healing process in most cases. The effects of immobilization and tissue healing are discussed in Chapter 5.

Active-Assistive

Active-assistive range of motion (AAROM) exercises are also performed actively by the client, with the clinician helping the motion to be safely and effectively performed either by manual or mechanical means. The clinician can help a client move the shoulder through abduction ROM by supporting at the wrist and elbow, aiding the client achieve the fullest motion available. The clinician may also use a set of over-the-door ropes and pulleys and have the client assist the abduction range of motion by mechanical means (Fig. 3–3).

Indications for AAROM are very similar to the use of AROM. AAROM exercises are indicated in a therapeutic exercise plan in the following cases:

1. When the client needs assistance to move the body part because of muscular weakness or for safety concerns (assuming no medical contraindications to motion exist)

Active-Assistive Range of Motion (AAROM)
Exercises performed actively by the client with the clinician assisting the body part through the available ROM.

FIG. 3–3
AAROM. By using over-the-door wall pulleys, the clinician can provide AAROM exercises to the client through mechanical means. The over-the-door wall pulleys can be utilized to perform PROM as well.

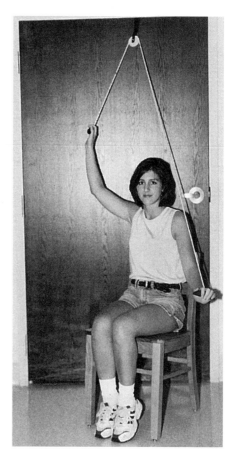

2. To promote use of the contractile elements of the muscle
3. To provide feedback from contracting muscles
4. To promote bone and soft tissue integrity
5. To promote circulation and prevent deep venous thrombosis (DVT) formation
6. To enhance coordination and motor skills
7. To learn new skill or movement patterns[1]

Limitations of performing AAROM exercises include:

1. The strength of an already strong muscle cannot be increased.
2. Coordination improvements will only be noted in specific exercise patterns performed.
3. AAROM is generally less effective in promoting use of contractile elements and promoting bone integrity than AROM.

Contraindications for the use of AAROM by the assistant are identical to those listed for the use of AROM:

1. When disruption of the healing process will occur
2. When undue harm may be caused to the client

Passive

Motions that are performed without any effort from the client as the clinician moves the client's body part through the available ROM are known as **passive range of motion** (PROM) exercises. Figure 3–4 demonstrates an assistant performing PROM on a client's shoulder moving through the available ROM. The client is not actively participating in the movement as the assistant moves the body part in a safe, controlled manner.

Passive range of motion exercises are indicated for use by the assistant in the following cases:

1. When a client is physically unable to move his or her own body part because of paralysis or coma
2. When a physician's order prohibits active motion, passive motion may be indicated to facilitate the healing process and prevent complications of immobilization
3. To assess joint limitations and joint integrity
4. To teach desired and/or proper motions during an exercise program
5. To prepare client for stretching activities
6. If client discomfort prevents the use of active motion[1]

Limitations of PROM include:

1. The inability to retard muscle atrophy
2. The inability to promote muscular strength and endurance

Passive Range of Motion (PROM)
Exercises performed without any effort from the client as the clinician moves the client's body part through the available ROM.

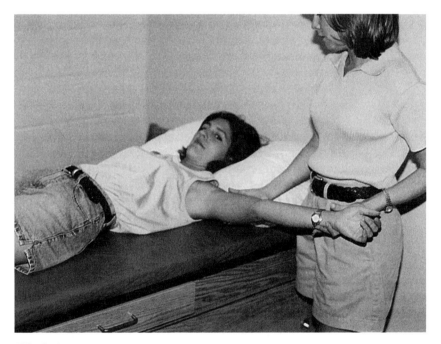

FIG. 3–4
PROM. The assistant may frequently have the opportunity to work with clients who are unable to actively perform range-of-motion exercises due to medical restrictions or due to a physical inability to move actively. PROM exercises are performed solely by the clinician, because the client is a passive participant.

3. Limited circulatory promotion
4. The inability of the client to fully relax, allowing true passive motion to occur

The limitations of PROM revolve around the premise that the muscle is not being actively used during the exercise. Strength gains (or prevention of strength losses) cannot be realized because the only method to promote strength gains is by producing active muscle contractions. Circulatory concerns are not fully addressed during passive activities because the active muscle contraction or "muscle-pumping" mechanism is absent to assist the return of venous blood. Active motion is more effective than PROM to promote circulatory concerns; however, if AROM is contraindicated, PROM may be the next best alternative.[1]

Contraindications for the use of PROM by the assistant are identical to those listed for the use of AROM:

1. When disruption of the healing process will occur
2. When undue harm may be caused to the client

Resistive

Resistive range of motion exercises are performed actively by the client moving through the available ROM with some form of resistance added to the movement. The resistance may be either mechanical (ankle weights) or manual (clinician applies the resistance directly to the client's moving body part). The indications, contraindications, and techniques for applying resistive techniques have been discussed in Chapter 2.

TECHNIQUES FOR APPLYING RANGE OF MOTION

The PTA will use ROM exercise as part of a therapeutic intervention program to achieve established goals for the client. The techniques for ROM activities can be performed in three different styles of movement, which include:

1. Anatomic planes
2. Combination movements
3. Functional patterns

Hand placement of the clinician will vary depending on the desired activity or movement to ensure safety of the client. When performing PROM exercises, the clinician must securely and comfortably support the entire body part during the motion. When performing AAROM, the clinician must give enough support to provide safety for the client, but also to grant adequate clearance to allow the client to move as much as possible. When performing AROM, the clinician may provide only verbal cuing and no physical assistance to the client when exercising. Box 3–1 summarizes the client preparation needed to safely and effectively perform ROM exercises. Figures 3–5 through 3–20A present the basic application techniques of ROM activities. The assistant—through proper knowledge of anatomy, myology (origins, insertions, actions of muscle), and functional activities of the extremities—will be able to apply ROM skills to any involved joint to achieve therapeutic goals.

FLEXIBILITY

Flexibility

A term indicating the ability to move a segment or a series of segments through the complete range of pain-free motion available.

Flexibility is defined as the ability to move a segment or a series of segments through the complete range of pain-free motion available.[20] Different activities

Text continued on page 77

Box 3-1

CLIENT PREPARATION FOR RANGE-OF-MOTION EXERCISES

The assistant should ensure client safety by performing the following preparatory steps before initiating ROM exercises:

1. From the evaluation, identify the proper motion technique to be performed (PROM, AAROM, AROM, resistive ROM).
2. Ensure that the client is positioned comfortably, allowing the fullest movement possible of the desired joint.
3. Explain to the client what you are about to do and why.
4. Remove restrictive clothing.
5. Proper body mechanics of the clinician is required for his or her safety.
6. Stabilize body segments that require support.
7. Describe the desired motion to the client that you want to produce. (For AAROM or AROM, you may need to demonstrate *passively* the desired technique to ensure proper performance and compliance. For PROM, instruct the client to completely relax and let you move the body part. Having the client focus on nonrelated tasks often helps them to relax and let you do the work).
8. Movement of the client's joint should be through the pain-free ROM. If pain is elicited, do not force joint into painful ROM because negative side effects such as muscle guarding or tissue damage may occur.
9. Motion by the assistant should be smooth, confident, and controlled. Repetitions vary depending on client tolerance and goals of the exercise session, but range from 10 to 20 repetitions.
10. Discuss the desired outcomes with the client during the treatment session. Involving the client in the treatment process generally increases client compliance.
11. Monitor the client for any negative responses. If negative situations arise, stop treatment and manage the new situation appropriately.
12. Progress as tolerated by the client *and* as designed in the plan of treatment.

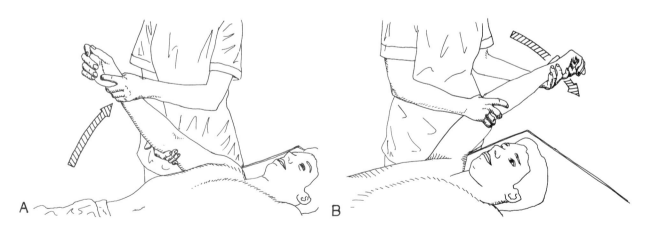

FIG. 3-5

Shoulder flexion ROM exercises. By grasping under the elbow and at the wrist (A), the assistant can move the shoulder through the available ROM and return to the starting position (B). Proper scapula stabilization and motion is desired to prevent impingement of the humerus under the acromial arch. The client may also be positioned sitting. (From Kisner & Colby, p 29, with permission.)

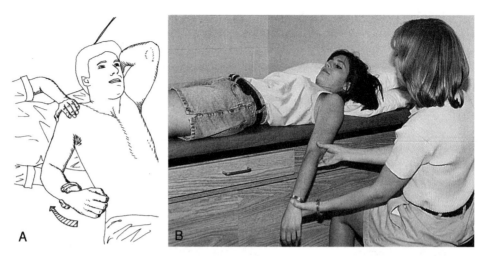

FIG. 3–6
Shoulder extension ROM exercises. Positioning the client in side lying (A) opposite the affected extremity will allow for easy access to grasp the wrist and stabilize at the shoulder girdle to move the humerus into extension. (From Kisner & Colby, p 29, with permission.) An alternate position (B) has the client supine with the affected extremity extended off the edge of the table grasping at the wrist and proximal humerus.

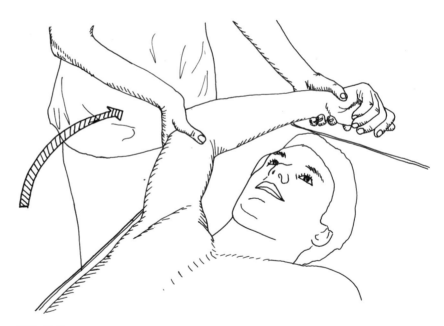

FIG. 3–7
Shoulder ABD/ADD ROM exercises. Positioning the client supine and grasping firmly at the wrist and elbow will allow for easy maneuvering into shoulder abduction and returning to starting point (adduction). Be keenly aware that the humerus externally rotates and the scapula upwardly rotates to complete full abduction. (From Kisner & Colby, p 30, with permission.)

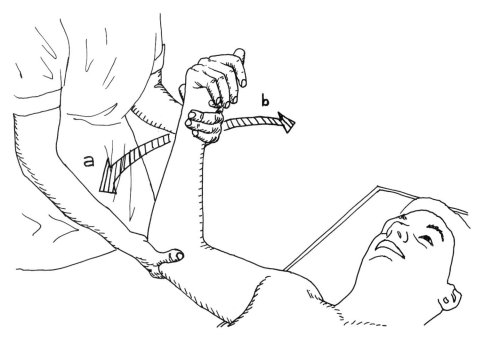

FIG. 3–8
Shoulder ER/IR ROM exercises. Stabilizing under the elbow and grasping the wrist securely as pictured will allow the assistant to easily perform internal rotation (A) and external rotation (B). (From Kisner & Colby, p 30, with permission.)

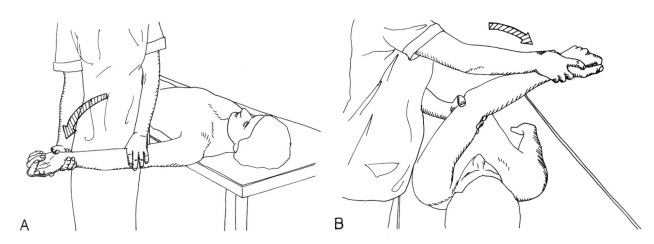

FIG. 3–9
Shoulder horizontal flexion and extension (Horizontal ADD/ABD) ROM exercises. The supine position allows for adequate scapular stabilization, allowing the assistant to move the client's humerus through horizontal extension (A) or horizontal flexion (B) by grasping the dorsal side of the wrist and the anterior surface of the elbow. (From Kisner & Colby, p 31, with permission.)

FIG. 3–10
Scapular ROM exercises. Positioning the client in side lying with the involved extremity superiorly facing the assistant allows for grasping of the scapula at the acromial arch
and the inferior angle. The client's arm should be relaxed
and supported appropriately by the assistant. The scapula
can be moved into the opposing motions of elevation/
depression, protraction/retraction and upward/downward
rotation easily, without changing hand placement or client
positioning.

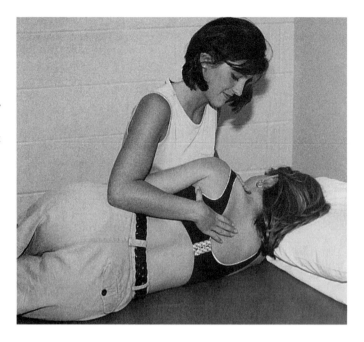

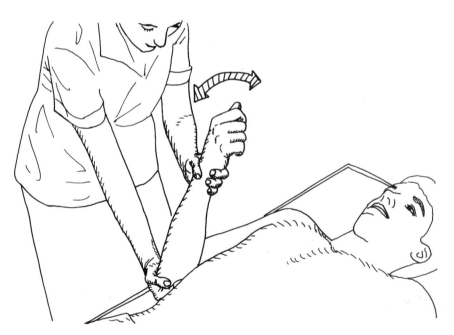

FIG. 3–11
Elbow flexion and extension ROM exercises. Position the client supine (alternate is
sitting) and stabilize under the elbow and grasp the anterior surface of the wrist to
move the elbow through the available ROM. (From Kisner & Colby, p 32, with
permission.)

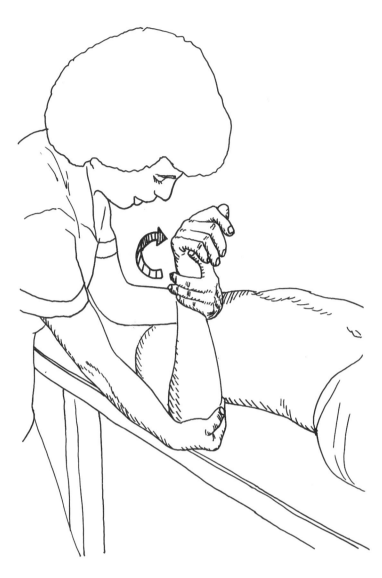

FIG. 3–12
Forearm pronation and supination ROM exercises.
Position the client supine (alternate is sitting) and stabilize under the elbow and grasp the anterior surface of the wrist. The assistant can roll the radius around the ulna, performing pronation and supination of the forearm. Ensure not to place increased stress on the wrist by performing the motion at the carpal bones. (From Kisner & Colby, p 33, with permission.)

require differing amounts of flexibility through the joints of the body or through a series of joints to successfully and safely perform the task. Easily pictured examples include the gymnast, divers, and ballet dancers. Participants in these activities place great flexibility demands on their bodies to perform the required elements of their sport. Previously in this chapter, factors limiting ROM were addressed, and now a discussion of the neurophysiological basis for flexibility is presented.

SENSORY ORGANS

The muscles and joints of the human body house many differing types of mechanoreceptors that provide feedback to the central nervous system. When activated, the mechanoreceptors provide an awareness or sense of what motion or type of activity is occurring. Two sensory organs found in skeletal muscle are of particular importance when discussing the availability of motion about a joint.

FIG. 3–13
Wrist flexion/extension and ulnar/radial deviation ROM exercises. Position the client supine (alternate is sitting) and stabilize by holding the forearm of the client with the elbow in a 90° flexed position. Grasp the hand of the client from the ulnar border and gently move the wrist through flexion/extension as well as ulnar/radial deviation. (From Kisner & Colby, p 34, with permission.)

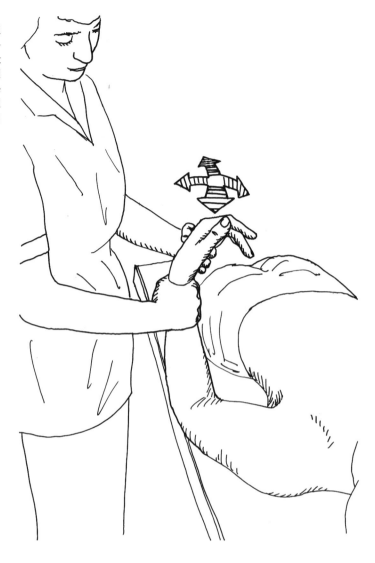

These sensory organs either limit or enhance methods to increase the flexibility of a joint.

Muscle Spindle

Muscle Spindle
The muscle spindle is found parallel to the muscle fibers responding to length changes and velocity of length changes. When activated, the muscle spindle will send impulses to the spinal cord initiating the stretch reflex, which in turn facilitates a contraction of the muscle being stretched.

The **muscle spindle** is found parallel to the muscle fibers and responds to length changes and velocity of length changes. When activated, the muscle spindle will send impulses to the spinal cord initiating the stretch reflex. The stretch reflex results in a contraction of the muscle being stretched. The stretch reflex principle is demonstrated by using a reflex hammer to quickly stretch the patellar tendon (Fig. 3–20B). Instruct the client to sit on an examination table with the knee relaxed at 90° of flexion. Using the hammer, strike just distal to the patella. The result should be a quick contractile response by the quadriceps muscle, producing knee extension. During flexibility exercises, if a muscle is stretched too quickly, the response of a stimulated muscle spindle will be to facilitate the muscle being stretched. Clinically, the assistant wants to avoid stimulation of the muscle spindle to promote relaxation of the muscular elements, allowing for lengthening to occur.[1,20]

Golgi Tendon Organ

The second sensory organ of importance in increasing flexibility is the **Golgi tendon organ** (GTO), which is found at the musculotendinous junction in series to the sarcomere or contractile units (Fig. 3–20C). The GTO senses length and tension changes developed within the muscle. The function of the GTO is to inhibit muscular contraction if the tension developed within the muscle becomes excessive, preventing damage that may be produced to the contractile elements. The inhibition of the muscle by the GTO produces a relaxation of the muscle. The GTO will activate in one of two fashions:

1. Through tension developed during an active contraction
2. Through tension and length changes developed during a passive stretch

Golgi Tendon Organ (GTO)
The GTO is found at the musculotendinous junction in series to the sarcomere or contractile units and senses length and tension changes developed within the muscle. When activated, the GTO sends an impulse to inhibit muscular contraction.

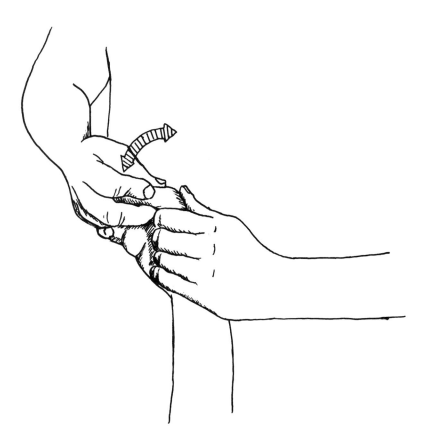

FIG. 3–14
Digit (MCP, IP) flexion/extension ROM exercises. Position the client in a sitting position and stabilize by holding the wrist and palm of the client's hand from the ulnar border. The thumb and index finger of the stabilizing hand can easily be moved to the client's involved digit to stabilize just proximal to the moving joint as the free hand of the assistant moves the joint by grasping distal to the joint. The wrist should be stabilized in a neutral position. (From Kisner & Colby, p 35, with permission.)

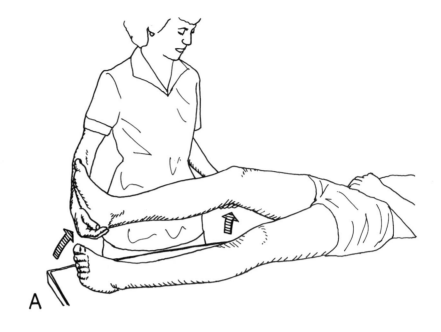

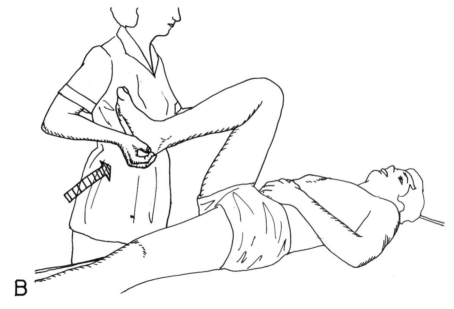

FIG. 3–15

Hip and knee flexion/extension ROM exercises. Positioning the client supine will allow the assistant to grasp the posterior surface of the heel and the knee (A) and be able to lift the lower extremity creating flexion at both the hip and knee (B). Positioning the client on his or her side allows the assistant to successfully hyperextend the hip through the available ROM. (From Kisner & Colby, p 37, with permission.)

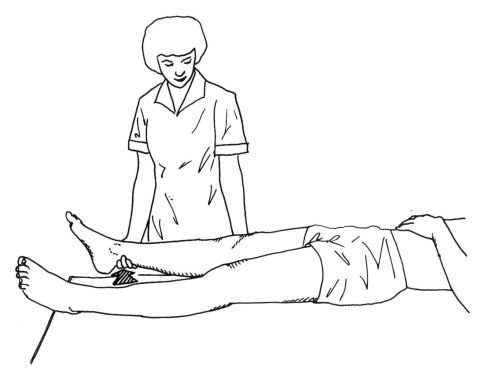

FIG. 3–16

Hip abduction/adduction ROM exercises. By grasping the posterior surface of the distal lower leg and the posterior knee in the supine position, the assistant can move the involved LE through the available ROM of hip abduction and return to an adducted position. The opposite leg may need to be in a position of abduction for full adduction on the involved side to be realized. Ensure to keep the lower extremity in neutral rotation by keeping the toes pointing straight up. (From Kisner & Colby, p 38, with permission.)

During an active contraction, if the tension in the muscle is sufficient enough to reach the GTO stimulus threshold, the activation of the GTO will cause the muscle to relax, resulting in a decrease in tension, thus preventing injury. If a passive stretch is held longer than 6 seconds, the GTO will be stimulated, resulting in a relaxation of the muscle and decreased resistance to passive stretching. However, if the assistant moves the body part too quickly, a stimulation of the muscle spindle will result, promoting a contraction of the muscle being stretched. Some evidence does exist that through a prolonged stretch, the GTO inhibition of the muscle will override the tendency of the muscle spindle to activate the muscle. Therefore, from a neurophysiological point of view, slow-velocity, longer-duration stretches will produce the best atmosphere for relaxation of the contractile elements of the muscle. See Table 3–1 for a review of the actions of the muscle spindle and the GTO.[1,20]

METHODS TO INCREASE FLEXIBILITY

The assistant may be given a goal by the evaluating PT to "restore lost function" or "increase ROM by 50 degrees." The challenge presented to the assistant is to effectively lengthen tissues that may be limited for one reason or another. (Chapter 4 discusses the mechanical changes occurring in skeletal tissue, and Chapter 5 discusses different types of joint contractures.) The following section will

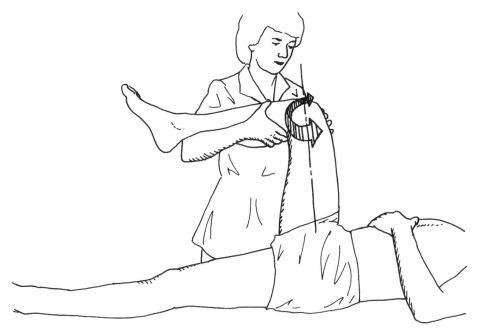

FIG. 3–17
Hip internal/external rotation ROM exercises. Position the client supine and bring the involved lower extremity into a 90-90 position of hip and knee flexion. Support at the knee joint laterally and grasp firmly the length of the lower leg with your forearm and hand. Internal/external rotation of the hip is now produced by swinging the lower leg inward (external rotation) and outward (internal rotation). Alternate method is to keep the client supine with hip and knee extended and gently roll the thigh medially or laterally. (From Kisner & Colby, p 39, with permission.)

discuss two primary methods available to the assistant to improve ROM or flexibility: (1) mechanical and (2) manual techniques.

Mechanical

Mechanical Elongation Techniques
Techniques for improving joint motion by the application of a mechanical device to the joint that is either a static or a low-load dynamic force to shortened tissue.

Mechanical elongation techniques for improving motion about a joint refer to the application of a mechanical device to the joint to apply a (1) static, (2) static progressive, or (3) low-load dynamic force to shortened tissue. Static devices may take the form of braces, splints, or casts that are applied to an involved joint holding the joint in a position of static elongation. The principle revolves around elongating shortened tissues, then securing the tissue in the lengthened position through the use of a rigid device. Connective tissue will remodel or reshape over time in response to the amount and type of physical stress that is applied to the tissue. The physiological process of remodeling occurs over longer periods of time as the tissues adapt to stress, compared to minutes of stress from brief intervention.[21] The connective tissue changes that occur from the immobilized lengthened state include:

1. An increase in the number of series sarcomeres
2. The length of the sarcomeres
3. A change in the length-strength relationship of the muscle[22]

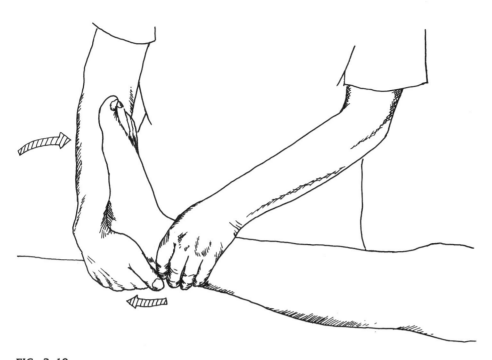

FIG. 3–18
Ankle dorsiflexion ROM exercises. Position the client supine and firmly grasp the posterior surface of the calcaneus in the palm of your hand, resting the client's plantar surface of the foot on your forearm. Simultaneously, pull down on the client's calcaneus and push up with your forearm producing dorsiflexion of the ankle. Full dorsiflexion of the ankle can not be realized in the supine position with the knee extended due to the two-joint nature of the gastrocnemius muscle, but this is a typical ROM position found when working with acute care clients. (From Kisner & Colby, p 39, with permission.)

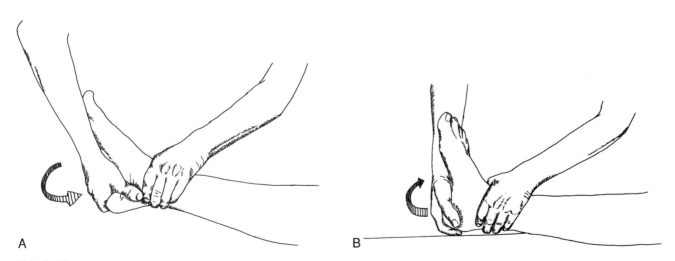

A   B

FIG. 3–19
Ankle inversion/eversion ROM exercises. Grasping the client's heel between the assistant's thumb and index finger will allow ease of moving the subtalar joint into a position of inversion (A) and eversion (B). (From Kisner & Colby, p 40, with permission.)

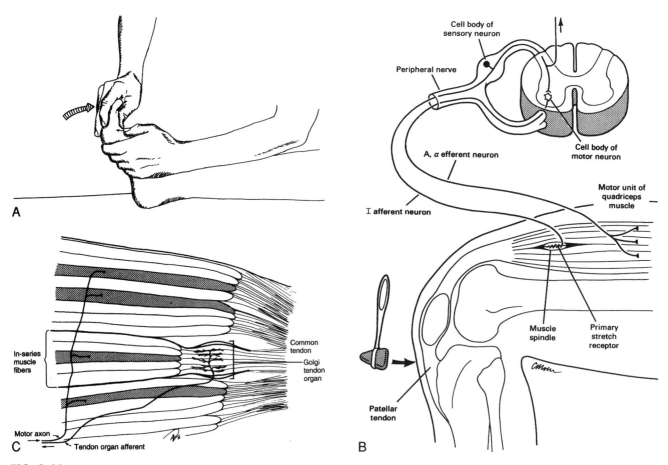

FIG. 3–20

(A) Great toe extension/flexion ROM exercises. Stabilize the client's foot with one hand across the dorsum and with your free hand move the distal toe joints through the available ROM. (From Kisner & Colby, p 40, with permission.) **(B) The muscle spindle.** Acting as a stretch receptor found within the muscle, the muscle spindle responds to the velocity of a stretch as well as the amount of length change during a stretch. Impulses are carried from the sensory organ along afferent neurons to the spinal cord. The return facilitory impulse is carried from the spinal cord along efferent motor neurons to the muscle. (From Smith, Weiss & Lehmkuhl, p 100, with permission.) **(C) The Golgi tendon organ (GTO).** Found at the junction of the muscle and the tendon in series (or in line) with the muscle fiber, the GTO senses tension build-up in the musculotendinous unit from either contracting forces or stretching forces. If the tension is sufficient enough, an impulse is transmitted from the sensory organ along afferent pathways to the spinal cord and an inhibitory impulse returns along efferent pathways to the muscle. (From Smith, Weiss & Lehmkuhl, p 97, with permission.)

Static Elongation: Serial Casting. One common type of static mechanical elongation used clinically is serial casting. When a client presents with soft-tissue limitations (e.g., increased Achilles tendon length limiting ankle dorsiflexion), a hard cast may be applied to the ankle in the position (dorsiflexion) that just reaches the passive limitation of the soft tissue (Achilles tendon). This cast will be worn for a set period (days to weeks), promoting a static stretching to the loaded soft tissue, and thus effectively lengthening the involved tissue. The cast will then be removed as the tissue reaches new lengths and a second cast will be applied to further stretch the involved tissue into a new length, thereby increasing ROM. This

_____ *Table 3–1* _____

ACTIONS OF THE MUSCLE SPINDLE AND THE GOLGI TENDON ORGAN			
Sensory Organ	Location	When is Organ Activated?	What is Response on the Muscle?
Muscle spindle	Parallel to sarcomere	Muscle stretched or lengthened quickly	Facilitation or contraction of the muscle
GTO	Musculotendinous junction (in series to the sarcomere)	During active contraction or passive stretching, sensing tension in the muscle	Inhibition or relaxation of the muscle

process will be repeated until the desired muscle or tendon length or joint ROM is achieved.[23] Typically, serial casting is used to treat:

1. Neurologically involved clients, such as:
   a. Children with cerebral palsy
   b. Clients with closed head injuries to increase ROM or abnormally reduce tone
2. Clients who have suffered burns:
   a. To prevent the development of severe joint contractures
   b. To prevent a loss of ROM
   c. To keep the client from scratching or injuring grafted areas

Phillips and Audet[24] presented a case study describing the effects of serial casting in managing knee flexion contractures in a client with cerebral palsy and concluded that serial casting is a useful adjunct in the treatment of knee flexion contractures in children with cerebral palsy. Johnson and Silverberg[25] reported on the use of serial casting in the management of an ankle plantar flexion contracture of a burned client presenting positive gains in ankle ROM over a 2-month period of time with the casts being changed two times per week. Although close monitoring of the healing process is indicated with the use of serial casting and burn care, these authors believe it is a successful conservative, cost-effective adjunct to burn management.

Static Progressive: Static Progressive Orthoses. Static progressive orthoses is a new concept in orthotic management and works by the same mechanical principles found in serial casting (static stretching). The inherent difference between serial casting and static progressive orthoses is that the device easily allows for progressive adjustments to be made by the clinician when positioning the joint. The same mechanical principles and benefits of static stretching are present promoting increased ROM, but the complexities of the cast application are eliminated as the progressive adjustments are made by simply manipulating the hinged mechanism on the orthoses.[21]

Ballistic Stretching
Technique designed to produce repetitive contractions of the agonistic muscle using a combination of muscle force and momentum to stretch the antagonistic muscle.

Static Stretching
Movement of a body part through ROM to the point of tissue resistance and holding for a set duration, promoting a lengthening of the shortened tissue.

Proprioceptive Neuromuscular Facilitation (PNF)
An adopted means of therapeutic exercise based on human movement and neurophysiological principles.

Low-Load Dynamic: Dynamic Orthoses. Dynamic mechanical devices are commonly seen in specialized braces that have a spring-loaded, hinged mechanism or rubber-band system that applies a low-load continuous force into the direction of joint limitation. The client wears the brace typically during sleep as adjunct to therapy to promote lengthening of pathologically shortened tissue. The brace applies a constant, low-load force over a short period (several hours) that has proved to be an effective method in producing plastic or permanent length changes in soft tissue as compared with manual short-duration stretching.[26] Devices are available for most extremity joints in the body, including the elbow, forearm, wrist, knee, and ankle (see Figs. 3–21 through 3–25). Empi, Inc., produces the Advance Dynamic ROM® Orthoses, which are designed as adjunctive tools to promote gains in ROM as clients wear the devices outside of normal clinical environments. In the current health-care environment that stresses cost-effectiveness and reliance on home programs, tools that the client can use outside of structured therapy sessions are desirable.

Manual

Lengthening of shortened tissue may also be accomplished by manual means. Manual techniques are often referred to in the literature in three forms: (1) ballistic stretching, (2) static stretching, and (3) proprioceptive neuromuscular facilitation (PNF). **Ballistic stretching** involves those techniques designed to produce repetitive contractions of the working muscle using a combination of muscle force and momentum to stretch the muscle. **Static stretching** is defined as moving a body part through ROM to the point of tissue resistance and holding for a duration of time, promoting a lengthening of the shortened tissue. Lastly, **proprioceptive**

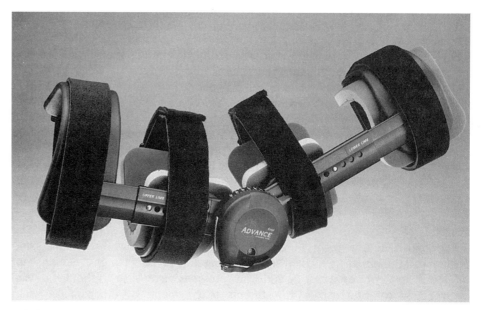

FIG. 3–21
Dynamic mechanical devices. Elbow—By using the Advance Dynamic ROM® orthosis, the therapist can design an adjunctive treatment session for the client to promote connective tissue lengthening while at home or asleep. (Reprinted by permission from Empi, Inc., St. Paul, MN.)

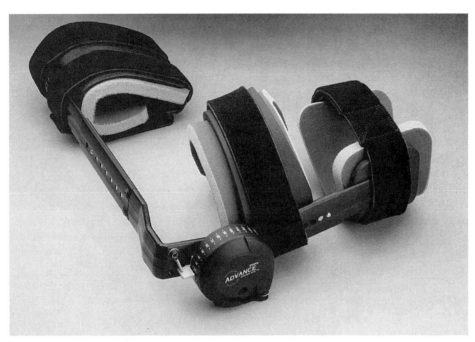

FIG. 3–22
Dynamic mechanical devices. Forearm—This orthosis will promote ROM gains in the functional positions of forearm supination or pronation. (Reprinted by permission from Empi, Inc., St. Paul, MN.)

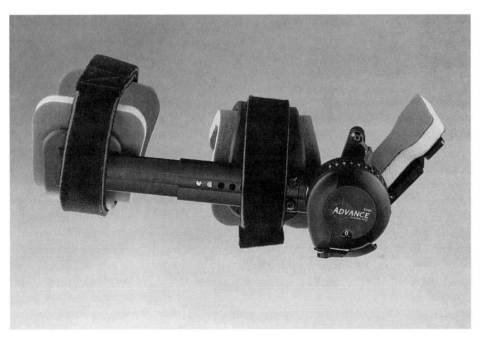

FIG. 3–23
Dynamic mechanical devices. Wrist—ROM limitations at the wrist will severely limit a client's functional abilities. (Reprinted by permission from Empi, Inc., St. Paul, MN.)

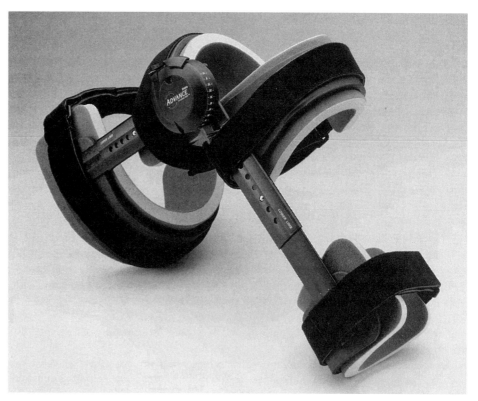

FIG. 3–24
Dynamic mechanical devices. Knee—The Advance Dynamic ROM® orthosis designed for the knee can improve the client's ability to successfully regain full ROM for normal gait skills. (Reprinted by permission from Empi, Inc., St. Paul, MN.)

neuromuscular facilitation (PNF) is an adopted means of therapeutic exercise based on human movement and neurophysiological principals.[1,20,27]

The terms *agonist* and *antagonist* are relevant during any discussion of muscular flexibility or lengthening techniques. A harmony must exist between the agonistic muscle and the antagonistic muscle so that when the joint is moving in the direction of the agonist, the antagonist muscle must fully relax to allow the full ROM. If the antagonist is contracting at the same time as the agonist, a state of cocontraction is reached producing limited or no motion about the joint. The potential for injury exists either to the agonist or antagonist if motion is forced during a state of cocontraction. The hamstring and quadriceps groups provide a good example of the harmony that must exist between an agonist and antagonist muscle. During active knee extension, the quadriceps work as the agonist moving the knee joint into full extension. The antagonist hamstrings must remain relaxed to allow the motion to occur. If the hamstrings do not relax, or are in a shortened state, then full knee extension cannot be achieved by the agonistic quadriceps group. Conversely, during active knee flexion, the hamstring group becomes the agonist and the quadriceps group becomes the antagonist and must remain relaxed to allow full knee flexion. It is important for the assistant to identify how a muscle is acting on a moving joint. Once properly identified, then the assistant can promote either the appropriate muscular contraction or relaxation to achieve the desired motion and results.

When stretching two joint muscles, the assistant must consider the action occurring at both of the involved joints. To achieve full lengthening of a shortened or tight two-joint muscle, the muscle must be lengthened over both joints. In the case of the hamstring group (performs active knee flexion and active hip extension), full knee extension with subsequent hip flexion will provide a lengthened state of the muscle over both involved joints (hip and knee). Conversely, the rectus femoris of the quadriceps group (performs knee extension and hip flexion) will be fully lengthened when the knee is fully flexed and the hip is extended. These opposing muscle groups of the hip and knee must work in concert to allow motion of the knee and hip.[8]

Ballistic Stretching. Ballistic stretching techniques are those designed to stretch the antagonistic muscle by repeatedly contracting the agonist in fast, quick, or even bouncing movements using momentum and agonistic muscular force to lengthen the opposing tissue. The applicability of this type of manual stretching technique is questionable when used by the PTA. Theoretically, there is potential for uncontrolled, excessive motion and the rapid, high-load stretching of the antagonist may result in a musculotendinous injury. Ballistic stretching, however, tends to be very functional in nature and is used frequently by athletes as a warm-up tool to prepare muscles for competition. If ballistic stretching is applied

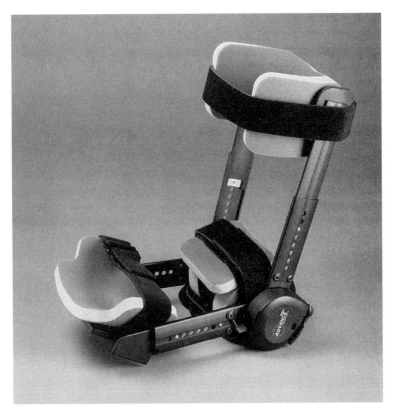

FIG. 3–25
Dynamic mechanical devices. Ankle—By wearing the dynamic orthosis while sleeping, the client can make the most efficient use of time to promote ROM gains from low-load, long-duration stretching. (Reprinted by permission from Empi, Inc., St. Paul, MN.)

in physical therapy treatments by the assistant, specific functional goals and care to prevent injury must be considered.[20]

Static Stretching. The second type of manual technique, static stretching, may be the most frequently used method of elongating shortened tissue in the physical therapy environment. As defined earlier in this section, static stretching is moving a body part through ROM to the point of tissue resistance and holding for a set duration, promoting a lengthening of the shortened tissue. Bandy et al.[27] agreed that this method is the most commonly used tool in physical therapy to promote flexibility gains, but they believe that adequate investigation into which technique can optimize gains in flexibility is lacking in the professional literature.

Performing static stretching maneuvers is very similar in nature to the previously mentioned positions and methods for ROM exercises. The significant difference is reaching a tissue limitation in the muscle. When the assistant moves the client's body part through the available ROM reaching a limitation, the body part is held in this position gently stretching the shortened tissue to promote flexibility gains. The assistant should not force or bounce the body part into a painful range or forcefully move through a tissue limitation. Damage to the tightened tissue may result, further promoting the shortening of the tissue. The assistant needs to be aware of the effects of pain on the involved structures. Generally, when a client is exposed to a painful stimulus, muscle tightening or guarding is produced to prevent the body part from moving into the painful ROM, thus protecting the body from injury. The assistant should promote a relaxed environment for the client and not elicit the pain response if true flexibility gains are desired.

Regarding the appropriate time to hold a static stretch, recent literature evidence suggests that the optimal time to hold the body part at the tissue limitation is 30 seconds. Bandy and Irion,[28] followed by a second investigation by Bandy et al.[27] demonstrated that a 30 second duration was superior in promoting flexibility gains than no stretching at all. They did not demonstrate any significant evidence that a 60-second stretch was superior to a 30-second stretch, therefore suggesting that a 30-second duration may be the ideal time frame to promote flexibility gains. Beaulieu[29] suggested that the 30 second time frame was critical in producing adequate relaxation of the muscle being stretched. Other researchers[30,31,32] have presented evidence that stretching durations as minimal as 9 to 20 seconds produce flexibility gains in muscular tissue. The clinical application for the assistant is not an intense focus on the exact duration of a stretch, but rather considering the quality of the stretch being provided. Research points to the fact that a static stretch must last more than 9 seconds, increasing to 30 seconds to be effective. However, each of the studies examined different types of tight muscles in the human body; therefore, generalizing an exact number for every clinical situation is erroneous. The assistant should promote a gentle force held over a duration of 10 to 30 seconds, which is enough to produce a relaxation of the tissues being stretched. As previously mentioned, if relaxation of the muscle being stretched does not occur, then injury might result.

Proprioceptive Neruomuscular Facilitation. Proprioceptive neuromuscular facilitation is a comprehensive concept of therapeutic exercise based on the theories of Knott and Voss developed over the last half century. Their work resulted in a systematic approach to strengthening, stretching, and motor re-education based on the science of human anatomy and neurophysiology. There are several texts[33,34] that describe in great detail the entire treatment approach of PNF. Many clinicians have modified elements of PNF treatment and techniques without fully appreciating the complexity and comprehensiveness of the PNF approach. The catch phrase of "diagonal patterns" is universally accepted as PNF as an entire treatment, but the comprehensive PNF approach is much more than simple movement patterns. This text presents a brief look at the stretching techniques and principles of PNF, in the knowledge that a great injustice is being done without covering the entire spectrum of the theories of Knott and Voss.

Neurophysiological Principles. Early work by Sherrington[35] provided the concepts of **facilitation** and **inhibition** in relation to how a muscle works neurophysiologically in response to a stimulus. An impulse that causes a motor unit to contract is a facilitory impulse. An impulse that prevents a motor unit from contracting is an inhibitory impulse. Clinically, the assistant will use facilitory techniques when the desired effect is to produce a contraction of a muscle for strengthening or stabilizing purposes, and inhibitory techniques when relaxation of a muscle is desired. The peripheral receptors (muscle spindle and GTO) described previously in this chapter are some of the primary influences on the motor units. The actions (or reactions) of the muscle spindle and the GTO will play a major role in either facilitory or inhibitory impulses that are sent to the muscle. Figure 3–26 is a schematic drawing reviewing the actions of the muscle spindle and the GTO in the facilitory and inhibitory processes.[20]

To develop the clinical tools of the PTA further, the understanding of the

Facilitation
The principle of an impulse causing a motor unit to contract.

Inhibition
The principle of an impulse preventing a contraction of a motor unit.

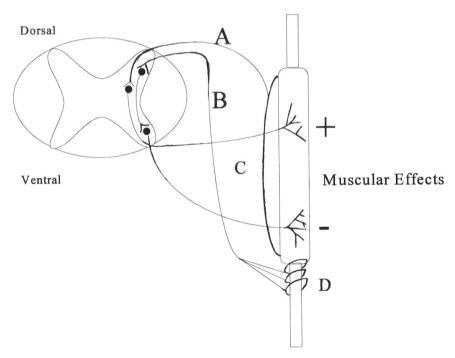

FIG. 3–26
Facilitory and inhibitory impulses from peripheral sensory organs. Afferent type Ia pathways (A) carry information from the muscle spindle (C) to the spinal cord and return the information via efferent fibers producing a facilitory (+) effect. Afferent type II pathways (B) carry information from the Golgi tendon organ (D) to the spinal cord and return an inhibitory effect (−) to the muscle via the efferent fibers.

Autogenic Inhibition
The basis for impulses from the muscle being stretched to produce a reflexive relaxation of the muscle. This is primarily mediated by the GTO.

Reciprocal Inhibition
The neurophysiological response that occurs when a facilitory impulse to the agonist triggers an inhibitory impulse to the antagonist.

neurological principles of **autogenic inhibition** and **reciprocal inhibition** is essential. Initially, when a muscle is being stretched, facilitory (muscle spindle) and inhibitory (GTO) impulses are generated. As the stretch is maintained, the inhibitory impulses from the GTO override the facilitory impulses of the muscle spindle, producing a relaxation of the muscle. The basis for impulses from the muscle being stretched to produce a reflexive relaxation of the muscle is referred to as autogenic inhibition. This mechanism serves as a protective mechanism to prevent injury of the muscle that is being stretched from a reflexive contraction.[1,20]

Previously mentioned in this chapter is the harmony that must exist between an agonist and an antagonist during the working phase of either muscle. The principle of reciprocal inhibition is demonstrated when an agonist receives a facilitory impulse from the spinal cord, and an inhibitory impulse is sent to the antagonist. The result is to produce a relaxation of the antagonist to allow movement by the agonist. This is also a protective mechanism encouraging the relaxation of the antagonist, to prevent injury when the agonist contracts causing a lengthening of the antagonist. This neurological wiring mechanism is used frequently as the basis of PNF techniques to produce the desired response or action. Figure 3–27 represents the principle of reciprocal inhibition.[20]

Proprioceptive Neuromuscular Facilitation Principles. Knott and Voss[33] outlined several principles when applying PNF techniques. As the PTA profession continues to grow and mature, the skilled assistant must begin to incorporate principles and rationale for procedure applications as opposed to technical

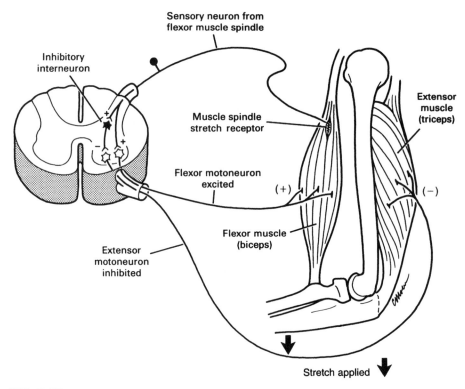

FIG. 3–27
Reciprocal inhibition. The process by which activation of an agonist muscle also produces an inhibition of the antagonist muscle. (From Smith, Weiss, & Lehmkuhl, p 102, with permission.)

application of learned skills. Knott and Voss stressed this point as the principles of PNF will superimpose any specific technique. The assistant must understand the therapeutic rationale of the procedure applications to ensure the safety of the client under his or her care. PNF principles are summarized as follows:

1. The client must be taught the correct pattern of movement.
2. Visual feedback helps the client learn new movement patterns.
3. Verbal cues must be simple and used to help the client learn movement patterns.
4. Firm and confident manual contact will help the client learn movement patterns.
5. The assistant should maintain proper body mechanics.
6. The amount of resistance or assistance provided by the clinician should be enough to promote smooth, coordinated movement from the client.
7. Rotational components in PNF patterns are critical to promote maximal contraction.
8. Selection of the proper technique is critical to obtained desired results.

Proprioceptive Neuromuscular Facilitation Techniques. Methods to increase flexibility are found within the described techniques of PNF. The original concepts described by Knott and Voss[33] and later by Sullivan et al.[34] were used in the treatment of movement disorders and dysfunction; however, many of the techniques have been applied to lengthen pathologically shortened tissues. The following techniques can be used with clients who have adaptive shortening of muscular or connective tissue to promote a functional lengthening. The patterns used may be performed in the classic PNF diagonal patterns or movement within anatomic planes. Some clinicians believe that PNF techniques are more effective and more comfortable for the client as compared with static manual stretching.[1,20]

Hold-relax (HR) is an isometric technique applied to a shortened muscle to improve ROM to one side of the joint. The primary neurophysiological basis for this technique lies in the autogenic inhibition produced from the increased tension in the holding (contracting) muscle followed by firing of the GTO producing an inhibition of the contracting muscle. Fatigue may also play a role in the ultimate relaxation of the muscle to be stretched. Moore and Kukulka[36] support that a brief window of inhibition (1 to 5 seconds) exists in the muscle after contraction. The assistant performs the procedure by comfortably positioning the client in such a manner that the tight body part is easily accessible to the assistant. The client is then asked to "hold" or "tighten" the muscle that is to be stretched, gradually increasing the tension in the muscle over a period of at least 10 seconds and then asked to "relax." The assistant then passively moves the body part into a new and greater ROM. The muscle that was performing the isometric hold is now placed on a stretch. Manual cuing by the assistant during the isometric phase consists of tapping the muscle belly that is being contracted. The procedure is repeated until further gains in ROM are not realized. The assistant must not produce pain with movement. Pain will cause a reflexive muscle guarding and limit increases in ROM.[1,20,33,34]

A variation of the HR technique is to have the client actively move the body part into the new and greater ROM instead of being passively moved by the assistant. This technique is performed in the same fashion as mentioned previously (under HR), except that after the client relaxes from the maximal isometric contraction, the assistant asks the client to "pull up" into a greater range. Manual cues by the assistant can include tapping the muscle belly that is being contracted. Painful arcs of motion should be avoided at all times. The element of reciprocal inhibition is added to the previous element of autogenic inhibition when performing this method of exercise. The maximal isometric contraction will produce an inhibitory impulse (autogenic inhibition) in the contracting muscle, and a second inhibitory impulse will be sent to the now relaxed muscle as it becomes the antagonist when the opposite side of the joint is being contracted (reciprocal inhibition) to move the body part into a new and greater ROM. If the hamstring group is the muscle that is identified as the tight structure, then the technique application of HR would be similar to the case presented in Box 3–2.[1,34]

A second PNF stretching technique is referred to as contract relax (CR). In this similar method, the same neurophysiological elements of autogenic inhibition and fatigue will play a role as mentioned in HR. The assistant will ask the client to "push or pull" instead of "hold" to produce a concentric contraction of the muscle to be stretched. From the starting position, the assistant will provide resistance to the concentric contraction, allowing movement of the muscle into a shortened range, then ask the client to "relax" as the assistant passively moves the body part into the lengthened position. In Box 3–2, simply replace the word "hold" with "push" and the procedure will be similar. The difference is an isometric contraction in the HR procedure versus a concentric contraction in the CR procedure.[1,20,33,34]

Box 3–2

HOLD-RELAX TECHNIQUES FOR TIGHT HAMSTRINGS

Explain to the client that you are about to perform a treatment technique to improve the flexibility of the hamstring muscle. Instruct the client to relax fully and to perform the tasks with his or her best effort when cued to do so. At no time should pain be elicited. Comfortably position the client supine on a treatment table and stand on the left side of the client. Firmly grasp the heel of the client in your left hand, freeing your right hand to give manual cues. By performing PROM into a straight-legged position, determine how much ROM is available for the client. Start the treatment technique to improve ROM about halfway through the available ROM by holding the client's leg and asking the client to "hold," tightening the hamstrings, and gently tap on the posterior surface of the thigh with your right hand to encourage proper contraction of the desired muscle. As the tension builds over a 6-second period and you are satisfied that a maximal contraction is reached, ask the client to "relax." On relaxation, with your left hand, slowly move the leg into a greater ROM, gently stretching the hamstrings. If you move too quickly, you may elicit the stretch reflex, which prodcues a facilitory impulse to the hamstrings. This is undesirable at this time. Repeat the procedure until you are satisfied that no more gains can be made during this treatment session.

Alternate method: Perform all procedures and commands in the same way, except that after the client is asked to "relax", ask the cleint to "pull up" into the greater ROM, ensuring that the motion is slow and controlled so as not to elicit the stretch reflex. Tapping on the anterior surface of the thigh will provide manual cues for proper muscular involvement. The cycle should repeat several times before the maximal ROM is reached.

Rhythmic rotation (RR) is a completely passive technique done by the assistant to produce ROM gains. It is particularly effective for clients with higher than normal tone. A rhythmic rocking or rotation tends to elicit an inhibitory response of the muscle.[37] The assistant should comfortably position the client with good access to the body part to be stretched. Care should be taken to avoid moving into a painful ROM. The instructions to the client should be "Relax. Let me move you." The body part should then be confidently and comfortably supported followed by a gentle, rhythmic rocking motion in an attempt to promote a full relaxation of the body part. As the relaxation is achieved, the assistant may passively move the body part into a new and greater ROM while continuing the application of the RR technique.[34]

Two final techniques adapted from the PNF literature include rhythmic stabilization (RS) and alternating isometrics (AI). Both techniques are isometric in nature and helpful in gaining ROM in joints in which significant muscle guarding or splinting is occurring. These techniques involve producing isometric contractions about a joint either in a simultaneous fashion (RS) or an alternating fashion (AI). The neurophysiological rationale follows the same premise of HR in that fatigue of the muscle may be encouraged as well as autogenic inhibition and reciprocal inhibition. The RS and AI techniques, in particular, require great skill and dexterity from the assistant as well as a good understanding of the procedure by the client.[34]

To perform an AI technique, the client is positioned comfortably and told, "Hold and don't let me move you." The assistant will resist an isometric contraction of one side of the involved joint, producing a maximal contraction (6 to 10 seconds) followed by a shift to the opposite side of the joint, producing a maximal isometric contraction without a rest period in between. Because of the continued isometric nature of this technique, the assistant must ensure that proper breathing techniques are followed by the client so as not to produce a Valsalva maneuver. The strength of each contraction is gradually increased during the exercise. After several alternating contractions have been performed, the client is allowed to rest and the assistant passively moves the body part into a newly lengthened ROM.[34]

When performing a rhythmic stabilization technique, the goal of the assistant is to produce a cocontraction about the involved joint. After positioning the client comfortably, the assistant tells the client, "Hold, and don't let me move you." By securely holding both sides of the involved joint, the assistant will encourage an isometric contraction by the client on each side of the joint simultaneously. The assistant can gradually increase the force of the isometric cocontraction and works to produce fatigue and relaxation of the muscles. A natural progression from a RS technique is moving immediately into an AI technique. Pain and discomfort should be avoided at all times because (1) this will not encourage the client to relax, and (2) the assistant will not be able to encourage movement into a new and greater ROM.[34]

The classic techniques described by Knott and Voss[33] were applied to diagonal patterns of movement. The described diagonal patterns or functional movement combinations tend to be similar to daily movement activities.[20] The brief description of techniques in this text may be applied in anatomic or functional positions. The assistant must be able to adapt the treatment skills being implemented to fit the client's needs and established goals. Figures 3–28 and 3–29 describe the combination of motions involved in PNF diagonal patterns. Two distinct patterns of movement are described, each for the upper and lower extremity and appropriately named either D1 or D2. Both patterns have a flexion and an extension component. Figures 3–30 through 3–33 demonstrate the manual application of the PNF diagonal patterns to the upper and lower extremities.

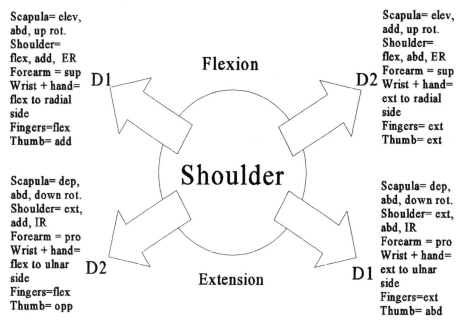

Scapula= elev, abd, up rot.
Shoulder= flex, add, ER
Forearm = sup
Wrist + hand= flex to radial side
Fingers=flex
Thumb= add

Scapula= elev, abd, up rot.
Shoulder= flex, abd, ER
Forearm = sup
Wrist + hand= ext to radial side
Fingers= ext
Thumb= ext

Flexion

D1   D2

Shoulder

Scapula= dep, abd, down rot.
Shoulder= ext, add, IR
Forearm = pro
Wrist + hand= flex to ulnar side
Fingers=flex
Thumb= opp

Scapula= dep, abd, down rot.
Shoulder= ext, abd, IR
Forearm = pro
Wrist + hand= ext to ulnar side
Fingers=ext
Thumb= abd

D2   Extension   D1

FIG. 3–28
PNF Diagonal patterns. UE.

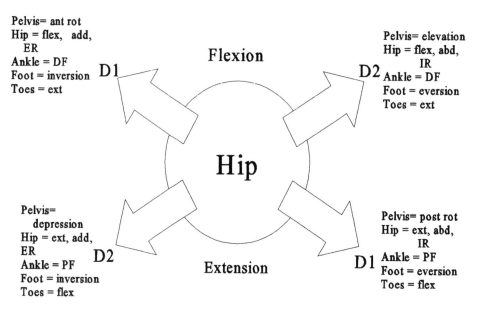

Pelvis= ant rot
Hip = flex, add, ER
Ankle = DF
Foot = inversion
Toes = ext

Pelvis= elevation
Hip = flex, abd, IR
Ankle = DF
Foot = eversion
Toes = ext

Flexion

D1   D2

Hip

Pelvis= depression
Hip = ext, add, ER
Ankle = PF
Foot = inversion
Toes = flex

Pelvis= post rot
Hip = ext, abd, IR
Ankle = PF
Foot = eversion
Toes = flex

D2   Extension   D1

FIG. 3–29
PNF Diagonal patterns. LE.

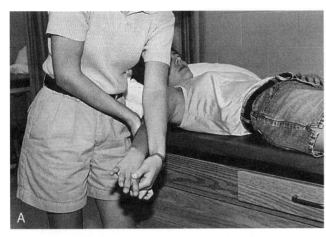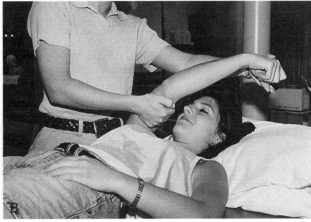

FIG. 3–30
Upper extremity PNF diagonal (D₁) pattern. (A) Shows the starting point of this UE pattern. As the client moves into the flexion component of the movement 1) the scapula elevates, abducts and upwardly rotates, 2) the shoulder flexes, adducts, and externally rotates, 3) the forearm supinates, and 4) the wrist and fingers flex to the radial side with the thumb adducting. The ending position is demonstrated (B) after all of the combination movements are completed. The extension component of this pattern is the exact opposite of the flexion components returning the extremity to the starting point (A).

 SUMMARY

The fullest motion available about a joint is referred to as ROM. Each joint has a differing amount, depending on the shape of the joint, the soft tissues that cross the joint, the age and gender of the individual, and the type of motion that is occurring. ROM activities confer many benefits. These benefits are dependent on the ability of the client to move through the available motion (AROM), on the need

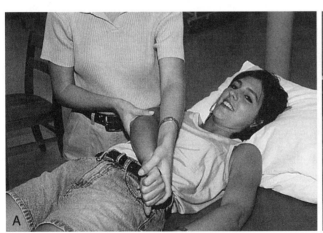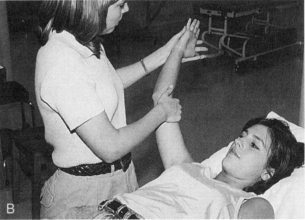

FIG. 3–31
Upper extremity PNF diagonal (D₂) pattern. (A) Shows the starting point of this UE pattern. As the client moves into the flexion component of the movement 1) the scapula elevates, adducts and upwardly rotates, 2) the shoulder flexes, abducts, and externally rotates, 3) the forearm supinates, and 4) the wrist and fingers extend to the radial side with the thumb extending. The ending position is demonstrated (B) after all of the combination movements are completed. The extension component of this pattern is the exact opposite of the flexion components returning the extremity to the starting point (A).

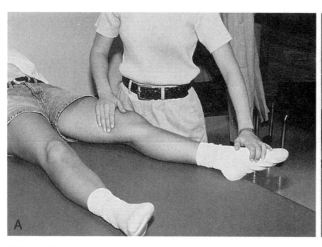
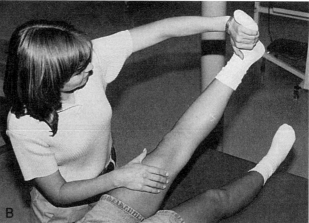

FIG. 3–32

Lower extremity PNF diagonal (D₁) pattern. (A) Shows the starting point of this LE pattern. As the client moves into the flexion component of the movement 1) the pelvis anteriorly rotates, 2) the hip flexes, adducts, and externally rotates, 3) the ankle and foot dorsiflex and invert, and 4) the toes extend. The ending position is demonstrated (B) after all of the combination movements are completed. The extension component of this pattern is the exact opposite of the flexion components returning the extremity to the starting point (A).

for assistance to perform the motion (AAROM), or on the inability to perform the movement (PROM). Indications, limitations, and contraindications for ROM activities were discussed. Flexibility means the ability to move a body segment or a series of segments through the fullest pain-free motion available. Different activities require differing amounts of flexibility to safely perform the task involved. The muscle spindle is a sensory organ found parallel to the sarcomere

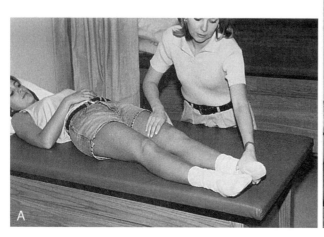
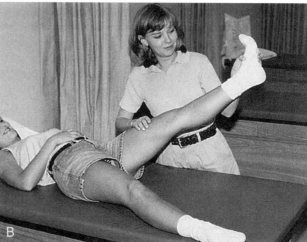

FIG. 3–33

Lower extremity PNF diagonal (D₂) pattern. (A) Shows the starting point of this LE pattern. As the client moves into the flexion component of the movement 1) the pelvis elevates (hip hike), 2) the hip flexes, abducts, and internally rotates, 3) the ankle and foot dorsiflex and evert, and 4) the toes extend. The ending position is demonstrated (B) after all of the combination movements are completed. The extension component of this pattern is the exact opposite of the flexion components returning the extremity to the starting point (A).

that senses speed of length changes in the muscle and responds by causing a contraction of the muscle. The GTO is a sensory organ found at the musculotendinous junction in series to the sarcomere that responds to the length and tension of the muscle producing a relaxation of the muscle when stimulated. Shortened tissues may be elongated by the assistant either by applying static or dynamic mechanical devices or by using various manual techniques. Ballistic stretching is designed to produce repetitive contractions of the agonistic muscle using a combination of muscle force and momentum to stretch the antagonistic muscle, but is not readily used by the PTA. Static stretching is performed when a body part is moved through the ROM to the point of tissue resistance, and held for a duration of time, promoting a lengthening of the shortened tissue. Lastly, PNF is an adopted means of therapeutic exercise based on human movement and neurophysiological principals that can be frequently used to promote a physiological lengthening of shortened tissue. Several techniques of manual flexibility techniques are presented in the chapter.

 ## REFERENCES

 1. Kisner, C, and Colby, LA: Therapeutic Exercise: Foundations and Techniques, ed 3. FA Davis, Philadelphia, 1996, p 24.
 2. Norkin, CC, and White, DJ: Measurement of Joint Motion: A Guide to Goniometry, ed 2. FA Davis, Philadelphia, 1995, p 6.
 3. Boone, DC, and Azen, SP: Normal range of motion of joints in male subjects. J Bone Joint Surg Am 61:756, 1979.
 4. James, B, and Parker, AW: Active and passive mobility of lower limb joints in elderly men and women. Am J Phys Med 68:162, 1989.
 5. Walker, JM, et al: Active mobility of the extremities in older subjects. Phys Ther 64:919, 1984.
 6. Roach, KE, and Miles, TP: Normal hip and knee active range of motion: The relationship to age. Phys Ther 71:656; 1991.
 7. Boone, DC, et al: Age and sex differences in lower extremity joint motion. Presented at annual conference of American Physical Therapy Association, Washington, D.C., 1981.
 8. Lippert, L: Clinical Kinesiology for the Physical Therapist Assistant, ed 2. FA Davis, Philadelphia, p 36.
 9. Miller, PJ: Assessment of joint motion. In Rothstein JM (ed): Measurement in Physical Therapy, Vol 7. Churchill Livingstone, New York, 1985, p 103.
10. Rheault, W, et al: Intertester reliability and concurrent validity of fluid based and universal goniometers for active knee flexion. Phys Ther 68:1676, 1988.
11. Robson, P: A method to reduce the variable error in joint range measurement. Annals of Physical Medicine 8:262, 1966.
12. Rothstein, JM, et al: Goniometric reliability in a clinical setting: Elbow and knee measurements. Phys Ther 63:1611, 1983.
13. Riddle, DL, et al: Goniometric reliability in a clinical setting: Shoulder measurements. Phys Ther 67:68, 1987.
14. Watkins, MA, et al: Reliability of goniometric measurements and visual estimates of knee range of motion obtained in a clinical setting. Phys Ther 71:90, 1991.
15. Mitchell, WS, et al: An evaluation of goniometry as an objective parameter for measuring joint motion. Scott Med J 20:57, 1975.
16. Gogia, PP, et al: Reliability and validity of goniometric measurements at the knee. Phys Ther 67:192, 1987.
17. Salter, RB: Textbook of Disorders and Injuries of the Musculoskeletal System, ed 2. Williams & Wilkins, Baltimore, 1983.
18. Salter, RB, et al: Clinical application of basic research on continuous passive motion for disorders and injuries of synovial joints. J Orthop Res 1:324, 1984.
19. Salter, RB, et al: The biological effects of continuous passive motion on the healing of full thickness defects in articular cartilage. J Bone Joint Surg Am 62:1232, 1980.
20. Prentice, WE: Rehabilitation Techniques in Sports Medicine, ed 2. Mosby, St. Louis, MO, p 38.
21. McClure, PW, et al: The use of splints in the treatment of joint stiffness: Biological rationale and an algorithm for making clinical decisions. Phys Ther 74:1101, 1994.

22. Williams, PE, and Goldspink, G: Changes in sarcomere length and physiological properties in immobilized muscle. J Anat 127:459, 1978.
23. Leahy, P: Precasting work sheet—An assessment tool: A clinical report. Phys Ther 68:72, 1988.
24. Phillips, WE, and Audet, M: Use of serial casting in the management of knee joint contractures in an adolescent with cerebral palsy. Phys Ther 70:521, 1990.
25. Johnson, J, and Silverberg, R: Serial casting of the lower extremity to correct contractures during the acute phase of burn care. Phys Ther 75:262, 1995.
26. Light, KE, et al: Low-load prolonged stretch vs. high-load brief stretch in treating knee contractures. Phys Ther 64:330, 1984.
27. Bandy, WD, et al: The effect of time and frequency of static stretching on flexibility of the hamstring muscles. Phys Ther 77:1090, 1997.
28. Bandy, WD, and Irion, JM: The effect of time of static stretch on the flexibility of the hamstring muscles. Phys Ther 74:845, 1994.
29. Beaulieu, JE: Developing a stretching program. The Physician and Sports Medicine 9(11):59, 1981.
30. Etnyre, BR, and Lee, EJ: Chronic and acute flexibility of men and women using three different stretching techniques. Research Quarterly 59:222, 1988.
31. Gajdosik, RL: Effects of static stretching on maximal length and resistance to passive stretch on short hamstring muscles. J Orthop Sports Phys Ther 14:250, 1991.
32. Raab, DM, et al: Light resistance and stretching exercise in elderly women: Effect upon flexibility. Arch Phys Med Rehabil 69:268, 1988.
33. Knott, M, and Voss, D: Proprioceptive Neuromuscular Facilitation: Patterns and Techniques, ed 2. Harper & Row, New York, 1968.
34. Sullivan, PE, et al: An Integrated Approach to Therapeutic Exercise: Theory and Clinical Application. Reston Publishing, Reston, VA, 1982.
35. Sherrington, C: The Integrative Action of the Nervous System. Yale University Press, New Haven, CT, 1947.
36. Moore, MA, and Kukulka, CG: Depression of hoffmann reflexes following voluntary contraction and implications for proprioceptive neuromuscular facilitation therapy. Phys Ther 71:321, 1991.
37. Semans, S: Bobath concept in treatment of neurological disorders. Amer J Phys Med Rehabil 46:732, 1966.

 # BIBLIOGRAPHY

Bandy, WD, and Irion, JM: The effect of time of static stretch on the flexibility of the hamstring muscles. Phys Ther 74:845, 1994.

Bandy, WD, et al: The effect of time and frequency of static stretching on flexibility of the hamstring muscles. Phys Ther 77:1090, 1997.

Beaulieu, JE: Developing a stretching program. The Physician and Sports Medicine 9(11):59, 1981.

Boone, DC, and Azen, SP: Normal range of motion of joints in male subjects. J Bone Joint Surg Am 61:756, 1979.

Boone, DC, et al: Age and sex differences in lower extremity joint motion. Presented at annual conference of American Physical Therapy Association, Washington, D.C., 1981.

Etnyre, BR, and Lee, EJ: Chronic and acute flexibility of men and women using three different stretching techniques. Research Quarterly 59:222, 1988.

Gajdosik, RL: Effects of static stretching on maximal length and resistance to passive stretch on short hamstring muscles. J Orthop Sports Phys Ther 14:250, 1991.

Gogia, PP, et al: Reliability and validity of goniometric measurements at the knee. Phys Ther 67:192, 1987.

James, B, and Parker, AW: Active and passive mobility of lower limb joints in elderly men and women. Am J Phys Med 68:162, 1989.

Johnson, J, and Silverberg, R: Serial casting of the lower extremity to correct contractures during the acute phase of burn care. Phys Ther 75:262, 1995.

Kisner, C, and Colby, LA: Therapeutic Exercise: Foundations and Techniques, ed 3. FA Davis, Philadelphia, 1996.

Knott, M, and Voss, D: Proprioceptive Neuromuscular Facilitation: Patterns and Techniques. Harper & Row, New York, 1968.

Leahy, P: Precasting work sheet—An assessment tool: A clincial report. Phys Ther 68:72, 1988.

Light, KE, et al: Low-load prolonged stretch vs. high-load brief stretch in treating knee contractures. Phys Ther 64:330, 1984.

Lippert, L: Clinical Kinesiology for the Physical Therapist Assistant, ed 2. FA Davis, Philadelphia., 1994, p 38.

McClure, PW, et al: The use of splinets in the treatment of joint stiffness: Biological rationale and an algorithm for making clinical decisions. Phys Ther 74:1101, 1994.

Miller, PJ: Assessment of joint motion. In Rothstein, JM (ed): Measurement in Physical Therapy, Vol 7. Churchill Livingstone, New York, 1985, p 103.

Mitchell, WS, et al: An evaluation of goniometry as an objective parameter for measuring joint motion. Scott Med J 20:57, 1975.

Moore, MA, and Kukulka, CG: Depression of hoffmann reflexes following voluntary contraction and implications for proprioceptive neuromuscular facilitation therapy. Phys Ther 71:321, 1991.

Norkin, CC, and White, DJ: Measurement of Joint Motion: A Guide to Goniometry, ed 2. FA Davis, Philadelphia, 1995.

Phillips, WE, and Audet, M: Use of serial casting in the management of knee joint contractures in an adolescent with cerbral palsy. Phys Ther 70:521, 1990.

Prentice, WE: Rehabilitation Techniques in Sports Medicine, ed 2. Mosby, St. Louis, MO, p 38.

Raab, DM, et al: Light resistance and stretching exercise in elderly women: Effect upon flexibility. Arch Phys Med Rehabil 9:268, 1988.

Rheault, W, et al: Intertester reliability and concurrent validity of fluid based and universal goniometers for active knee flexion. Phys Ther 68:1676, 1988.

Riddle, DL, et al: Goniometric reliabiity in a clinical setting: Shoulder measurements. Phys Ther 67:68, 1987.

Roach, KE, and Miles, TP: Normal hip and knee active range of motion: The relationship to age. Phys Ther 71:656; 1991.

Robson, P: A method to reduce the variable error in joint range measurement. Annals of Physical Medicine 8:262, 1966.

Rothstein, JM, et al: Goniometric reliability in a clinical setting: Elbow and knee measurements. Phys Ther 63:1611, 1983.

Salter, RB: Textbook of Disorders and Injuries of the Musculoskeletal System, ed 2. Williams & Wilkins, Baltimore, 1983.

Salter, RB, et al: The biological effects of continuous passive motion on the healing of full thickness defects in articular cartilage. J Bone Joint Surg Am 62:1232, 1980.

Salter, RB, et al: Clinical application of basic research on continuous passive motion for disorders and injuries of synovial joints. J Orthop Res 1:324, 1984.

Semans, S: Bobath concept in treatment of neurological disorders. Amer J Phys Med Rehabil 46:732, 1966.

Sherrington, C: The integrative action of the nervous system. Yale University Press, New Haven, CT, 1947.

Sullivan, PE, et al: An Integrated Approach to Therapeutic Exercise: Theory and Clinical Application. Reston Publishing, Reston, VA, 1982.

Walker, JM, et al: Active mobility of the extremities in older subjects. Phys Ther 64:919, 1984.

Watkins, MA, et al: Reliability of goniometric measurements and visual estimates of knee range of motion obtained in a clinical setting. Phys Ther 71:90, 1991.

Williams, PE, and Goldspink, G: Changes in sarcomere length and physiological properties in immobilized muscle. J Anat 127:459, 1978.

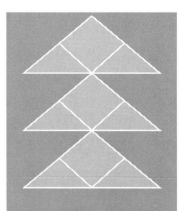

 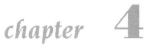

Mechanical Properties of the Human Body

OBJECTIVES

After completing this chapter, the PTA student will be able to:
1. Discuss the mechanical principles of stress and strain.
2. Relate the clinical significance of the stress-strain curve.
3. Explain the significance of mechanical elastic ranges and plastic ranges.
4. Discuss the different types of mechanical forces and the clinical application of each.
5. Discuss the properties of connective tissue.
6. Relate the tendency of fibrous components of connective tissue to be either elastic or plastic in nature.
7. Discuss the clinical significance related to the structural orientation of collagen fibers.
8. Discuss the composition and functions of skeletal bone.
9. List the categories of skeletal bone.
10. Discuss the blood supply and growing capacity of skeletal bone.
11. Discuss the role of weight bearing and activity in the modeling of bones.
12. State the clinical significance of Wolff's law.

Key Words

approximation
collagen fibers
compression forces
cortical (compact) bone
distraction
elastic range
elastin fibers
endochondral growth
mechanical failure
membranous growth
ossification
osteoblastic activity
osteoclastic activity
osteoporosis
plastic range
remodeling of bone
reticulin fibers
shear forces
strain (deformation)
stress (load)
stress-strain curve
tensile forces
trabecular (cancellous) bone
ultimate failure point
wolff's law
yield point

MECHANICAL FORCES: STRESS AND STRAIN

External forces applied to the human body regularly affect or deform the nature of internal structures. **Stress** is the term related to the magnitude of the force or load being applied to the internal structure. **Strain** is the term related to the amount of deformation that occurs to the structure in response to the stress applied. Clinically, external stresses may be skillfully applied to reshape, lengthen, or modify internal structures as needed to correct deformities, promote function, or alleviate pain. If the stress is too excessive and reaches a point at which it cannot be withstood by the internal structure, then **mechanical failure** occurs (**ultimate failure point**). The mechanical response of a selected internal structure to a deforming stress is graphically demonstrated in a **stress-strain curve** (Fig. 4–1). The stress-strain curve representation is different for every structure in the human body because each tissue has differing mechanical principles promoting or lessening the ability to withstand force. Some tissues (e.g., bone) may reach a point of mechanical disruption without much deformation, whereas other tissues (e.g., muscle) may be able to deform significantly before disruption occurs.[1,2]

ELASTIC AND PLASTIC PROPERTIES

The graphic representation of applied loads and the resulting deformation found in the stress-strain curve has several key components related to everyday practice of physical therapy. When applying therapeutic techniques, the PTA must have an understanding of the amount of force that may be safely applied to a structure before injury (mechanical failure) occurs. Also, the assistant should understand that the mechanical properties of internal structures dictate how the tissue will

Stress (Load)
The magnitude of the force or load being applied to a structure.

Strain (Deformation)
The amount of deformation that occurs to the structure in response to an applied stress.

Mechanical Failure
When load is excessive enough to physically disrupt the mechanical integrity of a structure. Examples include a bony fracture, a skin laceration, a ligament sprain, and a muscle strain.

Ultimate Failure Point
The representation on a stress-strain curve at which the tissue or internal structure is unable to withstand any greater stress without mechanical disruption or injury occurring.

Stress-Strain Curve
A graphic representation of the mechanical response of a selected tissue to the deforming load placed on the structure.

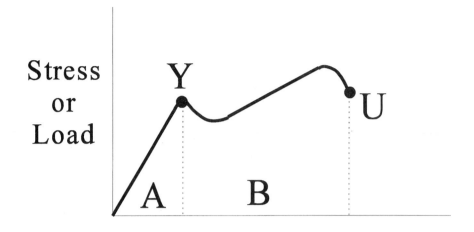

FIG. 4–1
Stress-strain curve. Also referred to as load-deformation curve. The elastic range (A) is demonstrated by the ability of the structure being loaded to return to the original length after the deforming load is removed. The plastic range (B) is noted by the ability of the structure being loaded to permanently obtain a new length after the deforming load is removed. The point of change between the elastic and plastic range is the yield point (Y) and the point where mechanical disruption occurs is the ultimate failure point (U).

Elastic Range
The ability of the structure being loaded to return to the original length after the deforming load is removed.

Plastic Range
The ability of the structure being loaded to permanently obtain a new length after the deforming load is removed.

Yield Point
The representation on a stress-strain curve at which the mechanical deformation occurring in a structure changes from elastic to plastic deformation.

respond to exercises, range of motion (ROM), or stretching techniques. Each tissue in the body has differing abilities to resist or to adapt to the applied deforming loads. The **elastic range** is demonstrated by the ability of the structure being loaded to return to the original length after the deforming load is removed. The **plastic range** is noted by the ability of the structure being loaded to permanently obtain a new length after the deforming load is removed. The point of change between the elastic and plastic range is defined as the **yield point.** The point at which mechanical disruption occurs is defined as the ultimate failure point. Clinically, when the assistant is applying stretching techniques to lengthen pathologically shortened tissue, the load must be of sufficient intensity and duration to achieve a plastic change in the tissue. If the stretching occurs only within the elastic range capabilities of the tissue, then the tissue being stretched will return to the original length after the stretch is removed.[1,2]

TYPES OF MECHANICAL STRESSES

The external forces applied to the human body and the ability of the body to resist or adapt to that load are characterized by differing applications of the loads. Application of stresses to human structures appear as three different mechanical properties: (1) compression forces, (2) tensile forces, and (3) shear forces. During active or passive motion in the human body, these mechanical principles occur singly or in combination. The composition of bone, muscular, and connective tissue imparts each with unique characteristics to resist, adapt, or combat these deforming and potentially destructive forces.[1,2]

Compression Forces

Mechanical **compression forces** or loads work to push one surface into another. The force is applied perpendicular to the articulating surface. Compression occurs regularly in lower-extremity joints during weight-bearing activities as well as during active contraction of muscular elements in the upper extremities. This mechanical process can also be used therapeutically (joint **approximation**) to promote weight bearing or joint cocontraction of the surrounding muscular elements. Figure 4–2 demonstrates the principle of approximation.[1,2] new length after the deforming load is removed.

Tensile Forces

Mechanical **tensile forces** work to pull apart opposing surfaces. The force is applied perpendicular to the articular surface. In a clinical practice, the principle promoted by tensile loads **(distraction)** can be used to reduce pain or enhance joint motion. Figure 4–3 demonstrates the principle of distraction.[1,2]

Shear Forces

Mechanical shear forces occur during the sliding of one surface over another. The force is applied parallel to the surface. Applying shear forces to connective tissue can be particularly destructive because the load applied quickly exceeds the ultimate failure point of the tissue. Clinically, mechanical shear forces occur when sliding a client over bed sheets or when moving a client across the tire of a wheelchair during a transfer. The ability of the skin tissue to withstand the shear force may be quickly exceeded, and injury to the exposed skin may result. Figure 4–4 demonstrates the principle of shear.[1,2]

During the clinical application of the mechanical elements of compression (approximation), tension (distraction), and shear, shear is usually a component force of either compression or tension when actions occur in the human body. The maximal compression or tensile force potentially applied is in a plane that is purely perpendicular to the opposing surface. If the deforming load is not in a pure perpendicular plane to the opposing surface, then an added element of shear will

Compression Forces
Forces applied perpendicular to the articulating surface pushing one surface against another.

Approximation
A therapeutic technique that moves one joint surface closer to the opposite surface.

Tensile Forces
Forces applied perpendicular to the joint surface, pulling opposing surfaces apart.

Distraction
A therapeutic technique causing separation of opposing joint surfaces.

Shear Forces
Forces applied parallel to the structure as one surface slides over another.

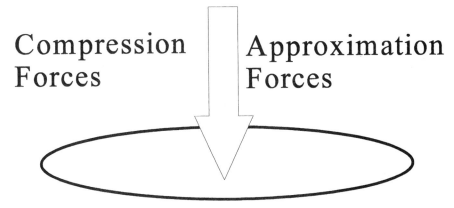

FIG. 4–2
Mechanical compressive forces. Loads that are applied in a perpendicular plane toward the articular surface. Also referred to as approximation.

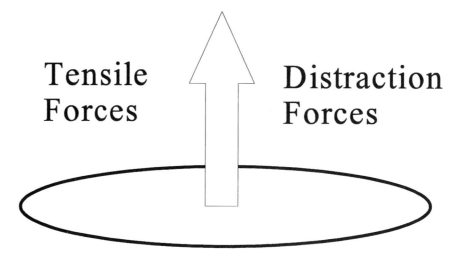

FIG. 4–3
Mechanical tensile forces. Loads that are applied in a perpendicular plane away from the articular surface. Also referred to as distraction.

occur (Fig. 4–5A). This principle is founded in the mechanics of physics and trigonometry and will not be discussed further; however, the assistant must understand that maximum compression or tension occurs in a perpendicular plane and other plane applications of force will have the added element of shear. The shear component is typically the factor behind tissue injury.[1,2]

 PROPERTIES OF CONNECTIVE TISSUE

CHARACTERISTICS OF CONNECTIVE TISSUE

Connective tissue categories include bone, tendons, skin, fascia, and ligaments. Each has a basic combination of structural components: (1) cellular component, (2) ground substance, and (3) fibrous component. The cellular component of the connective tissue contains fibroblasts and fibrocytes that serve to produce

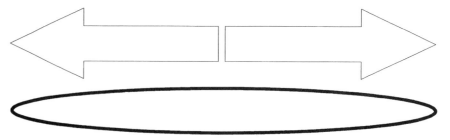

FIG. 4–4
Mechanical shear forces. Loads that are applied parallel to the articulating surface.

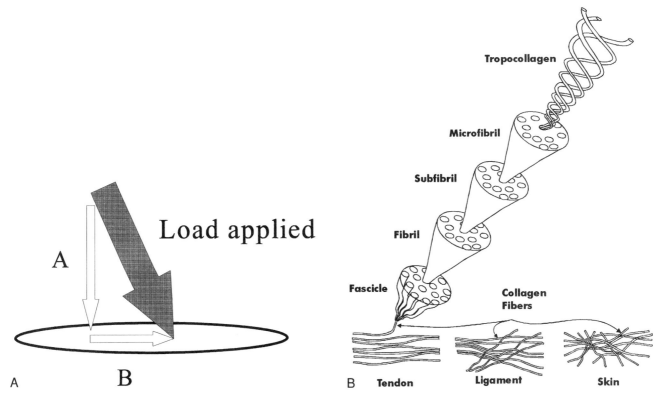

FIG. 4–5

(A) Real-life combination forces. Most forces applied in the human body are rarely in pure perpendicular planes. If this was to occur, the maximal compressive or tensile force would be transmitted, however, most loads occur in a oblique plane to the opposing surface resulting in a vector combination of the actual load applied. In this diagram, an oblique compressive force is really the net combination of a pure compression load (A) and a pure shear force (B). The resulting shear component has a potentially damaging element if the magnitude of shear is greater than the ability of the surface to withstand the force (ultimate failure point). **(B) Collagen fiber orientation.** This figure represents the building-block components of collagen fibers. The orientation of the fibers is demonstrated on a spectrum from very parallel in nature to a random organization. Tissues that have parallel collagen fibers (tendons) are able to withstand greater tensile forces in that same direction. Tissues that have collagen fibers in a random fashion (skin) are able to withstand tensile forces in multiple directions, but are not maximally effective in any one particular direction. (From Kisner and Colby, p 153, with permission.)

the fibers of the connective tissue as well as any specialized cells needed by the tissue. The ground substance is the fluid component of the tissue that serves the role of reducing friction among fibers, forming links between collagen fibers, resisting compressive forces, and filling spaces to help dissipate tensile forces. The fibrous component of connective tissue lends to the ability of the tissue to withstand applied loads and dictates the function of the tissue.[1,2]

The fibrous component of connective tissue consists of three different fibers: (1) collagen, (2) elastin, and (3) reticulin. **Collagen fibers** are large and coarse in nature, being found in bundles. They are best suited to withstand the effects of tensile loads. **Elastin fibers** are small and thin with a significant "elastic" component. These fibrous fibers have a great tendency to return to their original shape after a force is applied. **Reticulin fibers** simply provide bulk to the connective tissue. The mechanical behavior or function of connective tissue is determined by the proportions of collagen to elastin and the structural orientation of fibers.[1]

Collagen Fibers
Fibrous components of connective tissue that are large and coarse in nature, found in bundles, and best suited to withstand the effects of tensile loads.

Elastin Fibers
Fibrous components of connective tissues that are small and thin with a significant ability to return to their original shape after a force is applied.

Reticulin Fibers
Fibrous components of connective tissue that provide bulk to the tissue.

The orientation of connective tissue fibers plays a significant role in identifying the function of the tissue. Fiber orientation will be found along a spectrum from closely parallel in nature to a state of random orientation. The direction in which a particular fiber is oriented allows that fiber to withstand tensile forces (pulling apart) in the same direction. If all the collagen fibers found in a tissue are aligned from left to right in a parallel fashion, then that particular tissue would be very effective at withstanding forces that pull the tissue either to the left or right. However, the same tissue would be very ineffective at withstanding tensile forces that were coming from the top or bottom because the fibers would easily be pulled apart. The analogy is demonstrated by pulling on two ends of a piece of string. As tension is applied to the string along the direction of the fibers of the string, the string becomes taunt and resists deformation. If the stress is excessive, the string will break demonstrating the load needed to reach mechanical failure of the string. Now pull the individual fibers of the string in a perpendicular plane from the parallel orientation of the fibers (pull from the top if the string were laying flat on the table). The string should easily unravel and demonstrate a great inefficiency at withstanding the tensile forces from the perpendicular direction. The purpose of having collagen fibers oriented in one direction is to withstand extreme tensile forces in that same direction. Of course, this will sacrifice the ability of the tissue to withstand forces in other directions. Conversely, the purpose of having collagen fibers oriented in a random fashion is to withstand forces from a variety of directions. This tissue may not be able to withstand the maximal forces that parallel fibers could, but it is well prepared to deal with forces from many differing directions.

Collagen fibers resist tensile deformation and are responsible for the strength and stiffness of connective tissue. These fibers absorb most of the tensile stress in the body, quickly elongate under light loads, but with increasing tension will stiffen and resist deformation. Collagen fibers are five times stronger than elastin fibers. When found in tendons, collagen is oriented in a parallel fashion that can resist high-tension loads. When found in skin, the random order of collagen makes skin unable to resist maximal tensile forces, but quite effective in withstanding relatively lighter loads from a variety of directions. The collagen orientation found in ligaments, capsules, and fascia varies between the extremes of parallel alignment and random alignment. The more parallel the alignment of collagen, the more the tissue tends to function in the role of dissipating forces in one direction; the more random the alignment of collagen, the more the tissue tends to function in the role of dissipating forces from multiple directions (Fig. 4–5B).[1]

Elastin fibers provide for great extensibility and flexibility in connective tissue. These fibers can exhibit a great deal of elongation with small loads; however, elastin tends to fail abruptly without deformation. Functionally, if a tissue has a high percentage of elastin fibers, it will tend to be more flexible, but not particularly strong.[1]

Cortical (Compact) Bone
The outer wall or frame of bone.

Trabecular (Cancellous) Bone
The inner mesh of bone composed of thin, hard plates (trabeculae).

 PROPERTIES OF BONE

The human skeleton is a series of interconnecting bones that provide the framework for the body. Bone is composed of two types of tissue: cortical and trabecular. The outer wall, or frame of the bone, is referred to as **cortical (compact) bone,** whereas the inner sponge-like mesh is referred to as **trabecular (cancellous) bone.** Thin, hard plates called trabeculae form trabecular bone and serve as a storage site for calcium.[3] Salter[4] referred to bone in two capacities. The first role is that of an anatomic element providing the framework for the body, providing for rigid levers of motion, and providing for protection of vital structures. The second role is that of a physiological organ adding the roles of calcium storage and acting as an agent for red blood cell production.

CATEGORIES OF BONES

Skeletal bones fall into five general categories, each serving a different function and purpose. Long bones are greater in length than width. Each has an articular end that is either convex or concave in nature, possessing a hollow center called the medullary canal. The femur, tibia, and humerus are examples of long bones (Fig. 4–6). Short bones are generally cuboid in nature. The carpal bones of the hand and the tarsal bones of the foot are examples of short bones (Fig. 4–7). Flat bones are flat in nature with two plates of cortical bone sandwiching trabecular bone. The scapula and skull are examples of flat bones (Fig. 4–8). Irregular bones do not fit into other categories because they have nonuniform shapes. The vertebrae are good examples of irregular bones (Fig. 4–9). Lastly, sesamoid bones are round in nature and usually found in tendons. The role of the sesamoid bone is to protect the tendon or to improve the mechanical advantage of the tendon insertion. The patella is one example of a sesamoid bone that changes the mechanical advantage of a tendon attachment (Fig. 4–10).[2,5]

BLOOD SUPPLY TO BONES

Long bones possess an extensive vascular network that provides nutrition for growth, development, and repair of the bony tissue. Three distinct systems exist: (1) the metaphyseal and periosteal arteries, (2) the cortical capillary beds, and (3) the venous system. The metaphyseal arteries supply nourishment to the inner two-thirds of the cortex, whereas the periosteal arteries supply the outer third. An

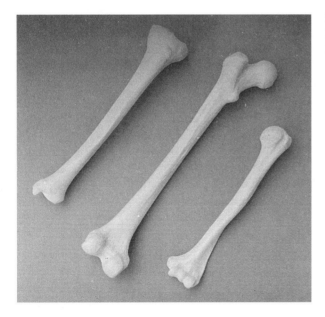

FIG. 4–6
Long bones. The femur, tibia, and humerus are all examples of long bones.

FIG. 4–7
Short bones. The carpal bones of the hand and the tarsal bones of the foot are examples of short bones.

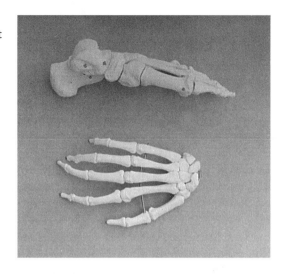

extensive capillary system exists within the cortex to distribute nutrients. This extensive blood supply assists in the healing process of fractured bones. Lastly, the venous system works to return venous blood. Typically, the flow of blood follows a pattern from inside to outside following from the medullary canal to the periosteal surface.[4]

Clinically, the healing of bones is easily predictable because of the typically sufficient and sometimes redundant supply of blood. Most bones will heal adequately within 4 to 8 weeks assuming there is no other metabolic or complicating disease. However, in the absence of adequate blood flow, healing may be significantly slowed or impaired. Some locations of bones provide for limited or unique vascular supplies, creating a potential situation that may result in limited healing after injury. The head of the femur and the navicular of the hand or foot are such examples. If the blood supply is disrupted as a result of fracture, then necrosis (death of bone) can easily occur.

FIG. 4–8
Flat bones. The scapula and skull are examples of flat bones.

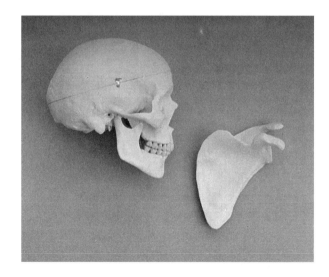

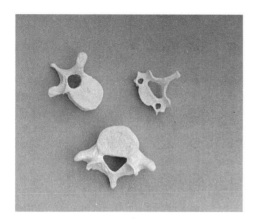

FIG. 4–9
Irregular bones. The vertebrae of the spine are example of irregular bones.

 BONE GROWTH

The nature of bone is dynamic and always changing. The growth of bones involves two differing processes depending on which direction of growth is needed. The bone itself is simply a cartilaginous foundation that has been embedded with calcium crystals.[3] This process is referred to as **ossification**. A bone grows in length by the addition of new bone deposits in the cartilaginous junctions near or at the ends of the long bone **(endochondral growth).** Conversely, a bone grows in width by a differing process. New bone deposits are added to the inner membrane layers, adding to the circumference of the overall bone **(membranous growth).**[2,4]

When a bone grows in length, an extension of the cartilaginous framework on the ends of the bone occurs. In long bones, endochondral growth can occur at either the articular cartilage or the epiphyseal (cartilage) plate. In short bones, growth occurs only at the articular cartilage. A balanced process by which new cartilage is formed extending the cartilaginous zone distally and ossification of the proximal end of the cartilaginous zone allows for longitudinal growth. Hormonal imbalances or malnutrition can disturb the balance needed for proper long bone growth.[4]

For a bone to grow in circumference, additional bone is added to the inside layers of the bone. New bone is deposited in the innermost membranous layers of the periosteum, causing an expansion in width of the bone. The skull, sternum, and part of the clavicle are produced from this type of bone growth. In children, the periosteal layer is significantly thick and produces new bone readily. This rapid capacity for growth is lost in adulthood as the periosteum thins. This is a partial explanation of why fractures heal faster in young children as compared with adults.[2,4]

Ossification
The process by which calcium crystals form in a cartilaginous network forming bone tissue.

Endochondral Growth
The process by which new bone deposits are added to the ends of long bones, providing for growth of the bone longitudinally.

Membranous Growth
The process by which new bone deposits are added to the inner membranous layers, providing for growth of the bone circumferentially.

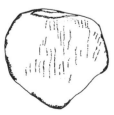

ANTERIOR SURFACE

SUPERIOR

INFERIOR

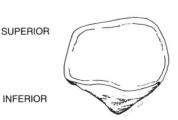

POSTERIOR SURFACE

FIG. 4–10
Sesamoid bones. The patella is an example of a sesamoid bone. (From Lippert, p 218, with permission.)

ADAPTATIONS OF BONE

REMODELING OF BONE

Remodeling of Bone
The process of reshaping or restructuring a bone.

Osteoblastic Activity
The cellular-level process concerned with the formation of bone tissue.

Osteoclastic Activity
The cellular-level process aiding in the absorption or removal of bone tissue.

Osteoporosis
A general term describing the reduction of bone mass sufficient enough to interfere with the mechanical support of the bone.

Wolff's Law
The phenomenon that describes the remodeling of bone occurring to the response to physical stresses placed on the bone.

Remodeling of bone is the process of reshaping or restructuring a bone. Even though the format for the shape of a bone is determined by genetics, the detailed form of the bone is a result of weight-bearing stresses and strains as well as musculotendinous loading.[6] This process occurs throughout the lifetime of normal bone by a simultaneous effort of **osteoblastic** bone formation and **osteoclastic** bone resorption. The need for reshaping the bones is prevalent in the continuing need to adjust to the stresses that are presented in everyday activities. The remodeling cycle typically sees one surface receiving osteoblastic efforts while the opposing surface receives osteoclastic manipulation. A state of bone balance is seen when osteoblastic activity is equal to that of osteoclastic activity. In the growth and development years, typically a positive bone balance is noted as bone formation exceeds bone resorption. However, a negative state of bone balance may result when osteoclastic activity is greater than osteoblastic activity. This is noted in **osteoporosis** pathologies (both disuse and hormonal in nature).[2,4]

WOLFF'S LAW

Physical stress or the absence of physical stress can influence the remodeling of bone. **Wolff's law** is the principle which explains that bone will be deposited along the lines of stress and resorbed if there is little or no stress. Cortical bone will thicken in areas of increased stress, such as on the concave surface of a curved bone. Trabecular bone will also align along the lines of stress. Developmentally, weight-bearing activities place stresses on the skeletal system, promoting the maturation and strengthening of the long bones. If a client has limited abilities to adequately weight-bear (e.g., those with spina bifida, muscular dystrophy, prolonged bedrest, or immobilization) during childhood, then the supporting bones of the lower extremities may not fully mature and become sufficiently strong enough to support the weight of the body. Clinically, weight-bearing activities that can be promoted through closed-chain exercises, standing frames, or joint approximation techniques will help promote strong, healthy bones. The absence of normal stress while the bones are developing may lead to a state of osteoporosis, and the potential for pathological fractures significantly increases.[4]

RESPONSE TO EXERCISE

Physical stresses that work to shape and align bone tissue come in the form of either weight-bearing activities or muscular forces.[3] Athletes tend to have greater bone density in comparison with their nonathletic counterparts. Marathon runners demonstrate an overall increase in bone density.[7,8] It has been demonstrated that unilateral or "one-sided" sports such as tennis result in a greater bone density in the dominant arm, and sports such as swimming (which lack a significant weight-bearing component) do not demonstrate a significant increase in bone mass.[9,10] Activities that produce little physical stress such as immobilization, bedrest, and space travel usually result in a loss in bone mass.[11,12] Riegger-Krugh[2] summarized the factors needed to promote an increase in bone mass as follows: (1) weight bearing and 2) intense activity. One mode without the other is generally ineffective. As stated previously, swimming is an intense exercise, but bone density increases are generally not observed. Weight-bearing activities alone, such as in the use of a tilt table with the client who has sustained a spinal cord injury, have little value to stimulate the increase in bone mass. (**Note:** This does not imply that the tilt table has no value. It is potentially beneficial for blood pressure regulation and management of spasticity.) The combination of intense activities and weight-bearing exercises will become clinically significant in the discussion of osteoporosis and the aging population in the following chapters of this text.

 ## SUMMARY

External forces or loads applied to the human body regularly affect or deform the nature of internal structures. Stress is the magnitude of the load being applied and strain the amount of deformation that occurs by the structure being loaded. The graphic representation of applied loads and the resulting deformation is known as the stress-strain curve. Each tissue in the body has differing abilities to resist or to adapt to the applied deforming loads. The elastic range is demonstrated by the ability of the structure being loaded to return to the original length after the deforming load is removed. The plastic range is noted by the ability of the structure being loaded to permanently obtain a new length after the deforming load is removed. Stresses and strains include compression (perpendicularly applied toward the surface), tensile (perpendicularly applied away from the surface), and shear (parallel to the surface) forces.

Connective tissue is constructed from a cellular component, ground substances, and a fibrous component. Collagen (which tends to resist tensile loads), elastin (which is elastic in nature), and reticulin fibers determine the respective strength or flexibility of connective tissue. The ratio of collagen to elastin and the orientation of fibers are also determining factors.

Bone is composed of two types: cortical (or compact) and trabecular (or cancellous) bone. The shape of the bone dictates the naming of the bone, including long, short, flat, irregular, and sesamoid. Ossification is the process by which calcium crystals are embedded in the cartilaginous framework to create bone. Bone grows in length by endochondral growth and in width by membranous growth. Remodeling of bone is the process of reshaping or restructuring a bone over time. Wolff's law is the principle which states that bone will be deposited along the lines of stress and resorbed in the case of no stress. Bones increase mass in response to intense activity and weight bearing. One component without the other leads to a generally ineffective means of increasing bone mass.

 ## REFERENCES

1. Kisner, C, and Colby, LA: Therapeutic Exercise: Foundations and Techniques, ed 3. FA Davis, Philadelphia, 1996, pp 143–155.
2. Riegger-Krugh, C: Bone. In Malone, TR, et al (eds): Orthopedic and sports Physical Therapy, ed 3. Mosby, St. Louis, MO, 1997, pp 5–43.
3. Aisenbrey, JA: Exercise in the prevention and management of osteoporosis. Phys Ther 67:1100, 1987.
4. Salter, RB: Textbook of Disorders and Injuries of the Musculoskeletal System, ed 2. Williams & Wilkins, Baltimore, 1983, pp 5–10.
5. Lippert, L: Clinical Kinesiology for the Physical Therapist Assistant, ed 2. FA Davis, Philadelphia, 1994, pp 13–15.

6. Frost, HM: Mechanical determinants of skeletal architecture. In Albright, JA, and Brand, RA (eds): The Scientific Basis of Orthopaedics, ed 2. Appleton and Lange, Norwalk, CT, 1987.

7. Aloi, JF, et al: Skeletal muscle mass and body composition in marathon runners. Metabolism 27:1793, 1978.

8. Dalen, N, and Olsson, KE: Bone mineral content and physical activity. Acta Orthop Scand 45:170, 1974.

9. Jacobson, PC, et al: Bone density in women: College athletes and older athletic women. J Orthop Res 2:328, 1984.

10. Nilsson, BE and Westlin, NE: Bone density in athletes. Clin Orthop 77:179, 1971.

11. Dietrick, JE, et al: Effects of immobilization upon various metabolic and physiologic functions of normal men. Am J Med 4:3, 1948.

12. Mack, PB, et al: Bone demineralization of foot and hand of Gemini-Titan IV, V, and VII astronauts during orbital height. Am J Roentgenol 100:503, 1967.

 ## BIBLIOGRAPHY

Aisenbrey, JA: Exercise in the prevention and management of osteoporosis. Phys Ther 67:1100, 1987.

Aloi, JF, et al: Skeletal muscle mass and body composition in marathon runners. Metabolism 27:1793, 1978.

Dalen, N, and Olsson, KE: Bone mineral content and physical activity, Acta Orthop Scand 45:170, 1974.

Dietrick, JE, et al: Effects of immobilization upon various metabolic and physiologic functions of normal men. Am J Med 4:3, 1948.

Frost, HM: Mechanical determinants of skeletal architecture. In Albright, JA, and Brand, RA (eds): The Scientific Basis of Orthopaedics, ed 2. Appleton & Lange, Norwalk, CT. 1987.

Jacobson, PC, et al: Bone density in women: College athletes and older athletic women. J Orthop Res 2:328, 1984.

Kisner, C, and Colby, LA: Therapeutic Exercise: Foundations and Techniques, ed 3. FA Davis, Philadelphia, 1996.

Lippert, L: Clinical Kinesiology for the Physical Therapist Assistant, ed 2. FA Davis, Philadelphia, 1994.

Mack, PB, et al: Bone demineralization of foot and hand of Gemini-Titan IV, V, and VII astronauts during orbital height. Am J Roentgenol 100:503, 1967.

Nilsson, BE, and Westlin, NE: Bone density in athletes. Clin Orthop 77:179, 1971.

Riegger-Krugh, C: Bone. In Malone, TR, et al (eds): Orthopedic and Sports Physical Therapy, ed 3. Mosby, St Louis, MO, 1997.

Salter, RB: Textbook of Disorders and Injuries of the Musculoskeletal System, ed 2. Williams & Wilkins, Baltimore, 1983.

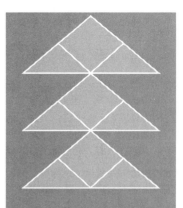

Tissue Response to Healing

Key Words

atrophy
collagen
continuous passive motion
contracture
fibroblastic (repair) cells
fibroplastic phase
granulation scar tissue
hyaline (articular) cartilage
inflammatory phase
musculotendinous unit
phagocytosis
remodeling phase
synovial fluid
synovial (diarthroidal) joint
synovial membrane (stratum synovium)
synovitis
weight bearing

Synovial (Diarthroidial) Joint
It is the most common joint found in the human body and is characterized by the ability to allow free motion. Synovial joints have articular cartilage and a joint capsule that secretes synovial fluid.

Synovial Membrane (Stratum Synovium)
The innermost layer of the joint capsule that secretes synovial fluid.

Hyaline (Articular) Cartilage
The cartilage that covers the articulating surfaces of the bones to prevent damage from the movement of the joint.

Synovial Fluid
The fluid that is secreted by the synovial membrane and serves to lubricate and nourish the joint surfaces of a synovial joint.

 SYNOVIAL JOINT STRUCTURE AND FUNCTION

ANATOMY OF A SYNOVIAL JOINT

The **synovial (diarthroidial) joint** is the most common type of joint found in the human body (Fig. 5–1). There is no direct union between the articulating bones; the joint gains its stability from either static (ligamentous) or dynamic (musculotendinous) elements. Free motion is allowed between the articulating surfaces, but may be limited by the static or dynamic support elements. The joint is surrounded by a strong fibrous capsule that seals and supports the joint. A joint cavity is produced from the sealing effect of the cavity around the joint. The outermost layer of the joint capsule (stratum fibrosum) is very dense in nature encircling the entire joint, poorly vascularized, and highly innervated. The role of the outer layer is to support the joint and to serve as a host for joint receptors, which give feedback to the central nervous system regarding the position of the joint in space. The innermost layer of the joint capsule is referred to as the **synovial membrane (stratum synovium)**. The synovial membrane is highly vascularized and poorly innervated, and it serves the primary role of secreting synovial fluid. The surfaces of the bones that articulate in the synovial joint are covered with a fine, smooth cartilage known as **hyaline (articular) cartilage.** The role of the hyaline cartilage is to provide a smooth gliding surface and to protect the moving surfaces of the joint from injury. The unique features of the joint, which make it the most important type of joint functionally in the human body include[1,2,3,4]:

1. Joint capsule and cavity
2. Articular cartilage covering the moving ends of the bones
3. Synovial membrane that secretes synovial fluid
4. No direct union of the articulating bones
5. Free motion of the joint

SYNOVIAL FLUID

Secreted from synovial membrane is a clear, pale yellow viscous liquid known as **synovial fluid.** Contained in the synovial fluid are specialized lubricants (hyaluro-

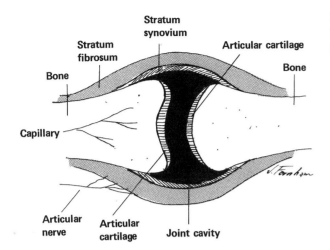

nate and lubrican) that serve to decrease friction between the capsule and the joint surfaces. Although there is typically only a small amount of synovial fluid (0.5 mL) present at any given time within the joint cavity, a second responsibility of synovial fluid is nourishment of the joint. Nutrients are passed from the vascular rich synovial membrane into the joint cavity via the synovial fluid, and waste products are eliminated in a reverse route from joint cavity to synovial membrane. Motion of the joint as well as weight bearing on the extremities help to passively circulate synovial fluid throughout the joint cavity to perform the lubrication and nutrition roles.[1,2,3,4]

 ## SCAR TISSUE FORMATION

The ability to regenerate actual tissue cells is present in the human body, but is limited to selected internal structures (liver and peripheral nerves are two examples) in the presence of mild to moderate tissue damage. Severe tissue damage or injury overwhelms the body's ability to regenerate tissue and demands a process of repair to restore the tissue to a state of wholeness. The body has specialized cells that form a collagenous glue to promote the repair process. The maintenance process of the body is a cycle composed of injury recognition, activation of repair cells, and finally, actual tissue repair.[5]

The collagenous glue needed for repair of tissue in the human body is referred to as **granulation scar tissue.** Only one inherent pattern of granulation scar tissue is found in the repair process. This single pattern adapts to each different anatomic tissue in need of repair (at least 14 varieties of collagen are found in the human body). Clinically, the scar tissue found in repaired epidermal tissue will be structurally similar to scar tissue found in repaired skeletal muscle, differing only in the adaptations made for the functional demands of the repaired structure. Mature scar tissue is composed of type I collagen, which works to adapt to the functional demands of the tissue being repaired. The result of the repair process is a tissue plug that mimics the surrounding structures. Unfortunately, the repaired site will never fully achieve strength or function equal to the original structures. However, the typical uncomplicated healing process will produce a functional substitution for the original structure. If the scar becomes excessive, function of the

Granulation Scar Tissue
The collagen-based glue in the human body that serves as a foundation for tissue repair.

structure is often compromised. Keeping scar tissue growth to a minimum is directly related to the normal return of function.[5]

 # PHASES OF HEALING

Tissue injury within the human body signals a predictable series of reparative events. The organized repair cycle is sequential in nature. When one cycle ends, the next event is triggered to begin. General timetables for each cycle of events are established, but they vary based on the extent of the tissue damage, presence of disease process, and health of the individual. The following factors influence the healing process[4]:

1. Infection
2. Persistent injury leading to chronic inflammation
3. Nutritional status
4. Diabetes
5. Corticosteroid
6. Blood diseases or lack of adequate healing nutrients
7. Location of injury and structures involved
8. Extent of injury (severity or involvement of other bodily systems)

The end result is the formation of a scar to repair the damaged tissue. Tissue injury may result from physical trauma and/or surgical intervention. The three distinct cycles include (1) the inflammatory phase, (2) the fibroplastic phase, and (3) the remodeling phase (Fig. 5–2).[5,6]

INFLAMMATORY PHASE

Inflammatory Phase
The phase of tissue healing that is responsible for cleansing and preparing the injured site for healing.

The purpose of the **inflammatory phase** of tissue healing is to cleanse and prepare the injured site for healing. Typically, all component processes of this phase of healing will occur within the first 48 to 96 hours after tissue injury. Factors that may extend the inflammatory phase include inadequate oxygen transport to injury site, severe tissue injury, other unrelated disease processes, and expansion of the injury site.[6]

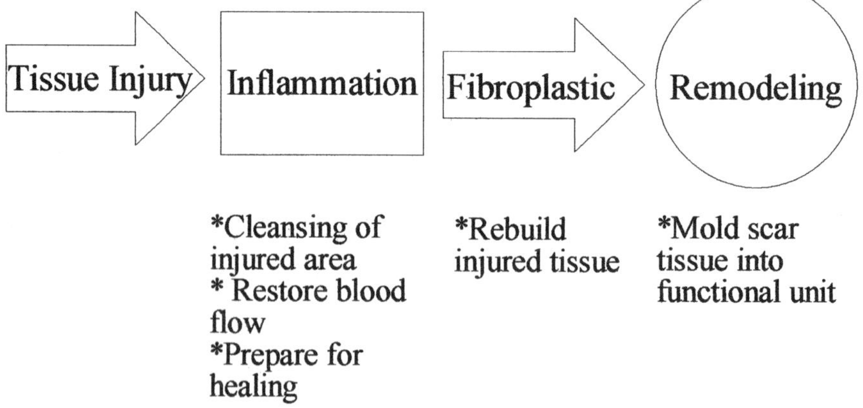

Tissue Injury ⟩ Inflammation ⟩ Fibroplastic ⟩ Remodeling

*Cleansing of injured area
* Restore blood flow
*Prepare for healing

*Rebuild injured tissue

*Mold scar tissue into functional unit

FIG. 5–2
Flow chart of the phases of healing.

Inflammation is a necessary component of the healing process. The initial clinical signs that present after tissue injury are a response by the vascular system. Actual blood vessels may be involved in the injury process, allowing whole blood to invade the injured area. This free blood will soon coagulate, forming a clot to halt the free flow of blood into the injury site. The clotting mechanism is actually a precursor for laying the foundation of future tissue regrowth. The injured cells respond by releasing histamine, causing vasodilation in surrounding noninjured blood vessels. This vasodilation allows an influx of serous blood bringing the necessary healing agents to begin the cleansing process. The presence of the whole blood exudate and the serous blood component in the injury site yields the initial classic clinical signs of inflammation: (1) pain, (2) heat, (3) redness, (4) swelling, and (5) loss of function.

Pain (*dolor* [L.]) is the unpleasant sensory experience as the result of tissue damage. *Heat* (*calor* [L.]) is the increase in tissue temperature that is felt upon palpation. *Redness* (*rubor* [L.]) is observed in the tissue surrounding the injury. *Swelling* (*tumor* [L.]) is most markedly observed as a distention of the tissue at the injury site. *Loss of function* (*functio laesa* [L.]) is observed as the functional status of injured tissue is limited or impaired.[5,7]

Excessive swelling found in a joint capsule during the inflammatory phase will produce a biased firing of the joint receptors to protect the injured joint. Studies have demonstrated that distension of the joint capsule will facilitate the agonistic muscle to pull the limb into a comfortable position, lessening the internal pressure of the involved joint. Conversely, the antagonistic muscle receives inhibitory impulses from the joint capsule, producing muscular atrophy.[8,9] This occurrence has significant clinical relevance when exercising with clients who have acute joint swelling (Box 5–1).

To prevent further damage during the inflammatory phase, protection of the joint is critical. Tissue injury may also disrupt inert structural components (bone, ligament, or capsule) that otherwise would serve to protect the joint from injury. The combination of pain and joint swelling will limit the ability of the muscles surrounding an injured joint to contract adequately to provide dynamic stability. Without the natural protection from the inert or dynamic structures, the potential to extend the injury is significant. Protection may take several forms, including (1) non–weight bearing in a lower-extremity injury, (2) external splinting as in a finger splint, or (3) taping of an acutely sprained ankle.[4,6]

The tissue injury disrupts the vascular system that transports oxygen to the injured structures. Oxygen is critical to the healing process. With the onset of acute ischemia and loss of blood, surrounding blood vessels are stimulated to produce sprouts that begin to infiltrate the injured area. Eventually, these new vessels unite forming a new capillary bed to furnish the tissue with the needed healing nutrients. Clinically, the injured tissue bed may appear pink to red as the capillary beds are filled with blood. Areas lacking revascularization will appear gray or dull and may even be cool to the touch. The newly formed capillary sites are very fragile and easily damaged. Care should be taken in the early stages of healing to adequately protect the tissue area. Aggressive early motion to an injured joint and certain physical agents (including hot packs) may damage the delicate blood vessels, thus delaying the healing process.[4,5,10,11]

As the inflammatory phase progresses, cleansing of the injury occurs. The process of **phagocytosis** is marked by the presence of white blood cells that enter the injured area, remove infectious agents, and destroy necrotic tissue. The newly developing vascular system assists in the removal of waste products during phagocytosis. The presence of white blood cells, in particular the macrophage

Phagocytosis
The process by which white blood cells enter the injured area removing infectious agents and promoting the destruction and removal of necrotic tissue.

Box 5–1

CLINICAL RELEVANCE OF EXERCISING AN ACUTELY INFLAMED JOINT

During the inflammatory phase of healing after an acute injury, swelling is typically noted. This swelling may involve the tissues adjacent to the injury site as well as infusing the joint capsule itself. Researchers have demonstrated that capsular distention produces an inhibitory impulse to the antagonistic muscle as the agonist "pulls" the joint into a comfortable position to relieve joint stress. Premature exercise of the antagonistic muscle will result in conflicting inhibitory and excitatory impulses as long as edema is present. Acute considerations prior to the onset of muscular strengthening should be the resolution of the acute swelling.

M.J. is an 18-year-old female basketball player who recently underwent an arthroscopic knee surgery for repair of a torn meniscus. She arrives for physical therapy ambulating on bilateral axillary crutches and has an elastic wrap around her left knee. As her therapy session begins, the assistant working with her notices that the left knee is significantly more swollen than the right and measures a circumferential difference at the joint line of 3 cm. The assistant also observes that the client holds the knee in a slightly flexed posture of approximately 15°. The first aspect of the plan of treatment for this client called for quad set exercises of which the client claims that "my left thigh just doesn't work like my right thigh." The assistant confirms that the client is having significant difficulty performing an adequate quad set.

Assuming that pain is not a limiting factor in this case, the signs observed by the assistant can be partially explained by the postsurgical joint swelling producing an inhibition of the quadriceps femoris muscle of the left leg. The hamstring muscle works to pull the knee into slight flexion to relieve the pressure within the joint capsule. Atrophy of the quadriceps femoris muscle will continue as long as the inhibitory impulses are being transmitted and thus make exercises to the quad difficult. In this scenario, a primary concern must be to apply therapeutic agents and techniques that will reduce the acute swelling and lessen the effects of the inhibitory impulses.

cells, begins to direct the repair process and to recruit fibroblasts (repair cells) to begin the next phase of healing.[4,5]

Clinical considerations for the inflammatory phase of healing include (1) protection of the injury site, (2) controlling the effects of acute inflammation, and (3) rest or immobilization of the injured area if necessary. Box 5–2 presents the classic method of management in an acutely inflamed joint. Also see Table 5–1 for a summary of characteristics, clinical signs, and interventions for each phase of healing.

FIBROPLASTIC PHASE

Near the end of the inflammatory phase, the macrophages encourage the invasion of fibroblastic cells into the injured tissue area, signaling the end of the first phase of healing and the onset of the second. The purpose of the **fibroplastic phase** of tissue healing is the rebuilding of the damaged structure. The primary acting agent, the **fibroblastic (repair) cells,** build on the foundation of healing laid down

Fibroplastic Phase
The phase of tissue healing that is responsible for rebuilding the damaged structure.

Fibroblastic (Repair) Cells
Repair cells that are prominent in the second phase of healing and are responsible for the production of collagen tissue and glycoaminoglycan (GAG).

___ **Box 5–2** _____

MANAGEMENT OF THE INFLAMMATORY PHASE OF HEALING

The acronym ICE (I = ice, C = compression, E = elevation) was the original guideline for treating an acutely injured structure. Over the years, the three-step process has grown to four (RICE) and now five letters (PRICE). PRICE represents the latest trend in acute management of the acute inflammatory response.

PRICE

P = Protection of the injured area is critical to prevent further, unnecessary injury.

R = Rest is required to allow the inflammatory process to begin, including the revascularization of the injured tissue.

I = Ice is applied to control swelling and to modulate pain.

C = Compression can be applied using elastic wraps or taping procedures to the injured region to assist with swelling control and the return of fluids.

E = Elevation above the heart will also assist with swelling control and the return of fluids.

---

by the blood clots and the white blood cells in the inflammatory phase. The responsibility of producing collagen molecules is directed at these repair cells. The collagen molecules gradually infiltrate the exudate framework that was formed by the blood clot at the injury site. Collagen fibers filling into a repair framework at the injury site is a mechanism that signals the production of scar tissue. Without adequate collagen production, the injury site will not heal. In human skin tissue, this process can be rapid. Closure of an open wound can occur in as little as 5 to 8 days after the initial injury.[6]

As **collagen** is produced to form scar tissue, the fibers are deposited in a random fashion. The new fibers are cross-linked and secured by a process known as hydrogen bonding. This bonding process is temporary and is nonspecific to the structures to which it will adhere. During this stage, the early formation of the scar tissue may unite with most of the surrounding tissue. If left unchecked, this adherence could severely limit functional abilities. During this phase, fibroblastic cells also produce glycosaminoglycans (GAG), which serve as spacing and lubricating agents between the collagen fibers. The greater content ratio of GAG to collagen may help to reduce excessive cross-linking and adherence to surrounding structures. Excessive cross-linking will result in an increased density of the connective tissue. Increased tissue density causes decreased mobility in the tissue.[5]

Two other events occur during the fibroplastic phase allowing for the rebuilding process to continue: (1) epithelialization and (2) wound contraction. Epithelialization is the process by which an open wound resurfaces itself, closing the area and preventing further contamination from the external environment. Skin cells migrate from the peripheral aspects of the wound inwardly, staying close to the highly vascular wound bed. Wound contraction is the process by which the wound is pulled together effectively shrinking the open defect and lessening the area needing to be repaired with scar tissue. This process is similar to a seamstress

Collagen
The building block of the repair process for damaged tissue. New collagen fibers are initially deposited in a random fashion, but it will adapt to the functional demands of the original tissue.

Table 5–1

PHASES OF HEALING			

Typical characteristics and clinical signs occur in each phase of healing. Depending on the literature reviewed, various names are given to each phase, but the characteristics remain the same. Alternative names are given below the descriptive names of phases referred to in this text.

	Inflammatory Phase **Acute Stage** **Protection Phase**	**Fibroplastic Phase** **Subacute Stage** **Controlled-Motion** **Phase**	**Remodeling Phase** **Chronic Stage** **Return-to-Function** **Phase**

Duration of phase
Characteristics
	0 to 4 days
	Acute response to injury
	Phagocytosis
	Cleansing of area
	Clot formation
	Capillary revasculariza-
	  tion begins
	Early fibroblastic activity
		4 days to 3 wk
		Collagen formation
		Hydrogen bonding
		Granulation tissue
		Extension of capillary
		  beds
			3 wk to 3+ mo
			Maturing process of
			  connective tissue
			Covalent bonding
			Remodeling of scar
			Collagen aligns to stress

Clinical signs	Redness Pain Swelling Heat Loss of function	Lessening of inflammatory signs	Inflammation is resolved

Clinical intervention	Protect area
	Rest area
	Control effects of
	  inflammation
	Immobilize as needed
	Perform compression
	Elevate part
		Promote healing
		Promote well-mobile scar
		Begin motion while
		  avoiding tissue irritation
		  or destruction
			Promote return to function
			  for the client
			Increase strength and
			  alignment of scar tissue

Source: Adapted from Kisner and Colby,[6] p 241.

gathering the edges of a quilting piece before sewing takes place to make a clean, even seam.[5]

Clinical considerations of the fibroplastic phase include (1) continuing to promote the healing process without extending the tissue damage, (2) promoting a mobile scar, and (3) beginning appropriate joint motion while carefully avoiding tissue irritation or tissue destruction. See Table 5–1 for a summary of characteristics, clinical signs and considerations for each phase of healing.

REMODELING PHASE

Remodeling Phase
The phase of tissue healing that is responsible for fitting the newly healed scar tissue to the surrounding tissue.

Near the end of the fibroplastic phase of healing, the tissue has been repaired and the collagen fibers have formed scar tissue replacing the original damaged tissue. Despite the abundance of collagen in the scar tissue, the functional strength of the new tissue is only 15% that of the original structures.[12] The purpose of the **remodeling phase** of tissue healing is to fit the newly healed scar tissue to the surrounding tissue. Return to function is optimal when remodeling of the scar occurs and is less optimal if remodeling does not occur. The maturing process of the scar tissue involves (1) the thickening of the newly formed collagen fibers,

(2) the strengthening of the bonds between fibers, and (3) the alignment of the collagen fibers to the functional lines of stress.[5,6]

Collagen production continues at a high rate in healing wounds. Soon into the remodeling phase, a process of collagen breakdown begins to replace the original immature collagen fibers with new thicker fibers. This process of formation (synthesis) and breakdown (lysis) continues in a balanced state (homeostasis) gradually leaving the injury site with newly produced, thicker collagen fibers. During the remodeling phase, if collagen synthesis and lysis is not in balance, abnormal scarring or hypertrophic scarring may result in a decreased functional return of the damaged tissue.[5]

The bonding process securing the cross-links in the collagen fiber orientation begins to change from the weaker hydrogen bonding to a more permanent covalent bonding (a bonding process consisting of sharing electrons between atoms in the tissue). During the early part of the remodeling phase (week 3 to week 10 postinjury), the collagen fibers will align to the lines of stress applied to the newly repaired tissue. Therapeutic interventions (soft-tissue mobilization, weight bearing, range of motion [ROM]) will promote the functional stresses needed to shape the new tissue and deter scar adherence to undesired structures. As the stronger covalent bonding becomes more prevalent in the collagen fiber cross-links (weeks 10 to 14 postinjury), the ability to easily remodel the scar is significantly decreased.[13]

Appropriate collagen alignment within scar tissue is critical to the return of functional movement. Although the mechanisms through which collagen fibers remodel are not fully understood, several concepts may explain the process through which scar tissue becomes a functional part of the injured tissue. The rapid turnover of collagen fibers in the remodeling phase is believed to allow the scar tissue to adapt to the functional demands of the original tissue. The original random orientation of immature collagen is replaced by mature collagen along the lines of functional stresses.[5]

Another explanation for collagen alignment may relate to the concept of scar tissue mimicking the original tissue. Dense connective tissue will encourage newly forming scar tissue to develop increased amounts of cross-links and short adhesions. Tissues with greater pliability will encourage less cross-links and longer adhesions. This theory proposes that tissue of greater density will have a greater influence over tissue with less density if the healing is occurring in adjacent structures. Clinically, if a bone and tendon are healing in close proximity, the scarring process within the tendon may tend to mimic more of the bony structure.[14]

Thirdly, it is believed that external and internal stresses applied to healing structures will align newly forming collagen along the lines of stress. Stresses can occur as a result of muscular tension, joint motion, soft-tissue mobilization, weight bearing, positioning and mobilization.[15]

Clinical considerations of the remodeling phase include (1) promoting the return to functional abilities for the client and (2) increasing the strength, function, and fiber alignment of scar tissue. See Table 5–1 for a summary of characteristics, clinical signs and considerations for each phase of healing.

CHRONIC INFLAMMATION

Chronic inflammation may occur in developing scar tissue that is repeatedly irritated or excessively stressed. The cycle of inflammation will continue as fibroblasts are activated at low-intensity levels. Collagen production will persist as destroyed mature collagen is replaced by immature new collagen. The effect to the involved structure is a weakening of the tissue at a cellular level. Clinically, the client will present with increased pain, swelling, stiffness, and muscle guarding surrounding the chronically inflamed area.[6]

 # HEALING RESPONSES OF SELECTED TISSUES

SYNOVIAL MEMBRANE

Synovitis
Inflammation of the synovial membrane.

The inflammatory response will present in synovial membrane tissue after injury or trauma. The primary response noted is a thickening of the synovial membrane with possible fibrosis of the tissue. This granulization of the membrane lining will alter the production and quality of synovial fluid. **Synovitis,** or inflammation of the synovial membrane, occurs in response to acute trauma or it may be chronic in nature. The healing process of the synovial membrane will occur as described in this chapter, with the exception that the clinical external inflammatory symptoms are not typically observed. The common complaint from the client is a tight sensation in the joint. This tightness is possibly related to the alteration of the quality of synovial fluid produced as well as the inability of the joint capsule to move easily upon demand.

Clinical considerations for management of acute synovitis follows the general healing principles of (1) controlling the effects of inflammation, (2) preventing further injury, (3) promoting the healing process. The acute inflammatory phase will last from 1 to 4 days and the entire healing process should be complete within 4 weeks from the onset of injury. If symptoms persist for more than 8 weeks, the synovitis may become chronic in nature with potentially destructive effects on the joint. Management of chronic synovitis may require a surgical removal (synovectomy) of the synovial membrane.[4]

SYNOVIAL FLUID

The chemical balance in synovial fluid accounts for its ability to act as a lubricant and a medium for nourishment transport. Alteration of the delicate chemical composition will directly affect the ability of the synovial fluid to perform its primary function. Direct injury to synovial fluid is rare unless a foreign agent producing an infection is introduced. Synovial fluid changes are typically seen as a result of inflammation to the synovial membrane. An increase in production of synovial fluid (10 to 20 times greater than normal) will expand the joint cavity. During the inflammatory process at the membranous level, an increase in white blood cells and reparative nutrients is found in the synovial fluid production, altering the balanced composition of lubricants. The viscosity of the newly produced synovial fluid decreases making motion and lubrication less effective within the joint. If this production is left unchecked or fails to be resolved with therapeutic measures, destruction of the joint surfaces is possible as a result of ineffective lubrication and poor nutrient exchange.[4]

JOINT CAPSULE

The healing response of the joint capsule after trauma is comparable to that of the synovial membrane: The capsule thickens or becomes more fibrous. Excessive thickening of the capsule can lead to decreased mobility of the joint. Acute swelling during the inflammatory phase can be destructive; expansion of the capsule and associated ligaments beyond their physiological capabilities produces an ineffective residual support mechanism. The normal healing process for joint capsule injury follows a 6 to 8 week time frame.[4]

MENISCUS

The meniscus (articular disk) is a very dense fibrous type of cartilage and are found in the knee, temporomandibular, sternoclavicular, distal radioulnar, and acromioclavicular joints. Injury to the meniscus can be a result of direct trauma or a rotational force applied to the joint. Frequently, a piece of the disk will separate from the main body. Meniscal tissue has a very poor blood supply and has no real neural innervation. The primary source of nourishment comes from the passive diffusion of nutrients from synovial fluid within the joint cavity. Healing of the meniscus is possible, but it is extremely slow and the tissue will be fragile during healing. Healing nutrients are slowly transported to the repair site via synovial fluid. If possible, healing of the meniscus should be encouraged. If the injured meniscus is removed from the joint surface, then a dense collagen fibrous scar may be produced from the remaining meniscus. The scar tissue formation is only a pseudoreplacement for the primary function of the articular disk (i.e., protection of the joint surface).[4,16,17]

ARTICULAR CARTILAGE

Normal articular cartilage, or hyaline cartilage, has relatively no blood or neural supply. Nourishment, as in the meniscus, comes from the passive transport by synovial fluid. Nutrients may also passively enter the cartilage from the bony attachment. This presents a unique atmosphere for healing of cartilage; protection or immobilization is medically encouraged in early stages of healing to prevent further injury. Clinically, it may be necessary to provide joint motion and weight bearing to ensure proper nourishment. Regeneration or repair of damaged articular cartilage is theoretically possible, if the proper conditions exist.[18] Clinically, the success rate of repair is very low. The healing phases will generally produce a thick, fibrocartilagenous scar that is structurally inferior to the damaged tissue.[4,6]

MUSCULOTENDINOUS UNIT

Tissue injuries to skeletal muscle and tendons are classified as strains. Because they have common functions, the muscle fibers and the tendon fibers are considered collectively as the **musculotendinous unit.** The muscle fibers serve as the dynamic element, whereas the tendons function as the static element uniting the muscle to the bone. Functions provided for by the musculotendinous unit include: (1) stabilizing a joint, (2) providing motor power for motion, and (3) absorbing forces. For proper function to occur clinically, both elements (static and dynamic) must be working in concert. Injuries to either element, or both elements concurrently, will disrupt the ability of the musculotendinous unit to perform effectively. The injuries can be either complete (grade III lesion) or incomplete (grade I: less than 50% of involved fibers, or grade II: more than 50% of involved fibers). Complete lesions require surgical intervention to suture the ruptured musculotendinous components followed by a 2- to 4-week period of

Musculotendinous Unit
The combination of the muscle and the tendon working in concert to provide common functions of stabilization, movement, and force absorption to the joints.

immobilization. Incomplete lesions will usually heal in 2 to 4 weeks without surgical intervention depending on the severity of the lesion. Because of the good vascular supply in muscle and tendons, the healing phases will typically progress over a 4- to 6-week period for complete resolution of the injury.[19]

During the phases of healing in musculotendinous elements, a fine balance between mobility and protection must be maintained. Normal stresses must be placed on healing structures to prevent adhesions to bony or fascial elements and promote the adaptation of scar tissue to the functional demands of skeletal muscle. If muscular stresses are excessive or injurious, further damage and inflammation may result in further scarring.[6]

LIGAMENTS

Ligamentous injuries (sprains) are graded similarly to musculotendinous elements. Grade I involves damage to less than 50% of involved fibers and no clinical instability is noted. Grade II involves damage to more than 50% of the involved fibers and clinical instability is noted. Grade III is a complete disruption of the supporting structure fibers with pathological instability of the joint resulting. Mild (grade I) injuries typically do not need surgical correction, whereas severe (grade III) injuries generally do need surgical repair. Grade II injuries may or may not require surgical intervention depending on the clinical presentation of the client's functional abilities, needs, and expectations.[19]

Healing of injury site in ligaments usually takes 6 to 12 weeks. Ligaments do not have the rich vascular supply of muscles. Longer periods of immobilization and protection may be indicated. In ligaments where adequate circulation remains after the injury, regeneration of the ligament can occur. Typically, the blood supply is disrupted in ligamentous injuries and scar tissue replaces the ligamentous tissue.[17] During the fibroplastic phase of healing, the immature connective tissue is extremely delicate and susceptible to reinjury. Controlled forces and motion can promote the alignment of collagen fibers and prevent the adherence to adjacent structures.[13]

The functional demands of repaired ligaments must be able to withstand deforming forces yet be able to relax when stress is removed. Typically, the orientation of the scar tissue fibers needs to be relatively parallel in nature (greater need for parallel fibers exists with tendons than with ligaments). A ligament that is repaired with scar tissue will never regain the same strength or function as the original tissue.[4,5,6]

BONE

The healing process of bone is similar in nature to the healing response of soft tissue. A major distinction between soft-tissue scar formation and callous formation of bone is the final building block. Eventually the callous formation is replaced with bony materials to provide the needed strength required by human bones. Immobilization of the fractured bone is necessary to stimulate the mechanisms of repair for bone. The healing time frame for the repair process of bone is typically 6 to 8 weeks, but healing may take as long as 12 weeks depending on the health of the individual and the severity of the injury.[20]

Of concern after a skeletal fracture is the typical soft-tissue injury from the actual fracture or from a surgical procedure to reduce the fracture. Soft tissue will heal and scar tissue is formed as described in this chapter; however, because of the immobilization needed for the bony fracture to heal, the soft-tissue scar may not mimic the injured tissue nor align along the lines of normal stress. Clinically, early nondestructive motion will allow remodeling of newly formed scar tissue. Great care should be taken to protect the healing fracture site.[6]

The scarring process can occur at the junction between ligament and bone as well as between tendon and bone. The orientation of the collagen fibers within the scar is more random, producing connective tissue with greater density, which is necessary to meet the structural demands that will be placed on the repaired tissues.[5]

 ## EFFECTS OF IMMOBILIZATION

Historically, rest and immobilization have been regarded as the gold standard for treatment of most musculoskeletal conditions. The early teachings of Hippocrates through the practice of the British orthopedic surgeon Hugh Owen Thomas have entrenched rest and immobilization in the practice of orthopedic medicine.[21] Orthopedic intervention regarding rest and immobilization (casting) versus mobility (open reduction, internal fixation with early mobility) began to change in the late 1950s moving away from the negative effects of immobilization and rest. Despite the advocation of rest and immobilization as an orthopedic modality, negative physiological effects to soft tissue and bone have been observed.[22,23] Immobilization and rest presents to the human body an absence of the normal physiological stresses and loads that shape normal development. Joints moved passively tend to have well-organized collagen fibers with the absence of adhesions. Joints that are not moved passively have significant amount of adhesions affecting the mobility and stability of resulting scar tissue.[5,24]

BONY CHANGES

The strength of bone is decreased with immobilization. Bony atrophy has been demonstrated with prolonged immobilization or bedrest.[25] Decreased strength in the junction between bone and ligament is also noted. Noyes et al.[26] demonstrated that the restoration of the strength in this bony junction was slow. Partial structural strength returned after 20 weeks of normal activity, and full strength was not realized until 12 months after immobilization.

CARTILAGINOUS CHANGES

Changes in the nature of articular cartilage can be detrimental to the proper function of a joint. Changes in the histological makeup of articular cartilage were observed by Enneking and Horowitz[27] upon examination of immobilized human knee joints. A resorption of articular cartilage and a subsequent replacement of the cartilage with fibrotic fatty tissue was observed. Degeneration of articular cartilage with immobilization was described by Salter et al.[28] as a result of ineffective synovial fluid exchange and nourishment. In this process, the synovial membrane adheres to the articular cartilage, preventing adequate nourishment and leading to eventual destruction of the articular surface.

COLLAGENOUS CHANGES

The primary difference noted in collagen is the orientation of the fibers. During the immobilization process and the absence of mechanical stresses, collagen continues to be produced but is synthesized in a random formation. This random orientation is referred to as cross-linking of fibers, which interferes with normal joint mechanics (Fig. 5–3). A loss of water content and GAG is also present, leading to poor interfiber lubrication, weaker bonds between collagen fibers, and an overall weakness in the tissue. Collagen fibers will tend to align along the lines of stress. Return to normal tensile strengths after immobilization is a very slow process that may take 5 to 12 months.[6,22,29]

The altered alignment state of collagen and loss of GAG after prolonged immobility have a direct effect on the mechanical stability of ligaments in the body. Scientific observations have noted a significant decrease in the ability of a ligament to withstand tensile loads after an immobilization period of 8 weeks. The ligamentous failure typically results in an avulsion fracture at the bony junction.[26]

MUSCULAR CHANGES

Atrophy
The wasting or decrease in the size of human tissue. It is often a result of decreased activity, disease process, or immobilization.

Disuse muscular **atrophy** is typically the result of immobilization.[30] The loss of muscular strength associated with postimmobilization atrophy has been documented extensively in the professional literature.[31,32]

Two primary reasons for the onset of disuse atrophy with immobilization include decreased neurological response and disruption of joint structures. A decrease in electromyogram activity is found in immobilized extremities suggesting that the nervous system does not readily activate motor units of the immobilized limb.[30] Also noted in the onset of disuse atrophy is the disruption of joint structures. Studies have demonstrated that joint capsule effusion as a result of injury produces a reflex inhibition of the associated musculature decreasing force output.[33]

JOINT MOTION CHANGES

The most common cause of knee motion limitation was described by Paulos et al.[34] as resulting from surgical intervention with subsequent immobilization. Re-

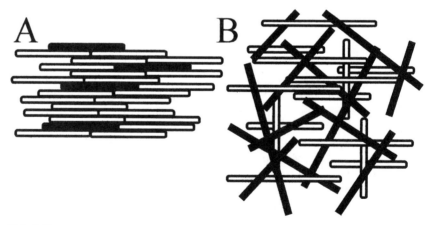

FIG. 5–3
Alignment of collagen fibers. (A) Alignment of collagen in a parallel fashion gives the tissue the ability to resist high tensile loads. (B) When alignment becomes random or cross-hatched during immobilization, the result is a decreased ability to resist tensile forces.

searchers have observed an increase in fibrotic fatty tissue within the suprapatellar and infrapatellar fat pads that encroached upon both cruciate ligaments, the joint surfaces, and eventually the entire joint cavity.[27] Prolonged immobility of the knee joint leads to a dysfunctional extension mechanism, which leads to abnormal joint motion. Abnormal joint motion typically results in subsequent degenerative changes.[34]

Contracture

A limitation of joint motion is defined as a **contracture.** The causes of joint contractures include (1) soft-tissue adhesions, (2) capsular adhesions, and even (3) extracelluar ossification. Research by Akeson et al.[35] described that the main structural change related to the formation of joint contractures is the increased collagen cross-linking in the connective tissue. Clinically, loss of motion in a joint can be either reversible or irreversible depending on the severity and extensiveness of the collagenous cross-links. Joint contractures will produce significant functional limitations and should be prevented from occurring.

Contracture
A limitation in joint motion.

 ## CLINICAL BENEFITS OF WEIGHT BEARING

With various pathologies that may result, a client may frequently be seen by the PTA during or just after a period of bedrest or immobilization. The effects on the structure of the human body discussed in this chapter are significant. Schneider and McDonald[36] examined the effects of prolonged bed rest on healthy individuals and concluded that the lack of weight-bearing activity produced changes in the skeletal system. In the study, despite proper nutrition, calcium supplements, and exercise, the healthy individuals placed on prolonged bedrest demonstrated a calcium mineral loss of 5% each month.

Clinically, the benefits of **weight bearing** are superior to most therapeutic interventions, if not medically contraindicated. The stimulus of gravity and the functional aspect of a client obtaining an upright standing posture should be included in every orthopedic rehabilitation program to promote healing, joint nourishment, and strengthening.

Weight Bearing
A therapeutic intervention used to promote healing by applying functional stresses to injured structures and to reverse the loss of nutrients in bones.

 ## CLINICAL BENEFITS OF RANGE OF MOTION

CONTINUOUS POSITIVE MOTION

Continuous passive motion (CPM) has been used to promote the concept of protected ROM early in rehabilitation efforts. Salter et al. pioneered the application of early controlled motion in animal studies demonstrating positive results in the healing of soft tissue, bone, and cartilage, as well as in the reduction of swelling and improvement of joint function.[28,37,38] Devices have been constructed to be applied to a variety of joints, including the shoulder, the knee, and the digits of the hand. The classic conditions in which CPM have been used include:

- Acromioclavicular reconstruction
- Total knee arthroplasties

Continuous Passive Motion (CPM)
The process of passively moving a joint through a protected ROM to promote healing and the reduction of adhesion formation after a surgical procedure.

Other conditions that may also benefit from the use of CPM include:

* Knee joint contractures
* Joint effusions
* Postimmobilization of joint fractures
* Tendon repairs
* Joint manipulations
* Burns involving peripheral joints
* Total shoulder arthroplasties[38,39,40,41]

The clinical benefits of CPM for the client include earlier ambulation, improved functional ROM, reduced joint swelling, promotion of healing, and reduction of pain.[42,43] Early ROM after surgery or immobilization helps to promote connective tissue strength, enhances nutrition of the joint, decreases the negative effects of adhesions, reduces edema, and restores normal kinematics of the involved joint.[44,45]

Considerations for use of CPM begin with the physician treating the client. Protocols and CPM use vary greatly. Some applications will be brief, lasting only a few hours per day for a few days. Other application protocols will be more aggressive, lasting 8 to 10 hours per day for many weeks. The application parameters should be determined by the supervising therapist in collaboration with the prescribing physician.

Commonalities of every CPM application include (1) positioning, (2) cycles, (3) ROM, (4) speed, and (5) duration. Positioning should be done according to manufacturer's guidelines for the particular machine in use. Generally, the mechanical axis of the machine will be aligned with the anatomic axis of the involved joint. Adjustments are made in the length of the machine to provide comfort and support to the client's involved limb. Test cycles should be performed each time a machine is applied to an extremity to ensure that the machine is moving in concert with the involved joint.

A cycle is the completion of the desired motion from one extreme of the available ROM to the other. When using a CPM device for a total knee replacement, one cycle begins in the extended position, moves up into the end range of flexion, and ends at the original extended position.

The available ROM is established either by tolerance of the client, parameters of the physician, or limitations of the device. When initially establishing how much ROM a device should move the client's extremity, the assistant should monitor the client's tolerance. The device will have a manual block or stop that establishes the amount of degrees the device will move. Forcing the extremity through a painful or intolerable ROM is potentially harmful. The method of establishing a pain-free cycle and then gradually progressing into degrees of greater ROM is typically tolerated more easily by the client.

The physician may specify a limited or desired target ROM of the CPM. Clients with total knee replacements may have a goal of full extension and 110° of flexion. Clients after total shoulder replacements may have a limitation of not greater than 90° of abduction. The device should have the adjustment capabilities to establish the desired arc of motion. Depending on the positioning of the client and the efficacy of the CPM device, the degrees moved on the device may not exactly correlate into the actual degrees moved on the extremity. A knee CPM limited to 90° of flexion may only take the knee to 75°. The assistant should use a standard goniometer to assess the effective ROM of the extremity while the device is moving through a cycle.

Limitations of certain machines will also affect the amount of ROM available passively to the client. Knee CPM devices typically move through an arc from 0° to

110°, but manufacturers may differ. If motion greater than this arc is desired, the CPM device will be structurally limited.

The speed of the CPM device is usually adjustable. The speed at which the device ascends and descends through the available ROM will assist in the tolerance of the client to the CPM modality. Initially, the slower speeds may help the client acclimate to the treatment. With familiarity of the CPM modality and decreased pain, the client may be able to tolerate increased cycle speeds. Salter described the ideal speed as one cycle every 45 seconds.[28]

The duration of the CPM applied to the extremity will vary according to physician protocols and levels of client tolerance. Studies have examined various application durations with differing results. Davis[42] demonstrated gains of earlier ambulation and greater ROM in clients with total knee replacements who had CPM application durations of longer than 18 hours, compared with an immobilized group over a 7-day period postoperatively. Stap and Woodfin[41] found ROM gains in clients with knee flexion contractures with application durations of 3 to 6 hours over a 7-week period. Gose[46] found positive gains in clients with total knee replacements in 1-hour sessions three times daily. Basso and Knapp[45] found similar results for their clients who used CPM for 5 hours per day and for the clients who used CPM for 20 hours per day. Because of the existing variety in application durations, all with positive results, further investigative research is warranted to establish the prime operating dosage for the use of CPM.

LOW-LOAD STRETCHING

Prevention of joint motion limitations is an ultimate therapeutic goal. MacKay-Lyons[47] stated that "daily range of motion exercises have become a standard prophylactic measure [to manage joint contractures, with] . . . limited effectiveness." Attempts to manage the cross-linking of collagen fibers is best accomplished with prolonged, mild tensile force.[48] The discussion of the different applications of low-load stretching is presented in Chapter 3.

 ## SUMMARY

The synovial joint is the most common articulation found in the human body and is characterized by the ability to allow free motion. It has articular cartilage covering the moving surfaces of the bones and has the presence of a joint capsule that secretes synovial fluid. Synovial fluid is secreted by the synovial membrane and serves to lubricate and nourish the joint surfaces of a synovial joint.

Granulation scar tissue provides the framework of the repair process for the human body. One pattern of scarring is derived from collagen fibers, which adapt or mimic the injured original structure. The phases of healing are sequential in nature and have predictive events. The inflammatory phase of healing cleanses the injured tissue and prepares the area for healing to occur. The fibroplastic phase encourages fibroblasts, or repair cells, to begin the production of collagen fibers, which are deposited in a random fashion in the blood exudate meshwork to begin repairing the injured tissue. The remodeling phase sees a continuation of collagen production forming a mature scar with a destruction of immature collagen. The newly formed scar readily adapts to the functional stresses applied during the remodeling phase until the strong covalent bonding process replaces the weaker hydrogen bonding process between the cross-linked collagen fibers. Scar tissue will mimic the original and surrounding tissues, although the process is not clearly understood. Clinically, therapeutic interventions during each phase of healing should be directed at the protection of injured tissue, promotion of the healing process, and prevention of adherence of scar tissue to undesired structures. The functional return of scar tissue is directly related to the number of cross-linked bonds. Tissues that must withstand greater forces require greater density and have more cross-links. Tissues that must have greater mobility require less density and have fewer cross-links.

Various tissues within the human body have unique healing attributes, but all generally follow the predictive phases of healing. If the inflammatory process becomes nonproductive as a result of repeated injury or stress, chronic inflammation may proliferate the injury site, thus leading to an overall weakening of the functional nature of the involved tissue.

Immobilization may or may not be of clinical benefit after tissue injury. Many structures in the human body require the stresses provided by muscular contraction or weight bearing to maintain adequate strength and viability. Prolonged immobilization may promote weakening of skeletal structures and lengthen the time needed for adequate rehabilitation. CPM and low-load stretching are used to lessen the effects of immobilization and promote functional return after tissue injury or surgical intervention.

REFERENCES

1. Norkin, CC, and Levangie, PK: Joint Structure and Function: A Comprehensive Analysis, ed 2. FA Davis, Philadelphia, 1992.
2. Lippert, L: Clinical Kinesiology for the Physical Therapist Assistant, ed 2. FA Davis, Philadelphia, 1994.
3. Moore, KL: Clinically Oriented Anatomy, ed 2. Williams & Wilkins, Baltimore, 1985.
4. English, T, et al: Inflammatory response of synovial joint structures. In Malone, TR, et al: Orthopedic and Sports Physical Therapy, ed 3. Mosby, St Louis, MO 1997.
5. Hardy, MA: The biology of scar formation. Phys Ther 69:1014, 1989.
6. Kisner, C, and Colby, LA: Therapeutic Exercise: Foundations and Techniques, ed 3. FA Davis, Philadelphia, 1996.
7. Taber's Cyclopedic Medical Dictionary, ed 18. FA Davis, Philadelphia, 1997.
8. Young, A, et al: Effects of joint pathology on muscle. Clin Ortho 219:21, 1987.
9. DeAndrade, et al: Joint distension and reflex muscle inhibition in the knee. J Bone Joint Surg Am 47:313, 1965.
10. Lotz, M, et al: Early versus delayed shoulder motion following axillary dissection. Ann Surg 193:288, 1981.
11. Paletta, FX, et al: Hypothermia and tourniquet ischemia. Plast Reconstr Surg 29:531, 1962.
12. Levenson, S: Practical applications of experimental studies in the care of primary closed wounds. Am J Surg 104:273, 1962.
13. Cummings, GS, and Tillman, LJ: Remodeling of dense connective tissue in normal adult tissues. In Currier, DP, and Nelson, RM (eds): Dynamics of Human Biologic Tissues. FA Davis, Philadelphia, 1992.
14. Madden, JW: Wound healing: The biological basis of hand surgery. Clin Plast Surg 3:3, 1976.
15. Arem AJ, and Madden, JW: Effects of stress on healing of wounds. I. Intermittent noncyclical tension. J Surg Res 20:93, 1976.
16. Maroudas, A, et al: The permeability of articular cartilage. J Bone Joint Surg Br 50(1):166, 1968.
17. Cailliet, R: Knee Pain and Disability. FA Davis, Philadelphia, 1972.
18. Radin, EL: The physiology and degeneration of joints. Semin Arthritis Rheum 2(3):245, 1972–73.
19. Keene, JS and Malone, TR: Ligament and muscle-tendon unit injuries. In Malone, TR, et al: Orthopedic and Sports Physical Therapy, ed 3. Mosby, St Louis, MO, 1997.
20. Salter, RB: Textbook of Disorders and Injuries of the Musculoskeletal System, ed 2. Williams & Wilkins, Baltimore, 1983.
21. Salter, RB: Motion vs. rest: Why immobilize joints? (Historical) Presidential address, Canadian Orthopaedic Association, Halifax, Nova Scotia, June 9, 1981. J Bone Joint Surg Br 64B:251, 1982.
22. Akeson, WH, et al: The connective tissue response to immobility: Biomechanical changes in periarticular connective tissue of the immobilized rabbit knee. Clin Orthop 93:356, 1973.

23. Noyes, FR: The functional properties of knee ligament and alterations induced by immobilization: A correlative biomechanical and histological study in primates. Clin Orthop 123:210, 1977.
24. Gelberman, RH, et al: Flexor tendon healing and restoration of the gliding surface: an ultrastructural study in dogs. J Bone Joint Surg Am 65:70, 1983.
25. Whedon, GD: Disuse osteoporosis: Physiological aspects. Calcif Tissue Int 36:sl46, 1984.
26. Noyes, FR, et al: Biomechanics of ligament failure: II. An analysis of immobilization, exercise, and reconditioning effects in primates. J Bone Joint Surg Am 56:1406, 1974.
27. Enneking, WF, and Horowitz, H: The intra-articular effects of immobilization on the human knee. J Bone Joint Surg Am 54:973, 1972.
28. Salter, RB, et al: The healing of articular tissues through continuous passive motion: Essence of the first ten years of experimental investigations. J Bone Joint Surg Br 64(6):640, 1982.
29. Woo, SL, et al: Connective tissue response to immobility: Correlative study of biomechanical and biochemical measurements of normal and immobilized rabbit knees. Arthritis Rheum 18:257, 1975.
30. Vaughan, VG: Effects of upper limb immobilization on isometric muscle strength, movement time, and triphasic electomyographic characteristics. Phys Ther 69:119, 1989.
31. Mendler, MH: Knee extensor and flexor force following injury. Phys Ther 47:35, 1967.
32. Stillwell, DM, et al: Atrophy of quadriceps muscle due to immobilization of the lower extremity. Arch Phys Med Rehabil 48:289, 1967.
33. Spencer, JD, et al: Knee joint effusion and quadriceps reflex inhibition in man. Arch Phys Med Rehabil 65:171, 1984.
34. Paulos, LE, et al: Infrapatellar contracture syndrome. Am J Sports Med 15:331, 1987.
35. Akeson, WH, et al: Collagen cross-linking alterations in joint contractures. Connect Tissue Res 5:15, 1977.
36. Schneider, VS, and McDonald, J: Skeletal calcium homeostasis and countermeasures to prevent disuse osteoporosis. Calcif Tissue Int 36:s151, 1984.
37. Salter, RB, et al: The biological effect of continuous passive motion on the healing of the full-thickness defects in articular cartilage: An experimental investigation in the rabbit. J Bone Joint Surg Am 62A:1232, 1980.
38. McCarthy, MR, et al: The clinical use of continuous passive motion in physical therapy. JOSPT 15:132, 1992.
39. Shankman, GA: Fundamental Orthopedic Management for the Physical Therapist Assistant. Mosby, St Louis, MO, 1997.
40. Covey, MH, et al: Efficacy of continuous passive motion devices with hand burns. J Burns Care Rehabil 9(4):397, 1988.
41. Stap, LJ, and Woodfin, PM: Continuous passive motion in the treatment of knee flexion contractures: A case report. Phys Ther 66:1720, 1986.
42. Davis, D: Continuous passive motion for total knee arthroplasty. Phys Ther 64:709, 1984.
43. Noyes, FR, and Mangine, RE: Early knee motion after open and arthroscopic anterior cruciate ligament reconstruction. Am J Sports Med 15:149, 1987.
44. Salter, RB, et al: Clinical applications of basic research on continuous passive motion for disorders and injuries of synovial joints: A preliminary report of a feasibility study. J Orthop Res 3:325, 1983.
45. Basso, DM, and Knapp, L: Comparison of two continuous passive motion protocols for patients with total knee implants. Phys Ther 67:360, 1987.
46. Gose, JC: Continuous passive motion in the postoperative treatment of patients with total knee replacement: A retrospective study. Phys Ther 67:39, 1987.
47. MacKay-Lyons, M: Low-load, prolonged stretch in treatment of elbow flexion contractures secondary to head trauma: A case report. Phys Ther 69:292, 1989.
48. Warren, CG, Lehmann, JF, and Koblanski, JN: Heat and stretch procedures: an evaluation using rat tail tendon. Arch Phys Med Rehabil 57:122, 1976.

BIBLIOGRAPHY

Akeson, WH, et al: Collagen cross-linking alterations in joint contractures. Connect Tissue Res 5:15, 1977.
Akeson, WH, et al: The connective tissue response to immobility: Biomechanical changes in periarticular connective tissue of the immobilized rabbit knee. Clin Orthop 93:356, 1973.
Arem, AJ, and Madden, JW: Effects of stress on healing of wounds. I. Intermittent noncyclical tension. J Surg Res 20:93, 1976.
Basso, DM, and Knapp, L: Comparison of two continuous passive motion protocols for patients with total knee implants. Phys Ther 67:360, 1987.

Cailliet, R: Knee Pain and Disability. FA Davis, Philadelphia, 1972.

Covey, MH, et al: Efficacy of continuous passive motion devices with hand burns. J Burn Care Rehabil 9(4):397, 1988.

Cummings, GS, Tillman, LJ: Remodeling of dense connective tissue in normal adult tissues. In Currier, DP, and Nelson, RM (eds): Dynamics of Human Biologic Tissues. FA Davis, Philadelphia, 1992.

Davis, D: Continuous passive motion for total knee arthroplasty. Phys Ther 64:709, 1984.

DeAndrade, JR, et al: Joint distension and reflex muscle inhibition in the knee. J Bone Joint Surg Am 47:313, 1965.

English, T, et al: Inflammatory response of synovial joint structures. In Malone, TR, et al: (eds): Orthopedic and Sports Physical Therapy, ed 3. Mosby, St Louis, MO, 1997.

Enneking, WF, and Horowitz, H: The intra-articular effects of immobilization on the human knee. J Bone Joint Surg Am 54A:973, 1972.

Gelberman, RH, et al: Flexor tendon healing and restoration of the gliding surface: An ultrastructural study in dogs. J Bone Joint Surg Am 65:70, 1983.

Gose, JC: Continuous passive motion in the postoperative treatment of patients with total knee replacement: A retrospective study. Phys Ther 67:39, 1987.

Hardy, MA: The biology of scar formation. Phys Ther 69:1014, 1989.

Keene, JS, and Malone, TR: Ligament and muscle-tendon unit injuries. In Malone, TR, et al: Orthopedic and Sports Physical Therapy, ed 3. Mosby, St Louis, MO, 1997.

Kisner, C, and Colby, LA: Therapeutic Exercise: Foundations and Techniques, ed 3. FA Davis, Philadelphia, 1996.

Levenson, S: Practical applications of experimental studies in the care of primary closed wounds. Am J Surg 104:273, 1962.

Lippert, L: Clinical Kinesiology for the Physical Therapist Assistant, ed 2. FA Davis, Philadelphia, 1994.

Lotz, M, et al: Early versus delayed shoulder motion following axillary dissection. Ann Surg 193:288, 1981.

MacKay-Lyons, M: Low-load, prolonged stretch in treatment of elbow flexion contractures secondary to head trauma: a case report. Phys Ther 69:292, 1989.

Madden, JW: Wound healing: The biological basis of hand surgery. Clin Plast Surg 3:3, 1976.

Maroudas, A, et al: The permeability of articular cartilage. J Bone Joint Surg Br 50(1):166, 1968.

McCarthy, MR, et al: The clinical use of continuous passive motion in physical therapy. JOSPT 15:132, 1992.

Mendler, MH: Knee extensor and flexor force following injury. Phys Ther 47:35, 1967.

Moore, KL: Clinically Oriented Anatomy, ed 2. Williams & Wilkins, Baltimore, 1985.

Norkin, CC, and Levangie, PK: Joint Structure and Function: A Comprehensive Analysis, ed 2. FA Davis, Philadelphia, 1992.

Noyes, FR: The functional properties of knee ligament and alterations induced by immobilization: A correlative biomechanical and histological study in primates. Clin Orthop 123:210, 1977.

Noyes, FR, and Mangine, RE: Early knee motion after open and arthroscopic anterior cruciate ligament reconstruction. Am J Sports Med 15:149, 1987.

Noyes, FR, et al: Biomechanics of ligament failure. II. An analysis of immobilization, exercise, and reconditioning effects in primates. J Bone Joint Surg Am 56A:1406, 1974.

Paletta, FX, et al: Hypothermia and tourniquet ischemia. Plast Reconstr Surg 29:531, 1962.

Paulos, LE, et al: Infrapatellar contracture syndrome. Am J Sports Med 15:331, 1987.

Radin, EL: The physiology and degeneration of joints. Semin Arthritis Rheum 2(3):245, 1972–73.

Salter, RB: Motion vs. rest: Why immobilize joints? (Historical) Presidential address, Canadian Orthopaedic Association, Halifax, Nova Scotia, June 9, 1981. J Bone Joint Surg Br 64B:251, 1982.

Salter, RB: Textbook of Disorders and Injuries of the Musculoskeletal System, ed 2. Williams & Wilkins, Baltimore, 1983.

Salter, RB, et al: Clinical applications of basic research on continuous passive motion for disorders and injuries of synovial joints: A preliminary report of a feasibility study. J Orthop Res 3:325, 1983.

Salter, RB, et al: The biological effect of continuous passive motion on the healing of the full-thickness defects in articular cartilage: an experimental investigation in the rabbit. J Bone Joint Surg Am 62A:1232, 1980.

Salter, RB, et al: The healing of articular tissues through continuous passive motion. Essence of the first ten years of experimental investigations. J Bone Joint Surg Br 64B(6):640, 1982.

Schneider, VS, and McDonald, J: Skeletal calcium homeostasis and countermeasures to prevent disuse osteoporosis. Calcif Tissue Int 36:s151, 1984.

Shankman, GA: Fundamental Orthopedic Management for the Physical Therapist Assistant. Mosby, St Louis, MO, 1997.

Spencer, JD, et al: Knee joint effusion and quadriceps reflex inhibition in man. Arch Phys Med Rehabil 65:171, 1984.

Stap, LJ, and Woodfin, PM: Continuous passive motion in the treatment of knee flexion contractures: A case report. Phys Ther 66:1720, 1986.

Stillwell, DM, et al: Atrophy of quadriceps muscle due to immobilization of the lower extremity. Arch Phys Med Rehabil 48:289, 1967.

Taber's Cyclopedic Medical Dictionary, ed 18. FA Davis, Philadelphia, 1997.

Vaughan, VG: Effects of upper limb immobilization on isometric muscle strength, movement time, and triphasic electromyographic characteristics. Phys Ther 69:119, 1989.

Warren, CG, et al: Heat and stretch procedures: an evaluation using rat tail tendon. Arch Phys Med Rehabil 57:122, 1976.

Whedon, GD: Disuse osteoporosis: Physiological aspects. Calcif Tissue Int 36:s146, 1984.

Woo, SL, et al: Connective tissue response to immobility: Correlative study of biomechanical and biochemical measurements of normal and immobilized rabbit knees. Arthritis Rheum 18:257, 1975.

Young, A, et al: Effects of joint pathology on muscle. Clin Ortho 219:21, 1987.

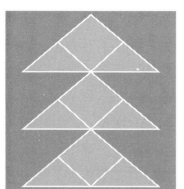

chapter 6

Normal Aging

Key Words

activities of daily living
aging
dementia
excess disability
information processing
kinesthesia
muscle atrophy
nerve conduction velocity
osteoporosis
proprioceptive sensation
total lung capacity
vital capacity

 ## STEREOTYPES OF AGING

Stereotypes and assumptions have created an inaccurate description of the aging process in western societies. Most are based on falsehoods or distorted concepts but are generally accepted as natural law. Growing old has been associated with losing one's hearing, one's vision, one's ability to walk, and one's mind and having one's hair turn grey. Attitudes and values about aging are often passed from generation to generation with each subsequent generation modifying values to meet the needs of that generation. The value of an extended family under the same roof today in the United States has significantly less worth than it did 200 years ago. Along with the decline in the value placed on the extended family is an increase in the institutionalization of elderly persons. Nursing home placement has become an accepted means of dealing with aging in our culture. Many eastern cultures would view this institutional process as cruel and disrespectful. Osa Jackson[1] views aging as a natural process with certain norms and expectations that are typically different than accepted stereotypes. She also stresses the importance for clinical personnel of understanding how the aged view the physical therapy process.

In the traditional medical model, the client has been viewed by the medical professional as having a diagnosis with certain norms and expectations that accompany the particular diagnosis. When excessive or differing symptoms present, thus limiting the functional abilities of the client that may not be related to the actual diagnosis, the medical model is limited to explain the cause of the added dysfunction. **Excess disability** is noted when there exists more loss of function than can be explained by the disease process alone.[1] Box 6–1 presents a case related to the concept of excess disability. The physical therapist assistant should treat the client as a whole person not simply treat the orthopedic condition.

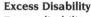
Excess Disability
Excess disability is noted when there exists more loss of function than can be explained by the disease process alone.

 ## NORMAL AGING

As time passes, many life events are experienced that affect human development on many levels. **Aging** is defined as changes in a living system that occur over time and is a complex field of study that involves the social, psychological, and physical

Aging
The changes in a living system that occur over time involving social, psychological, and physical aspects.

Box 6–1

EXCESS DISABILITY

R.S., an 86-year-old man, recently underwent an open reduction, internal fixation of his left hip and splinting for a compacted fracture of his left distal radius sustained in a fall as he was getting out of his car on a rainy afternoon. He had been in generally good health, but he had progressive peripheral neuropathies of unknown etiology that began to rob him of his balance and lower-extremity coordination. His rehabilitation course was prefaced by the orthopedic surgeon who told his family, "His bones are strong and he will heal quickly." After spending 3 weeks in an acute care setting followed by 6 weeks in a rehabilitation setting, R.S. became increasingly depressed and was slow to recover. The orthopedic surgeon could not explain the slow results in simple orthopedic terms, even though the surgery and bones were healing well.

From the point of view of the orthopedic surgeon, R.S. had a simple "broken hip and wrist", but in the view of R.S., his hip hurt, and he had to use a walker. He was also losing his independence, his home, the ability to drive, and he was outliving most of his friends and peer support groups. Several of R.S.'s friends had physical therapy during their hospitalizations, not long after which, his friends died. Rehabilitation was not viewed by R.S. as an opportunity to improve, but as a messenger of death. In this scenario, "a simple broken wrist and hip" should have been easily overcome in the eyes of a younger individual, but in the eyes of an aging individual, this same scenario was a precursor to losing overall independence.

aspects of our clients.[2] Some have vainly attempted to avert aging through chemicals, herbs, plastic surgeons, and exercise gurus. Ponce De Leon believed in a magic fountain several centuries ago that would preserve his youth. The attitude toward aging in the western hemisphere has generally been negative, and an emphasis has been placed on being young and healthy.

SOCIOLOGICAL

Cultural attitudes are placed on the process of aging. Chronological events occur with certain expectations, such as the ability to drive a car when one turns 16 or the ability to vote when turning 18 or retiring at age 65. The definition of adulthood or measure of maturity has no established chronological time frame. Western societies place a great emphasis on the chronological age of a person, despite the great differences among individuals at like ages. This is easily demonstrated by observing a 12-year-old prepubescent boy and a 12-year-old female adolescent. The 12-year-old girl is typically more mature and beginning to model herself after young adults, whereas the 12-year-old boy is generally more immature and modeling himself after fellow children. Also well demonstrated is the fact that most aging Americans have the motivation and ability to work effectively past age 65, yet are forced into mandatory retirement. Lewthwaite[3] says that social factors, including beliefs on aging of family and friends or attitudes toward exercise, can undermine motivational efforts of clients in a rehabilitation setting. Generalizations about cultural attitudes toward aging in western societies include:

Young is beautiful.
Fitness is desirable.
Disability is undesirable.
Retirement is nonproductive.
Growing old means having to rely on other people for help (losing independence).

PSYCHOLOGICAL

Psychological factors complicate cultural attitudes, presenting questions of self-worth and loneliness in the aging individual. When a society places value on youth, many people develop their sense of well-being along those societal values. When youth is lost, attitudes of the individual may become negative possibly, leading to unhealthy conditions. Psychological factors that may concern your aging client include:

Change in Living Status
Change in Peer Support Groups
Death of Partner or Spouse
Onset of Disability
Fear of Being Institutionalized
Outliving an Offspring
Losing Ability to Drive a Car
Using a Walker
Fear of Falling
Fear of Being Dependant on Others

Motivation (or lack thereof) may often be related to the psychological perceptions of the aging individual in any given situation. In working with geriatric clients, the assistant must appreciate that each individual has a unique life story and personal motivators forming attitudes of the client toward the current medical condition. If the assistant is not attentive to the client's social and psychological needs, then an opportunity to interact with and understand the motivations of the client may be missed. Box 6–2 presents an example of understanding how cultural attitudes and individual motivators can effect an individuals health.

PHYSICAL

Normal physical effects of aging involve most of the organ systems of the body including the cardiopulmonary, musculoskeletal, and nervous systems. Collectively, these elements are part of the normal aging process for an individual in the absence of disease, but in no way constitute absolutes for every individual. A challenge to all clinicians lies in realizing that each individual ages in a unique fashion or manner. The physical effects of normal aging include:

Respiratory Changes
Bony Changes
Central Nervous System Changes
Cardiac Changes

___ **Box 6–2** _____

CULTURAL ATTITUDES AND INDIVIDUAL MOTIVATION

I once treated an 86-year-old male client who was by societal standards "crippled" with degenerative arthritis affecting his hands, elbows, shoulders, hips, knees, and ankles. He had been a cattle rancher most of his life and had lost his wife of 50 years three summers earlier. His farm was small and modest with 40 head of cattle grazing all around. Everyday he had gotten out of bed and cared for the animals, although the pace was slow compared to that of a younger man. Despite caring for the farm adequately, the son had convinced the father to sell the cattle and "take it easy for a while." I began seeing him several months after this event because his arthritis began to create motion limitations in his knees and feet. His life had become sedentary, creating an ample opportunity for the arthritis to advance and for his motivation to regress. The gentleman bragged to me that he had never been in a hospital nor seen a doctor until his son convinced him to give up his cattleman's life.

The self-worth of this individual came from caring for the ranch and animals. Personal motivation to get out of bed in the mornings was lost and his health condition began to decline. This is not meant to be a scientific summary of preventing debilitation in the aging population, but an awareness that the psychological motivators of a client must be appreciated.

Muscular Changes
Sensory Changes

It is beyond the scope of this textbook to discuss in detail every researched aspect of the aging process, but the following summarize the major components related to orthopedic rehabilitation.

Respiratory Changes

Total Lung Capacity
The total amount of air contained in the lungs after a maximal inspiration.

Respiratory changes are often demonstrated by a loss of efficiency through (1) a reduction in the total lung capacity, (2) decreased vital capacity, and (3) thickening of the support membranes between the alveoli and the capillaries.[2] **Total lung capacity** is the total amount of air contained in the lungs after a maximum inspiration, and **vital capacity** is the amount of air that can be maximally inspired after a maximal expiration. These capacities are usually measured in milliliters (mL) through the use of volumetric respiratory devices.[4] When thickening occurs between the alveoli and the capillary beds, a decreased efficiency of gaseous exchange and an overall decrease of oxygenization in the blood are noted. As we age, we gradually become less efficient in oxygen intake into the lungs and oxygen exchange into the bloodstream. This can lead to shortness of breath, dizziness, confusion or loss of consciousness in affected clients.

Vital Capacity
The amount of air that can be maximally inspired after a maximal expiration.

Bony Changes

Osteoporosis
A state of bone loss or "porous bones."

A bony change that is commonly seen in the aged includes the loss of bone mass, which results in porous, lighter, and mechanically inefficient bones. **Osteoporosis,** which translated means "porous bones," is a popular phrase used by the news media today and is one of the most significant fears of the aging population. There has been a great deal of debate over the cause of this condition that places those affected at greater risk for fractures and deformity. The actual process of bone loss is a combination of decreased osteoblastic (new bone deposits) formation and an increase in the osteoclastic (bone absorption) resorption of bone, the end result being a decrease in mass of the bone matter. Salter[5] puts more of the blame for bone loss on the osteoclastic activity or the reabsorption of the bone than on the osteoblastic deficits. Along with a positive family history, the triad of inactivity, poor diet (calcium intake), and hormonal changes (deficiency of estrogen) have surfaced as the leading factors involved in the onset of osteoporosis.[6] Clinically, osteoporosis is rarely identified until a specific pathology is noted. For example, an 83-year-old client with hip fracture may be told by her physician that her osteoporosis may have been the cause of the fracture, but she insists that she has never had osteoporosis before. This scenario may be common when dealing with the aging population, and the assistant must be able to adequately describe the aging process and the effects of bone loss on the skeletal system.

Central Nervous System Changes

Normal central nervous system changes have been popularly, but incorrectly, associated with memory loss, forgetfulness, and **dementia** or the impairment in some or all aspects of intellectual functioning in a person who is fully alert.[7] Facts about normal aging and the brain include a physical decrease in the weight of the brain but do not include any of the previously mentioned misconceptions. The brain loses thousands of cells daily, but the vital areas related to speech, memory, and thinking are spared.[8] **Information processing** is the ability of the brain to receive a stimulus, identify the stimulus, select a response, and then plan and execute the motor response (Fig. 6–1). The clinician may often see the manifestations of aging on the central nervous system as (1) a decreased ability to perform speed-related tasks, (2) a decreased rate of learning new skills, and (3) a difficulty with balance and fine motor skills. Light[9] stated that the delays in motor response in the elderly are related to central nervous system processing limitations rather than to physiological deficits in the peripheral nervous system. It has been documented, however, that a decrease in **nerve conduction velocity,** or the speed at which a nerve transmits an impulse, is noted by 10% to 15% in elderly persons compared with younger persons.[10] The Arndt-Schultz principle can be used as a guideline for clinical discrepancies in information processing among aged clients:

1. The elderly require a higher level and/or a longer period of stimulation before the threshold for initial physiological response is reached.
2. The physiological response in the aged is rarely as big, as visible, or as consistent as is noted in the younger age groups.[11]

As the PTA interacts with the client during rehabilitation, disbanding geriatric aging myths is critical. In the absence of a disease process, a client will be slightly slower in neural-processing skills but still be able to learn, interact, and recall events just as the client did in his or her youth. Box 6–3 gives some suggestions for successful interaction with the geriatric population.

Dementia
The impairment in some or all aspects of intellectual functioning in a person who is fully alert.

Information Processing
The ability of the brain to receive a stimulus, identify the stimulus, select a response, and then plan and execute the motor response.

Nerve Conduction Velocity
The speed at which a nerve transmits an impulse.

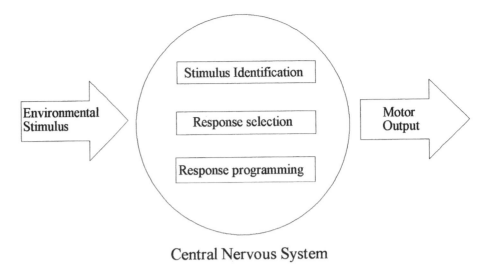

FIG. 6–1
Information processing. The ability of the brain to receive a stimulus, identify the stimulus, select a response and then plan and execute the motor response.

Cardiac Changes

Cardiac capacities change with the aging process. Generally, the ability of the heart to respond or adapt to extra workloads is decreased.[2] It is unclear whether this change is a deconditioning response as cardiac output declines and peripheral resistance to blood flow increases, or an inherent part of aging. Clients will often be seen with an increased heart rate (90 to 120 bpm) even though they may have been lying in bed waiting to be taken to therapy. The ability for the heart rate to adapt quickly to changing postures is poor. As the client remains supine in bed for most of the day, the client's heart may have difficulty adjusting to the demands of

---

Box 6–3

SUGGESTED INTERACTING TECHNIQUES WITH GERIATRIC CLIENTS: PROCESSING AND LEARNING

1. Make the client aware of your presence by touching. Initially, the client may not hear you.
2. Perform activities that are meaningful for your client.
3. Speak clearly, calmly, and in a normal conversational tone (avoid shouting).
4. Give specific, not abstract, examples.
5. Provide a positive learning environment (keep distractions to a minimum).
6. Set your client up for success, not failure.
7. Build on successes.
8. Give positive feedback, and avoid condescending tones.
9. Be patient. Give time for clients to respond in *their* time, not yours.
10. Actively demonstrate the task during instruction.

upright activities. The increased demand for oxygen in the working muscles during gait combined with the heart's decreased ability to circulate blood may produce dizziness, confusion, or loss of consciousness. It is always a good policy to sit and speak with the client before initiating other activities to ensure that they have become acclimated to an upright posture.

Muscular Changes

Muscular changes take two forms in the aging population: (1) **muscle atrophy** (decrease in the muscle mass), and (2) the decreased ability of the muscle to adapt to stress and generate force.[12] Does inactivity or aging produce muscular weakness and atrophy? Thompson[13] stated that the muscle atrophy process in aging is a combination of the reduction in the total number of muscle fibers and the decrease in the size of the muscle fibers, type II fibers being the most affected. Several authors[14,15,16] have published studies identifying that the number of muscular motor units decreases in older adults. Hopp[12] also found that decreasing strength in aging individuals was related to the inability to recruit motor units resulting in a decreased maximal voluntary contraction for those over age 60. However, in studies by Fiatarone et al.[17] and Brown,[18] the force-generating ability of aging skeletal muscles were shown to be significantly improved through the use of resistance training, even though Brown believed that there was inadequate data to support the use of resistance training in the geriatric population. The argument of inactivity with aging versus normal aging producing muscular changes is a "chicken and the egg"–type debate that cannot easily be conceded. Clinically, most aging clients will be affected by muscular atrophy and weakness either from normal aging or inactivity, and possibly a combination of both.

> **Muscle Atrophy**
> A decrease in muscle mass.

The ability of the muscle to adapt to stress and repair itself decreases with age. Adequate rest periods are critical to the rebuilding and repairing phase of the muscle for all physical therapy clients, but the need for adequate rest periods during therapeutic intervention for geriatric clients may be greater. Health-care professionals often squeeze clients into crowded schedules, particularly when the client is institutionalized, paying little regard to their physiological needs. A typical day for a hospitalized client may begin poorly as a result of a difficult night's rest. Nursing may have measured vital signs and turned the client every 2 hours during the night shift. The occupational therapist probably arrived at 6 a.m. to begin **activities of daily living** (ADLs) skills, followed by breakfast and morning rounds by the physician. The PTA then enters the client's room as the physician is leaving to begin the morning gait training session. The client might be exhausted before lunchtime because of inadequate rest periods. The assistant should remember that if the geriatric client is pushed beyond his or her physiological limits, the stress can cause muscular, tendinous, or ligamentous damage. Ensure that adequate rest periods are incorporated into part of the treatment plan.

> **Activities of Daily Living (ADLs)**
> The tasks performed in everyday life, such as dressing, eating, and bathing.

Sensory Changes

Sensory changes in hearing, taste, smell, proprioception, and vision seen in the aged population usually occur gradually and may be subtle upon examination. These sensory changes can often be misinterpreted as forgetfulness, dementia, or uncooperativeness. Communication deficits may be the result of subtle hearing changes. It has been published that the incidence of hearing disturbances is five times greater in residents of nursing homes as compared with the general population.[19] The hearing loss pattern is characterized by the inability to distinguish higher frequency sounds in both ears. Most people with hearing loss will develop coping mechanisms for the gradual loss of this vital sensory component. A person with hearing loss may adapt by avoiding situations in which fine hearing skills are needed. Examples of situations that the client with hearing loss may seek to avoid are (1) large crowds or (2) places with distracting noises.[2] As the assistant working with the older client, identification of potential communication deficits due to hearing loss is critical in performing rehabilitation. Be aware whether the client uses a hearing aid and ensure that the hearing aid is in proper working order to obtain the best functional performance by your client.

The loss of the sense of smell and taste may present slowly over time and can lead to subtle changes in the behaviors of the geriatric client. These losses may be attributed to medication interaction or the aging process and can lead to a decrease in appetite and malnutrition. The assistant may encounter the client who says that "the food just doesn't taste right" and refuses to eat. The experience of eating is associated with the senses of smell, taste, and sight. If food is regularly unappealing to the senses, eventually the client may simply choose not to eat, and this may be interpreted as the client's forgetting to eat. The challenge to the dietician in the health-care team is to prepare meals that have a variety of smells and textures that enhance the experience of eating. Another potential hazard regarding the loss of smell or taste may present when the client lives alone. The client with a smelling and taste impairment may lose the ability to detect if food has become spoiled or rotten. Routinely marking dates on items in the refrigerator is a simple way to help adapt to this loss of sensation.[2]

The loss or decrease of **proprioceptive sensations,** which includes both position sense (awareness of posture in space) and **kinesthesia** (awareness of body movement) can greatly affect the safety and treatment of elderly clients.[20] The ability to appropriately integrate visual, vestibular, and proprioceptive information is critical in the process of maintaining balance.[21] If a client presents with a decreased ability to perceive small postural deviations or shifts, this can alter the sense of standing balance or the performance of gait and places the client at greater risk for falls. Proprioceptors are specialized sensory organs that provide feedback from the extremities and trunk to the central nervous system, alerting the body to its postural position in space. Proprioceptive awareness is critical in maintaining upright posture and in adapting to uneven surfaces. Quoniam et al.[22] demonstrated that age-related differences exist in the processing of proprioceptive inputs, finding slower and smaller amplitude adjustments for postural sways in the elderly subject as compared with a younger subject. If balance deficits are identified, then client education must be centered around the safe and effective management of the sensory loss for preventing falls. According to Shumway-Cook et al.,[23] falls are a major health problem among the geriatric population. In people over age 65, 35% experience one or more falls annually resulting in potentially devastating consequences. Also in this same age group, 40% of all hospital admissions are related to injuries suffered in falls.[24] Normal sensory changes over time may be a factor leading to an increased probability of falling. This aspect of aging is discussed in detail later in the text, when the special needs of the geriatric client are presented.

Normal visual changes occur with the aging process. Ophthalmologists often claim that no one escapes their services and that they will either get the client when they are young or when they are old. Depth perception and the ability to focus are usually affected as the cornea flattens. The vestibular ocular reflex is used to fix the eyes during head movement; with aging, distortion of this vital reflex can impair ADLs, including ambulation.[25,26] Di Fabio and Emasithi[27] believe

Proprioceptive Sensation
The awareness of posture in space and the awareness of body movement.

Kinesthesia
The awareness of body movement.

that there has been little systematic investigation of how the aged integrate sensory input to accommodate to visual disturbances. Clinically, when working with a client, ensure that clean, corrective lenses are worn properly and keep objects out of the path, limiting the potential for falls. Remain alert that the depth perception of the client may be impaired, leading to an unsteady gait.

FUNCTIONAL EXPECTATIONS

Functional expectations for the aging population are shaped and defined by cultural and individual attitudes. Van Sant[28] in her research on life-span development relates the following:

> To be "immature" or "past your peak" is to be devalued. From a life-span perspective, maturity is just a passing point in time, to be valued no more than infancy, the middle-aged years, adolescence, or any other age period.

Too often our culture associates disease, effects of pathology, or simple inactivity with the aging process. The PTA's attitudes toward aging will be reflected in his or her interactions with and treatments of the aged. Lewthwaite[3] believes that successful physical therapy outcomes are directly related to the attitudes and interaction between the clinician and the client. Aging is a natural process of change and adaptation over an entire life span. Aging affects every living creature on earth, and despite vain efforts, cannot be reversed. The health professional should not embrace the negative connotations surrounding the aging process. When working with the geriatric population, the assistant should be aware of the aging process and how it may affect treatment outcomes. Prevention and wellness is a different aspect of aging that society is now beginning to incorporate. Good health can be carried into our golden years without the negativism of "getting old" if society places a positive value on aging.

SUMMARY

Excess disability is a term used to identify an existence of greater loss of function that can otherwise be described by the disease process alone. Aging is the normal change that occurs within a living system and involves social, psychological, and physical aspects. Cultural and psychological attitudes toward aging may affect the outcomes of your treatments. Normal physical changes are predictable, but not inclusive to every client of who will be treated by a PTA. To promote a positive rehabilitation experience, the PTA must not associate normal physical changes with pathologies or negative attitudes.

REFERENCES

1. Jackson, O: Neuro-orthopedics and geriatric rehabilitation: Balance, flexibility, coordination improving function for older persons, using a feldenkrais method. Northeast Seminars, East Hampstead, NH, 1997.
2. Hollander LL: Normal aging. In Logigian, MK (ed): Adult rehabilitation: A team approach for therapists. Little, Brown & Co, Boston, 1982.
3. Lewthwaite R: Motivational considerations in physical activity involvement. Phys Ther 70:808, 1990.
4. Kisner, C, and Colby, LA: Therapeutic Exercise: Foundations and Techniques, ed 3. FA Davis, 1996, p 656.

5. Salter, RB: Textbook of Disorders and Injuries of the Musculoskeletal System: Williams & Wilkins, Baltimore, 1983.

6. Aisenbrey, JA: Exercise in the prevention and management of osteoporosis. Phys Ther 67:1100, 1987.

7. Jackson, O: Brain function, aging, and dementia. In Umphred, DA (eds): Neurological Rehabilitation, ed 3. Mosby, St Louis, 1995, p 723.

8. Brody, H, and Vijauashankar, N: Anatomical changes in the nervous system. In Finch, CE, and Hayflick, L (eds): Handbook of the Biology of Aging. Van Nostrand Reinhold, New York, 1977.

9. Light, KE: Information processing for motor performance in aging adults. Phys Ther 70:820, 1990.

10. Birren, JE: Handbook of aging and the individual. University of Chicago Press, Chicago, 1973.

11. Licht, S: Therapeutic Heat and Cold. Elizabeth Licht, New Haven, CT, 1960.

12. Hopp, JF: Effects of age and resistance training on skeletal muscle: a review. Phys Ther 73:361, 1993.

13. Thompson, LV: Effects of age and training on skeletal muscle physiology and performance. Phys Ther 74:77, 1994.

14. Campbell, MJ, et al: Physiological changes in aging muscles. J Neurol Neurosurg Psychiatry 36:174, 1973.

15. Brown, WF, et al: Methods for estimating numbers of motor units in biceps brachialis muscles and losses of motor units with aging. Muscle Nerve 11:423, 1988.

16. Tomlinson, BE, and Irving, D: The numbers of limb motor neurons in the human lumbosacral cord throughout life. J Neurol Sci 34:213, 1977.

17. Fiatarone, MA, et al: High-intensity strength training in nonagenarians: Effects of skeletal muscle. JAMA 263:3029, 1990.

18. Brown, M: Resistance exercise effects on aging skeletal muscles in rats. Phys Ther 69:46, 1989.

19. National Center of Health Statistics. Vital Health Statistics: Prevalence of Selected Impairments. Health Resource Administration, Public Health Service, Rockville, MD, Series 10, No. 99, 1975.

20. Schmitz, TJ: Sensory assessment. In O'Sullivan, SB, et al (eds): Physical Rehabilitation: Assessment and Treatment, ed 3. FA Davis, 1994, p 91.

21. Woollacott, MJ, and Shumway-Cook, A: Changes in posture control across the life span: A systems approach. Phys Ther 70:799, 1990.

22. Quoniam, C, et al: Age effects on reflex and postural responses to propriomuscular inputs generated by tendon vibration. J Gerontol Biol Sci 50:B155, 1995.

23. Shumway-Cook, A, et al: Predicting the probability for falls in community-dwelling older adults. Phys Ther 77:812, 1997.

24. Sattin, RW, et al: The incidence of fall injury events among the elderly in a defined population. Am J Epidemiol 131:1028, 1990.

25. Paige, GD: Senescence of human visual-vestibular interactions, 1. Vestibulo-ocular reflex and adaptive plasticity with aging. J Vestib Res 2:133, 1992.

26. King, OS, et al: Control of head stability and gaze during locomotion in normal subjects and patients with deficient vestibular function. In Berthoz, A, et al (eds): The Head-Neck Sensory Motor System. Oxford Press, New York, 1992, p 568.

27. Di Fabio, RP & Emasithi, A: Aging and the mechanisms underlying head and postural control during voluntary motion. Phys Ther 77:458, 1997.

28. Van Sant, F: Life-span development in functional tasks. Phys Ther 70:788, 1990.

 # BIBLIOGRAPHY

Aisenbrey, JA: Exercise in the prevention and management of osteoporosis. Phys Ther 67:1100, 1987.

Birren, JE: Handbook of Aging and the Individual. University of Chicago Press, Chicago, 1973.

Brody, H, and Vijauashankar, N: Anatomical changes in the nervous system. In Finch, C, and Hayflick, L (eds): Handbook of the Biology of Aging. Van Nostrand Reinhold, New York, 1977.

Brown, M: Resistance exercise effects on aging skeletal muscles in rats. Phys Ther 69:46, 1989.

Brown, WF, et al: Methods for estimating numbers of motor units in biceps brachialis muscles and losses of motor units with aging. Muscle Nerve 11:423, 1988.

Campbell, MJ, et al: Physiological changes in aging muscles. J Neurol Neurosurg Psychiatry 36:174, 1973.

Di Fabio, RP, and Emasithi, A: Aging and the mechanisms underlying head and postural control during voluntary motion. Phys Ther 77:458, 1997.

Fiatarone, MA, et al: High-intensity strength training in nonagenarians: Effects of skeletal muscle. JAMA 263:3029, 1990.

Hollander, LL: Normal aging. In Logigian, MK (ed): Adult Rehabilitation: A Team Approach for Therapists. Little, Brown & Co, Boston, 1982.

Hopp, JF: Effects of age and resistance training on skeletal muscle: A review. Phys Ther 73:361, 1993.

Jackson, O: Brain function, aging, and dementia. In Umphred, DA (ed): Neurological Rehabilitation, ed 3. Mosby, St Louis, MO, 1995, p 723.

Jackson, O: Neuro-orthopedics and geriatric rehabilitation: Balance, flexibility, coordination improving function for older persons, using a feldenkrais method. Northeast Seminars, East Hampstead, NH, 1997.

King, OS, Seidman, SH, Leigh, RJ: Control of head stability and gaze during locomotion in normal subjects and patients with deficient vestibular function. In Berthoz, A, et al (eds): The Head-Neck Sensory Motor System. Oxford Press, New York, 1992, p 568.

Kisner, C, and Colby, LA: Therapeutic Exercise: Foundations and Techniques, ed 3. FA Davis, Philadelphia, 1996, p 656.

Lewthwaite, R: Motivational considerations in physical activity involvement. Phys Ther 70:808, 1990.

Licht, S: Therapeutic heat and cold. New Haven, CT, 1960.

Light, KE: Information processing for motor performance in aging adults. Phys Ther 70:820, 1990.

National Center of Health Statistics: Vital Health Statistics: Prevalence of Selected Impairments. Health Resource Administration, Public Health Service, Rockville, MD, Series 10, No. 99, 1975.

Paige, GD: Senescence of human visual-vestibular interactions. 1. Vestibulo-ocular reflex and adaptive plasticity with aging. J Vestib Res 2:133, 1992.

Quoniam, C, et al: Age effects on reflex and postural responses to propriomuscular inputs generated by tendon vibration. J Gerontol Biol Sci 50: B155, 1995.

Salter, RB: Textbook of Disorders and Injuries of the Musculoskeletal System. Williams & Wilkins, Baltimore, 1983.

Sattin, RW, et al: The incidence of fall injury events among the elderly in a defined population. Am J Epidemiol 131:1028, 1990.

Schmitz, TJ: Sensory assessment. In O'Sullivan, SB, and Schmitz, TJ (eds): Physical Rehabilitation: Assessment and Treatment, ed 3. FA Davis, Philadelphia, 1994, p 91.

Shumway-Cook, A, et al: Predicting the probability for falls in community-dwelling older adults. Phys Ther 77:812, 1997.

Thompson, LV: Effects of age and training on skeletal muscle physiology and performance. Phys Ther 74:77, 1994.

Tomlinson, BE, and Irving, D: The numbers of limb motor neurons in the human lumbosacral cord throughout life. J Neurol Sci 34:213, 1977.

Van Sant, F: Life-span development in functional tasks. Phys Ther 70:788, 1990.

Woollacott, MJ, and Shumway-Cook, A: Changes in posture control across the life span: A systems approach. Phys Ther 70:799, 1990.

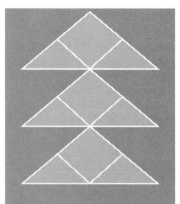

 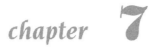

Concepts of Mobilization

OBJECTIVES

After completing this chapter, the PTA student will be able to:

1. Describe the role of peripheral joint mobilization in orthopedic treatment.
2. Discuss the role of the PTA in the delivery of joint mobilization techniques.
3. Compare osteokinematics with arthrokinematics during selected range of motion of the extremities.
4. Identify normal arthrokinematics including the roll, spin, and glide.
5. Relate the clinical importance of the convex-concave rule.
6. Identify normal arthrokinematics during selected movements of the extremity joints.
7. Discuss the clinical relevance of the closed-packed position of a joint.
8. Identify what is meant by the concept of end-feel.
9. Compare and contrast the clinical dosages of peripheral joint mobilization.
10. State the indications and contraindications of peripheral joint mobilization.
11. Demonstrate safe and effective joint mobilization techniques to selected peripheral joints.

Key Words

accessory motions (joint play)
arthrokinematics
capsular restriction pattern
closed-packed position
convex-concave rule
end-feel
joint congruency
manipulation
manual therapy
mechanical axis
mobilization
osteokinematics
ovoid joints
resting position (loose-packed)
roll
sellar (saddle) joints
slide (glide)
spin
swing

HISTORY OF MOBILIZATION

Manual therapy is the concept of musculoskeletal evaluation and treatment in physical therapy that applies the principles of kinesiology, histology, neurophysiology, and pathophysiology. Passive movement techniques, mobilization, and manipulations are used to promote the well-being of clients.[1,2,3] Several historical figures have shaped the modern-day concepts used in manual therapy, including Cyriax, Mennell, Kaltenborn, and Maitland. All of these icons have pioneered the use of the human hand to restore lost function to the human body. In 1951, Mennell[4] commented about the role of the human hand in the healing process:

> Beyond all doubt the use of the human hand, as a method of reducing human suffering, is the oldest remedy known to man; historically no date can be given for its adoption.

In addition to these pioneers, credit can be given to Dr. Andrew Taylor Still and the osteopathic school of thought that has melded the roles of manual manipulative treatment with modern medicine (Box 7–1). Skilled evaluations and techniques, such as soft-tissue mobilization, massage, manual traction, joint manipulation, joint mobilization, and therapeutic exercise, have been incorporated into the practice of modern-day manual therapy. Manual therapy techniques in orthopedic treatments have been effective in the hands of skilled clinicians,

Manual Therapy
The concept of musculoskeletal evaluation and treatment in physical therapy that applies principles of kinesiology, histology, neurophysiology, and pathophysiology to promote the well-being of clients. Passive movement techniques, mobilization, and manipulations are used to restore lost function, reduce pain, or lessen the effects of muscle spasms.

Box 7–1

OSTEOPATHIC HISTORICAL CONTRIBUTIONS TO THE ART OF JOINT MOBILIZATION[10]

Dr. Andrew Taylor Still was a practicing physician living in Kansas when all three of his children contracted meningitis and ultimately died. As a physician, he was greatly frustrated by the lack of knowledge and ability of current medicine to save the lives of his three children and was determined to find answers to his questions. He spent many hours studying the exhumed remains of native-Americans, paying close attention to the anatomy and relationships among bones, nerves, and arteries. After a "divine revelation," he claimed he had found the cause of all human disease. The "law of the artery" claimed that all pathologies were a direct result of interference with blood flow through arteries that carried vital nutrients to a body part. Still founded the first osteopathy school located in Kirksville, Missouri in 1892, and by 1920, the U.S. Congress had granted equal rights to osteopaths and medical doctors. Gradually, the osteopathic profession became aware of deficiencies in the law of the artery and began to implement changes towards traditional medicine with the practice of joint manipulation.

providing positive outcomes for clients with somatic (body) pain.[5] This chapter introduces a component of the entire practice of manual therapy: peripheral joint mobilization. The clinical application of mobilization will be as an adjunct to orthopedic interventions and to identify the role of the PTA in the delivery of mobilization techniques.

ROLE OF MOBILIZATION IN ORTHOPEDIC TREATMENT

Mobilization is a low-velocity passive movement performed by the clinician to an affected joint within or at the limits of joint range of motion (ROM) at a speed slow enough that the client can stop the movement. The techniques may be oscillatory or sustained; physiological or accessory movements of the joint are used with the goal being to increase tissue mobility or decrease pain. **Manipulation** is a sudden high-velocity technique at the end of ROM that cannot be stopped by the client. Manipulations are designed to release pathologically adhered or limited tissues to increase joint ROM. The techniques are rapid and forceful and may be performed when the client is awake or under anesthesia. Proper joint function, anatomy, and pathology must be considered when performing mobilization or manipulation techniques to treat conditions such as stiffness, hypomobility, or pain.[5,6]

Mobilization techniques can be used safely to stretch capsular structures in restoring normal joint mechanics and lessening pain. If applied skillfully and when indicated, mobilization techniques will enhance joint capsule mobility with less trauma to the joint capsule than occurs during passive stretching. Using mobilization as an adjunctive treatment in orthopedic management will enhance the clinician's ability to restore lost motion to the structural elements of the human skeletal system. Previous discussions of modalities designed to enhance contractile element flexibility included passive stretching, proprioceptive neuromuscular

Mobilization
A low-velocity passive movement performed by the clinician to an affected joint within or at the limits of joint ROM, applied at a speed slow enough to allow the client to stop the movement.

Manipulation
A sudden high-velocity technique applied at the end of ROM that cannot be stopped by the client. This technique is designed to release pathologically shortened or adhered structures.

facilitation, and active inhibition techniques. Di Fabio[5] performed an extensive review of the professional literature relating to manual therapy, mobilization, and manipulation. He summarized that there exists "clear evidence that manual therapy can be an effective modality when used to treat patients who have somatic pain syndromes." Furthermore, the literature revealed that "there may be a difference in [the] efficacy . . . between manipulation and mobilization therapy." Although there were studies showing positive results with mobilization used as a treatment technique, there was a significantly greater percentage of reliable research investigations that cited manipulation techniques as effective in treating pain and joint limitations. Di Fabio believed that additional research efforts are needed to establish mobilization as an effective primary treatment modality in the profession of physical therapy and orthopedic medicine.[5,6]

Role of the Physical Therapist Assistant

In identifying the role of the PTA in the delivery of mobilization skills, two issues will be investigated: legal and practical. The first issue of legality must concern the licensing practice act of the state in which the assistant practices. Some states still do not have legal rules and regulations covering the service delivery of PTAs in general, and certain states have laws that limit the performance of specific PTA-related skills or tasks. Each state is unique in its definition of skilled services. Some states have fought battles with other medical professions over the terms and use of mobilization and manipulation. The terms "manipulation," "manipulative therapy," and "mobilization" have often been used interchangeably in the literature. The Practice Affairs Committee of the Orthopaedics Section of the American Physical Therapy Association took the following position: "manipulation implies a variety of manual techniques which is not exclusive to any specific profession."[7] Commonalities of state practice acts include (1) that the PTA must be supervised by the physical therapist and (2) that the PTA cannot perform or interpret initial evaluations. Farrell and Jensen[7] critically assessed the role of manual therapy in the profession of physical therapy identifying six approaches (Cyriax, Mennell, Osteopathic, Maitland, Kaltenborn, and McKenzie) by philosophical basis, concepts, evaluation history, physical assessment, interpretation of data, and treatment strategies. The concept of joint mobilization was used consistently within the scope of treatment strategies along with common interventions of friction massage, exercise, client education, traction, and myofascial techniques. These latter terms have all been accepted treatment to be implemented by the PTA. Therefore, mobilization as a treatment modality should also be a legally accepted role of the PTA.

The possible confusion surrounding assistants performing mobilization as a treatment comes from the use of mobilization as an evaluative term and not a treatment modality. This text will not present mobilization as an evaluative tool, but as a physical technique identified in the plan of treatment by the supervising therapist to be performed by the assistant to enhance the outcomes of orthopedic intervention. It is imperative that the assistant identifies the appropriate legalities of PTA practice in his or her respective state and resolves potential conflicts surrounding the treatment aspect of mobilization before performing these techniques.

A second issue that must be addressed when the assistant performs mobilization techniques is the practical nature of acquiring the clinical skills to be an effective clinician. In a 1970 study by Stephens,[8] it was found that nearly 60% of the responding physical therapy programs in the Untied States were not instructing students on the principles of manual (manipulative) therapy. By 1988, the inclusion of joint mobilization into physical therapy curricula was demonstrated when Ben-Sorek and Davis[9] found that 38% of responding programs actually integrated a class in joint mobilization theory and 60% had mobilization offered as a subcomponent in another course. The curricular design and knowledge base of physical therapy programs regarding joint mobilization has changed significantly over the past two decades because this is an expected element in all physical therapy educational programs. However, this knowledge has not been universally adopted into the philosophies of all PTA programs. A trend in the 1990s has been for PTA programs to include mobilization education in their academic curricula to meet the market demands of PTA clinicians needing these orthopedic skills and the increasingly comprehensive requirements of national accrediting standards dictating competent entry-level clinicians.

For the assistant to be an integral part of the orthopedic team, the clinical skills of joint mobilization must be learned and practiced to effectively perform the plan of treatment. The PTA must demonstrate proper knowledge of anatomy, physiology, and arthrokinematics or the knowledge of joint motion to safely perform any physical therapy intervention procedure, including peripheral mobilization techniques. There are numerous continuing educational courses conducted each year in which clinicians can acquire or enhance mobilization skills. Professional development and lifelong learning is critical for all clinicians to aspire to, because if they are not sharpening their skills, it is likely that others are passing them by.

 ## JOINT MOTION: ARTHROKINEMATICS AND OSTEOKINEMATICS

Arthrokinematics

The description of the motion of the joint surfaces within a joint when a bone moves through a ROM.

Osteokinematics

The biomechanical description of the motion of the bone as it swings through a ROM.

Swing

The direction that the bone is moving around the mechanical axis.

Mechanical Axis

The line through the moving bone perpendicular to the stationary bone.

Arthrokinematics as described by Grimsby[2] is the description of the motion of the joint surfaces. **Osteokinematics** is the description of the motion of the bone. Collectively, both fields make up the study of human kinesiology, which is the study of human movement. As clinicians, the observed external movement of the human body is described in osteokinematic terms: *flexion, extension, abduction, adduction, internal rotation, external rotation, radial deviation,* or *ulnar deviation.* The assistant can document that the client's right shoulder actively moved through partial ROM from 0° of flexion to 90° of flexion. In this description of the client's motion, the clinician has described what the bones were doing: the humerus moved through a 90° arc swinging anteriorly in what is the motion of shoulder flexion. The osteokinematic term of importance is **swing,** or simply the direction that the bone is moving around the mechanical axis. Kessler and Hertling[10] defined the **mechanical axis** as the line through the moving bone perpendicular to the stationary bone (Fig. 7–1). It is important for the assistant to understand that while osteokinematic movements are being observed, specific and predictable arthrokinematic activities are occurring inside the joint. Arthrokinematic discussion will begin to describe the actions of the joint during the osteokinematic movement. It is expected that when reading the remainder of this chapter, the PTA student has a good understanding of osteokinematic and biomechanical principles related to the human body. A detailed discussion of osteokinematics can be acquired from reading a relevant kinesiology textbook (see Lippert, L: Clinical Kinesiology for the Physical Therapist Assistant, ed 2. FA Davis, Philadelphia, 1994). The shape of the joint and accessory motions will be some of the most important determining factors in analyzing the movement of the joint surfaces.

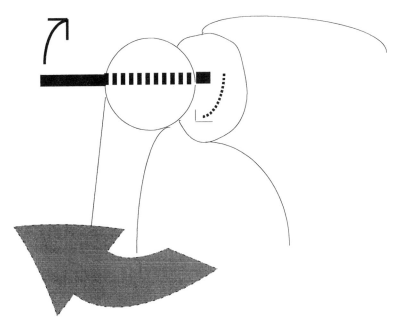

FIG. 7–1
Mechanical axis. As a bone swings about a joint, the mechanical axis remains perpendicular to the joint surface. This figure represents a shoulder moving through an abduction swing. At any point in time, the mechanical axis remains perpendicular to the joint surface.

JOINT CONGRUENCY

Shapes of Joints

Joint congruency is defined as how well opposing joint surfaces match. This is an important concept to appreciate when performing mobilization techniques. The amount of motion that occurs around a joint is largely dependent on the shape and congruency of the particular joint surfaces. Two primary surface shapes are presented in the discussion of mobilization: ovoid and sellar.[10] **Ovoid joints** consist of two surfaces: one is concave and one is convex (Fig. 7–2A). **Sellar (or saddle) joints** are recognized by the unique trait of possessing a convex and a concave surface on each opposing joint surface (Fig. 7–2B). Examine how a saddle sits on the back of a horse or how Pringles™ potato chips stack together. The horse's back (or bottom chip) is convex from left to right and concave from front to back while the bottom surface of the saddle (or the top chip's bottom surface) is concave from left to right and convex from front to back.

Loose-versus Closed-Packed Position

The joint is said to be in a **resting position (loose-packed)** when there exists the greatest amount of intracapsular space, the supporting soft tissue is as relaxed as possible, and the joint surfaces are noncongruous. The **closed-packed position** occurs when the joint intracapsular space is as small as possible, the supporting soft tissue is as tight as possible, and there exists maximal joint surface congruency (Table 7–1).[2,10] Movement of a joint toward the closed-packed position involves

Joint Congruency
The degree to which joint surfaces match.

Ovoid Joints
Joints consisting of two surfaces: one is concave and the opposite is convex.

Sellar (Saddle) Joints
Joints possessing a convex and a concave surface on each opposing joint surface.

Resting Position (Loose-Packed)
Joint position that occurs when there exists the greatest amount of intracapsular space, the supporting soft tissue is as relaxed as possible, and the joint surfaces are noncongruous.

Closed-Packed Position
Joint position that occurs when the joint intracapsular space is as small as possible, the supporting soft tissue is as tight as possible, and there exists maximal joint surface congruency. The potential for injury is greater if mobilizations are performed in a close-packed position.

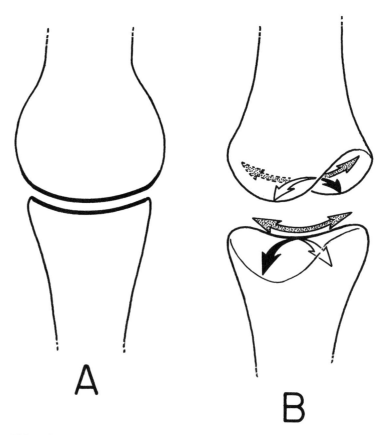

FIG. 7–2
Ovoid and sellar joints. In an ovoid joint (A), opposing surfaces of the joint are matching concave and convex surfaces. In a sellar (saddle) joint (B), opposing surfaces have both a concave and a convex surface on each articulating surface. One surface will be concave in one direction with a convex surface in the opposite direction. The opposing joint surface will be convex and concave to fit congruently. (From Kisner & Colby, p 185, with permission.)

compression forces (Fig. 7–3) or the approximation of the joint surface. Movement away from the closed-packed position involves tensile forces or distraction of the joint surfaces (Fig. 7–4). Once the closed-packed position of the joint is realized, very little, if any, active motion may occur further in that direction.[10] Another concept that may help to identify the loose-versus closed-packed position is in relation to stability versus mobility. In a closed-packed position, the joint has reached maximum stability. Conversely, in a loose-packed position, the joint has reached maximum mobility. This is one reason why the starting point for application of mobilization techniques is in the resting position of the joint; this promotes maximum mobility and avoids extreme compressive and potentially injurious forces on the joint surfaces.

ACCESSORY MOTIONS

Specific terms and definitions have been used in the study of arthrokinematics to describe the activity of the joint surfaces during movement. The concept of

Table 7–1

COMPARISON OF LOOSE- AND CLOSED-PACKED POSITIONS FOR
SELECTED JOINTS OF THE EXTREMITIES

Joint	Loose Packed*	Closed Packed
Glenohumeral	About 55° abduction and 30° degrees flexion	Combination of Horizontal extension and external rotation
Elbow	About 70° flexion	Full extension
Wrist	Neutral flexion and extension	Full extension with radial deviation
MCP of hand	Less than full extension	Full flexion
IP of hand	Less than full extension	Full extension
Hip	Slight flexion, abduction and external rotation	Internal rotation with extension and abduction
Knee	About 25° flexion	Extension with external rotation
Talocrural	Slight plantar flexion	Full dorsiflexion

Source: Adapted from Kessler and Hertling,[10] p. 533.

*Although there is variation among literature, loose packed is any point of least joint congruency.

accessory motion (joint play) has been defined by several authors (Mennell, Williams, and Warwick), but the working definition that will be used in this text is presented by Kessler and Hertling,[10] who stated that **accessory motions (joint play)** are joint surface movements which are not under voluntary motor control and are essential for normal joint function. These necessary motions are readily seen in the loose-packed position of a joint. In a loose-packed position, the joint surfaces are non congruent and there is laxity of the joint capsule and support structures. The motions will occur throughout the entire ROM, allowing for normal kinematics. If normal accessory motion is lost, a joint will prematurely compress into the closed-packed position, thus restricting movement.

Accessory Motions (Joint Play)
Joint surface movements that are not under voluntary motor control and are essential for normal joint function.

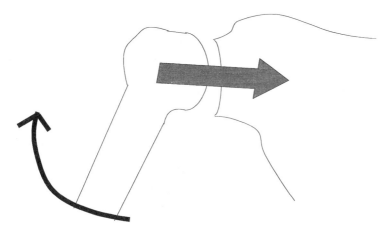

FIG. 7–3
Joint compression. Surface compression occurs as the joint moves toward a closed packed position.

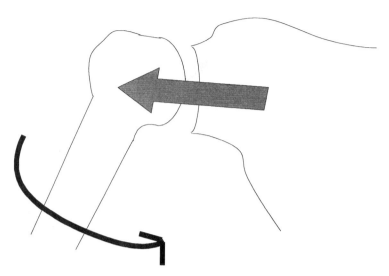

FIG. 7–4
Joint distraction. Surface distraction occurs as the joint moves away from a closed packed position.

Roll, Spin, and Glide

Arthrokinematic terms related to accessory motion for normal joint motion to occur include the following: role, spin, and slide (glide). When performing joint mobilization techniques, it is critical that the clinician understand how the joint surfaces are moving in relationship to each other to properly apply the mobilizing forces and to avoid damaging the articular surfaces. The convex-concave rule will guide the clinician in properly performing mobilization techniques safely. The following paragraphs present the important concepts that the PTA must understand to provide safe and effective joint mobilization.

    The arthrokinematic terms of roll, slide, and spin are simple mechanical principles. The mechanical definitions of these terms is presented, and then a practical discussion and clinical application follow. **Roll** occurs when points at constant intervals on the moving surface contact points at the same intervals on the opposing surface (Fig. 7–5). **Slide (glide)** occurs when a single point of one surface contacts multiple new points on the opposing surface (Fig. 7–6). **Spin** is a variation of a slide when a rotation about a single axis is noted by half of the moving surface sliding in one direction with the opposite half of the same surface sliding in the opposite direction (Fig. 7–7). This spinning motion usually occurs in combination with other joint accessory motions.[6,10]

    The technical definitions of arthrokinematic accessory motions periodically leave some students in a quandary. It is sometimes difficult for the PTA student to relate mechanical engineering principles to applications in the physical therapy environment. A description of these terms and concepts in a practical fashion follows that, hopefully, will be more easily understood. Imagine riding a bicycle over pavement. Picture what the front wheel is doing as it is moving over the paved surface. The wheel is rolling over the paved surface as each point on the moving surface (wheel) encounters a new point at the same distance on the stationary (paved) surface. This is an example of a roll.

    Now picture the locking up of the rear wheel on the bicycle as the cyclist has to suddenly stop. As children, most have enjoyed leaving "rubber" on the pavement

Roll

The accessory motion that occurs in which points at constant intervals on the moving surface contact points at the same intervals on the opposing surface.

Slide (Glide)

The accessory motion that occurs when a single point of one surface contacts multiple new points on the opposing surface.

Spin

The accessory motion that occurs when a rotation about a single axis is noted by half of the moving surface sliding in one direction with the opposite half of the same surface slides in the opposite direction.

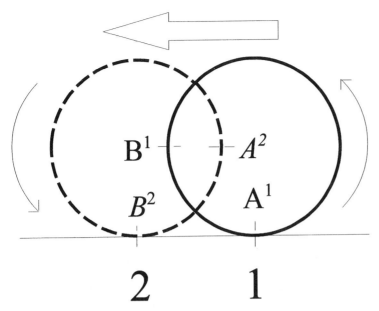

FIG. 7–5
Accessory motion: Roll. As one surface rolls over a stationary surface, points at constant intervals on the moving surface contact points at the same intervals on the opposing surface. The point (A) on the ball contacts point (1) on the stationary surface. As the ball rolls, point (B) contacts point (2) on the stationary surface.

in these gallant efforts. The rear wheel is now sliding across the pavement. The same point on the locked wheel (moving surface) is contacting many new points on the pavement (stationary surface). This is an example of a slide or a glide.

Examining two carousel horses directly opposite each other on a merry-go-round will demonstrate the principle of spin. As the spin occurs around the center of the ride (mechanical axis), the opposing horses are always facing opposite directions. When one horse is facing directly north, the counterpart will be facing directly south. If the horses were able to break free of their restrictions, they would

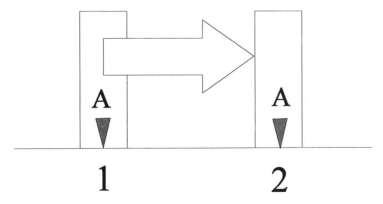

FIG. 7–6
Accessory motion: Slide or glide. As one surface slides over another, a single point (A) on the moving surface contacts multiple new points (1, then 2) on the opposing surface.

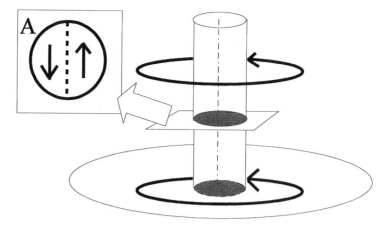

FIG. 7–7
Accessory motion: Spin. Spinning occurs about a single axis and is noted by half of the moving surface sliding in one direction with the opposite half of the same surface sliding in the opposite direction (A). The action is compared to that of a spinning top.

continue to travel in the opposing directions. Figure 7–8A presents three examples of joint spin in the human body. Preserve those mental images as you try to apply the movement concepts to the articular surface, and remember that the movements are significantly more subtle with smaller arcs of movement in the human body, yet still important to the overall functioning of the joint.

In a normal joint, pure rolling or sliding does not occur. The actual motion is a combination of both the roll and the slide depending on the congruency of the articular surfaces. The more congruent the joint surfaces tend to be, the greater the tendency of the sliding component to be greater than the rolling component. Conversely, the more incongruent the joint surfaces tend to be, the greater the tendency for the rolling component to be greater than the sliding component. If excess rolling occurs, the joint will dislocate (Fig. 7–8B). If excess sliding occurs, impingement of the joint will be seen clinically (Fig. 7–8C). Articular surface compression occurs on the side to which a bone rolls; articular distraction occurs on the opposite side of the same stationary surface. When applying mobilization techniques clinically, the sliding technique in a loose-packed position will produce less potentially injurious compressive joint forces compared with long-lever arm-stretching techniques aimed at the joint capsule. Although effective, the long-lever arm-stretching technique is not be addressed in this text because great skill and technique are required for application.

Concave-Convex Rule

Concave-Convex Rule
The rule that is used to identify the direction of the moving surfaces in a joint.

The **concave-convex rule** identifies the direction of the moving surfaces in a joint during normal physiological motion. The implications of this rule help to make the clinical connection between observed osteokinematic motions and arthrokinematic motions. The PTA must, first, identify the component surfaces (concave or convex) of the moving joint and, second, identify which surface is the moving surface and which is the stationary surface. After these components have been identified, the assistant can properly identify the directions of the accessory motions within the moving joint. The convex-concave rule has two premises:

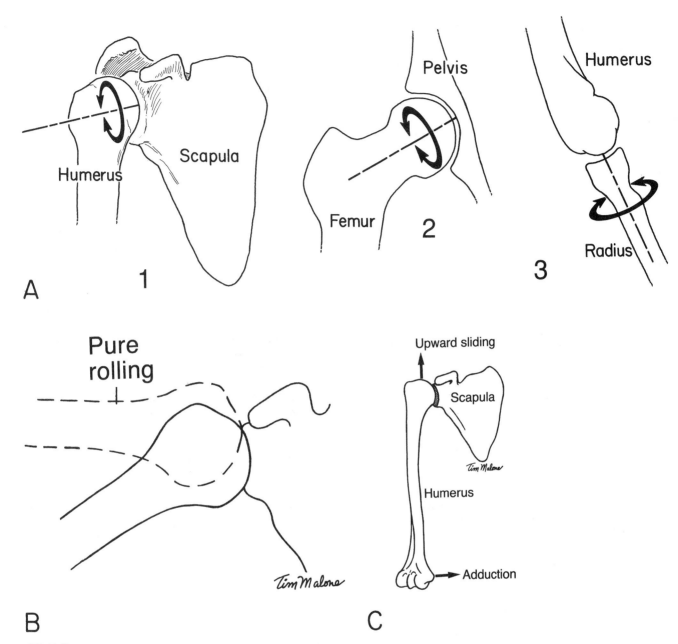

FIG. 7–8

(A) Spin in the body. During flexion and extension, the humerus rotates in the glenoid fossae (A). During flexion and extension, the femur rotates in the acetabulum (B). During supination and pronation of the forearm, the radius spins on the humerus (C). (From Kisner & Colby, p 189, with permission.) **(B) Joint dislocation.** Clinically, if excessive rolling is seen arthrokinematically, then joint dislocation will result. If the head of the humerus rolls excessively in any direction, the joint will dislocate from under the acromial arch. Dislocation typically occurs from a traumatic event, but can also be a result of faulty arthrokinematics. Often, after a traumatic dislocation, the structural integrity and faulty arthrokinematics will make the client prone to successive dislocations. (From Norkin & Levangie, p 72, with permission.) **(C) Joint impingement.** Clinically, if excessive sliding is seen arthrokinematically, then joint impingement will result. If the head of the humerus slides excessively in an upward direction, impingement under the acromial arch will occur. Most impinement syndromes seen clinically are the result of faulty arthrokinematics. (From Norkin & Levangie, p 71, with permission.)

FIG. 7–9
Convex-concave rule. The rule states that when a convex surface moves on a stationary concave surface (A), the roll occurs in the same direction of the swing of the bone and that the slide at the joint surface occurs in opposite direction. When a concave surface moves on a stationary convex surface (B), the roll and slide occur in the same direction as the swing of the bone. (From Kisner & Colby, p 187, with permission.)

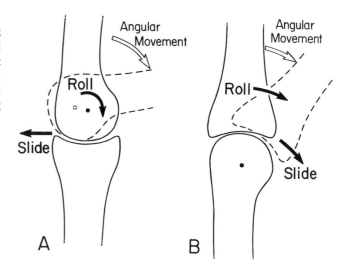

1. When a concave surface moves on a stationary convex surface, the roll and slide occur in the same direction as the swing of the bone.
2. When a convex surface moves on a stationary concave surface, the roll accompanies the direction of the swing of the moving bone and the slide occurs in opposite directions (Figs. 7–9 and 7–10).

These predictable arthrokinematic events can be applied by the assistant to observed osteokinematic movements (Box 7–2).

The therapeutic intervention of mobilization attempts to reproduce the normal glide that occurs arthrokinematically in the joint during movement. Before any mobilization technique is performed for the treatment of a limitation or impairment, the assistant must understand the relationships of the moving structures within the joint both osteokinematically and arthrokinematically. Appropriate directions of mobilization are indicated to restore lost function or motion. If the

FIG. 7–10
Rolling and swing of the bone. Part of the convex-concave rule includes the principle that the roll component during joint accessory motion always occurs in the same direction as the swing of the bone. This principle remains true for either a moving convex (A) or concave (B) surface. (From Kisner & Colby, p 186, with permission.)

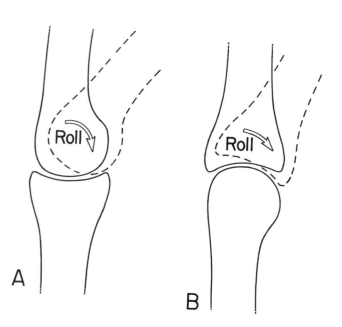

Box 7–2

CLINICAL CORRELATION BETWEEN OSTEOKINEMATIC MOVEMENTS AND ARTHROKINEMATIC MOVEMENTS

A PTA intern is working with a client on her clinical rotation with a diagnosis of right shoulder impingement syndrome. The client, a 46-year-old male factory worker, complains of a general aching pain in his right shoulder most of the day. The pain will improve if he doesn't use his arm or lift it over his head at work. If he lifts his right arm over his head, he will experience a quick, stabbing pain. Soon after that pain has resolved, the aching will intensify. The client has been receiving treatment of moist heat and ultrasound to the right shoulder three times a week. With treatment, the client notes that he feels better, but he still has the sharp pain if he lifts his arm over his head.

This observant intern then discusses the situation with her supervising PT. The intern believes that the impingement and irritation to the soft tissue under the acromial arch may be a result of a faulty sliding (arthrokinematic) mechanism between the humerus and the glenoid fossae. From an osteokinematic view, the intern observes the abduction of the humerus or the swinging of the bone in a frontal plane superiorly. Arthrokinematically, the intern understands that if the bone is swinging superiorly, then the roll must be occurring in the same direction. The intern also remembers her anatomy and describes the structure of the glenohumeral joint: The humerus is convex, and the glenoid fossae with the addition of the glenoid labrum is concave. If the moving bone (osteokinematics) is the humerus, then the convex surface is the moving surface (it is assumed for this illustration that the scapula is the stationary surface; however, indeed there is actual movement occurring at both surfaces [scapular elevation and upward rotation] to complete full abduction). Therefore, according to the convex-concave rule, if the convex surface is moving on a stationary concave surface, the roll and the slide must occur in opposite directions. Because the swing of the bone is superior and the roll is also accordingly superior in direction, then the intern understands that inferior gliding must occur arthrokinematically.

The PTA intern concludes that the use of modalities is helping relieve the acute irritation to the subacromial structures; however, if the faulty mechanics are not addressed, the situation will continue to inhibit full function and motion for this client.

assistant applies a mobilizing force in an inappropriate or incorrect direction, the level of impairment or dysfunction may increase.

DEGREES OF MOBILITY

Hypermobility, Hypomobility, and Grading Scale

Kaltenborn and Evjenth[11] have identified a grading scale for describing the amounts of accessory motion in a joint. Some authors have questioned the scientific validity and reliability of properly assessing joint play, placing more

Table 7–2

RELATIVE SCALE FOR JOINT PLAY WITH RECOMMENDED THERAPEUTIC INTERVENTIONS		
Joint Play	**Description**	**Intervention**
Hypomobile	0 Ankylosed	Surgery; no PT
	1 Considerable decreased motion	Mobilization; avoid exercise due to poor mechanical axis that may produce other dysfunction
	2 Slight decreased motion	Mobilization; self-mobilization
Normal	3 Normal	No intervention needed
Hypermobile	4 Slight increased motion	Postural correction; taping; stabilization exercise
	5 Considerable increased motion	Postural correction; corsets, collars; Stabilization exercise
	6 Pathologically unstable	Surgery; no PT needed

Source: Adapted from Kaltenborn and Evjenth,[11] p 182; and Grimsby, p 11.

emphasis on clinical experience versus reproducible measurements.[3] The physical therapy profession has classically attributed the term *hypermobile* to define excessive movement and the term *hypomobile* to define limited movement. This grading reference has limitations as clinical experience and subjective opinion may play a role in the "objective" measurement of accessory motion. Grimsby[12] has further imposed upon the joint play assessment scale appropriate therapeutic interventions for identified levels of hypermobility or hypomobility. The scale ranges from 0 as an ankylosed (immobile) joint, 1 and 2 as degrees of hypomobility, 3 as normal, 4 and 5 as degrees of hypermobility, and 6 as a pathologically unstable joint (Table 7–2).

Physical therapists during the evaluation of a client should use a consistent scale to determine the degree of mobility of a joint. In the current arena of health-care efficacy, reproducibility, and justification of intervention, it is important that a grading scale for observed degrees of joint mobility be included in client documentation. Despite the inherent arguments outlined in the previous paragraph, physical therapy professionals are mandated to provide justification for intervention in terms of reimbursement and ethical behavior. By using a consistent, valid grading scale (see Table 7–2), the physical therapy professional can improve interrater reliability, improve outcome collection data, and eventually improve reimbursement and efficacy issues.

END-FEELS

Normal and Pathological

End-feel as originally described by Cyriax[13] (Box 7–3) is the concept of the type of resistance in a joint perceived by the examiner during a physiological passive range-of-motion test. Many authors have identified, modified, or created descrip-

End-Feel
The resistance in a joint perceived by the examiner during a physiological passive range-of-motion test.

__ Box 7–3 __

CLASSIC END-FEELS[10,13]

- **Bony:** Abrupt, as when moving the normal elbow into full extension.
- **Capsular:** Firm, leathery feeling such as when forcing the normal shoulder into full extension or external rotation.
- **Soft-tissue approximation:** Soft feeling, as when fully flexing the normal elbow or knee.
- **Muscular:** Rubbery feeling felt at the end of a passive straight-leg raise.
- **Empty:** Examiner feels no restriction to motion; movement is stopped by the insistence of the client due to pain.
- **Muscle spasm:** Fairly abrupt stoppage of motion with a possible rebounding effect; pain may accompany point of restriction.
- **Boggy:** Soft, mushy feeling that typically accompanies joint effusion.
- **Internal derangement:** Pronounced, springy, rebounding feeling at end of motion; noncapsular pattern is noted and typically results from a loose body in joint or meniscal derangement.

tive lists of end-feels, both normal and pathological, based on the type of tissue identified as the resistance to the passive motion. Presented in this text for the PTA is a classification system of end-feels originally presented by Kaltenborn, but modified for ease of clarification by Riddle.[3] The advantage of using the Riddle system is that the terms are operational in nature and do not imply that a specific tissue is producing the end-feel. This can be of benefit to the PTA student by simply explaining the limitation that is perceived to the supervising physical therapist and not trying to identify the nature of the exact restriction.

The resistance felt by the clinician falls into one of three categories: (1) soft, (2) firm, or (3) hard. Soft end-feel is a gradual increase in the resistance at the end of ROM. Firm end-feel is an abrupt increase in resistance at the end of ROM. Hard end-feel is an immediate stoppage to movement at the end of ROM. These classifications can be applied to either normal ROM limitations (such as the firm end-feel felt at end of motion during a passive straight-leg raise) or pathological limitations (such as the firm end-feel felt during the midrange of motion in a client who has suffered a cerebrovascular accident and exhibits elbow flexion hypertonicity). Table 7–3 presents normal and pathological operational end-feels. When applying peripheral mobilization techniques, the assistant must have a working knowledge of normal and pathological end-feels to avoid injuring the client.

DOSAGES OF MOBILIZATION TREATMENTS

Clinically, the PTA will use one of the two following techniques to mobilize a peripheral joint: (1) a sustained traction (or distraction) motion that occurs perpendicular to the articulating joint surface, and (2) a slide or glide that occurs parallel to the articulating joint surface (Fig. 7–11). The mobilization techniques are applied to the articular surfaces to:

1. Stretch supporting tissues for the restoration of normal accessory motion
2. Reduce pain
3. Reduce muscle guarding per the plan of treatment

Table 7-3

OPERATIONAL END-FEELS	
Soft End-Feel	Gradual increase in the resistance at the end of ROM.
	Normal: Flexing the elbow or knee through the fullest ROM.
	Pathological: Resistance felt in midrange of a severely swollen knee, limiting full ROM.
Firm End-Feel	Abrupt increase in resistance at the end range of motion.
	Normal: End-range straight-leg raise or shoulder external rotation.
	Pathological: Resistance felt in shoulder abduction of a client with adhesive capsulitis.
Hard End-Feel	Immediate stoppage to movement at the end range of motion.
	Normal: Fullest extension of the elbow.
	Pathological: Unstable displaced fracture of the elbow limiting motion in mid-ROM.
No End-Feel	Cases may occur in which nothing is felt by the examiner, but the client relates pain and discomfort. Cyriax terms this as an "empty end-feel."

The techniques can either be static or dynamic in nature. Static mobilization is described by Kaltenborn and Evjenth[11] as a sustained glide or distraction technique held for a brief period (10 to 60 seconds). Dynamic mobilization consists of an oscillatory motion occurring in a sliding manner. An oscillation is a repeated, alternating, controlled motion applied by the clinician (Fig. 7–12). Maitland[14] identified a grading (dosage) scale of mobilization oscillations (2 to 3 per second) consisting of five grades (Fig. 7–13A). The scale depends on the relative magnitude of the oscillation and where in the accessory motion availability the oscillation is applied. Kaltenborn[11] also presented a dosage scale relative to sustained translatory joint-play techniques (Fig. 7–13B). This scale depends on the magnitude of stress placed on the joint capsule.

FIG. 7–11
Mobilizing forces applied by the clinician.
The clinician will either apply a mobilizing force through traction separating the joint surfaces (A) or by sliding one surface over another (B).

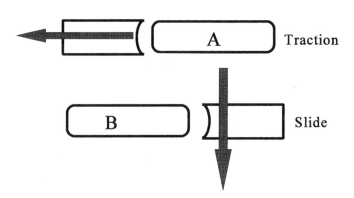

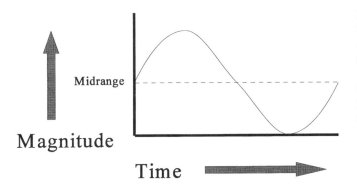

FIG. 7–12
One oscillation. An oscillation is a rhythmic, controlled, alternating motion applied by the clinician. The clinician stabilizes the proximal aspect of the joint then oscillates (mobilizes) the distal aspect of the joint in a fashion parallel to the joint surface. This figure represents the magnitude of a potential oscillation in relation to midrange of accessory motion over time.

Maitland's or Oscillation Grades

- Grade I is a low-amplitude, rhythmic oscillation performed at the beginning of available motion primarily for the introduction of mobilization to the client, for the reduction of pain or muscle guarding.
- Grade II is a high-amplitude, rhythmic oscillation performed within the available motion, but not extending to the limitation. This graded technique is used primarily for pain control and the reduction of muscle guarding.
- Grade III is a high-amplitude, rhythmic oscillation performed within the available motion reaching the motion limitation. This grade is primarily used to increase tissue mobility and reduce joint limitations. Clinically, this grade is typically well tolerated after muscle guarding and pain has been resolved or lessened.
- Grade IV is a low-amplitude, rhythmic oscillation performed at the end of the available motion reaching the motion limitation. This grade is primarily used to increase tissue mobility and reduce joint limitations. Clinically, this end-range oscillation can be very effective, but can also increase soreness if performed excessively and may cause undue discomfort to the client.
- Grade V is a thrust or high-velocity technique beyond the tissue limitation designed to break tissue adhesions. This is considered a manipulation force and will not be discussed further in this textbook. Manipulation force is beyond the

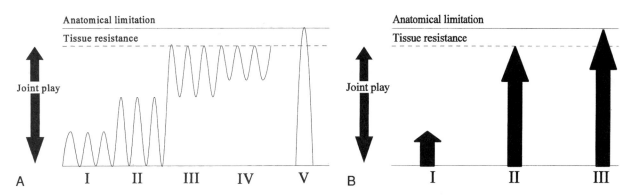

FIG. 7–13
(A) Mobilization grades by Maitland[14]. The classic grades or dosages by Maitland are presented in graphic form. The clinician moves the distal aspect of the joint in a rhythmical gliding oscillation through the selected availability of joint accessory motion. Each grade is designed to produce differing therapeutic results. **(B) Mobilization grades by Kaltenborn[11].** Where the Maitland dosages are dynamically moving through the various ranges of joint play, the Kaltenborn dosages differ in nature by being static or sustained. The distraction or gliding force is applied in a sustained manner to the limits of the designated joint play. Specific therapeutic goals are achieved with each different application.

scope of practice for the PTA, and it is also often beyond the legal scope of practice for many physical therapists as well. There continues to exist significant professional controversy over the use of manipulations.

Kaltenborn's or Sustained Grades

- Grade I is referred to as loosening. No stress is placed on the joint capsule by the sustained distracting or gliding force. This grade is used for pain relief.
- Grade II is referred to as tightening. The slack of the joint capsule is eliminated as enough stress is applied to the joint capsule by the sustained distraction or glide to tighten the tissues around the joint. This grade is used as an assessment technique to determine sensitivity of joint tissue. This grade can be used intermittently to reduce pain or preserve integrity of joint play when ROM is contraindicated.
- Grade III is referred to as stretching. Stress applied to the joint capsule is of sufficient magnitude to stretch the capsule and surrounding periarticular tissue.

This grade is used as a therapeutic means to increase joint accessory motion.

Clinical Implications of Oscillatory and Sustained Grades

Therapeutic goals are similar for the different dosage guidelines designed by Maitland and Kaltenborn. Both approaches address techniques designed to reduce pain, assess joint play, increase joint accessory motion, and decrease tissue limitations. Maitland I and II are comparable in nature to the goals of Kaltenborn I. Both approaches are designed to stay within the limits of joint play without stretching the joint capsule at the end of tissue or capsule limitations. Maitland III and IV and Kaltenborn II are designed to reach tissue limitation. Maitland V and Kaltenborn III both exceed tissue limitation remaining under anatomic limitations to stretch joint structures and increase joint play. The amount of external force applied to the joint by the clinician to produce desired therapeutic results should be respectively similar for each comparable grading level (comparing similar Maitland to Kaltenborn grades).[6,11,14]

The significant difference in the dosage application of peripheral mobilization is the dynamic or static nature of each technique. The clinical application will vary depending on the response of the client. In any application for pain, the client may prefer one technique over another. Client comfort and confidence in a technique must be addressed to produce adequate relaxation for pain reduction. Maitland I or II and Kaltenborn I are effective at reducing pain. Kaltenborn I may also be varied to do intermittent sustained techniques to produce similar results. The response of the client will dictate the intensity and frequency of the treatment application.[6,11,14]

When trying to increase joint play because of tissue adherence or limitation, plastic deformation of the connective tissue is desired to allow increased mobility and functional ROM. As discussed in previous chapters, the best method to promote plastic changes in connective tissue is to apply low-load, long-duration stretches. The Kaltenborn III technique may be the best suited application to achieve this goal. However, sustained grade III application, at times, may produce discomfort in the client and increase reflexive muscle guarding. Therefore, intermittent application of the sustained III technique may work equally as well.[6,11,14]

If the goal is to prevent loss of ROM in a joint, application of Maitland II or

Kaltenborn II may produce the best results. These techniques will promote the mechanical lubrication of the joint by passively moving the joint surfaces, but will not significantly stretch the joint capsule. Joint nourishment and movement within the available ROM is critical for preventing loss of ROM and contracture formation.[6,11,14]

INDICATIONS AND CONTRAINDICATIONS OF PERIPHERAL JOINT MOBILIZATION

Indications for the use of peripheral mobilization techniques include musculoskeletal conditions that cause restrictions of accessory motions, which result in pain or functional limitation of joint motion. The PTA must perform only those techniques that have been identified by the supervising physical therapist per the plan of treatment. Once the proper techniques have been identified, the assistant must skillfully apply the proper dosage with knowledge of the anatomy of the involved joint, the convex-concave rule, the pathophysiology of the client's condition, and the goals of the treatment program.

Contraindications for peripheral joint mobilization as described by Kessler and Hertling[10] fall into two categories: (1) absolute and (2) relative. Absolute contraindications include bacterial infection, neoplasm, joint hypermobility, and recent fracture. Relative contraindications include joint effusion or inflammation, degenerative joint disease, rheumatoid arthritis, osteoporosis, derangement of joint, and pregnancy (Table 7–4). If the PTA ever has any questions or doubts regarding the applicability of a therapeutic mobilization treatment, the supervising physical therapist should be consulted before the treatment is initiated.

CLINICAL APPLICATION OF PERIPHERAL JOINT MOBILIZATION

The remainder of this chapter presents visual and instructional applications of common mobilization techniques for the peripheral joints. Mobilization application for the spine and temporomandibular joint are not, however, described in this

Table 7–4

INDICATIONS AND CONTRAINDICATIONS OF PERIPHERAL JOINT MOBILIZATION	
Absolute	Bacterial infections
	Neoplasm
	Joint hypermobility
	Recent fracture
Relative	Joint effusion
	Degenerative joint disease (either acute or if causing a bony block)
	Rheumatoid arthritis
	Osteoporosis
	Derangement of the joint
	Pregnancy

textbook. Each joint is grouped to identify the following aspects of proper peripheral mobilization techniques:

1. Joint surface and motion considerations
2. Identifying resting position, closed-packed position, and capsular restriction pattern
3. Suggested mobilization directions to improve restricted movement
4. Proper client positioning
5. Positioning of the clinician with proper hand placement

Capsular Restriction Pattern
A characteristic combination of restricted movements unique to each joint possibly identifying capsular involvement in producing joint limitations.

A new term introduced in this section is **capsular restriction pattern**. A capsular pattern is a characteristic combination of restricted movements unique to each joint. The limitations can be observed clinically through ROM assessment, which can identify the possible capsular involvement producing the functional limitation.

Peripheral joint mobilization skills should be practiced extensively before therapeutic intervention is attempted on actual clients. When done properly, mobilization techniques may be beneficial to the overall outcome of your client. If done improperly, tissue damage, pain, and disruption of the healing process is possible.

GENERAL CONCEPTS

Initiating treatment should begin only after appropriate guidelines and parameters have been established by the supervising physical therapist. The client should be placed in the appropriate position to allow access to the extremity that is to be mobilized. The client should be encouraged to relax and not "help" with the procedure, and also to give appropriate verbal feedback related to pain levels and comfort. Stabilization of the joint should occur at the proximal aspect of the joint. This can be accomplished in several manners:

1. Manually by the clinician
2. Manually by a PT technician
3. Structurally from a belt or table

The goal of stabilization is to avoid directing undue stresses to surrounding joints. The mobilizing force should be applied as close as possible to the proximal joint component. For comfort of the client, use as large a mobilizing surface as possible (broad surface of the hand). Mobilizing forces (traction or glide) should be directed appropriately to the targeted surface or treatment plane (Fig. 7–14). The glide force should be applied in the same direction that would normally occur as determined by the convex-concave rule. The entire bone should glide across the opposing surface, not be used as lever. Lever arm stretching will produce joint roll with surface compression in the direction of the roll. Excessive joint compression may result in articular damage.[6]

Clinically, mobilization techniques should not produce acute pain. If pain occurs during treatment, stop the procedure and contact the supervising therapist. Treatment soreness may result after mobilization, but it should not last longer than 24 hours. If persistent soreness occurs, consult with the supervising therapist. As part of the rehabilitation program, warming the target tissue before mobilizing through gentle exercise, modalities, or therapeutic massage may help relax the client. After a mobilizing session, exercises designed to promote use of the new ROM should be encouraged.

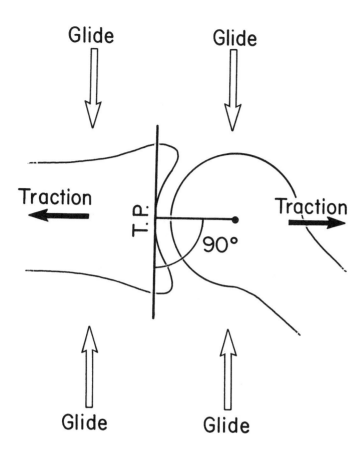

FIG. 7–14
Treatment plane.
The mobilizing forces should be targeted at the treatment plane on the concave surface, which lies at a right angle from the mechanical axis of rotation on the convex surface. Joint traction is applied perpendicular, and joint glides are applied parallel, to the treatment plane. (From Kisner & Colby, p 17, with permission.)

Shoulder Girdle

Glenohumeral Joint

Joint surface and motion considerations: Convex humeral head, concave glenoid fossa. The roll moves in the same direction as the humerus, and the glide occurs in opposite directions. For full glenohumeral motions to occur, the scapula, acromioclavicular (AC), and sternoclavicular (SC) joints must also be addressed. (**Note:** Care should be taken when mobilizing the glenohumeral joint because this joint can be easily dislocated anteriorly in some clients.)

Resting position: Combination of 55° abduction, 30° horizontal flexion.

Closed-packed position: Combination of horizontal extension and external rotation.

Capsular pattern: External rotation is most limited followed by abduction.

Mobilizing forces: Traction (Fig. 7-15) is used for pain control or increasing general mobility.

  1. Force is applied laterally away from glenoid fossa or through long axis of the humerus.
  2. **Client position:** Supine, shoulder in resting position. Stabilize scapula with belt, table, or body weight.
  3. **Hand placement:** Place in client's axilla, thumb anteriorly, fingers posteriorly. Free hand supports the humerus.

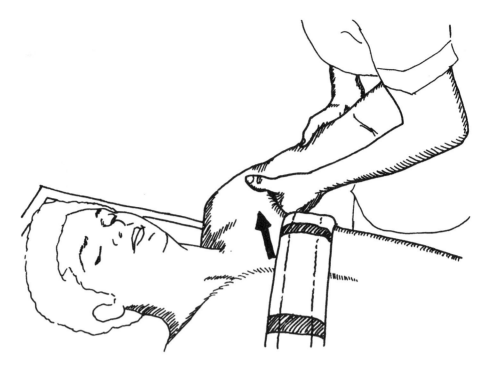

FIG. 7–15
Glenohumeral joint traction. Used for pain control or increasing general mobility. (From Kisner & Colby, p 200, with permission.)

Mobilizing forces: Caudal glide (Fig. 7–16) is used to increase abduction.
   1. Force is applied from superiorly placed hand by moving the head of the humerus inferiorly.
   2. **Client position:** Same as when applying traction
   3. **Hand placement:** Place web space of hand just distal to acromial arch. Free hand supports the medial humerus.
Mobilizing forces: Posterior glide (Fig. 7–17) is used to increase flexion and internal rotation.
   1. Force is applied from anterior surface by moving the humeral head posteriorly.
   2. **Client position:** Same as when applying traction.
   3. **Hand placement:** Place ulnar border of hand just distal to joint line anteriorly, fingers pointing superiorly. Free hand supports the humerus laterally.
Mobilizing forces: Anterior glide (Figs. 7–18A and 7–18B) is used to increase extension and external rotation.
   1. Force is applied from posterior surface by moving the humeral head anteriorly.
   2. **Client position:** (A) Same as when applying traction. (B) Alternate position is prone.
   3. **Hand placement:** (A) Place in client's axilla with thumb anteriorly and fingers posteriorly; free hand also positioned with thumb anteriorly and fingers posteriorly just distal to acromial arch. (B) Place ulnar border of hand just distal to posterior joint line. Free hand supports the humerus at the elbow.

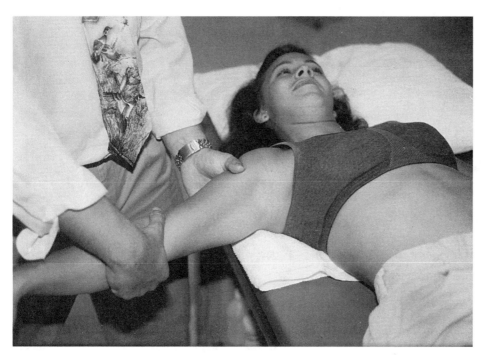

FIG. 7–16
Glenohumeral joint caudal glide. Used to increase abduction.

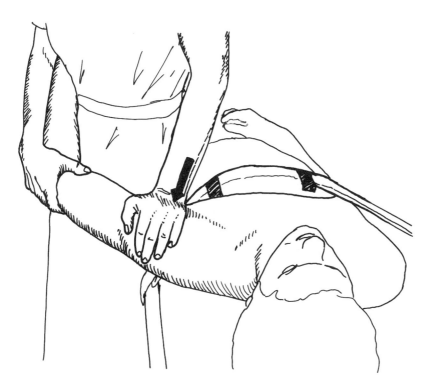

FIG. 7–17
Glenohumeral joint posterior glide. Used to increase flexion and internal rotation. (From Kisner & Colby, p 203, with permission.)

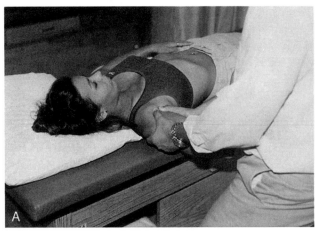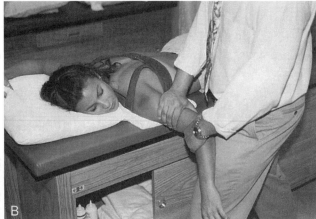

FIG. 7–18A & B. Glenohumeral joint anterior glide. Used to increase extension and external rotation.

Acromioclavicular Joint

Joint surface and motion considerations: The AC joint allows for upward and downward rotation of scapula; full glenohumeral motions are limited if the AC joint is involved.

Resting position: Arm at side.

Closed-packed position: Upward rotation of the scapula and horizontal flexion of the humerus.

Capsular pattern: Pain demonstrated in horizontal flexion.

Mobilizing forces: Anterior glide (Fig. 7–19) is used to increase overall mobility of joint.

1. Force is applied anteriorly by thumb of clinician.
2. **Client position:** Seated.
3. **Hand placement:** Place thumb posterior to distal clavicle. Free hand stablizes the scapula.

Alternate method: If difficulty is experienced in moving the distal clavicle anteriorly with the mobilizing thumb, try this alternate method:

1. Force is applied posteriorly by fingers at anterior aspect of acromial arch.
2. **Client position:** Same as above.
3. **Hand placement:** Same as pictured in Figure 7–19 except right hand is stabilizing force and left hand is mobilizing force. Fingers and thumb of right hand stabilize the clavicle anteriorly and superiorly (do not touch any part of the scapula with stabilizing hand). Digits of left hand grasp acromial arch anteriorly and posteriorly and slide arch posteriorly. The net effect of posterior movement of the acromion is an anterior glide of the clavicle at the AC joint.

STERNOCLAVICULAR JOINT

Joint surface and motion considerations: The SC joint allows for elevation and depression of the clavicle, forward and posterior swing of the clavicle, and long-axis rotation of the clavicle; full glenohumeral motions are limited if the SC joint is limited.

Resting position: Arm at side.

Closed-packed position: Maximum rotation and elevation of the clavicle; full abduction of the humerus.

Capsular pattern: Pain occurs at extreme of motions.

Mobilizing forces: Posterior glide (Fig. 7–20) is used to increase scapular retraction.
1. Force is applied posteriorly by thumb to proximal clavicle.
2. **Client position:** Supine.
3. **Hand placement:** Place thumb over proximal clavicle with index finger supporting thumb.

Mobilizing forces: Superior glide (see Fig. 7–20) is used to improve scapular depression.
1. Force is applied superiorly by index finger to proximal clavicle.
2. **Client position:** Supine.
3. **Hand placement:** Place thumb over proximal clavicle with index finger placed inferior to the clavicle.

Mobilizing forces: Anterior glide (Fig. 7–21) is used to increase scapular protraction.
1. Force is applied anteriorly (lifting) by fingers to proximal clavicle.
2. **Client position:** Supine.

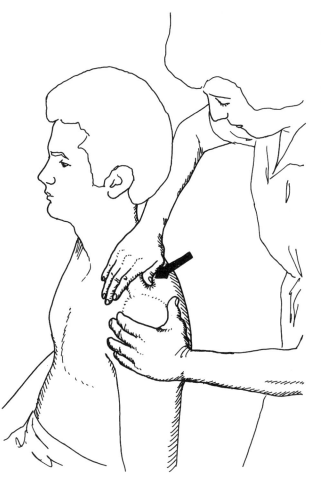

FIG. 7–19
Acromioclavicular joint anterior glide. Used to increase overall mobility of joint. (From Kisner & Colby, p 206, with permission.)

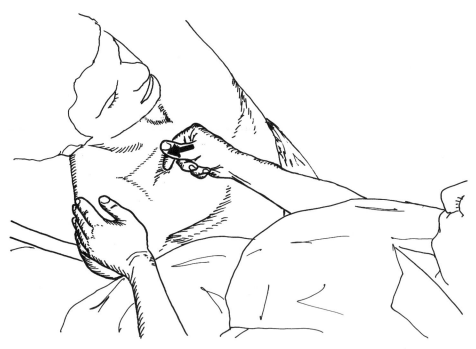

FIG. 7–20
Sternoclavicular joint posterior and superior glide. Used to increase scapular retraction (posteriorly) or used to improve scapular depression (superiorly). (From Kisner & Colby, p 206, with permission.)

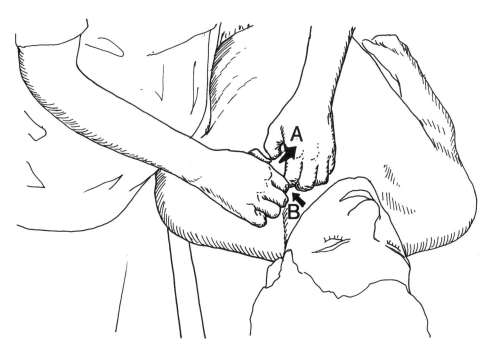

FIG 7–21
Sternoclavicular joint anterior and inferior glide. Fingers lift clavicle for anterior glide (A) used to increase scapular protraction, and depress clavicle (B) for inferior glide used to increase scapular elevation. (From Kisner & Colby, p 207, with permission.)

3. **Hand placement:** Place fingers superior and posterior to the proximal clavicle. Thumb stabilizes inferior to the proximal clavicle.

Mobilizing forces: Inferior glide (Fig. 7–21) is used to increase scapular elevation.

1. Force is applied inferiorly by fingers to the proximal clavicle.
2. **Client position:** Supine.
3. **Hand placement:** Place fingers superior to the proximal clavicle. Thumb stabilizes inferior to the proximal clavicle.

Elbow and Forearm

Humeroulnar Joint

Joint surface and motion considerations: Concave trochlear notch, convex trochlea. The roll and the glide occur in the same direction when the ulna is moving.

Resting position: 70° flexion, 10° supination.

Closed-packed position: Extension.

Capsular pattern: Greater flexion limitation than extension.

Mobilizing forces: Traction (Fig. 7–22) is used to increase flexion or extension.

1. Force is applied inferiorly to the proximal ulna.
2. **Client position:** Supine, elbow in a flexed position.
3. **Hand placement:** Placed fingers anteriorly over the proximal ulna. Thumb stablizes posterior to the proximal ulna. Free hand stabilizes the humerus.

Radioulnar Joint (Proximal)

Joint surface and motion considerations: Convex radial head, concave radial notch (ulna). The roll and the glide occur in opposite directions when the radius is moving.

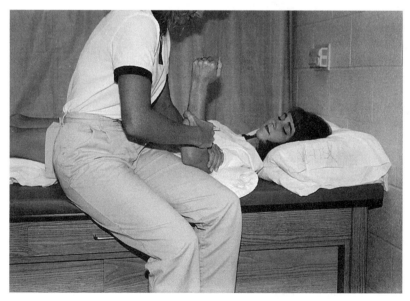

FIG. 7–22
Humeroulnar joint traction. Used to increase flexion or extension.

Resting position: 70° flexion, 35° supination.

Closed-packed position: 5° supination.

Capsular pattern: Greater limitation of supination than pronation.

Mobilizing forces: Glide (Fig. 7–23) is applied dorsally to increase pronation and volarly to increase supination.

1. Force is applied either dorsal or volar to the radial head.
2. **Client position:** Seated, elbow in a comfortable position.
3. **Hand placement:** Fingers and thumb grasp radial head over the proximal forearm. Thumb stabilizes posterior to the proximal ulna. Free hand stabilizes the ulna.

Radioulnar Joint (Distal)

Joint surface and motion considerations: Convex ulnar head, concave ulnar notch (radius). The roll and the glide occur in same directions as the radius moving around the ulna.

Resting position: 10° supination.

Closed-packed position: 5° supination.

Capsular pattern: Little limitation of motion, but pain at extremes of supination or pronation.

Mobilizing forces: Glide (Fig. 7–24) applied dorsally to increase supination and volarly to increase pronation.

FIG. 7–23
Radioulnar joint (proximal) glide. Mobilized dorsally to increase pronation and volarly to increase supination.

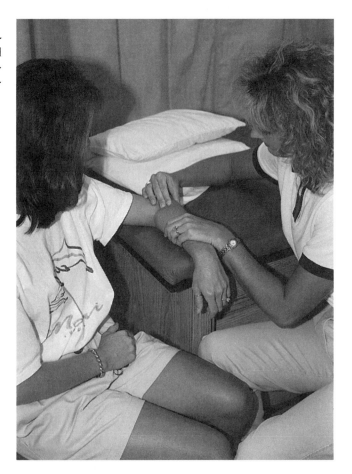

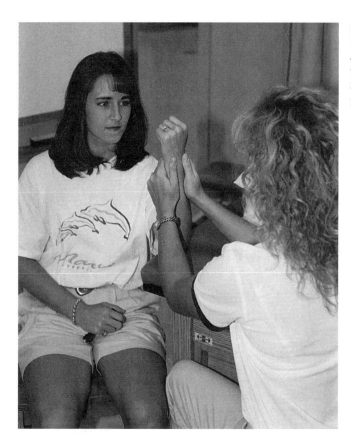

FIG. 7–24
Radioulnar joint (distal) glide. Mobilized dorsally to increase supination and volarly to increase pronation.

1. Force is applied in either a dorsal or volar direction to the distal radius.
2. **Client position:** Seated.
3. **Hand placement:** Fingers and thumb grasp the distal radius over the distal forearm. Free hand stablizes the ulna.

Wrist

Radiocarpal Joint

Joint surface and motion considerations: Convex proximal row of carpal bones, concave distal radius and articular disk. The roll and the glide occur in opposite directions when the wrist and hand moves on the radius. This is a very complicated joint for analyzing motion arthrokinematically because of intricate articulations of the ulna, the radius, the ulnar articular disk, and all the carpal bones. This text addresses the major motions of flexion, extension, and ulnar and radial deviation.

Resting position: Neutral with slight ulnar deviation.

Closed-packed position: Extension with radial deviation.

Capsular pattern: Both flexion and extension limitations equally.

Mobilizing forces: Traction (Fig. 7–25) is used for pain control and to improve general mobility.

1. Force is applied distally, distracting the articular surfaces.

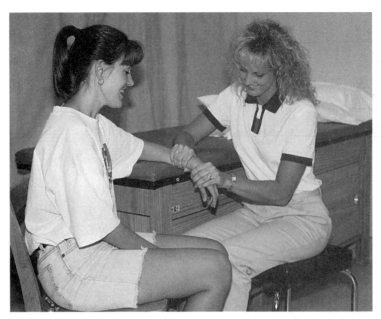

FIG. 7–25
Radiocarpal joint traction and glides. Traction used for pain control and to improve general mobility. Glides used dorsally to increase flexion and volarly to increase extension. Ulnar glides are used to increase radial deviation and radial glides are used to increase ulnar deviation. Hand placement is similar for traction and glide forces. All glide forces (dorsal, volar, ulnar, and radial) are accomplished from similar hand placement.

    2. **Client position:** Seated.
    3. **Hand placement:** Grasp around wrist just distal to the radiocarpal joint. Free hand stabilizes the radius.
Mobilizing forces: Glides (see Fig. 7–25) are used in a dorsal direction to increase flexion and in a volar direction to increase extension. Ulnar glides are used to increase radial deviation, and radial glides are used to increase ulnar deviation.
    1. Force is applied in a volar, dorsal, ulnar, or radial direction from the same hand placement of clinician.
    2. **Client position:** Seated.
    3. **Hand placement:** Grasp around wrist just distal to the radiocarpal joint. Free hand stabilizes the radius.

Hand and Digits

Metacarpophalangeal and Interphalangeal Joints of the Digits

    1. **Joint surface and motion considerations:** There are numerous combinations of carpal and metacarpal mobilization techniques. Presented here are several of the commonly used mobilizations. These should not be taken as a comprehensive list for mobilization of the hand and digits. The distal end of each proximal (metacarpal or phalangeal) bone is convex, and the proximal end of each distal

bone is concave. Each (metacarpophalangeal (MCP) and interphalangeal (IP) joint is constructed similarly, and the same techniques can be applied to each joint. The roll and the glide occur in the same direction as the distal bone moving on the proximal bone.

2. **Resting position:**

First carpometacarpal (CMC) joint: neutral

First MCP joint: slight flexion

Second through fifth MCP joints: slight flexion and ulnar deviation

First through fifth IP joints: slight flexion

Closed-packed position:

First CMC joint: full opposition

First MCP joint: full extension

Second through fifth MCP joints: full flexion

First through fifth IP joints: full extension

Capsular pattern:

Trapeziometacarpal joint: abduction and extension greatly limited

MCP joints: greater flexion limitation than extension

IP joints: greater extension limitation, but flexion is also limited

Mobilizing force: Traction (Fig. 7–26) is used for pain control and to improve general mobility.

1. Force is applied along longitudinal axis of digit, distracting joint surfaces.

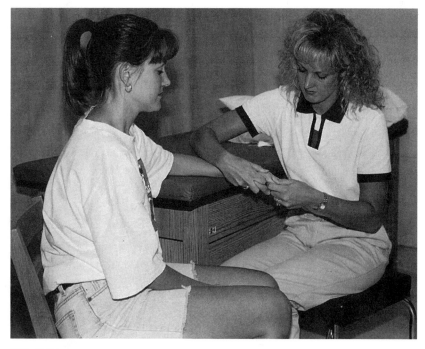

FIG. 7–26

Metacarpophalangeal and interphalangeal joints of the digits traction and glides. Traction used for pain control and to improve general mobility. Glides volarly to increase flexion and dorsally to increase extension. Ulnar and radial glides can be used at the MCP to increase abduction or adduction. All glide forces (dorsal, volar, ulnar, and radial) are accomplished from similar hand placement.

2. **Client position:** Seated.
3. **Hand placement:** Grasp distal articulating bone as close as possible to the joint. Free hand stabilizes the proximal articulating bone.

Mobilizing force: Glide (see Fig. 7–26) in a volar direction to increase flexion and in a dorsal direction to increase extension. Ulnar and radial glides can be used at the MCP joints to increase abduction or adduction.

1. Force is applied by thumb to the proximal aspect of the bone to be mobilized in appropriate direction. Rotational (spin) mobilization can also be done along longitudinal axis to aid in obtaining final degrees of motion.
2. **Client position:** Seated.
3. **Hand placement:** Grasp distal articulating bone as closely as possible to the joint. Free hand stabilizes the proximal articulating bone.

Hip

1. **Joint surface and motion considerations:** The femoral head is convex, and the acetabulum concave. The roll and the slide occur in opposite directions when the femur moves on the acetabulum.
2. **Resting position:** Flexion 30°, abducted 30°, and slightly externally rotated.
3. **Closed-packed position:** (A) Internal rotation, extension, and abduction, or (B) flexion to 90°, abduction, and external rotation.
4. **Capsular pattern:** Internal rotation and abduction greatly limited; flexion and extension less limited.

Mobilizing force: Traction (Fig. 7–27) is used to relieve hip pain and improve general mobility.

1. Force is applied through a long-axis traction (not to be done if client has knee dysfunction).
2. **Client position:** Supine.
3. **Hand placement:** Grasp proximal to malleoli with both hands.

FIG. 7–27
Hip joint distraction. Utilized to relieve hip pain and improve general mobility.

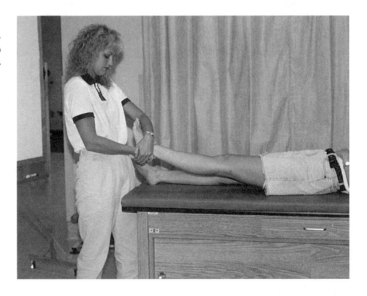

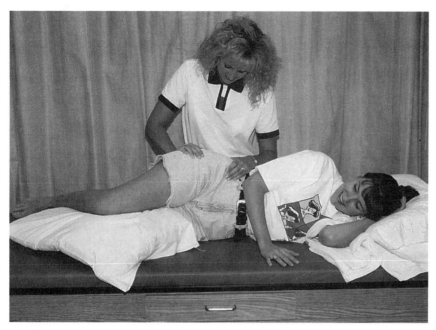

FIG. 7–28
Hip joint anterior glide. Utilized to increase extension and external rotation.

Gently lean caudally using your body weight as the mobilizing force. A belt can be used to assist in gripping the client's lower extremity. Ensure that you gently apply and gently release this force.

Mobilizing force: Anterior glide (Fig. 7–28) is used to increase extension and external rotation.

1. Force is applied as clinician moves femoral head anteriorly from a posterior force.
2. **Client position:** Side-lying.
3. **Hand placement:** Position palm of hand posterior to the greater trochanter. Free hand stabilizes the pelvis.

Mobilizing force: Posterior glide (see Figure 7-29) is used to increase flexion and internal rotation.

1. Force is applied as clinician moves femoral head posteriorly from an anterior force.
2. **Client position:** Supine, hip and knee flexed with belt supporting the knee
3. **Hand placement:** Position palm of hand on the anterior thigh. Free hand supports the femur.

Knee

Joint surface and motion considerations: The tibial plateau and menisci are concave, and the femoral condyles are convex. The roll and slide directions depend on an open-chain versus a closed-chain environment. When the tibia moves on the femur, the roll and slide occur in the same direction as the tibia. When the femur moves on the tibia, the roll and slide occur in opposite directions.

Resting position: Flexion 25°

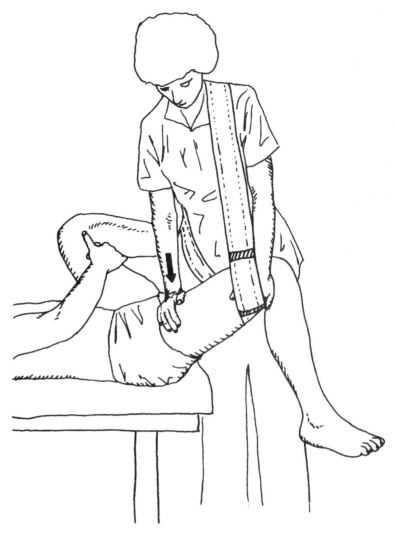

FIG. 7–29
Hip joint posterior glide. Utilized to increase flexion and internal rotation. (From Kisner & Colby, p 220, with permission.)

Closed-packed position: Lateral rotation and extension.
Capsular pattern: Greater flexion limitation than extension.
Mobilizing force: Traction (Fig. 7–30) is used for general mobility and pain control.
1. Force is applied along long axis of the tibia.
2. **Client position:** Seated with knee in a relaxed position.
3. **Hand placement:** Grasp distal end of tibia and fibula.
Mobilizing force: Glide (Fig.7–31) in the anterior direction (tibial) to promote increased extension and apply glide in the posterior direction (tibial) to promote increased flexion. Mobilizing the tibia on the femur in either direction is easily accomplished from the same client position and same hand position.
1. Force is applied either anteriorly or posteriorly gliding the tibia over the femur.
2. **Client position:** Hook lying position.

3. **Hand placement:** Grasp proximal tibia with both hands just distal to knee joint. Thumbs point to the patella, and fingers wrap around to posterior aspect of the tibia.

Mobilizing force: Glide (Fig. 7–32) in the posterior direction (femoral) to promote increased extension.

1. Force is applied in a posterior direction from the palm of the hand.
2. **Client position:** Supine, knee in slight flexion with a support under the proximal tibia.
3. **Hand placement:** Place palm of hand over anterior distal femur. Free hand stabilizes the tibia.

Patellofemoral Joint

Joint surface and motion considerations: Proper patellar mobility is necessary for full knee flexion and normal quadriceps femoris function. This is a pseudojoint, not a true synovial joint, that can greatly impact the treatment of knee pathologies. The patella glides inferiorly and superiorly in the femoral groove during flexion and extension of the knee.

Mobilizing force: Glide (Fig. 7–33) patella distally to improve knee flexion.

1. Force is applied from web space of hand to superior pole of patella in an inferior direction parallel to the femur.
2. **Client position:** Supine, knee relaxed.
3. **Hand placement:** Place web space of hand along superior pole of patella. Ensure that the motion is parallel to the femur and does not compress the patella against the femoral groove.

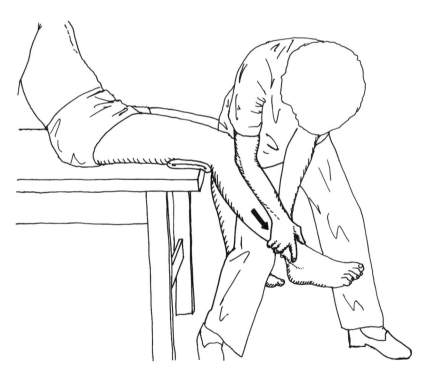

FIG. 7–30
Knee joint distraction. Used for general mobility and pain control. (From Kisner & Colby, p 223, with permission.)

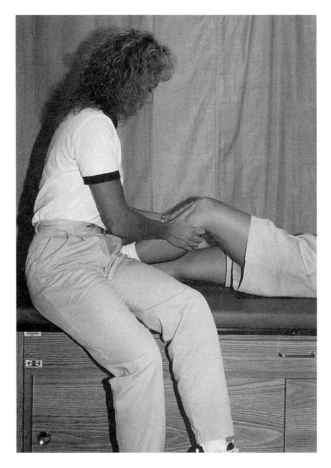

FIG. 7–31
Knee joint glide (open chain). By gliding the tibia anteriorly or posteriorly from the hook lying position, open chain mobilization of the knee joint occurs. Glides in the anterior direction (tibial) promote increased extension and glides in the posterior direction (tibial) promote increased flexion.

Mobilizing force: Glide (Fig. 7–34) in a medial and lateral direction to improve patellar mobility.

1. Force is applied to medial or lateral border of patella
2. **Client position:** Supine, knee relaxed.
3. **Hand placement:** Grasp patella with both thumbs on one side and both index fingers on opposing side.

Ankle

Talocrural Joint (Ankle Mortise)

Joint surface and motion considerations: Convex dome of the talus, concave tibia and fibula (mortise). Roll and glide occur in opposite directions.
Resting position: Plantar flexion 10°, neutral inversion and eversion.
Closed-packed position: Dorsiflexion.
Capsular pattern: Limitations of both dorsiflexion and plantar flexion.
Mobilizing force: Traction (Fig. 7–35) is used for pain control and improving general mobility.

1. Force is applied by distracting the talus inferiorly.
2. **Client position:** Supine.
3. **Hand placement:** Grasp dorsum of foot with both hands just distal to ankle mortise joint. Thumbs stabilize on the plantar surface of the foot.

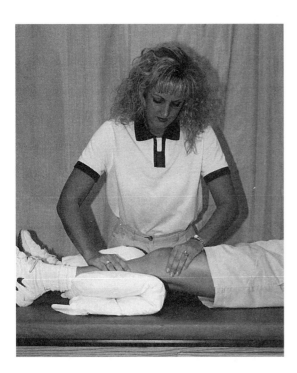

FIG 7–32
Knee joint glide (closed chain). A posterior glide of the femur on the tibia will improve extension in a closed chain environment.

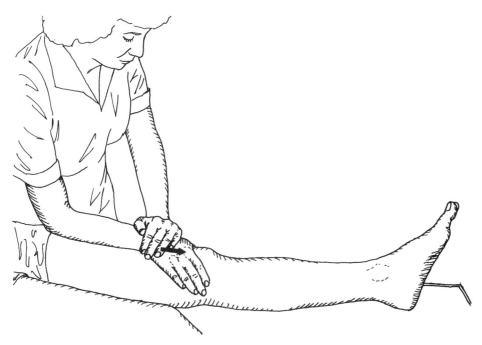

FIG. 7–33
Patellofemoral inferior glide. Utilized to improve knee flexion. (From Kisner & Colby, p 225, with permission.)

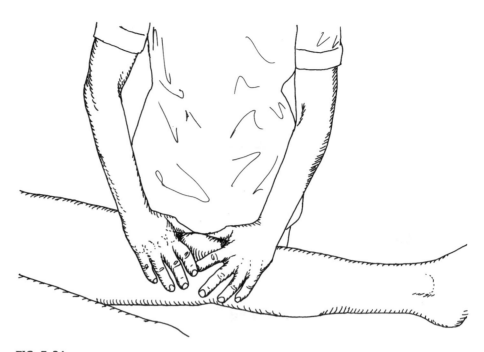

FIG. 7–34
Patellofemoral medial-lateral glide. Utilized to improve patellar mobility. (From Kisner & Colby, p 226, with permission.)

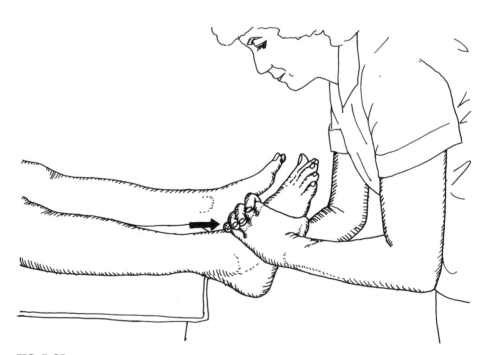

FIG. 7–35
Talocrural joint traction. Used for pain control and improving general mobility. (From Kisner & Colby, p 229, with permission.)

Mobilizing force: Glide (Fig. 7–36) anteriorly to improve plantar flexion.

1. Force is applied from the posterior aspect of the calcaneus, gliding the talus in an anterior direction.
2. **Client position:** Supine, ankle in resting position.
3. **Hand placement:** Grasp calcaneus with palm of hand. Free hand stabilizes over anterior distal tibia close to the ankle joint.

Alternate method (not pictured): Glide anteriorly to improve plantar flexion. Force is applied on the posterior aspect of the calcaneus, gliding the talus in an anterior direction (or toward the floor).

1. **Client position:** Prone, ankle in resting position.
2. **Hand placement:** Rest hand on posterior aspect of the calcaneus with palm of mobilizing hand. Free hand stabilizes under the tibia on the anterior surface.

Mobilizing Force: Glide (Fig. 7–37) posterior to increase dorsiflexion.

1. Force is applied in a posterior direction, gliding the talus posteriorly on tibia.
2. **Client position:** Supine.
3. **Hand placement**: Place web space of hand across the dorsum of the foot close to the talocrural joint. Free hand stabilizes distal tibia.

Subtalar Joint

Joint surface and motion considerations: Functionally, the subtalar joint is a bicondylar joint. Posteriorly, the concave talus rests on the convex calcaneus. Anteriorly and medially, the convex talus rests on a

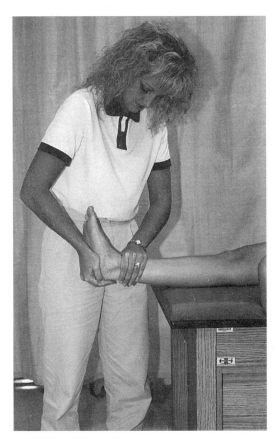

FIG. 7–36
Talocrural joint anterior glide. Utilized to improve plantarflexion.

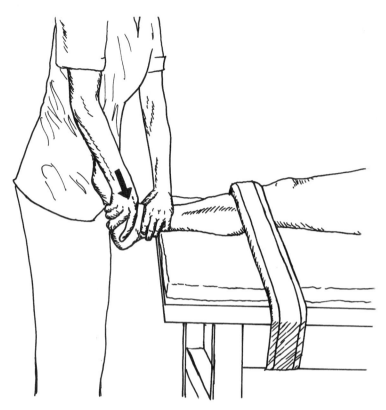

FIG. 7–37
Talocrural joint posterior glide. Utilized to increase dorsiflexion. (From Kisner & Colby, p 229, with permission).

concave calcaneus. The roll and glide at the joint occurs in opposite directions posteriorly, but in the same direction anteriorly. To successfully evert the subtalar joint, the posterior surface of the calcaneus must glide medially and the anterior surface laterally.

Resting position: Subtalar neutral.

Closed-packed position: Inversion.

Capsular pattern: Significant inversion limitation.

Mobilizing force: Traction (Fig. 7–38) is applied to improve general mobility for inversion and eversion as well as pain control.

  1. Force is applied longitudinally, distracting the calcaneus from the talus.

  2. **Client position:** Supine.

  3. **Hand placement:** Grasp the posterior calcaneus. Free hand stabilizes the anterior distal tibia.

Mobilizing force: Glide (Figs. 7–39 and 7–40) medially to improve eversion, and laterally to improve inversion.

  1. Force is applied through the heel of your hand aimed at the medial or lateral surface of the calcaneus gliding parallel to the plantar surface of the foot.

  2. **Client position:** Medial glide on posterior aspect of calcaneus, client is prone; lateral glide on posterior aspect of calcaneus, client is side-lying with involved side down.

3. **Alternate position (not pictured):** Client is prone with knee flexed to 90°.
4. **Hand placement:** Place heel of hand against the medial or lateral aspect of the calcaneus posteriorly depending on direction of mobilization. Fingers wrap around the posterior calcaneus for stability. Free hand stabilizes the distal tibia.

Foot

Tarsal, Metatarsal, and Phalangeal Joints

Joint surface and motion considerations: As with the bones of the hand, there are many combinations of mobilization techniques at the transverse tarsal, forefoot, and digits. It is beyond the scope of this text to cover each technique.

Resting position:
   First through fifth MTP joints: extension 10°
   First through fifth IP joints: slight flexion

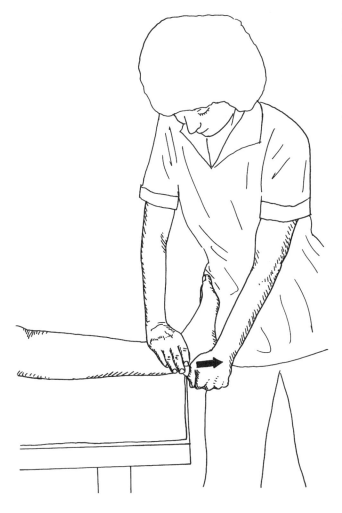

FIG. 7–38
Subtalar joint traction. Utilized to improve general mobility for inversion and eversion as well as pain control. (From Kisner & Colby, p 229, with permission.)

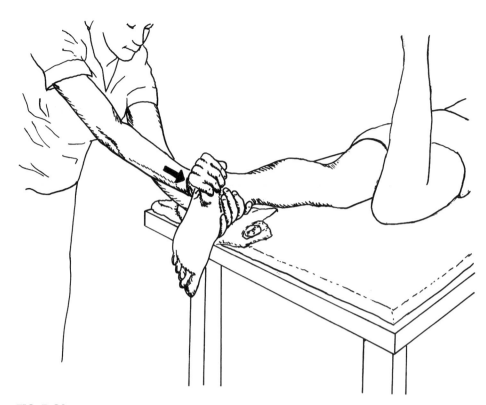

FIG. 7–39
Subtalar joint medial glide. Utilized to improve eversion. (From Kisner & Colby, p 230, with permission.)

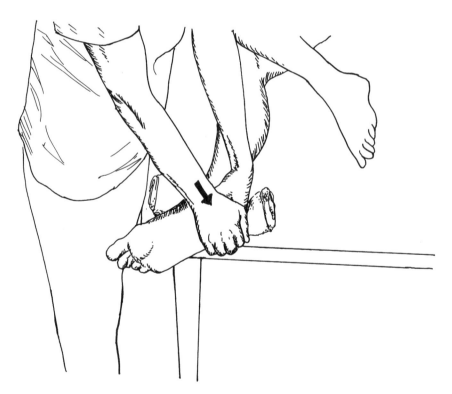

FIG. 7–40
Subtalar joint lateral glide. Utilized to improve inversion. (From Kisner & Colby, p 230, with permission.)

Closed-packed position:
    First through fifth MTP joints: full extension
    First through fifth IP joints: full extension
Mobilizing force: The digits of the foot are mobilized and stabilized in a similar fashion to that of the digits of the hand.

 # SUMMARY

Manual therapy is the therapeutic approach of musculoskeletal evaluation and treatment in physical therapy that applies principles of kinesiology, histology, neurophysiology, and pathophysiology. Passive movement techniques, mobilization, and manipulations are used to promote the well-being of clients, restore lost function, reduce pain, or lessen the effects of muscle spasms. Mobilization is a low-velocity, passive therapeutic technique performed by the clinician to an affected joint within or at the limits of joint ROM, using a speed slow enough to allow the client to stop the movement. Manipulation is a sudden, high-velocity technique at the end of ROM that cannot be stopped by the client and is designed to release pathologically adhered or shortened structures. The PTA must identify the legal and practical aspects of delivering manual techniques in an orthopedic environment. Each state has varied rules and regulations permitting or prohibiting the application of peripheral mobilization techniques by the assistant. Controversy in the profession of physical therapy continues as to the exact role of the PTA in administering joint mobilization treatment.

Arthrokinematics is the description of the motion of the joint surfaces, and osteokinematics is the description of the motion of the bone. Osteokinematic terms include swing of the bone and the mechanical axis of rotation. Joint congruency is how well opposing joint surfaces match. The two primary shapes of human joints are ovoid and sellar. The resting position (loose-packed) exists when there is greatest amount of intracapsular space. Mobilization is performed with the joint in a loose packed position. The closed-packed position is when the joint intracapsular space is as small as possible. Accessory motions (or joint play) are joint surface movements that are not under voluntary motor control, but are essential for normal joint function. The roll, spin, and glide are accessory motion components. The convex-concave rule of joint surface movement is used to identify the direction of glide in relation to the swing of the bone. The roll always occurs in the same direction as the swing of the bone.

Degrees of mobility exist in a spectrum ranging from severely hypomobile (ankylosed) to severely hypermobile (pathologically unstable). Evaluating the extent of mobility is an evaluative function performed by the physical therapist. End-feels are what is perceived by the examiner as limitations to passive motion. Many differing classifications of end-feels exist, but they generally fall into operating classes of soft, firm, or hard.

Peripheral mobilization is performed by doing joint oscillations or sustained techniques. The application can be done by gliding parallel to the joint surface or by performing joint distraction in a perpendicular manner. Mobilizations are indicated to increase the mobility of pathologically restricted tissues, reduce muscle spasm, or relieve painful somatic conditions. Maitland described a grading scale (I to V) depending on the magnitude of the oscillation and on where it is applied in the ROM. Kaltenborn described a sustained mobilization grading scale (I to III) classifying as loosening, tightening, and stretching. Contraindications are presented for the application of mobilization techniques. Application techniques for the peripheral joints are presented to include joint surface and motion considerations, resting position, closed-packed position, capsular pattern, application of mobilizing force, client position, and hand placement of the clinician.

 # REFERENCES

1. Farrell, JP, and Jensen, GM: Foreword: Manual therapy. Phys Ther 72:842, 1992.
2. Grimsby, O, and Power, B: Basic Manual Therapy for Physical Therapy Assistants: A Course Workbook, ed 2. The Ola Grimsby Institute. San Diego, CA, 1995.
3. Riddle, DL: Measurements of accessory motion: Critical issues and related concepts. Phys Ther 72:865, 1992.
4. Mennell, JM: Manual Therapy. Charles C Thomas, Springfield, Il, 1951.
5. Di Fabio, RP: Efficacy of manual therapy. Phys Ther 72:853, 1992.
6. Kisner, C, and Colby, LA: Therapeutic Exercise: Foundations and Techniques, ed 3. FA Davis, Philadelphia, pp 183–233, 1996.
7. Farrell, JP, and Jensen, GM: Manual therapy: A critical assessment of role in the profession of physical therapy. Phys Ther 72:843, 1992.
8. Stephens, E: Manipulative therapy in physical therapy curricula. Phys Ther 53:40, 1973.
9. Ben-Sorek, S, and Davis, CM: Joint mobilization education and clinical use in the United States. Phys Ther 68:1000, 1988.
10. Kessler, RM, and Hertling, D: Management of Common Musculoskeletal Disorders: Physical Therapy Principles and Methods, ed 3. Lippincott, Philadelphia, 1996.
11. Kaltenborn, FM, and Evjenth, O: Manual mobilization of the extremity joints: basic examination and treatment techniques, ed 4, Olaf Norlis Bokhandel Universitesgaten, Oslo, Norway, 1989.
12. Grimsby, O: Fundamentals of manual therapy: a course workbook. Sorlandets Institute, San Diego, CA, 1985.
13. Cyriax, JH: Textbook of orthopaedic medicine: diagnosis of soft tissue lesions, 8th ed. Bailliere Tindall, London, England, 1982.
14. Maitland, GD: Peripheral Manipulation, ed 2. Butterworth, Boston, 1977.

 # BIBLIOGRAPHY

Ben-Sorek, S, and Davis, CM: Joint mobilization education and clinical use in the United States. Phys Ther 68:1000, 1988.

Cyriax, JH: Textbook of Orthopaedic Medicine: Diagnosis of Soft Tissue Lesions, ed 8. London, England: Bailliere Tindall, 1982.

Di Fabio, RP: Efficacy of manual therapy. Phys Ther 72:853, 1992.

Farrell, JP, and Jensen, GM: Manual therapy: a critical assessment of role in the profession of physical therapy. Phys Ther 72:842, 1992.

Grimsby, O: Fundamentals of Manual Therapy: A Course Workbook. Sorlandets Institute, San Diego, CA, 1985.

Grimsby, O, and Power, B: Basic Manual Therapy for Physical Therapy Assistants: A Course Workbook, ed 2. The Ola Grimsby Institute, San Diego, CA, 1995.

Kaltenborn, FM, and Evjenth, O: Manual Mobilization of the Extremity Joints: Basic Examination and Treatment Techniques, ed 4. Olaf Norlis Bokhandel Universitesgaten, Oslo, Norway, 1989.

Kessler, RM, and Hertling, D: Management of Common Musculoskeletal Disorders: Physical Therapy Principles and Methods, ed 3. Lippincott, Philadelphia, 1996.

Maitland, GD: Peripheral Manipulation, ed 2. Butterworth, Boston, 1977.

Mennell, JM: Manual Therapy. Charles C Thomas, Springfield, IL, 1951.

Riddle, DL: Measurements of accessory motion: Critical issues and related concepts. Phys Ther 72:865, 1992.

Stephens, E: Manipulative therapy in physical therapy curricula. Phys Ther 53:40, 1973.

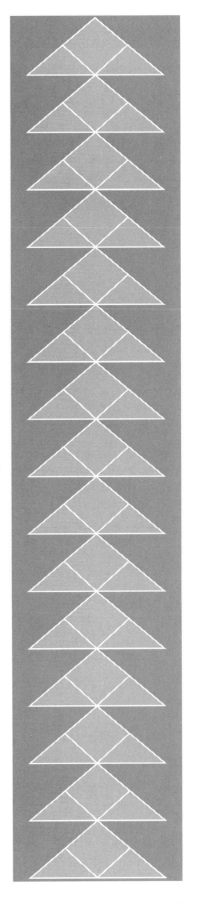

part **II**

MANAGEMENT OF ORTHOPEDIC INJURIES

Introduction to Part II

Emily Gordon, a fragile-looking woman in her eighties, fractured her hip one week ago. She is sitting in your office for evaluation and treatment. Next to her is Rachel Spencer, a twenty-year-old athletic-looking woman. Rachel also has a week-old hip fracture. Their diagnoses are the same. Both have had this injury for the same period of time. Both are women, and they are waiting for you to provide them with the best rehabilitation. However, they are very different.

Carole Bernstein Lewis, PT, GCS, MSG, MPA, PhD
Aging: The Health Care Crisis Challenge[1]

The health-care profession should give highest priority to designing skilled interventions based on an individual client's anxieties, feelings, and concerns about his or her diagnosis, injury, or disease. This demonstrates respect for the client as a person. In practice, however, the health-care system frequently resembles an operational machine that inputs a disease, mixes a "diagnosis" with protocol and treatment "approaches," and produces an outcome. Unique considerations that present in different phases of the client's life are often ignored or overlooked. The concerns of parents who have just been told that their newborn child has a hip injury are significantly different from those of an athlete who has just been told he or she has a hip injury. I believe that it is important for the physical therapy professional to treat the client, not the condition. By doing so, health care becomes a little less institutionalized and automated.

The life-span development approach has been adopted for the second part of this textbook. To my knowledge, this is a first attempt to place orthopedic management into "client" categories rather than categories of the anatomic joint. Each chapter in this section, is organized by clients' concerns in relation to life phase. In addition, conditions are further subdivided into the following categories:

- Description of the condition
- Clinical presentation of the client
- Evaluation tools and methods used by the PT
- Clinical management of the client

The description of the condition includes definitions, incidence, etiology, and pathophysiology of the condition. The clinical presentation describes typical signs and symptoms. The clinical management of the client describes treatment considerations for each condition, including appropriate indications and contraindications. New exercise or treatment concepts may be presented and detailed for students to learn. Evaluative tools and methods used by the PT are taken from the Preferred Practice Patterns adopted by the American Physical Therapy Association.[2] This information has been incorporated to facilitate an understanding of, and appreciation for, the various techniques applied by the professional PT in the development of the diagnosis and prognosis of the client. The student should have a solid knowledge of these elements before trying to master the information presented in this section.

Every effort was made in this text to present a comprehensive examination of orthopedic conditions that are commonly treated by the PTA. The Clinical Orthopedics for the Physical Therapist Assistant is not, however, a comprehensive textbook applicable to every orthopedic client that the PTA may encounter in the clinical setting. It should be used instead as a springboard for future learning and investigation by the student. I hope that the information presented in this textbook challenges your thought process, encourages you to develop as a clinician, and ultimately, promotes the development of professionalism among PTAs.

Steven G. Lesh, MPA, PT, SCS, ATC
Assistant Professor of Physical Therapy
Arkansas State University

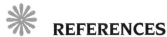

REFERENCES

1. Lewis, CB: Aging: The Health Care Challenge. FA Davis, Philadelphia, 1985.
2. Guide to Physical Therapist Practice. Phys Ther 77:1163, 1997.

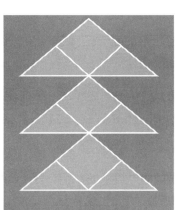

chapter **8**

Pediatric Clients

Outline

Needs of the Client: Promotion of
    Normal Development
Needs of the Family: Promotion of
    Education and Participation
Acquired Conditions
    Skeletal Fractures
    Juvenile Rheumatoid Arthritis
    Growth Disorders
    Osteochondropathies
Congenital Conditions
    Congenital Amputations
    Developmental Dysplasia of the
        Hip
    Equinovarus
    Limb-Length Discrepancies

Key Words

acquired

ankylosis

arthritis

arthrodesis

autoimmune response

congenital

dislocation

dysplasia

equinovarus

exacerbations

iridocyclitis

moiré topography

osteochondrosis

osteogenesis

remissions

rheumatoid

scoliosis

subluxation

synovectomy

OBJECTIVES

After completing this chapter, the PTA student will be able to:
1. Discuss the rehabilitation concerns and needs of pediatric clients and their families.
2. Identify communication methods that will improve the quality of educating pediatric clients, parents, and families.
3. Describe the incidence, etiology, and pathophysiology of the conditions presented in this chapter.
4. Identify the evaluation tools and methods used by the physical therapist to form a diagnosis, prognosis, and plan of treatment for the client conditions described in this chapter.
5. Describe the clinical management of the client conditions described in this chapter.
6. Discuss the expected physical therapy outcomes for the client conditions described in this chapter.

Where once pediatric orthopedics was little more than splinting of deformities caused by wholly preventable birth defects or malnourishment syndromes, it is now touched by the wonders of modern medicine. . . .[1]

Jules M. Rothstein, PhD, PT
Editor, Pediatric Orthopedics
American Physical Therapy Association

 NEEDS OF THE CLIENT: PROMOTION OF NORMAL DEVELOPMENT

A child with a recently healed fractured arm enters a physical therapy clinic with her parents. The small child suffered the injury about 5 weeks ago when she fell from a tree in the backyard while playing. The cast had just been removed at the doctor's office, and the skin of the arm is dry, chaffing, and has a mild odor. The father is greatly concerned that his only daughter cannot move her elbow, because she tells him that there is "a lot of stiffness and it hurts to move." The mother has fears and anxieties surrounding the long-term effects of the injury to her daughter's left elbow. The mother asks the physical therapist, "Will Jamie ever be normal again?"

One significant question often presented to health-care professionals by families of pediatric clients with medical conditions is, "Will they ever be normal?" This brief question contains many implications, possibilities, definitions, concerns, opinions, and statistical comparisons. Infants and young children are the future generation, full of promise and potential. Society often views pediatric injuries and conditions as setbacks and disappointments as harbingers that these children's potential promise may not be reached. The young mother carried the baby for 9 months, expecting her first healthy, baby boy, instead finds an infant with a congenital hip problem that may affect his future. The father of the young athletic superstar has the child's future professional baseball career planned, but the plan may need to be revised when the child falls from a bicycle, fracturing his wrist and elbow. The father's dream may never materialize.

When an infant or child is diagnosed with an illness or physical limitation, there is a pressure of concern and uncertainty carried by the client and family. The health-care provider must have the ability to identify the needs of the client as well as the family, and provide accurate intervention and appropriate information.

The physical therapy team should focus on the promotion of normal development when identifying the needs of the pediatric client. Young children are some of the most resilient and rapid healers across the generational life span. Often, if left alone (and the condition is not excessively severe), the pediatric client will run, play, and interact normally. The orthopedic condition will heal and resolve in time. However, conditions present that may prevent the child from running, walking, and interacting in a normal fashion that effectively limit the growth and development of the client. The challenge for the rehabilitation team is to promote the normal developmental process of interaction, weight bearing, and mobility for the pediatric client. This will help to encourage the innate healing abilities of the pediatric client and prevent long-term complications from a lack of physical development.

When orthopedic conditions present that are either **congenital** or **acquired** in nature, identification of immediate, short-term and long-term goals and needs must be established. Immediate needs include:

1. Stabilization of injuries or deformities through nonsurgical immobilization or surgical fixation
2. Promotion of a positive healing environment by encouraging healing and preventing re-injury

Short-term goals may include:

1. Prevention of secondary complications by addressing range of motion (ROM), strength, and functional mobility of the noninvolved structures
2. Promotion of normal development through selected therapeutic interventions (Figs. 8–1 and 8–2)
3. Education of the client and client's family in therapeutic program

Congenital
Orthopedic condition that is present at birth.

Acquired
Orthopedic condition that is not hereditary, innate, or present at birth. The occurrence or nonoccurrence of an event results in the acquired condition.

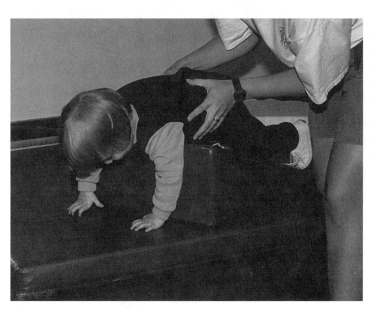

FIG. 8–1

Promoting normal development: Developmental sequence. Therapeutic activities such as lying prone on elbows or prone on a wedge help to promote head control and proximal stability of the shoulder girdle. Other activities include (1) the all-fours position, (2) creeping, (3) crawling, (4) half kneeling, (5) tall kneeling, and (6) standing. The developmental sequence should be addressed in the neurological component of the PTA curriculum and is not covered in detail in this text.

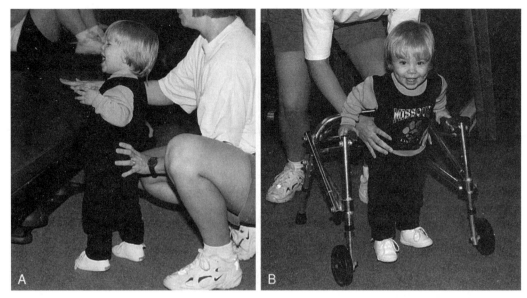

FIG. 8–2
Promoting normal development: Weight-bearing. When a pediatric client can obtain an upright, weight-bearing position (A), many benefits are promoted including: (1) proximal joint stability, (2) balance and righting reactions, (3) pregait motor skills, (4) weight-bearing stimulus for bone development, (5) providing CNS proprioceptive feedback from the muscles and joint receptors, and (6) promoting a positive body image (B).

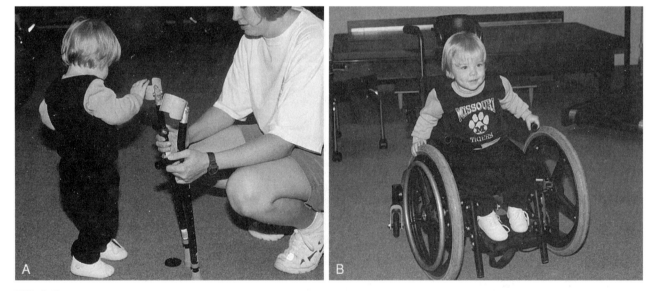

FIG. 8–3
Promoting normal function and mobility. Pictured are various assistive devices that can promote normal function and mobility for the pediatric client, including forearm crutches (A) and a wheelchair (B). Figure 8–2B shows a retro walker that can also be used to promote mobility for the pediatric client. The properly fit wheelchair cannot only promote mobility for the pediatric client, but can help to limit or reduce deformities through the use of various wedges, straps, and supports.

Long-term goals may include:

1. Restoration of normal function and mobility (Fig. 8–3)
2. Independent management of long-term complications or secondary conditions
3. Promotion of positive self-image of the client.

Interacting with and treating the pediatric client is often an enjoyable clinical experience for the PTA. Children communicate in the present moment, oblivious to future concerns. Most often, the anxieties that factor into the rehabilitative process are introduced, understandably, by the parents and families.

 ## NEEDS OF THE FAMILY: PROMOTION OF EDUCATION AND PARTICIPATION

Over the past 20 years, the health-care industry has seen an increased use of pediatric early intervention programs in the prevention of long-term complications and the reduction of associated costs. The physical therapy team has unique skills that benefit the treatment of the pediatric population. These interventions have had a positive impact on the management of costly and complicated pediatric orthopedic conditions.[2] Most pediatric early intervention programs require client and family education. Rehabilitation efforts must include the parents and families to ensure effective delivery of services and promotion of goals. If the parents and families are unable or unwilling to promote the rehabilitation process in the home, efforts of the rehabilitation team may often become increasingly difficult or eventually impossible.

In a study by Cochrane et al.,[2] the researchers identified that the two most important perceived needs when working with a pediatric client were (1) the need for a family assessment and (2) effective communication with the family. These needs were paramount to the effectiveness of the interdisciplinary team's efforts, the early intervention process, and the client assessment and evaluation. Discouragingly, these researchers found that many students in physical therapy curriculums "received minimal or no exposure to family-related [pediatric] content" and concluded that the development of family assessment and intervention educational material was of the greatest priority for professional interaction with pediatric clients.[2]

Needs and concerns of the parents and families of the pediatric orthopedic client must be addressed. Methods of integrating educational efforts related to the orthopedic condition and the needs of the client's family include:

1. Using videotapes for informational and educational purposes
2. Providing adequate written and electronic information about the rehabilitation program goals and roles of the parents in the process.
3. Promoting active participation in the rehabilitation process in treatment or class sessions fostering open discussion and communication.
4. Encouraging participation in a condition-specific support group if available (if not available, considering forming one).[2]

Parental stresses—perceived or real—that accompany the pediatric client's condition can impact the rehabilitation process. The pediatric client cannot be treated in a vacuum. The needs of the parents must also be addressed. Inclusive efforts by the rehabilitation team will eventually lead to increased participation and effective outcomes.

ACQUIRED CONDITIONS

Children are active, inquisitive, and adventurous. Often, these mischievous traits will lead the child into a situation or an environment that results in injury. Acquired orthopedic conditions can be the result of direct trauma as in a broken bone, but acquired orthopedic conditions may also be the primary or secondary result of a disease process. Arthritic joint destruction in juvenile rheumatoid arthritis or spinal deformity during the adolescent growth period are classified as acquired conditions.

SKELETAL FRACTURES

Activity or unforeseen circumstances may result in injury to the skeletal system of the growing pediatric client. Injuries to bones can take many shapes, forms, and severity and may lead to various clinical implications. The mechanical properties and the growth attributes of skeletal bone were presented in Chapter 4, and the healing capabilities and the effects of immobilization on bone were discussed in Chapter 5. This chapter identifies the unique bone-healing characteristics of the pediatric client, classifies types of injuries, and discusses medical management of the acquired condition.

Osteogenesis
The formation and development of bone.

Fractures in the bones of children have several unique characteristics (Box 8–1).[3] Pediatric clients have skeletal fractures more often than adults. Rapid healing of fractures is also a common trait for the younger clients. The periosteum is stronger and demonstrates greater **osteogenesis** than adult bones. The presence of some fractures in children may only develop a temporary deformity as the bone development process remodels the apparent deformity over time, or through the growth of the bone at the epiphyseal plate. Torn ligaments and associated injuries to the joint capsule are more frequently seen in adult clients. The ligaments of a pediatric client tend to be resilient.

Damage to the epiphyseal or growth plate can occur in pediatric fractures. Salter[3] claimed that an epiphyseal injury should be considered if the fracture was near either end of a long bone, with dislocations of a joint, or ligamentous injuries.

Box 8–1

UNIQUE CHARACTERISTICS OF PEDIATRIC FRACTURES

The rapid healing of a fracture to the skeletal bone is demonstrated by the comparative rate of recovery or union of a fractured bone. In a newborn infant, a fractured femur may heal in as little as 3 weeks. In an 8-year-old child, the same fracture may take 8 weeks to unite. In an adult, the fractured femur may take as long as 20 weeks to unite completely. The amazing ability of pediatric bones to heal is also demonstrated by the potential for spontaneous correction of deformities. If a small child sustains a fracture that creates a mild deformity, over time, as the osteoblastic and osteoclastic activity work to shape the bone, the deformity may no longer be present. With time, the bone should also lengthen from epiphyseal growth, further reducing the apparent deformity. The spontaneous reduction of a deformity, though possible, usually does not occur in adults.

In childhood, the strength of a ligament is greater than that of the epiphyseal plate. The clinical implications of injury to the growing ends of the bone are severe. Premature closure of the growth plate may produce disability from uneven limb lengths well into adulthood.[3]

Clinical Presentation

A client may present with various types of skeletal fractures. The Salter-Harris classification system of fractures[3] describes the relationships of the fractured bones, the mechanism of injury, and prognosis for the fracture (Fig. 8–4).

Type I: A complete separation of the epiphysis occurs without any other fracture occurring to the bone. This fracture is a result of a shearing force and is typical in infants and newborns. There is a very good prognosis because of excellent vascular supply and easy stabilization of fracture through a closed reduction.

Type II: This is the most common type of fracture seen. A complete separation of the epiphysis is noted, and a small piece of the metaphysis is also fractured. The mechanism of injury is from bending or shear forces and is typically seen in older children. The outer surface of the bone, the periosteum, is ruptured on the convex side of the injury, but it remains intact on the concave side of the injury. Prognosis, as with type I, is very good if the blood supply remains intact and the fracture was easily reduced through a closed reduction.

Type III: This is a rare type of injury that occurs from the joint surface of the long bone, traveling deep into the bone and making a right angle, which separates the fragment from the rest of the bone at the growth plate. Typically, this type of fracture is only seen in the distal tibia as a result of intra-articular shear forces. The prognosis is good if the open reduction procedure stabilizes the fragment and does not jeopardize the blood supply.

Type IV: A second type of intra-articular fracture similar to type III. Instead of separating the fragment from the bone at the epiphyseal plate, the fracture line continues deep into the bone, splitting it past the metaphysis. This can be seen in the distal humerus as the lateral epicondyle is separated from the bone. The prognosis for a type IV injury is poor. Skillful surgery must be performed to secure and stabilize the bone with the concern that the vascular supply is not compromised.

Type V: A crush injury produces this uncommon type of fracture. An uneven compressive force collapses one side of the long bone through the epiphysis. The injury can be seen in crush injuries to the knee and ankle and generally has a poor prognosis because the growth plate will prematurely close.

Fractures can also be described in relation to[3,4]:

1. **The site of the fracture:** Being proximal, midshaft, or distal.
2. **The degree of the fracture:** Being either complete or incomplete.
3. **The direction of the fracture line:** Being horizontal or transverse, oblique or diagonal, and possibly spiral or rotational.
4. **The position of the bony fragments:** Displaced, nondisplaced, angulated, overriding, or avulsed.

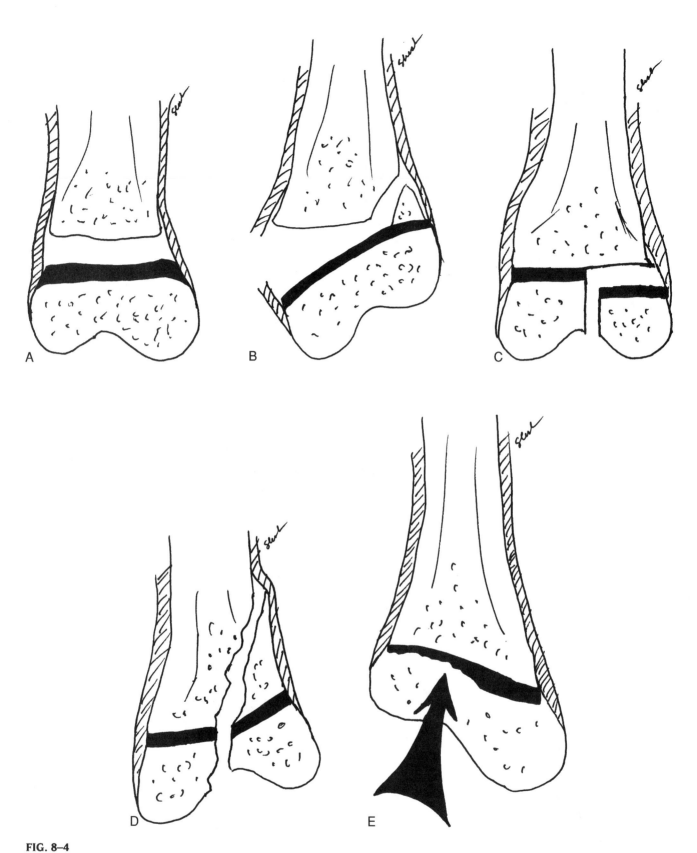

FIG. 8–4
Salter-Harris fracture classifications. Drawn are representations of the classes of epiphyseal fractures. Type I (A), type II (B), type III (C), type IV (D), and type V (E).

5. **The opened or closed state of the fracture:** An open fracture has the bony elements exposed through the skin, and a closed fracture has intact skin.
6. **The degree of complications:** Uneventful course means no complicating factors, but the course could be eventful if the bones fail to heal (nonunion).

Evaluation: Tools and Methods

The physical therapist will address areas concerned with demographics and history of the current condition. A relevant systems review should include the following:

1. **Cardiopulmonary:** endurance, and capacity for overall conditioning
2. **Integumentary:** status of skin related to surgeries or immobilizations
3. **Musculoskeletal:** ROM, muscle strength, joint integrity, posture;
4. **Neuromuscular:** sensory assessment.

Assessment of the functional status of the pediatric client should address transfer skills, gait skills, balance, and the need for assistive or protective devices.[5]

Clinical Management

Immobilization is the primary method of medical management for a bone that has been fractured. Immobilization can come from the use of plaster casts, splints, or surgical fixation (either internal or external). Use of physical therapy traditionally begins after the removal of the immobilization devices. Specific rehabilitation techniques will vary depending on the location of the fracture. There are general rehabilitation principles common to every rehabilitation team effort.

After the evaluation by the supervising physical therapist, a plan of treatment should be identified that will promote the expected outcomes for the individual client (expected outcomes are presented below). Treatment interventions may include any combination of the following and are dependent on healing constraints as to when they may be safely implemented:

1. **Endurance activities:** The use of treadmills, ergometers, or stationary bikes may be implemented as conditioning activities.
2. **Range of motion:** ROM exercises (active range of motion [AROM], passive range of motion [PROM], active assistive range of motion [AAROM], resistive ROM), stretching, or flexibility exercises may be included.
3. **Muscle strengthening:** Using free weights, ankle weights, resistive tubing, wall pulleys, or exercise machines can promote the return of muscular strength.
4. **Gait and locomotion:** Gait training may be needed using an appropriate assistive device on all appropriate surfaces (level, uneven, stairs and curbs).
5. **Balance and coordination:** Exercises specifically designed to promote balance and coordination for the lower or upper extremities are often needed. Closed kinematic chain exercises are often appropriate.
6. **Joint mobility:** (If prescribed in the plan of treatment) Peripheral joint mobilization techniques can improve accessory joint play and help to restore normal arthrokinematics.
7. **Pain management:** The use of ice, electrical stimulation, and soft-tissue mobilization are all indicated for the relief of pain.
8. **Self-care and activities of daily living (ADLs):** Promotion of self-care skill and exercises needed to build dexterity or mobility to promote ADLs is indicated.
9. **Adaptive, supportive or protective devices:** After removal of the immobiliza-

tion device, a removable orthotic or protective device may be needed to ensure continued healing or prevent future injury.

10. **Education:** Promotion of an understanding of the risk factors associated with fractures and a promotion of an awareness of the rehabilitative goals and processes.

The expected physical therapy outcomes related to managing a pediatric client with a fracture include[5]:

1. Promoting an improved health-related quality of life
2. Promoting optimal function
3. Reducing the risk of future disability from the fracture
4. Promoting an understanding of the risk factors that may jeopardize optimal health status.

After the child has been successfully immobilized and the healing of the bones has occurred, physical therapy intervention for most cases is minimal, lasting usually no longer than 1 month. In extreme cases of disability produced from the fracture or with other complicating conditions not related to the fracture, longer durations may be necessary, until functional outcomes are achieved.

JUVENILE RHEUMATOID ARTHRITIS

Rheumatoid
A general term for acute or chronic conditions characterized by inflammation, muscle soreness, and stiffness and pain in joints and associated structures.

Arthritis
Inflammation of the joint with the possible symptoms of pain, swelling, and change in structure of the involved joint.

Autoimmune Response
A response that occurs when the body's own immune defense mechanisms (lymphocytes) are unable to distinguish normal cells from infectious or destructive antigens. Destruction of healthy tissue is the end result of the disease process.

Ankylosis
State of immobility of a joint.

The most common pediatric **rheumatoid** disease in North America is juvenile rheumatoid arthritis (JRA). This crippling disease is one of the major causes of pediatric disability, and as many as 10% of afflicted clients will grow to adulthood with a severe functional impairment.[6] The etiology of JRA is unknown, but there exists many theories related to the onset of the disease, including infectious agents and genetic predisposition. The incidence of the disease is 14 in 100,000 individuals, with young girls being affected twice as often as young boys in all cases. The age of onset is before the client's 16th birthday, and complete remission of all types of JRA is seen in 75% of cases.[7]

The inflammatory **arthritis** disease process promotes destruction of the involved joints. An **autoimmune response** occurs, causing destruction of tissue when lymphocytes are unable to distinguish antigens from healthy tissue. Lysosomal enzymes and collangenase are released in the joint capsule and proliferate the synovial membrane cells. The articular cartilage softens and becomes structurally weak, possibly leading to bony destruction. Intra-articular pressure increases from the presence of joint effusion and synovial thickening. The surrounding support structures of the joint begin to become more fibrotic and soft-tissue contractures result. If unchecked, the disease may lead to an **ankylosis** of the joint.

Clinical Presentation

Three distinct types of JRA are classified depending on the onset of the disease, the number of afflicted joints, and the clinical manifestation: (1) pauciarticular (or oligoarticular), (2) polyarticular, and (3) systemic juvenile arthritis (Still's disease). Over half of the pediatric clients with chronic arthritic symptoms have fewer than four or five joints affected by the disease. These clients are classified with the mildest form of JRA: pauciarticular juvenile arthritis. The typical onset is under the age of 10 years, with a peak occurring at 1 to 2 years. Males are generally more affected than females (5:1), and the disease manifestation is typically asymmetrical in nature. Most of these clinical cases have one or two involved joints (knee, ankle, or elbow are most common). If the joint involvement does not spread for a period of 1 year from the onset of the disease, the likelihood of the disease spreading at that point is minimal. One-half of these cases will have spontaneous recovery within 5 years. One major complication of the pauciarticular variety of JRA is the possible development of **iridocyclitis** and the onset of vision impairment or blindness.[3,6,7]

Iridocyclitis
A chronic inflammation of the iris in the eye.

The polyarticular form of JRA affects primarily young girls (3:1 over boys) at any age less than 16 years with the most common age of onset being from 1 to 3 years. As the name implies (*poly* means "many"), many joints are involved in the arthritic process, and this type of JRA accounts for 30% to 40% of all cases of JRA. In addition to the symmetrical involvement of the knees and ankles, the feet, wrists, hands, and neck are also involved. The prognosis is relatively good for remission if the onset of the symptoms is rapid. However, if the onset of joint symptoms is relatively insidious, the prognosis for recovery is worse. Polyarticular JRA will generally remain active for several years. A major confounding aspect of the disease, in conjunction with the administration of corticosteroids to control the inflammatory process, is the retardation of skeletal growth and maturity.[3,6,7]

Systemic juvenile arthritis (Still's disease) is uncommon (10% of all cases), but clients with this disease present with severe symptoms and serious implications. The disease affects young boys and girls alike before age 5 years. The principal clinical presentation includes the involvement of multiple body systems. Elevated temperature may precede the onset of joint pain and irritation. A recurrent rash may appear on the trunk and proximal extremities. Anemia, liver and spleen enlargement, and pericarditis may occur. The clinical course of the disease is characterized by periods of **exacerbation** and **remission**. About half of the diagnosed cases will experience progressive involvement of the joints, eventually leading to moderate to severe disability. Seventy percent of the pediatric clients affected with Still's disease will experience remission of the active disease process after 10 years. However, the disabling conditions will most likely persist.[3,6,7]

Exacerbation
An aggravation of symptoms or an increase in the severity of a disease process.

Characteristic bony changes may occur in all affected rheumatoid joints. Osteoporosis, decreased joint space, changes in bony outlines, and loss of bony alignment can all be seen radiographically (Fig. 8–5).[8]

Remission
The lessening of the severity of a disease process or the complete abatement of symptoms.

Evaluation: Tools and Methods

A baseline examination is the first priority of the supervising physical therapist because of the chronic and potentially progressive nature of juvenile arthritis. Subsequent evaluations will be used to judge progressions or regressions and the effects of treatment on the disease. Evaluation components will include a history, an assessment of pain, swelling, ROM, muscle strength, posture, gait, functional status, endurance, need for orthotics or adaptive equipment, and functional mobility. ROM and strength evaluation should include the spine and extremities. Joints are examined for the presence of the signs and symptoms of chronic irritation (effusion, synovial thickening, heat and redness). Pain can be differentiated between pain at rest, pain during activities, and a description of what increases or decreases pain. Functional mobility should consider at least (1) the proficiency of completing a task, (2) the quality of movement, (3) speed or rate of performance, and (4) overall endurance to complete the activity.[5,7]

Clinical Management

General management considerations include first and foremost that JRA is an individual disease affecting one client at a time, and therefore, the treatment plan

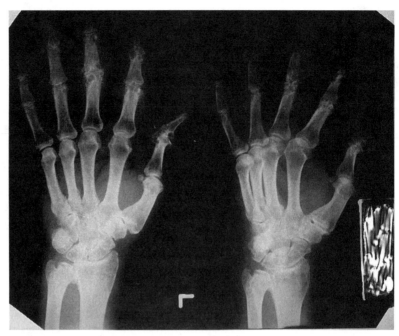

FIG. 8–5
Arthritic hand. Pictured are two different left hands with varying degrees of arthritic changes. The hand pictured on the left has mild joint deterioration noted in the third proximal interphalangeal (PIP) joint as well as the interphalangeal (IP) joint of the thumb. The hand pictured on the right has moderate deformity and arthritic changes of the IP and MCP joints of the first, second and third digits.

should be individualized to meet that specific client's needs and abilities. Goals of the intervention team should include:

1. Decreasing joint inflammation
2. Relieving pain
3. Achieving or maintaining maximal function
4. Educating client and family to promote awareness of expected disease progression

The program should balance concerns of lifelong health, adequate rest, and joint protection while working to achieve the established therapeutic goals.[5,7]

Medications typically achieve the goals managing pain and decreasing inflammation. Anti-inflammatory medications (aspirin, ibuprofen) and disease-modifying antirheumatic agents (hydroxycloroquine [Plaquenil], gold salts) help to control the effects of the disease. Therapeutic heat modalities including whirlpool, moist hot packs, or paraffin bath may help relieve joint pain, stiffness, and protective muscle guarding. Deep-heating agents such as ultrasound and diathermy are contraindicated because they can increase joint inflammation and cause epiphyseal plate damage. Transcutaneous electrical nerve stimulation application may be beneficial for pain control, which may result in increased tolerance for functional activities. Biofeedback may be of benefit in helping the chronically weak client learn proper muscle activation while promoting maximal effort during exercise. Cryotherapy, if tolerated by the client, could reduce pain through its physiological effects. Application of cold could increase joint stiffness.[7,9]

The physical therapy team plays a critical role in the achievement of the third and fourth goals (i.e., promotion of maximal function, education of the client and family regarding disease progression). During an acute exacerbation of the arthritis, ROM and strengthening should be focused on the prevention of the loss of motion (AROM, AAROM, PROM, isometric, and contract-relax exercises). Byers[10] investigated the effect of ROM exercises on joint stiffness. Her conclusions were that ROM exercises performed either in the morning before getting out of bed or performed the previous night 15 minutes before going to bed were effective at reducing joint stiffness and increasing ROM. Resistive exercises and stretching should be avoided as to prevent an increase in symptoms. During periods of remission, the addition of resistive exercises and stretching should be added cautiously to discourage symptom exacerbation. Prolonged steroid use may limit the structural integrity of the joint capsule, and therefore its ability to withstand stretching or mobilizing forces, so the clinician should exercise caution in prescribing this medication.[7,11]

Gait training should focus on the minimization of gait deviations and the maximization of gait efficiency. The client's primary lower-extremity deformities may include hip flexion contractures, femoral anteversion, genu valgum, knee flexion contractures, tibial torsion, pes cavum, or leg-length discrepancies. Gait cadence may be slow and deliberate with a small stride length. If lower-extremity joints are inflamed, then there may be asymmetrical movement patterns if both limbs are not equally involved. Assistive devices and orthotic management are indicated to promote gait efficiency and reduce abnormal stresses on the involved joints. Custom shoes for painful feet should be considered.[7,11,12]

Client and family education must include the identification of characteristic periods of exacerbation and remission. The client and family should be able to identify the symptoms associated with each period, and understand the treatment implications for each. During periods of exacerbations, rest and energy-conservation techniques should be encouraged. Joint protection through the use of night splints or assistive devices may be indicated. Prone positioning for 20 to 30 minutes should be encouraged to help reduce hip flexion contractures, and the use of pillows under the knee should be discouraged because this can cause knee flexion contractures.[7,11]

The occurrence of deconditioning in the chronically ill pediatric client has been well documented in the professional literature.[13,14,15] Some have speculated that the level of deconditioning is directly related to the level of joint involvement. As the arthritic involvement intensifies, the activity of the client becomes low or hypoactive, and the deconditioning process begins.[13] Giannini and Protas[15] demonstrated, in a comparative examination between clients with JRA and clients without JRA, that tolerance to exercise was lower in the JRA group; however, the lower tolerance was not related to the severity of the disease process. They suggested that deconditioning will occur in the JRA client due to hypoactivity, but that all JRA clients have the potential to exercise aerobically. Clinically, the rehabilitation team should individually evaluate the ability of the client with JRA to participate in aerobic exercises to prevent deconditioning.

Overall body conditioning should be included in the client's home exercise program and educational considerations. During an acute onset of symptoms, the client may become sedentary due to the severity of the pain. However, during a period of mild or no symptoms, the client should be encouraged to be as active as possible. Activities that have a significant weight-bearing component (e.g., such as walking, running, jumping) may be avoided to prevent the onset of acute symptoms. Non–weight-bearing activities, such as aquatic therapies and a stationary bike, may be beneficial. Harkcom et al.[16] found that aerobic activity three times per week benefited the arthritic women in his study. The amount of physical activity the pediatric client with JRA is able to perform is directly dependent on the severity and extent of the disease process.[7]

Possible surgical management of the client with JRA includes hip and knee arthroplasty, **synovectomy**, surgical releases of contracted soft tissue, and possibly an **arthrodesis**. The physical therapy team will be involved postsurgically implementing a similar therapeutic program to achieve the same therapeutic goals.[3,7]

The expected physical therapy outcomes related to managing a pediatric client with JRA include [5]:

1. Improving the health-related quality of life
2. Promoting improved functional skills
3. Reducing risk of further disability from identified limitations
4. Promoting an understanding of factors that may contribute to jeopardizing health status
5. Promoting an understanding of strategies to prevent further disability

The expected time frame for outcome achievement can range significantly, depending on the severity of the disease and extent of the disability. A minimum course of intervention could be 4 months, but may extend to as many a 10 months of periodic care, assessment, and intervention.

GROWTH DISORDERS

An otherwise normal child may begin to develop structural problems and conditions as a result of growth. A child's height doubles between ages 2 and 18 years. This growth period can place tremendous stress and strain on the skeletal frame, joints, tendons, muscles, and the central nervous system. Often, the onset of puberty initiates the rapid growth of an individual; however, some growth-related dysfunctions may occur in late childhood as well. Two relatively common pediatric growth disorders will be discussed: (1) idiopathic scoliosis and (2) slipped capital femoral epiphysis.

Idiopathic Scoliosis

The spine has normal anterior and posterior curvature reflected as a cervical lordosis, thoracic kyphosis, and lumbar lordosis. The anterior and posterior curves dynamically add structure and support to the axial skeleton. However, when abnormal lateral curves are noted, the deformity is called **scoliosis**. The word scoliosis comes from the Greek word skolíōsis, meaning "curved or crooked." A scoliotic curve can be either structural or nonstructural. A structural or irreversible scoliosis will not reduce when the client is positioned supine or when asked to forward flex. A rotational component of the vertebrae typically accompanies a structural scoliosis. A nonstructural or reversible scoliosis will straighten or reduce when the client is positioned supine or asked to flex forward. A nonstructural scoliosis will not have a rotatory component and is typically a secondary effect of another condition. Poor posture, leg-length discrepancies, and muscle spasms of the spinal column muscles can produce a nonstructural scoliosis.[3,17]

The presence of a lateral curve in the spine of a pediatric client may have a compensatory effect on the rest of the body. If the appearance of the shoulders is level and directly over the pelvis, the scoliosis is a compensated curve. The main,

Synovectomy
The surgical removal of a diseased synovial membrane.

Arthrodesis
The surgical immobilization of a joint.

Scoliosis
The presence of abnormal lateral curvature in the spine. It can be of a structural or nonstructural nature.

primary, or largest curve develops a secondary or compensatory curve to keep the shoulders level. If the shoulders are not level and are structurally offset from the pelvis, the curve is uncompensated (Fig 8–6). A curve is identified to the right or left by the direction of the convex surface of the curve. The apex of the curve is named by the vertebrae that are at the peak of the lateral curve either to the left or the right (Fig. 8–6). Suspected curves are measured either radiographically or through **Moiré topography**. The curve is graded by degrees, with a mild deformity considered to be greater than 10°, a moderate deformity greater than 20°, and a severe deformity greater than 30°.[3,17]

The term *idiopathic* means that there is no known etiology for the onset of scoliosis; however, some hereditary traits have been identified. Three age-dependent onsets of idiopathic scoliosis can affect an otherwise healthy pediatric client: 1) infantile, 2) juvenile, and 3) adolescent. Infantile scoliosis affects newborns to 3-year-olds. Juvenile scoliosis affects young children from ages 3 to 10 years. Lastly, adolescent scoliosis, the most common type, which accounts for 70% to 80% of all scoliosis cases, affects children older than 10 years. Idiopathic scoliosis predominantly affects girls, and infantile scoliosis is more common in young boys. Any combination of cervical, thoracic, thoracolumbar, or lumbar curve is possible, but the most common statistical scoliosis deformity is a right thoracic curve. The frequency of the idiopathic scoliosis with curves greater than 20° in the general population is 1 to 3 cases in 1000 people.[3,17]

Clinical Presentation. The onset of the scoliosis is slow and generally asymptomatic. Without close examination, the development of the deformity may go unnoticed by either the client or the client's parents for several years. External symptoms exhibit as unequal shoulder height, one longer pant's leg, or scapular winging. If the client has not received intervention previous to these deformities being noticed, then the structural deformity has been well established, necessitating medical intervention.

Evaluation: Tools and Methods. Early intervention and screening by the rehabilitation team have significantly aided in the identification of the onset of idiopathic scoliosis in the pediatric population. Screening in all children has significantly reduced the amount of invasive spinal surgeries needed to correct severe deformities. The primary screening tools used are the forward bend test in which the examiner examines the spine externally for the presence of abnormal deviations or "rib humps" (Fig. 8–7). Other evaluation tools include leg-length measurements, palpation, posture assessment, gait assessment, ROM, strength, spinal mobility assessment, and functional status. Pulmonary function tests are warranted in severe curves because of rib cage restrictions and decreased chest wall expansion.[5]

Clinical Management. Scoliosis is caused by a growth dysfunction of the spine, leading to structural deformity. For the client who presents with idiopathic scoliosis, medical intervention is necessary to prevent the progression of the deformity. Conservative or surgical management are two accepted pathways of treatment, depending on the severity of the lateral curvature.

Conservative Management. Conservative management of idiopathic scoliosis is often the first-line management. Mild curves are usually not directly treated but are monitored for progression by a health-care professional. Moderate and severe curves can be treated conservatively. Orthotic management and lateral electrical stimulation are the two most common conservative modalities.[3,17]

Moiré Topography
A noninvasive technique by which light is projected through grids onto the back of the client to assess topographical asymmetry. Advantage of use is the avoidance of exposure to x-rays.

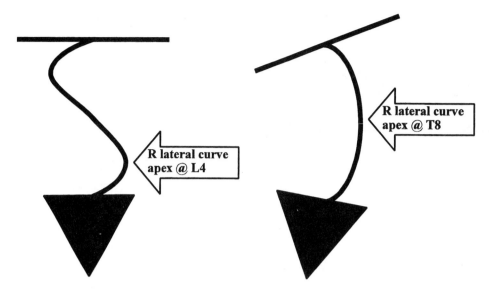

FIG. 8–6

Scoliosis. A lateral curve is said to be compensated if the shoulders are level and even with the pelvis (left). A lateral curve is said to be uncompensated if the shoulders are not level and offset from the pelvis (right). The curve is named right or left according to the direction of the convex surface. The apex is the lateral most vertebrae or the peak of the lateral curve.

Orthotic bracing has been a well-established modality used in slowing the progression of idiopathic scoliosis for the better part of the twentieth century. The primary goal of orthotic management is the slowing of progression, not the reversal of the deformity. This is often a misconception of the client when the orthotic is applied. Historically, the Boston and Milwaukee braces have been associated with conservative management, but the modern-day orthotist uses various custom-fitted, close-fitting, rigid devices and shells grouped into the broad category of thoracic-lumbosacral orthosis ([TLSO]; Fig. 8–8). If the cervical region needs rigid support as well, extensions on the orthosis make the device a CTLSO. These custom-fitted orthotics are generally worn 23 hours per day (minus one hour for personal hygiene needs) over a course of several years. The critical time period is during the growth phases of the individual.[3,17]

Functional electrical stimulation is delivered to the paraspinal muscles on the convex side of the primary curve as a method used to retard progression of the spinal deformity. Originally fashioned by an orthopedic surgeon named Bobechko, the theory proposed that intermittent stimulation of great enough amplitude would cause a force contraction on the convexity to slow down or even reverse progression. Standard surface electrodes can be positioned accordingly on the convex side of the deformity while the client is asleep. As a substitution for orthotic management, electrical stimulation is appealing. The client is not forced to wear a cumbersome orthosis throughout the day. However, some studies have identified that the use of lateral electrical stimulation as a single intervention is ineffective in almost 60% of the cases studied.[18,19] The use of electrical stimulation as the only intervention may not be as effective as bracing; however, outcome studies using a combination of orthotic management and electrical stimulation could be warranted.

Physical therapy exercise intervention in conservative management of idiopathic scoliosis is still controversial.[20] Exercise alone has very little, if any, chance of successfully reducing a moderate or severe spinal deformity.[17] The use of exercise in scoliosis management has been misidentified as curative. In fact, the inclusion of flexibility exercises and strengthening exercises should be identified not as a means of reducing the abnormal curve, but as a means of maintaining posture and function. Goals of a general scoliosis exercise program include:

1. Development of postural awareness
2. Determination that there is adequate chest-wall mobility for breathing
3. Promotion of proper length and strength relationships of spinal and extremity musculature
4. Promotion of spinal mobility for functional activities
5. Promotion of normal function and activity of the client

Various flexibility, strengthening, conditioning, and stabilizing exercises should be identified in the physical therapist's plan of treatment. Specified treatment parameters should then be implemented by the PTA and a home exercise program provided to the client.

The expected physical therapy outcomes for managing a client with scoliosis include[5]:

1. Improved health-related quality of life
2. Optimal functioning
3. Prevention of further deformity.

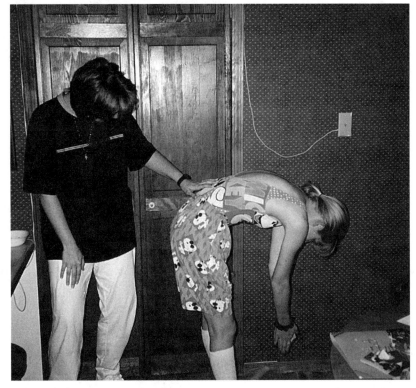

FIG. 8–7
Scoliosis screening. By having the client forward flex at the spine and hips, keeping the palms of the hands together, the examiner can look for spinal symmetry or the presence of a "rib hump" where one side of the thoracic spine sits higher than the opposite side.

FIG. 8–8
Orthotic management for idiopathic scoliosis. The use of rigid trunk orthoses has been common in the conservative management of idiopathic scoliosis. The client wears the custom-fit orthosis for several years during the peak growth time to limit progression of the spinal deformity.

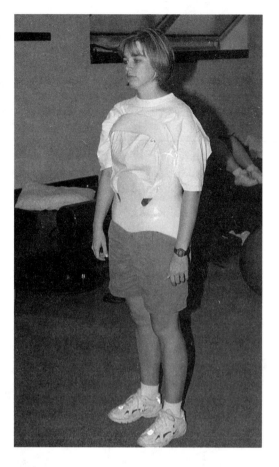

Depending on the severity of the lateral curve when identified, the course of physical therapy intervention will vary from as little as one or two educational visits to up to 12 months of rehabilitative intervention after major spinal surgery.

Surgical Management. Surgical management is indicated when the curve reaches 40° and the client is still growing, or when the client has stopped growing, but the curve is in excess of 50°. Surgical goals are to (1) straighten the spine as much as possible without causing other damage, (2) balance the trunk and pelvis, and (3) promote stability of the spine by fusing the affected area. Surgical intervention uses various rods and stabilizing devices in combination with bone grafts to promote the goal of fixation and stabilization. After successful surgery, the client is usually immobilized in a TLSO for added stability. As with any spinal surgery, there is risk of damage to the neural elements.[17]

Postsurgical physical therapy intervention will include a baseline assessment of posture, ROM, mobility, leg length, muscle strength, respiratory function, and functional status. Treatment includes the following[17]:

1. Breathing exercises
   a. To promote rib cage expansion
   b. To promote effective coughing
   c. For pulmonary hygiene (postural drainage used as needed).

2. Functional mobility exercises
    a. Log rolling when moving from supine to sit to prevent excessive spinal movement
    b. Lower-extremity strengthening, as needed, for functional skills
    c. Transfer training
    d. Gait training as needed
3. Client education
    a. To promote knowledge of proper use of the external orthotic device (TLSO).

Slipped Capital Femoral Epiphysis

The hip joint is subject to a significant amount of force during normal weight-bearing activities. The positioning of the femur into the acetabulum at an oblique angle encourages a shear force that potentially can damage the integrity of the proximal head of the femur. In growing pediatric clients, an epiphyseal growth plate is found proximally in the head of the femur to allow for growth in length proximally and is subject to injury from excessive stresses. A pediatric orthopedic condition relative to growth is referred to as slipped capital femoral epiphysis (adolescent coxa vara). The excessive shear forces cause the neck of the femur to "slip" upwardly and anteriorly in relation to the epiphysis. This can either be a gradual event or a sudden traumatic event.[3]

Young male clients beginning at age 9 years or the onset of the adolescent growth period are highly susceptible to having this condition. Typically the onset begins only in one hip, but about 30% of the cases are bilateral. Two male body types are at risk for the occurrence of a slipped capital femoral epiphysis: (1) very tall, thin, and rapidly growing; or (2) short, stocky, and overweight. The etiology of the disease is not completely understood but may be related to rapid growth that extends the epiphyseal plate, hormonal imbalances, and excessive shear forces at the proximal hip. If the shifting is sudden, the potential for vascular damage is great with a resulting necrosis of the femoral head.[3]

Clinical Presentation. The most common initial symptom of the client that fits the at-risk profile is mild to moderate discomfort in the affected hip. Often the pain is referred to the ipsilateral knee. When knee pathology is ruled out, the pain is often diagnosed as "growing pains." As the slipping progresses, a mild Trendelenburg gait may develop and noted external rotation of the involved lower extremity is seen.[3]

Evaluation: Tools and Methods. Suspected diagnosis comes from clinical observation of gait, anthropometric characteristics, posture, ROM, and client history. If the physical therapist passively flexes the hip, an associated external rotation of the femur will be noted as the client demonstrates marked limitations of hip internal rotation. The physician will confirm the diagnosis with a radiographic examination. The initial evaluation should also include a complete history and status of current condition, functional status analysis, and appropriate systems (cardiopulmonary, integumentary, musculoskeletal and neuromuscular) review as needed.[3,5]

Clinical Management. Conservative management of this pediatric client with slipped capital femoral eiphysis includes the avoidance of further damage or remodeling of the affected hip joint and the preservation of the blood supply to the head of the femur. Surgical stabilization with orthopedic pins is usually indicated. After successful stabilization, the client should not bear weight on the affected lower extremity for several months while healing progresses. Initially, gait training is warranted to ensure effective non–weight-bearing patterns and the prevention of damage to the repaired hip. ROM and strengthening exercises to the surgically repaired hip are introduced by the rehabilitation team when sufficient healing has occurred. Gait training at this point will focus on the minimization of the Trendelenburg gait, if present.[3]

The structural changes within the hip joint resulting from the movement of the neck of the femur on the capital epiphysis may produce long-term implications for the client. The altered kinematics may predispose this client to degenerative changes at the joint surface itself. The client should be educated about this possible scenario and encouraged to engage in non–weight-bearing conditioning activities (swimming) as opposed to stressful impact activities (running). The lifelong maintenance of the strength and stability of the hip will help minimize the potential for degenerative changes in adulthood.[21]

The expected physical therapy outcomes for managing a client with a slipped capital epiphysis include[5]:

1. Promoting an improved health-related quality of life
2. Promoting a return of maximal function
3. Promote an understanding of risk factors
4. Preventing further disability

Length of intervention may last from 1 month to 1 year, depending on the severity of the condition.

OSTEOCHONDROPATHIES

Osteochondrosis
A condition causing degenerative changes in the epiphyseal plates of bones during periods of rapid growth. The process may mature to a state of avascular or aseptic necrosis of the bone with very slow healing and repair.

The general condition causing degenerative changes in the epiphyseal plates of bones is referred to as **osteochondrosis**. The condition typically appears during periods of rapid growth from ages 3 to 10 years. There is much debate in the professional literature as to the exact etiology of osteochondrosis. Many theories clearly identify that the degenerative changes are a result of avascular necrosis in the epiphyseal plate, although it is unclear why this occurs. Many specific disorders are identified by the particular bony part that is affected by the degenerative changes. Legg-Calvé-Perthes, Scheuermann's, and Osgood-Schlatter diseases are all examples of orthopedic pediatric conditions related to osteochondrosis.[3]

Legg-Calvé-Perthes Disease

Osteochondrosis of the femoral head is the most common and most serious of the pediatric avascular conditions. It commonly occurs in boys (4:1 over girls) between the ages of 3 and 11 years, is bilateral in 15% of the cases with positive familial tendencies. There is some indication that the very physically active male client may be more susceptible to this condition. The pathophysiology of Legg-Calvé-Perthes disease exhibits as necrosis of the epiphyseal plate with subsequent collapse and destruction of the subchondral bone. The head of the femur flattens (coxa plana) in the acetabulum making the arthrokinematics of the hip joint ineffective. The healing process is slow as the blood supply gradually returns peripherally, then migrating centrally. Long-term implications of the condition include degenerative arthritis, subchondral fractures, and joint subluxation.[3,22]

Clinical Presentation. The client may not initially seek assistance from a health-care professional because the early symptoms of the destructive process are silent. When symptoms do present, they include hip pain, but more often knee pain, hip joint effusion from synovitis, and an antalgic gait pattern. There may be a limitation of hip abduction and internal rotation with disuse atrophy present about the hip. If a Trendelenburg gait is noticed, this is most likely indicative of degenerative changes occurring at the joint surface. Radiographic examination confirms the diagnosis of Legg-Calvé-Perthes disease.[3,22]

Evaluation: Tools and Methods. Evaluation data may include:

1. General demographics of the client
2. An accurate history of current condition, including growth and development record
3. Current functional status
   a. Gait, locomotion, balance
   b. Assessment of assistive and adaptive devices used
4. Appropriate systems review
   a. **Cardiopulmonary:** aerobic capacity and endurance
   b. **Integumentary:** status of skin relative to bracing or casting
   c. **Musculoskeletal:** ROM, strength, posture, joint integrity
   d. **Neuromuscular:** reflexes, sensory, pain[5]

Clinical Management. The older the child is at the time of onset (after age 8 years), the less likely the outcomes will be completely successful. If the child is younger than age 5 years, the prognosis is very good. Clinical management of the condition centers on the prevention of orthopedic deformity of the femoral head and protection of the hip joint to allow for the gradual revascularization. Although some orthopedic surgeons believe that no intervention is warranted—because no conclusive evidence suggests that immobilization affects outcomes—an immobilization process that relieves weight bearing on the lower extremity is indicated. The pediatric client is placed in abduction plaster casts or splints that hold the hip in a stable position to promote healing and prevent further deformity. Surgical intervention, including femoral or innominate osteotomy procedures, is reserved for older clients who were not successfully managed conservatively.[3,22]

Physical therapy management of the pediatric client with Legg-Calvé-Perthes disease is indicated after the successful healing of the fragile femoral epiphysis. When the hip joint is stabilized and deformity is minimized, the client needs intervention to minimize gait deviations through the reduction of soft-tissue contractures and the promotion of adequate hip strength. Normal joint kinematics need to be promoted to reduce excessive stress and strain on the joint surfaces. Client and family education is necessary to learn strategies to protect the hip joint and minimize degenerative changes into adulthood.

According to the Preferred Practice Patterns,[5] physical therapy outcomes include:

1. Improved health-related quality of life for the client
2. Optimal return of function
3. An understanding of current condition's risk factors
4. Prevention of further disability

These outcomes should be achieved in less than 16 weeks for nonsurgical cases, but may require as much as 12 months of intervention in surgically repaired cases.[5]

Scheuermann's Disease

Osteochondrosis of the thoracic spine is named Scheuermann's disease. Avascular necrosis of the anterior portion of three to four adjacent thoracic vertebrae results in a premature closing of the anterior epiphyseal plates while the posterior halves continue to grow. The result is an adolescent kyphosis or an anterior wedging to the affected vertebrae (Fig. 8–9). It is a fairly common adolescent condition affecting males and females equally. There is a mild hereditary factor. The etiology is unknown, but the condition may be related to microtrauma or vascular compromise.[3]

Clinical Presentation. This condition is typically identified in school or by the parents because the client is noticed to have "rounded" shoulders. The initial onset of the condition, like most of the osteochondropathies, is asymptomatic. Once the external signs are identified, the avascular process to the anterior portion of the vertebrae is well estabished. Eventually, the client may complain of an aching sensation in the upper spine. On visual examination, there is a noted thoracic kyphosis with a secondary hyperlordosis.[3]

Evaluation: Tools and Methods. The adolescent client with Scheuermann's disease may never be referred for physical therapy unless the symptoms during the growth periods become unmanageable. The physical therapist should take a comprehensive history followed by an evaluation of the client's functional status, relevant systems review and posture.[5]

Clinical Management. The prognosis for this condition is very good, because all symptoms will resolve when the adolescent client stops growing. However, the fixed spinal kyphotic deformity remains. Physical therapy agents may be used during the painful stage; however, deep thermal agents should be avoided because of the potential for disruption of the growth plates. Postural awareness exercises may be indicated in decreasing the progression of the kyphotic condition. An external TLSO (such as a Milwaukee brace) may be modified to help limit the progression of the condition during growth periods.
The expected physical therapy outcomes include[5]:

1. Improved health-related quality of life
2. An understanding of how to prevent future disabilities

The intervention for this client may be as little as one outpatient visit for education and home exercise program instruction or up to several months for pain-control intervention.

Osteochondritis Dissecans

The convex surfaces of some joints are susceptible to avascular necrosis processes. Osteochondritis dissecans occurs when a small piece of subchondral bone separates from the distal end of the epiphysis and floats freely in the joint. The knee and elbow joints are most commonly involved by this relatively uncommon condition. The process typically occurs in older male adolescents and has an unknown etiology. There may be a familial tendency, but trauma may also cause the avascular necrosis and resulting separation of bone.[3]

Clinical Presentation. It is possible that the necrosis process affecting a small section of the subchondral bone heals in time, and never detaching. The client

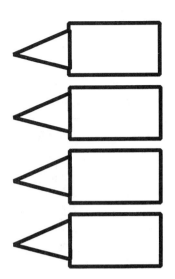 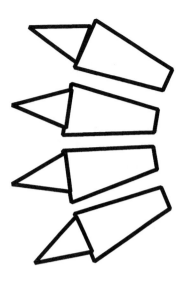

FIG. 8–9
Scheuermann's disease. As the avascular process of osteochondrosis of the thoracic spine progresses, the result is a collapse and wedging of the anterior aspect of the thoracic vertebrae. An adolescent kyphosis is exhibited.

may remain relatively asymptomatic with only intermittent aching in the involved joint and no joint motion limitations. However, if the necrosis process results in a bone fragment separation, the free-floating piece is referred to as a "joint mouse." In addition to the aching and irritation that results from the disruption of the bone, the client will complain of intermittent locking and catching of the joint as the joint mouse becomes wedged in the joint during movement. Arthroscopic examination usually confirms the presence of a joint mouse and the original defect.[3]

Evaluation: Tools and Methods. In either surgical or nonsurgical intervention, the physical therapist should obtain a complete history of current condition followed by a relevant systems review. The musculoskeletal review should include ROM, strength, and functional status assessments, and the integumentary review should address the status of the surgical incision or the presence of edema or joint effusion.[5]

Clinical Management. The prognosis for a client with osteochondritis dissecans is very good if the client is young and still growing and if the involved area is on a non–weight-bearing aspect of the joint surface. If the client is older with epiphyseal plates nearly closed and the affected area involves a weight-bearing surface, the potential for long-term degenerative changes is possible. If the client does not present with a joint mouse, the goal of treatment is to promote a positive non-weight-bearing atmosphere for healing. The rehabilitation team may instruct the client in a non–weight-bearing gait pattern with appropriate assistive device to allow the necrotic tissue to remain intact while healing. If the necrotic patch becomes isolated, surgical repair or removal is necessary. After surgical intervention, the rehabilitation team will address postsurgical concerns of edema, pain, ROM, strength, with return to functional activities as appropriate. If the avascular defect was significant in size, the client must be educated in the prevention of future disability from degenerative joint disease.

According to the Preferred Practice Patterns,[5] the expected physical therapy outcomes for managing a client with osteochondritis dissecans include:

1. Promote improved health-related quality of life
2. Promote optimal function
3. Promote an understanding of how to prevent future disabilities

Nonsurgical interventions may require a minimal number of outpatient visits with client education and a home exercise program emphasized by the physical therapy team. Surgical intervention may require up to 3 months of skilled intervention to achieve expected outcomes.

Osgood-Schlatter Disease

The tendon insertion of the patellar tendon into the tibial tuberosity is the site for an osteochondrosis pathology common in skeletally immature active males. The repeated, stressful traction force on the developing epiphysis adjacent to the tibial tuberosity results in a partial avulsion of the bony prominence. Subsequent to the avulsion, the avulsed portion becomes necrotic.[3]

Clinical Presentation. The active client will complain of sharp pain with certain activities, localized at the irritated tibial tuberosity. Kneeling on the affected knee, running, jumping, and any direct impact to the anterior lower knee will reproduce the painful symptoms. On visual inspection, a noted anterior deformity of the tibial tuberosity is observed and most likely is tender to palpation. On x-ray, the involved area is visibly separated from the anterior aspect of the tibia (Fig. 8–10).

Evaluation: Tools and Methods. When the client with Osgood-Schlatter disease presents to the rehabilitation team, the physical therapist will evaluate the client. The components of the examination should include a history of the disease and demographics of the client, functional status, and relative systems review. The musculoskeletal examination should focus on pain, ROM, strength, joint integrity, gait and balance. The client may have noted discomfort in the affected area with palpation and resistive assessments.[5]

Clinical Management. Although the painful symptoms do not quickly resolve, the tibial tuberosity will completely ossify in 2 to 3 years, depending on the age of onset. After skeletal maturity is reached, the symptoms resolve, but the anterior deformity remains. In extreme cases, the avulsion does not ossify and remains mobile with persistent symptoms of pain and instability. Management includes limiting the acute symptoms of irritation and inflammation that are occurring during the avulsion process. Activity is not halted, but modification is encouraged to minimize discomfort. Stressful running and repetitive jumping should be limited during acute symptoms. Isometric quadricep femoris exercises can replace isotonic strengthening exercises when discomfort persists. Cryotherapy works well in reducing acute painful symptoms. Taping of the patellar tendon or the use of patellar supportive straps helps to decrease the pull on the involved tibial tuberosity (Fig. 8–11).

The expected physical therapy outcomes for managing a client with Osgood-Schlatter disease include[5]:

1. An improved health-related quality of life
2. Return of optimal function

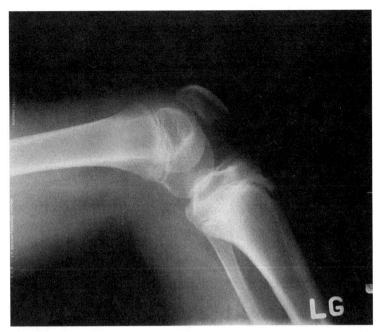

FIG. 8–10
X-ray of a client with Osgood-Schlatter's disease. Radiographic examination will reveal a widening space between the tibial tuberosity and the tibia. With the extreme force application from the quadriceps tendon, the tuberosity is literally suffering an avulsion from the bone.

3. An understanding of the disease process and risk factors
4. Prevention of further disability.

Most clients will successfully be treated conservatively for 2 weeks to 2 months under the supervision of the rehabilitation team.

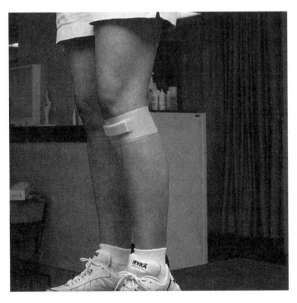

FIG. 8–11
Patellar taping for Osgood-Schlatter's disease. The use of a small felt bar, prewrap, and white athletic tape can splint the patellar tendon effectively to reduce acute symptoms of Osgood-Schlatter's disease. Through small modification of activities, the client should be able to participate in all desired activities.

CONGENITAL CONDITIONS

Orthopedic dysfunctions or deformities that are present at the birth of an infant are classified as congenital orthopedic conditions. One of the greatest parental fears during the 9 months while awaiting birth of their child is the thought that the newborn may be delivered with a dysfunction or deformity. Some conditions, such as congenital amputations, may be readily visible just after the delivery, whereas other, such as development dysplasia of the hip, may not appear for several months. The psychosocial demands, anxieties, and uncertainties can be addressed by the skillful and compassionate rehabilitation team in providing accurate, reliable, and realistic information about the condition. The rehabilitation team should become a valued resource for the new parents in terms of therapeutic handling, positioning, and development to effectively manage the congenital orthopedic condition.

CONGENITAL AMPUTATIONS

The loss of a limb or a limb present with an abnormality at birth can be traumatic to both the pediatric client and the parents. Acquired amputations are more common than congenital amputations, but each has its own unique psychosocial adjustment period. The child that loses a limb from a traumatic event will often have a grieving process over loss of the limb, and possibly guilt or anger will accompany the condition. If the amputation is congenital, the child may never experience loss; however, the parents of the child may demonstrate the feelings of loss, guilt, or anger for the child. May[23] claims that "most congenital amputations result from prenatal or birth deficits" and goes on to state that many "amputations will require subsequent surgical amputation for conversion of the anomaly to enable better prosthetic fitting." Not only must the parents and the pediatric client endure the birth with subsequent awareness of the anomaly, but are potentially faced with further revisions and corrective surgeries.[23]

Clinical Presentation

Anomalies that are present at birth can involve either the upper or lower extremities. Below-the-elbow (BE) congenital amputations are the most common, yet various combinations of anomalies and amputations involving all body parts are plausible. Surgical intervention to improve the function of the abnormal limb is sometimes required. The presence of a congenital amputation may also lead to secondary complications as the pediatric client begins to grow and develop. Overgrowth phenomenon presents as the child with a congenital amputation grows normally. The residual bone grows excessively in width involving congenital amputations of the humerus, fibula, tibia, and femur. A "pincer-like" contour may eventually develop as overgrowth occurs with the radius in relation to the ulna in terminal BE amputations, or the overgrowth of the ulna may result in a subcutaneous projection. In pediatric clients that present with congenital joint disarticulations, a possible lack of growth in residual limb may create a new limb-length discrepancy in comparison to the nonaffected limb.[22,23]

Evaluation: Tools and Methods. The physical therapist should follow a systematic evaluation plan for preprosthetic and prosthetic concerns of the pediatric client with a congenital or revised amputation. The component parts of the evaluation should include demographic data gathering and evaluation of

(1) medical history, (2) skin integrity, (3) length of residual limb, (4) shape of residual limb, (5) ROM, (6) muscle strength, (7) neurological screening, and (8) functional status of the client. Table 8–1 describes detailed subcomponents of the physical therapist's evaluation methods for the pediatric client with a congenital amputation.[5,23]

Clinical Management. Management of the pediatric client with a congenital deformity will be specific to the client's age and development. Use of various prosthetic appliances for either the upper or lower extremity that can be custom-fitted may significantly promote improved mobility and function. However, in some extreme cases, as when an entire extremity is absent, the pediatric client may find that the use of a prosthesis actually decreases function: The extreme energy demands needed to manipulate a full-extremity prosthesis may be too great for such clients. Development of motor and cognitive skills will help dictate when the child is ready to be challenged with the use of a prosthesis. An upper-extremity prosthesis may be fitted to the client when he or she begins normal bilateral hand activity as early as 3 to 6 months. Likewise, a prosthesis may be fitted when the client demonstrates the efforts to pull to a standing position (6 to 14 months). Careful fitting, monitoring, and education by the rehabilitation team will promote effective and successful implementation of prosthetic appliances into the pediatric client's everyday life. Figures 8–12 and 8-13 present the use of prosthetic devices to promote function for clients with congenital amputations. May[23] provides an in-depth analysis of the functional use of prosthetic devices in the management of amputations.

The expected physical therapy outcomes related to managing a client with an amputation include[5]:

1. Improved health-related quality of life
2. Optimal return to function
3. Improved safety of client
4. Prevention of future disabilities

The expected time to achieve these outcomes should be less than 6 months; however, the pediatric client with an amputation will experience frequent reassessments as growth dictates assistive and prosthetic device refitting or revisions.

DEVELOPMENTAL DYSPLASIA OF THE HIP

Developmental dysplasia of the hip (DDH) is a condition that describes a wide range of hip dysfunctions in the pediatric client from neonatal hip instability to adolescent fixed hip dislocation.[24] Salter[3] claims that DDH is "one of the most challenging and most important [pediatric] abnormalities of the musculoskeletal system. [U]nless treated early and well, [DDH] leads inevitably to painful crippling degenerative arthritis of the hip in adult life. Indeed, at least one third of all degenerative joint disease of the hip in adults is caused by the sequelae of [DDH]."

Hip dysfunction and **dysplasia** in pediatric clients is a fairly common condition. The incident of occurrence is 1.5 in 1000 live births and tends to involve the left hip slightly more than the right hip. Bilateral involvement occurs in more than half of the diagnosed cases. Females are affected eight times more often than males. The incidence of DDH is greater in pediatric clients who have other congenital conditions, including equinovarus and abnormal muscular tone.[3,25,26]

Dysplasia
The abnormal development of tissue.

Table 8–1

PREPROSTHETIC EVALUATION GUIDE

General Medical Information	Cause of amputation (disease, tumor, trauma, congenital)
	Associated diseases and symptoms (neuropathy, visual disturbances, cardiopulmonary disease, renal failure, congenital anomalies)
	Current physiological state (postsurgical cardiopulmonary status, vital signs, OOB, pain)
	Medications
Skin	Scar (healed, adherent, invaginated, flat)
	Other lesions (size, shape, open, scar tissue)
	Moisture (moist, dry, scaly)
	Sensation (absent, diminshed, hyperesthesia)
	Grafts (location, type, healing)
	Dermatologic lesions (psoriasis, eczema, cysts)
Residual Limb Length	Bone length (transtibial limbs measured from medial tibial plateau; transfemoral limbs measured from ischial tuberosity or greater trochanter)
	Soft tissue length (note redundant tissue)
Residual Limb Shape	Cylindrical, conical, bulbous end, or the like
	Abnormalities ("dog ears," adductor roll)
Vascularity (Both Limbs if Amputation Cause is Vascular)	Pulses (femoral, popliteal, dorsalis, pedis, posterior tibial)
	Color (red, cyanotic)
	Temperature
	Edema (circumference measurement, water displacement measurement, caliper measurement)
	Pain (type, location, duration)
	Trophic changes
Range of Motion	Residual limb (specific for remaining joints)
	Other lower extremity (gross for major joints)
Muscle Strength	Residual limb (specific for major muscle groups)
	Other extremities (gross for necessary function)
Neurologic	Pain [phantom (differentiate sensation or pain), neuroma, incisional, other causes]
	Neuropathy
	Cognitive status (alert, oriented, confused)
	Emotional status (acceptance, body image)
Functional Status	Transfers (bed to chair, to toilet, to car)
	Balance (sitting, standing, reaching, moving)
	Mobility (ancillary support, supervision, closed and open environments, steps, curbs)
	Home and family situation (caregiver, architectural barriers, hazards)
	Activities of daily living (bathing, dressing)
	Instrumental activities of daily living (cooking, cleaning)
Other	Vital signs
	Preamputation status (work, activity level, degree of independence, lifestyle)
	Prosthetic goals (desire for prosthesis, anticipated activity level, lifestyle)
	Financial (available means to pay for prosthesis)
	Prior prosthesis (if bilateral)

Source: May,[23] p 73, with permission.

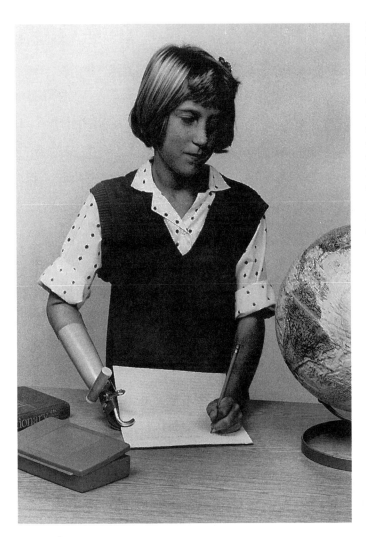

FIG. 8–12
Upper extremity prosthesis to improve function. Prosthetic devices can significantly improve upper extremity function if the energy cost of utilization is not extreme. (Courtesy of Hosmer Dorrance Corp., Campbell, CA.) (From May, BJ: *Amputations and Prosthetics: A Case Study Approach*. FA Davis, Philadelphia, 1996, p 215, with permission.)

Dislocation of the hip in the pediatric client is probably a combination of genetic attributes and environmental factors. The exact etiology of the disease is unknown and debated among scholars. A possible explanation is genetic predisposition to dislocation of the hip. Another explanation may be the release of hormones by the mother during pregnancy. The newborn may be susceptible to the hormones that relax the mother's ligaments of the pelvis to widen the birth canal for delivery, making the newborn's ligaments about the hip structurally lax. A third explanation is that the fetal position of the baby during gestation has promoted extreme flexion of the hip and the subsequent extension after delivery can dislocate an immature hip. Most newborns (1 in 80) demonstrate undue hip joint laxity that spontaneously becomes stable within the first 2 months of life. This would suggest that handling at birth and in the first few months after birth could create a situation in which the hip dislocates leading to DDH.[3,27]

The condition of DDH that creates increasing dysfunction for the pediatric client is not the original dislocation insult of the hip, but the subsequent secondary changes that develop. With persistent dislocation or **subluxation** of the hip, degenerative changes are produced in the supporting structures in and around the hip joint. Possible secondary changes include (1) abnormal development of the

Dislocation
The temporary displacement of a bone from its normal position in a joint.

Subluxation
A partial or incomplete dislocation.

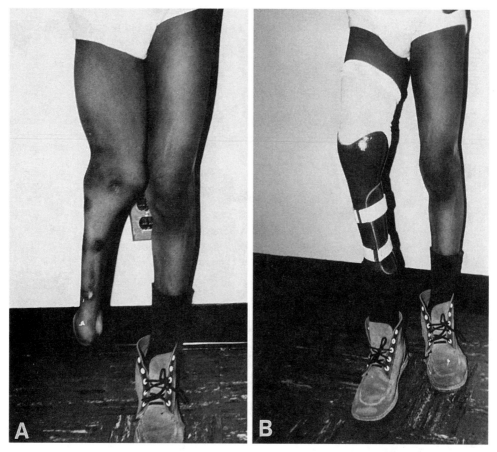

FIG. 8–13
Lower extremity prosthesis to improve function. Pictured in (A) is a congenital Syme's amputation of the right lower extremity; pictured in (B) is the prosthetic device used to promote functional gait activities. (From May, BJ: *Amputations and Prosthetics: A Case Study Approach.* FA Davis, Philadelphia, 1996, p 223, with permission.)

hip joint (hip dysplasia), (2) hypertrophy of the joint capsule, (3) joint contracture, (4) muscular shortening of all muscles that cross the joint (especially the hip flexor and the adductor groups), and (5) degenerative arthritis.[3]

Clinical Presentation

The newborn infant (0 to 3 months) will not have any visual clinical signs and the presence of a hip dislocation must be identified through manual or other diagnostic means. The older infant and toddler (3 months to 2 years) may present with an apparent leg-length discrepancy on the affected lower extremity and have had a significant delay in the ability to crawl or walk. A marked adduction contracture is most likely present. Pain and discomfort may be associated in the involved hip. In addition to the previous clinical signs, the client whose dislocation remained undetected until after age 2 years will present with significant gait deviations associated with a dislocated hip. If the involvement is unilateral, the child will demonstrate a Trendelenburg gait. If the involvement is bilateral, the gait deviation may resemble the waddling of a penguin as the client shifts the trunk over each affected limb to stabilize the lower extremity during the stance phase of gait.[3]

Evaluation: Tools and Methods

The early detection of the potential hip dislocation in newborns is the key to preventing the onset of DDH. If dislocation is prevented, or identified and treated early, then the hip joint will develop normally with the avoidance of the secondary conditions that arise from DDH. Evidence suggests that early detection within the first 3 months of life is critical in preventing the development of any secondary complications. The condition may be treated if detected after three months, but the clinical outcomes are less positive.[3,27]

Screening should occur at intervals at birth and early infancy. The evaluation tools that can be used include visual observation, manual examination with special tests, radiography, and diagnostic ultrasound. Salter[3] claims that the "abnormality is never obvious," and stresses that the condition must be sought out "by careful examination of every infant." The Barlow, Ortolani, Dupuytren (telescoping), and Galezzi tests and the passive abduction test are all used in the physical examination to identify a dislocated hip. Radiographic examination (Fig. 8–14) or diagnostic ultrasonography are used to confirm the diagnosis of a hip dislocation if manual special tests are positive.[3,5,28,29]

Clinical Management

To manage a client with DDH successfully, the rehabilitation team must consider the age of the client and when the hip dislocation was identified. For any client

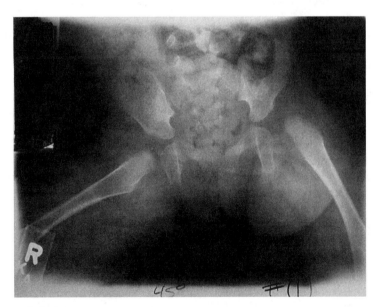

FIG. 8–14
X-ray of client with a congenital hip dislocation. Notice on the radiographic examination the different positioning of the proximal aspect of the femur in this pediatric client. The client's left hip is dislocated and positioned superiorly. If this condition remains undetected, the client will most likely develop significant dysfunction in the future.

identified with a hip dislocation, initial management must be the relocation of the hip into the acetabulum and ensuring future stability of the lax hip joint. The most favorable time frame for reduction and stabilization of the hip joint is in the first 3 months of life. The joint is usually easily reduced, and the stability is promoted by the use of a splint or a spica cast. The client remains in the splint or cast for 3 to 4 months, allowing the joint capsule of the hip to tighten and thus preventing future dislocation. Intervention by physical therapy professionals during this management is minimal: Once the child is removed from the splint, normal developmental progression resumes without much difficulty or limitation.[3,27,30]

The client that is not identified until between ages 3 and 18 months still has a very good prognosis, but the process of reducing the hip and ensuring long-term stability is more difficult and time consuming. The onset of secondary complications during this time frame necessitate the management of developed soft-tissue contractures around the hip joint. Sustained, low-load traction is indicated to reduce the contracture of the adductor group before the reduction of the hip joint. If the soft-tissue structures are not managed, the likelihood is low that the hip will remain stable. The traction units are now available for implementation in the home by the parents of the client to reduce prolonged hospitalization. Additional psychological benefits occur when the client is able to remain in the home maintaining as normal a routine as possible.[31] After successful reduction management of the soft-tissue contractures, the dysfunctional hip joint must be reduced either manually (closed-reduction) or surgically (open-reduction). After successful reduction, the client is placed in a plaster spica cast for a minimum of 6 months lasting to a maximum of 18 months. The cast is changed every 1 to 2 months for reexamination and hygiene purposes. After the cast is removed and hip joint stability assured, physical therapy is implemented to promote muscle-strength balance in the lower extremities, developmental activities, gait training, and the use of assistive devices as needed. The success of this age group relates directly to the early identification of the hip dysplasia. Positive outcomes lessen for the client that is identified closer to age 18 months compared with the child identified at 3 months. The overall success rate is 80% for clients that are identified in the 3- to 18-month age group.[3,27]

If the identification of a congenitally dislocated hip does not occur until after age 18 months, more severe secondary complications of DDH are already affecting the client. The success rate of managing the secondary complications is very low for this age group. Contractures of the hip are generally resistant to sustained traction, and reversal may occur only after surgical release of the contracted muscles, tendons, and soft tissue. Closed-reduction results are poor. The poorly developed acetabulum does not accept the placement of the head of the femur. Multiple surgeries are often needed to rebuild the shape and integrity of the hip joint. Postsurgical immobilization in a spica cast or splint is required to help maintain the integrity of the repaired hip joint. Physical therapy intervention after immobilization is designed to promote muscle strengthening of the hip joint muscles, gait training, postural exercises, and use of assistive devices as needed. Educating the client and family about the disease process, positioning, and postsurgical handling is essential. The ultimate goal of physical therapy intervention is the promotion of normal function. The success rate in achieving a stable hip joint in these clients is less than 50%. It is more likely that the client will have continued onset of secondary complications of DDH including degenerative joint disease.[3,27]

The expected outcomes of physical therapy intervention vary depending on the client's age when the condition was identified. Another factor to be considered is the extent of medical intervention, whether it be conservative or surgical. At the minimum, the expected outcomes include[5]:

1. An improved health-related quality of life
2. Optimal function
3. An understanding of risk factors
4. Prevention of further disability.

Severity of the condition will determine the length of skilled intervention. It may range from 1 month to 1 year. If subsequent surgical interventions are warranted, a second intervention period will be necessary.

EQUINOVARUS

Talipes **equinovarus** is commonly known as "clubfoot." This congenital orthopedic deformity is easily identified on visual inspection, but sometimes less effectively managed. The foot is in a combination position of forefoot adduction, supination, excessive calcaneal varus, and medial tibial torsion. The involved joints include the talocalcaneal, talonavicular, and calcaneocuboid joints. Some form of clubfoot is found in 2 of every 1000 live births. In more than half of all cases, the clubfoot is bilateral. Infant boys are affected twice as often as infant girls, and there does exist a mild familial tendency. The deformity is present early in the gestational cycle of fetal development with subsequent soft-tissue contractures of the posterior and medial lower leg muscles. The soft-tissue contractures lead to bony deformation of the ankle and foot even before the infant is delivered.[3,22,32]

Equinovarus
A combination of pes equinus and pes varus. During ambulation, the client's heel does not contact the ground and the sole of the foot is inwardly turned.

Clinical Presentation

At delivery, the classic clubfoot position is easily identified by the physician delivering the newborn. The soles of the feet are inwardly pointed, and there is resistance to passively placing the feet and ankle in a neutral or normal position.

Evaluation: Tools and Methods

The evaluation of the foot primarily centers on the severity of the deformity. This is determined by manual examination determining the resistance to passive reduction of the deformity (assessing the end feel). If there is significant resistance to reduction of the deformity, the condition is deemed severe. An apparently severe visual deformity may only be mildly involved if there is minimal resistance to passive reduction.[3]

Clinical Management

Early management of the identified equinovarus will usually lead to a functional lower limb in childhood and into adulthood. Orthopedic management for clients with a clubfoot is the gradual reduction of the deformity. This is accomplished through serial casting or splinting. Beginning at about age 1 month, plaster casts are applied weekly to facilitate the gradual lengthening of shortened tissue and promote normal bony relationships. Within the first 3 months of intervention, conservative splinting will result in a 60% success rate. The remaining percentage of clients are often resistant to the serial casting approach, because the deformity recurs when the cast or splint is removed. Clients who do not respond to serial casting will require surgical correction, with subsequent casting and night splinting continuing for up to 3 years of age.[3,33]

Physical therapy intervention for these clients typically arises after the successful reduction and stabilization of the congenital deformity. The client may have been significantly delayed in normal weight-bearing activities on the lower extremity, and therapeutic goals will be identified to promote normal gait, weight shifts, and functional activities on the lower extremities. Education of the client and parents is critical to ensure effective carryover of intervention at home. The parents may be required to regularly assess skin status and apply orthopedic braces and footwear. The correct application and utilization of night splints will assist in the prevention of recurrence of the condition. In some facilities, the physical therapy team will be involved in the education process of the client's parents related to the appropriate care and handling of the client while in the casts or splints.

The expected physical therapy outcomes for the client with talipes equinovarus include[5]:

1. An improved health-related quality of life
2. Optimal function of the client
3. An understanding of risk factors
4. Prevention of further disability.

Length of intervention will range from 1 month to 1 year depending on the severity of the condition.

LIMB-LENGTH DISCREPANCIES

Leg-length discrepancy is a common orthopedic problem. This condition occurs during the growth periods of human life and can be a result of many different pathologies. Poliomyelitis was once the leading cause of juvenile limb-length discrepancies. The Salk and Sabin vaccines helped eradicate most cases of acute infectious polio that once affected many pediatric clients in this country. Limb deficits may be acquired, congenital, or developmental in nature. Traumatic fractures or bony infections may prematurely close the growth plate of a long bone in an adolescent client resulting in an unequal leg length. Small differences in the length of the lower extremities are common and are usually managed conservatively. Larger deficits can create secondary orthopedic disturbances necessitating surgical intervention.[34,35]

Clinical Presentation

A client with unequal lengths of the lower extremities may have secondary orthopedic concerns leading to pain and dysfunction. A deficit of greater than 2 cm may produce a pelvic obliquity, scoliosis, and gait deviations. The length imbalance may produce abnormal stresses to the affected hip, knee, and patella. Gait deviations may include circumduction, or hip hiking of the lower extremity opposite the shorter limb. Lateral trunk shifting over the shorter limb may also occur. The abnormal mechanics and stresses produced may result in pain in the spine, hip, knee, or ankle.[34]

Evaluation: Tools and Methods

The measurement of the length of the limb from the anterosuperior iliac spine (ASIS) to the medial malleolus is compared bilaterally (see Fig. 8–15). The evaluating therapist must ensure that any apparent deficit is not a result of pelvic rotation or obliquity. A leg-length discrepancy can be confirmed by placing the client in the hook-lying position and observing the height of one knee compared with the opposite knee (Fig. 8–16).[36]

Clinical Management

Nonsurgical Intervention. For clients with small length differences in the lower extremity, conservative treatment is indicated. The use of shoe inserts placed between the heel and the sole of the shoe of the affected limb works well for small deficits (about 1 cm). For larger deficits of up to 6 cm, the shoe worn on the affected limb may have the sole built up by an orthotist to effectively correct the length deficit.

Surgical Intervention. When a leg-length discrepancy greater than 6 cm produces significant dysfunction or deformity in the client, surgical lengthening of the affected limb may be indicated. The *Ilizarov procedure for limb lengthening* has been developed by European orthopedic surgeons and has recently been introduced in the United States (Box 8–2). The Ilizarov procedure includes the application of an external fixation device that holds the surgically separated or traumatically fractured bone apart (Fig. 8–17). Distraction of the two ends of the bone occurs across a small gap where healing occurs. Simard et al.[35] state that there are advantages to lengthening a deformed bone using an external fixation device, which include the following: (1) new bone growth is immediate as the bone crosses the distraction gap, (2) the new bone quickly resembles the current bone, and (3) the procedure is effective in either pediatric or adult clients. Complications that may result from the procedure include: (1) muscle contracture, (2) joint subluxation, (3) neurological involvement or insult, (4) infection at the pin sites, and (5) psychological adjustment to wearing the external fixation device for up to 2 years until sufficient healing and lengthening have occurred.

Physical therapy management of the pediatric client who is undergoing a surgical limb-lengthening procedure include (1) client and parent education about the surgical procedure and the rehabilitation expectations, (2) baseline assessment of the client to all unaffected extremities (ROM, strength, and sensation), (3) addressing functional considerations for gait and mobility, (4) assistive devices if needed, and (5) conditioning program to all unaffected limbs. During the time when the client is wearing the external fixation device, proper care of the skin to prevent infection is necessary. After the removal of the device, the physical therapy team will readdress all of the same concerns mentioned previously. Particular emphasis will be placed on the length and strength of the muscles to promote functional use of the newly lengthened extremity.[35]

The physical therapy expected outcomes for management of a limb-length discrepancy may vary dramatically depending on whether the intervention is conservative or surgical. The minimal expected outcomes include[5]:

1. Improved health-related quality of life
2. Optimal function
3. An understanding of the risk factors
4. Prevention of further disability.

Depending on the severity of the condition and the type of intervention, treatment may last from one visit to 2 years.

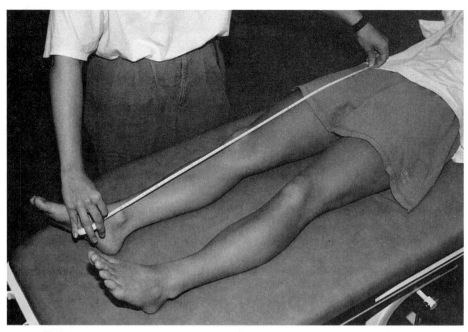

FIG. 8–15
Measuring leg length discrepancies. By measuring from the ASIS to the medial malleolus, the evaluating physical therapist can determine if a bony leg length discrepancy exists. There is an expected variance for all lower extremities, and deficits less than 2 cm are usually treated conservatively or not at all.

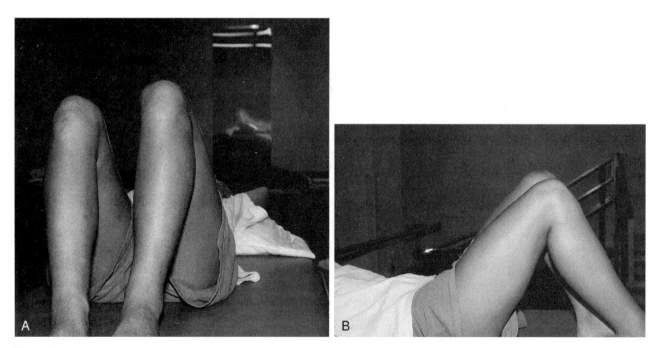

FIG. 8–16
Determining nature of leg length discrepancies. Placing the client in the hook-lying position will help identify the nature of a leg length discrepancy. If the affected knee is taller from a caudal view, then the tibia most likely is longer than the opposite tibia (A). If the affected knee is taller from a lateral view, then the femur most likely is longer than the opposite femur (B).

Box 8-2

THE USE OF EXTERNAL FIXATION AND DISTRACTION OSTEOGENESIS

The method of stimulating bone growth by applying distraction to the bone held by an external skeletal device was pioneered in Europe by Gavriil Abramovich Ilizarov. The technique was developed during World War II in response to the large number of cases of bony deformities and osteomyelitis seen in soldiers returning from battle. The premise of the theory to stimulate new bone growth was that the external fixation device would hold the two bones stable with a small gap between the bones. A fibrovascular framework would then bridge the gap between the two ends of the bone. Eventually, the fibrovascular framework is filled with osteoblasts to create new bone. As the bone growth is sufficient and stable, the external fixation device is moved slightly further apart to place more distraction on the repair site. The healing process continues as new bone is formed and the external fixation device is gradually separated. The end result is a well-healed bone of greater length.

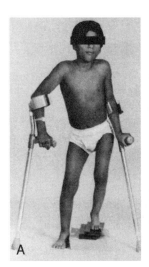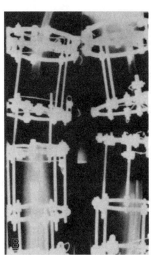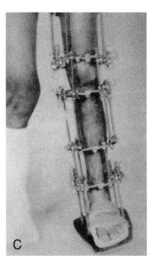

FIG. 8-17

External fixation device used for limb lengthening. Pictured is a child, age 10, with a paralytic shortening of the left leg due to acute infectious poliomyelitis. Leg length discrepancy was 7.5 cm (A). External fixation devices were applied stimulating lengthening of the tibia and femur (B, C). Eventually, this child achieved functionally equal length limbs. (From Simard S: The Ilizarov Procedure: Limb Lengthening and Its Implications. *Physical Therapy* 1992; 72:30, with permission of the American Physical Therapy Association.)

SUMMARY

When working with pediatric clients, the rehabilitation team must work to identify the immediate, short-term, and long-term needs of the client. Immediate needs include the stabilization of injuries or deformities and the promotion of a positive healing environment. Short-term needs include the prevention of secondary complications, the promotion of normal development, and the provision of education to the client and family. Long-term consideration must include the restoration of normal function and mobility, the independent management of long term complications, and the promotion of a positive self-image for the client. Families need to be educated about the orthopedic condition and encouraged to be active participants in the rehabilitation process. There are often concerns about long-term disability or dysfunction, and familial apprehensions. The rehabilitation team can assist families through education, and referral to agencies or support groups that can assist.

Acquired conditions discussed in this chapter include fractures, JRA, growth disorders, and osteochondroses. The healing characteristics of the pediatric client who has sustained a fracture as well as the classifications of fracture types and medical management were presented. Unique characteristics of fractures in pediatric clients include the frequency of injury compared to adults, the rapid healing process, and the ability to remodel deformities. The potential to injury of the epiphyseal plate in children is substantial and has significant growth implications for the client. Management of the condition includes immobilization followed by a therapeutic intervention program to promote mobility and a return to function.

Scoliosis is an abnormal lateral curvature of the spine. Early detection of the deformity is critical in effectively managing the progression of the curve. Treatment can be conservative using bracing, exercises, and electrical stimulation, or the condition can be corrected and stabilized through surgery.

Juvenile rheumatoid arthritis is the most common pediatric rheumatoid disease in North America and is one of the major causes of pediatric disability. The autoimmune inflammatory process promotes the destruction of the involved joints. Three distinct types of JRA are classified depending on the onset of the disease, the number of affected joints, and the clinical manifestation, which includes (1) pauciarticular or oligoarticular, (2) polyarticular, and (3) systemic juvenile arthritis or Still's disease. Discussions of the clinical presentations, goals, and therapeutic interventions for clients with JRA were presented.

Slipped capital femoral epiphysis is a pediatric orthopedic condition that occurs during adolescent growth periods. Excessive shearing forces cause the neck of the femur to "slip" upwardly and anteriorly in relation to the epiphysis. Physical therapy intervention occurs postsurgically for gait training, ROM, and strengthening to the involved hip.

Osteochondropathies are a general condition causing degenerative changes in the epiphyseal plates of growing bones. The primary factor identifying the degenerative changes is a state of avascular necrosis of unknown etiology. Legg-Calvé-Perthes disease affects the hips of active, growing males. Scheuermann's disease, or adolescent kyphosis affects the anterior growth plates of the thoracic vertebrae. Osteochondritis dissecans occurs when a small piece of subchondral bone separates from the bone as a result of avascular necrosis. Commonly seen in the knee or elbow, the small piece then becomes a loose body in the joint. Osgood-Schlatter disease affects the tibial tuberosity of growing, active males. The osteochondropathies have a wide-ranging prognosis from little or no disability to significant disability into adulthood.

Congenital conditions discussed in this chapter include congenital amputations, developmental dysplasia of the hip, equinovarus, and limb-length discrepancies. Amputations can be congenital or acquired affecting almost any appendage in the body. The pediatric client may never experience loss with a congenital amputation; however, the parents of the child may demonstrate the psychological feelings of loss, guilt, or anger for the child. Some amputations will require subsequent surgical amputation for conversion of the anomaly to enable better prosthetic fitting. The use of prosthetic devices should be identified by the rehabilitation team for the promotion of improved function for the client.

Developmental dysplasia of the hip (DDH) is a cumulation of secondary degenerative and adaptive conditions from a recurrent hip dislocation early in the life of a pediatric client. Early screening for dysfunction usually identifies dislocation of the hip and leads to early intervention and positive outcomes. Treatment at any age consists of managing secondary conditions, reducing the dislocated hip and promoting stability of the joint. The older the child when the condition is identified, the less favorable the outcomes from treatment.

Talipes equinovarus is commonly known as "clubfoot." It is a congenital orthopedic deformity that is visually identified at birth. Conservative management consists of serial casting and splinting to reduce the deformity. Surgical intervention is required for resistant cases, which generally have less successful outcomes than those cases that are successfully managed conservatively.

Limb-length discrepancies can occur from congenital abnormalities or from acquired deficits, such as a fracture to the epiphyseal plate. The discrepancy manifests during growth periods of the pediatric client and can lead to secondary complications that produce pain and dysfunction. Most LLDs are treated conservatively with shoe or heel lifts, but surgical intervention, such as the Ilizarov procedure, are indicated in severe, dysfunctional cases.

 REFERENCES

1. Rothstein, JM: Pediatric Orthopedics. American Physical Therapy Association, Alexandria, VA, 1992, p 3.
2. Cochrane, CG, et al: Preparation of physical therapists to work with handicapped infants and their families: current status and training needs. Phys Ther 70:372, 1990.
3. Salter, RB: Textbook of Disorders and Injuries of the Musculoskeletal System. Williams & Wilkins, Baltimore, 1983.
4. Shankman, GA: Fundamental Orthopedic Management for the Physical Therapist Assistant. Mosby, St Louis, MO, 1997.
5. Guide to Physical Therapist Practice. Phys Ther 77:1163, 1997.
6. Cassidy, JT, and Petty, RE: Juvenile rheumatoid arthritis. In Textbook of Rheumatology, ed 2. Churchill Livingstone, New York, 1990.
7. Rhodes, VJ: Physical therapy management of patients with juvenile rheumatoid arthritis. Phys Ther 71:910, 1991.
8. Ansell, BM: Joint manifestations in children with juvenile chronic polyarthritis. Arthritis Rheum 20:204, 1977.
9. Behrens, BJ, and Michlovitz, SL: Physical Agents: Theory and Practice for the Physical Therapist Assistant. FA Davis, Philadelphia, 1996.
10. Byers, PH: Effect of exercise on morning stiffness and mobility in patients with rheumatoid arthritis. Res Nurs Health 8:275, 1985.
11. Kisner, C, and Colby, LA: Therapeutic Exercise: Foundations and Techniques, ed 3. FA Davis, Philadelphia, 1996.
12. Lechner, DE, et al: Gait deviations in patients with juvenile rheumatoid arthritis. Phys Ther 67:1335, 1987.

13. Giannini, MJ, and Protas, EJ: Exercise response in children with and without juvenile rheumatoid arthritis: A case-comparison study. Phys Ther 72:365, 1992.
14. Bar-Or, O: Pathophysiology factors which limit the exercise capacity of the sick child. Med Sci Sports Exerc 18, 276, 1986.
15. Giannini, MJ, and Protas, EJ: Aerobic capacity in juvenile rheumatoid arthritis patients and healthy children. Arthritis Care and Research 4:131, 1991.
16. Harkcom, TM, et al: Therapeutic value of graded aerobic exercise training in rheumatoid arthritis. Arthritis Rheum 28:32, 1985.
17. Cassella, MC, and Hall, JE: Current treatment approach in the nonoperative and operative management of adolescent idiopathic scoliosis. Phys Ther 71:897, 1991.
18. Sullivan, JA, et al: Further evaluation of the scolitron treatment of idiopathic adolescent scoliosis. Spine 11:903, 1986.
19. Axelgaard, J, and Brown, JC: Lateral surface stimulation for the treatment of progressive idiopathic scoliosis. Spine 8:242, 1983.
20. Lonstein, JE, and Winter, RB: Adolescent idiopathic scoliosis: nonoperative treatment. Orthop Clin North Am 19:239, 1988.
21. Kessler, RM, and Hertling, D: Management of Common Musculoskeletal Disorders: Physical Therapy Principles and Methods, ed 3. Lippincott, Philadelphia, PA, 1996.
22. Wheeless CR: Wheeless' Textbook of Orthopaedics. [http://www.medmedia.com/med.htm]. 1996.
23. May, BJ: Amputations and Prosthetics: A Case Study Approach. FA Davis, Philadelphia, 1996.
24. Haugh, PE: An evaluation of the adequacy of health visitor education for neonatal hip screening. J Adv Nurs 20:815, 1994.
25. Echternach, DK: Hip problems in children and adolescents. Churchill Livingstone, New York, 1990.
26. Beaty, JH: Congenital Abnormalities of Hip and Pelvis. Mosby, St Louis, MO, 1992.
27. Jamali, M, and McCoy, KL: Developmental dysplasia of the hip: new terminology for an old problem in young patients. Advance 9(18):8, 1998.
28. Magee, DJ: Orthopedic Physical Assessment. WB Saunders, Philadelphia, 1994.
29. Phillips, WE: Ultrasonography of developmental displacement of the infant hip. Applied Radiology 6:25, 1995.
30. Hampton, S, Reed, B, and Nixon, W: Diagnosis of congenital dislocated hips. Radiol Technol 59(3):211, 1988.
31. Hayes, MB: Traction at home for infants with developmental dysplasia of the hip. Orthopedic Nursing 14(1):33, 1995.
32. Tiberio, D: Pathomechanics of structural foot deformities. Phys Ther 68:1841, 1988.
33. Cusick, BD: Splints and Casts: Managing foot deformity in children with neuromotor disorders. Phys Ther 68:1903, 1988.
34. Simard, S, et al: The ilizarov procedure: limb lengthening and its implications. Phys Ther 72:25, 1992.
35. Tachdjian, M: Pediatric orthopaedics. WB Saunders, Philadelphia, 1990.
36. Hoppenfeld, S: Physical Examination of the Spine and Extremities. Appleton-Century-Crofts, Norwalk, CT, 1976.

 BIBLIOGRAPHY

Ansell, BM: Joint manifestations in children with juvenile chronic polyarthritis. Arthritis Rheum 20:204, 1977.
Axelgaard, J, and Brown, JC: Lateral surface stimulation for the treatment of progressive idiopathic scoliosis. Spine 8:242, 1983.
Bar-Or, O: Pathophysiology factors which limit the exercise capacity of the sick child. Med Sci Sports Exerc 18, 276, 1986.
Beaty, JH: Congenital Abnormalities of Hip and Pelvis. Mosby, St Louis, MO, 1992.
Behrens, BJ, and Michlovitz, SL: Physical Agents: Theory and Practice for the Physical Therapist Assistant. FA Davis, Philadelphia, 1996.
Byers, PH: Effect of exercise on morning stiffness and mobility in patients with rheumatoid arthritis. Res Nurs Health 8:275, 1985.
Cassella, MC, and Hall, JE: Current treatment approach in the nonoperative and operative management of adolescent idiopathic scoliosis. Phys Ther 71:897, 1991.
Cassidy, JT, and Petty, RE: Juvenile rheumatoid arthritis. In Textbook of Rheumatolog, ed 2. Churchill Livingstone, New York, 1990.
Cochrane, et al: Preparation of physical therapists to work with handicapped infants and their families: current status and training needs. Phys Ther 70:372, 1990.

Cusick, BD: Splints and Casts: Managing foot deformity in children with neuromotor disorders. Phys Ther 68:1903, 1988.

Echternach, DK: Hip Problems in Children and Adolescents. Churchill Livingstone, New York, 1990.

Giannini, MJ, and Protas, EJ: Aerobic capacity in juvenile rheumatoid arthritis patients and healthy children. Arthritis Care and Research 4:131, 1991.

Giannini, MJ, and Protas, EJ: Exercise response in children with and without juvenile rheumatoid arthritis: A case-comparison study. Phys Ther 72:365, 1992.

Guide to Physical Therapist Practice. Phys Ther 77:1163-1650, 1997.

Hampton, S, et al: Diagnosis of congenital dislocated hips. Radiol Technol 59(3):211, 1988.

Harkcom, TM, et al: Therapeutic value of graded aerobic exercise training in rheumatoid arthritis. Arthritis Rheum 28:32, 1985.

Haugh, PE: An evaluation of the adequacy of health visitor education for neonatal hip screening. J Adv Nurs 20:815, 1994.

Hayes, MB: Traction at home for infants with developmental dysplasia of the hip. Orthopedic Nursing 14(1):33, 1995.

Hoppenfeld, S: Physical Examination of the Spine and Extremities. Appleton-Century-Crofts, Norwalk, CT, 1976.

Jamali, M, and McCoy, KL: Developmental dysplasia of the hip: new terminology for an old problem in young patients. Advance 9(18):8, 1998.

Kessler, RM, and Hertling, D: Management of Common Musculoskeletal Disorders: Physical Therapy Principles and Methods, ed 3. Lippincott, Philadelphia, 1996.

Kisner, C, and Colby, LA: Therapeutic Exercise: Foundations and Techniques, ed 3. FA Davis, Philadelphia, 1996.

Lechner, DE, et al: Gait deviations in patients with juvenile rheumatoid arthritis. Phys Ther 67:1335, 1987.

Lonstein, JE, and Winter, RB: Adolescent idiopathic scoliosis: nonoperative treatment. Orthop Clin North Am 19:239, 1988.

Magee, DJ: Orthopedic Physical Assessment. WB Saunders, Philadelphia, 1994.

May, BJ: Amputations and Prosthetics: A Case Study Approach. FA Davis, Philadelphia, 1996.

Phillips, WE: Ultrasonography of developmental displacement of the infant hip. Applied Radiology 6:25, 1995.

Rhodes, VJ: Physical therapy management of patients with juvenile rheumatoid arthritis. Phys Ther 71:910, 1991.

Rothstein, JM: Pediatric Orthopedics. American Physical Therapy Association, Alexandria, VA, 1992.

Salter, RB: Textbook of Disorders and Injuries of the Musculoskeletal System. Williams & Wilkins, Baltimore, 1983.

Shankman, GA: Fundamental Orthopedic Management for the Physical Therapist Assistant. Mosby, St Louis, MO, 1997.

Simard, S, Marchant, M and Mencio, G: The Ilizarov procedure: Limb lengthening and its implications. Phys Ther 72:25, 1992.

Sullivan, JA, et al: Further evaluation of the scolitron treatment of idiopathic adolescent scoliosis. Spine 11:903, 1986.

Tachdjian, M: Pediatric Orthopaedics. WB Saunders, Philadelphia, 1990.

Tiberio, D: Pathomechanics of structural foot deformities. Phys Ther 68:1841, 1988.

Wheeless, CR: Wheeless' Textbook of Orthopaedics. [http://www.medmedia.com/med.htm]. 1996.

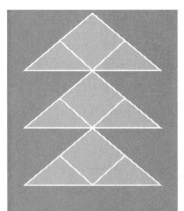

chapter 9

Clients with Injuries from an Active Lifestyle

Key Words

allograft
arthroplasty
arthrosis
autograft
bankart lesion
ecchymosis
hemarthrosis
hill-sachs lesion
kinesthesia
mechanoreceptor
myositis ossificans
nonsteroidal anti-
*   inflammatory drug*
pitting edema
proprioception
splinting

The best preparation for tomorrow is to do today's work superbly well.

Sir William Osler

CONCERNS OF THE ACTIVE INDIVIDUAL: RETURN TO COMPETITION OR LIFESTYLE

Mark is a 21-year-old football player at the local college. He injured his left ankle in a game on the previous Saturday afternoon. It is now Monday, and he enters the outpatient clinic using a pair of wooden axillary crutches, carefully avoiding placing any weight on his injured leg. After the supervising PT evaluated the injury, you were given a plan of treatment that included using cryotherapy and compression to the left ankle for 20 minutes and were directed to instruct Mark in an ankle range of motion (ROM) home program. As you are applying the cryocompression pump to Mark's left ankle, you notice that there is a moderate amount of swelling surrounding his lateral malleolus and some discoloration is beginning distally in the foot. As Mark shivers when the cold pump is placed on his foot and ankle, he asks you if he will be able to play this coming Saturday. He goes on to exclaim that this game is homecoming and the team that they are playing is their biggest rival. Mark continues to press you for an answer.

Luckily for Mark, he is young and healthy. His only concern in life at this time is when can he put himself in harm's way again on the football field. Injuries are a part of athletic competition. Often it is not a question of whether an athlete will get hurt, but when the athlete will get hurt. Contact sports, such as football, rugby, or hockey, at times will produce graphic, dramatic injuries (Fig. 9–1). The participant may be away from the sport for a brief period of time while the injury heals. The injury may require surgery. Possibly the injury may keep the athlete from ever participating in the activity of their choice again. Noncontact sports, such as running or gymnastics, may not produce the same violent injuries, but the net effect for the participant is the same (Fig. 9–2).

The rehabilitation team has a unique obligation to the client with an active

FIG. 9–1
Injuries are a part of competition. The athlete who participates in high-risk sports is moving at high velocities and colliding during the competition. Sports such as football often result in injury to the participant.

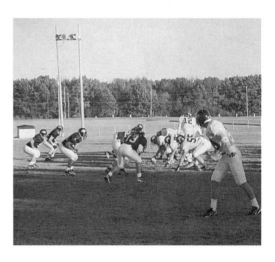

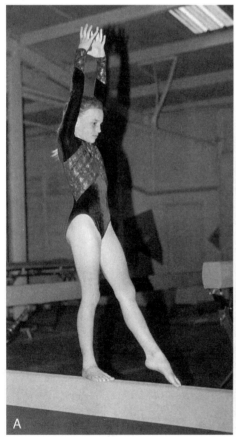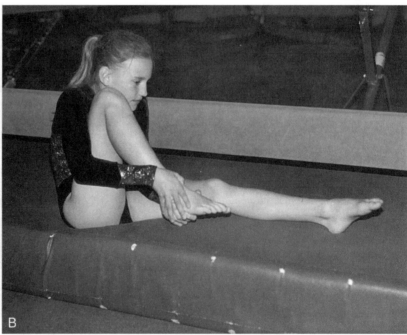

FIG. 9–2
No injury is small to the participant. Even noncontact sports such as gymnastics (A) will produce injuries that have the same limiting effects on the participant as do violent collision injuries. No injury is small to an athlete if it prevents participation in the sport (B).

lifestyle. Promoting participation and getting the client "better" quickly must be balanced with preventing the client from reinjury. There is a fine line between preparing the client to resume playing the sport and releasing the client from therapy prematurely. Aggressive rehabilitation protocols may move an injured participant back into competition quickly. Critics of aggressive rehabilitation protocols claim that such protocols may impose certain long-term, deleterious effects on a client who lacks the medical knowledge to make an informed choice. Proponents of aggressive approaches claim that life is too short and that the athletic season will be over if the client must wait 6 to 8 weeks for an ankle sprain to heal. However, these concerns must be weighed against the objective of promoting the lifelong health of the client.

There is no perfect answer that applies to every situation. The best approach in rehabilitating the active client (or any client) is individualization. Some clients may return quickly from an injury, and the same injury to a second individual may keep the client out of competition for months. For example, a fractured ring finger can be an injury that would result in a football wide receiver being out of his game for 6 weeks as the broken bone heals. This client would be unable to successfully catch a ball that was thrown his way. However, an offensive lineman teammate of the wide receiver can also sustain the same fractured ring finger and may never miss a practice. The offensive lineman can play with a silicone game cast on his wrist and hand, protecting the injury, because he does not need to catch a ball that is thrown to him. Injuries are specific to the individual, and the rehabilitation program designed by the team should meet the needs of that individual.

 SPRAINS

CLASSIFICATIONS OF SPRAINS

A sprain is an injury to a ligament in the body. The ligament sustains a load or force sufficient to produce a mechanical disruption of the structural fibers. The damage can be graded depending on the extent of the injury in relation to the fibers torn. A mild sprain is classified as a grade I injury resulting in only a small amount of the fibers being damaged. Pain and swelling is mild, with no disruption of the structures. A moderate sprain is classified as a grade II injury resulting in damage to about half of the ligamentous structure. Pain is moderate to severe, and swelling is significant with some loss of motion noted. A mild increase in joint accessory motion is noted with a grade II lesion. A severe sprain is classified as a grade III injury resulting in a complete mechanical disruption of the integrity of the supporting ligament. Pain is minimal to moderate (usually less than a grade II), swelling is significant, and a marked loss of function is noted. The healing requirements of the ligament are presented in Chapter 5.[1,2,3]

A sprain can affect nearly any joint in the body and is usually the result of a sudden, unexpected traumatic event. Conservative, but functional management of most acute sprain injuries is possible to promote the recovery of the client and enable return to the activity of choice. The remainder of this chapter explains common sprain injuries treated by PT professionals.

SHOULDER COMPLEX SPRAINS

The bones, muscles, tendons, and ligaments that make up the shoulder girdle are a finely coordinated, intricately operating series of dependent components collaborating to achieve motion of the upper extremity. If one component fails to accomplish its design task, then limitations or impairments of the entire complex will result. The working elements of the clavicle, scapula, and the dynamic stabilizers all function to produce the end result of humeral motion. If one of these elements is lost, the hand may not be able to reach the desired position. Joints that are susceptible to sprain in the shoulder complex include the sternoclavicular (SC) joint and the acromioclavicular (AC) joint (Fig. 9–3). Rehabilitation approaches for injuries to either joint are similar in nature. The following section discusses the more frequently injured joint, the AC joint.

Acromioclavicular Joint

The AC joint is the articulation of the distal end of the clavicle with the acromion of the scapula. A small articular joint disk is present. The two significant structural ligaments providing stability for the joint include (1) the AC ligaments and (2) the coracoclavicular ligaments. The superior and inferior AC ligaments reinforce the weak joint capsule, limiting horizontal movement. The coracoclavicular ligaments do not directly attach to the AC joint but grant significant stability by securing the clavicle to the scapula. The lateral portion (trapezoid) and the medial portion (conoid) of the coracoclavicular ligament work to prevent a superior dislocation of the clavicle on the acromion. Injuries to the AC joint are typically caused by a traumatic fall directly onto the lateral tip of the shoulder.[4,5]

Clinical Presentation. For sprains of the AC joint, the following grading system is used[3]:

Grade I: mild sprain involving only the AC ligaments, with no displacement of the clavicle noted

Grade II: AC ligaments disrupted, sprained coracoclavicular ligaments still intact, and mild upward displacement of distal clavicle noted

Grade III: AC and coracoclavicular ligaments are completely disrupted, significant displacement of the clavicle in relation to the scapula is noted; surgical stabilization is likely needed

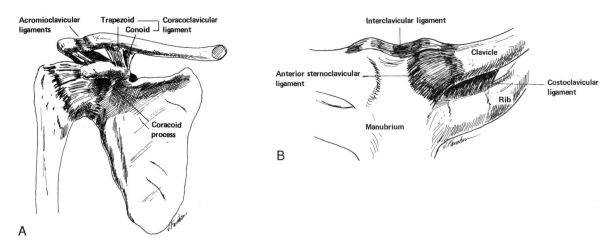

FIG. 9–3
Shoulder girdle joints and ligaments. (A) Ligaments and the relationship of the AC joint to the shoulder girdle. (B) Ligaments and the relationship of the SC joint to the shoulder girdle. (From Norkin & Levangie, p 214 & 217, with permission.)

Table 9–1

REHABILITATION OF THE CLIENT WITH AN ACROMIOCLAVICULAR SPRAIN	

Grade I Sprain

Week 1	Use cryotherapy to reduce inflammation and pain.
	Immobilize arm in sling to prevent further injury.
	Introduce AROM of the hand and elbow to prevent loss of motion in adjacent joints, and Codman's pendulum exercises to injured arm (see Figure 9–4).
Week 2	As symptoms resolve, increase AROM of involved shoulder.
	Discontinue use of sling.
	Gradually return to ADLs as tolerated.

Grade II Sprain

Week 1	Use cryotherapy to reduce inflammation and pain.
	Immobilize arm in sling to prevent further injury and encourage healing of sprained ligament.
Week 2	Introduce Codman's pendulum exercises and ROM to involved shoulder
	Encourage use of involved upper extremity in ADLs
	Avoid any strenuous activity for 6 to 8 wk

Grade III Sprain

Week 1	Discuss surgical or conservative approach with client. If client uses shoulder for high-demand activities, surgical stabilization may be needed. Discuss the deformity present as a result of the dislocated distal clavicle.
	If conservative management is chosen, use cryotherapy and oral painkillers as prescribed by the physician.
	Immobilize arm in sling to prevent further injury.
Weeks 2–4	Gradually encourage ADLs with involved upper extremity.
	Gradually introduce Codman's and ROM exercises.
	By end of week 4, full motion should be achieved. Avoid stressful activities for 6 to 8 wk, and reintroduce functional activities as tolerated.

The client will have moderate discomfort and may not be able to actively elevate the humerus with an acute AC sprain. Tenderness to palpation over the distal clavicle and AC joint is noted.

Evaluation: Tools and Methods. The supervising PT should take a complete history, including the mechanism of injury. Observation may reveal a superior displacement of the clavicle if the injury is at least a grade II. Assessment of ROM, pain, strength, and functional status should be documented. The evaluation may also include examination of the SC joint, the clavicle, and the neck and upper extremity to rule out other associated, but undetected injuries.

Clinical Management of the Client. The management of the client with an AC sprain is guided by the degree of injury. In general, a conservative approach is most often used. A brief period of protective immobilization is accompanied by modalities to reduce inflammation. A gradual introduction of ROM exercises followed by strengthening and functional activities is encouraged, as tolerated by the client. Table 9–1 presents an outlined protocol for the rehabilitation of an acute AC sprain by severity of injury (Fig. 9–4).[3,5]

FIG. 9–4
Codman's pendulum exercises. Have the client lean over a table supporting the body weight with the noninvolved upper extremity. Dangling the involved limb with gravity assisting provides a gentle, sustained mobilization that will begin to restore motion. With the involved arm relaxed, have the client swing the trunk and hips, creating a pendulum motion of the involved arm. Swing the arm passively in a sagittal plane or a frontal plane. This should be a relaxing exercise that does not produce pain. As the client progresses, a small weight can be placed in the hand during this exercise.

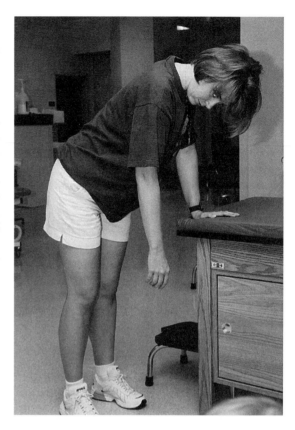

The expected physical therapy outcomes for managing a client with an AC sprain include[6]:

1. Improved functional skills and the optimal return of function
2. Reduced risk of further disability from identified limitations
3. An understanding of the risk factors that may contribute to jeopardizing health status
4. An understanding of strategies to prevent further disability

The expected time frame for achieving the outcomes is brief. The client who sustained a grade I or grade II lesion should easily return to normal activities of daily living (ADLs) within 2 weeks. A longer period of time (6 to 8 weeks) may be needed for sufficient healing to occur for athletes that performed specialized activities with the injured shoulder (e.g., throwing motions for a football quarterback). Special attention to the mechanics of throwing must be considered for these clients. Surgically repaired cases may take 2 to 3 months to heal before full function is restored.

HAND AND DIGIT SPRAINS

Ligamentous injury to the digits of the hand can temporarily limit function and mobility for the client. Structurally, the metacarpophalangeal (MCP) and interphalangeal (IP) joints have supporting capsular collateral ligaments limiting valgus or varus forces (Fig. 9–5). These ligaments can easily be damaged in sports

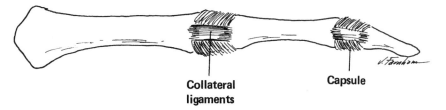

FIG. 9–5
Collateral ligaments of the digits. The medial and lateral supporting structures of the digits include the collateral capsular ligaments that support the MCP, PIP, and DIP. (From Norkin & Levangie, p 276, with permission.)

participation as the finger is accidentally placed at an injurious angle with a force great enough to result in ligament damage. The next section details the management of a common sprain of the digits: skier's thumb. Management of sprains to the other MCP and IP joints of the digits is very similar.

Skier's Thumb

Historically this condition has been called a gamekeeper's thumb. The injury was common among individuals that regularly kept and gathered wild game. However, a more recent name defining a sprain of the ulnar collateral ligament (UCL) of the thumb MCP joint is a skier's thumb. A fall onto an extended upper extremity with a ski pole in the hand of the client may result in a sprain to the UCL of the thumb (Fig. 9–6). The mechanism of injury is forced abduction (Fig. 9–7).

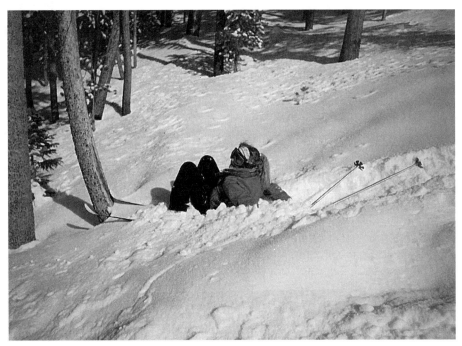

FIG. 9–6
Skier's thumb. Holding a ski pole in the hand of the skier may keep the thumb in an extended, abducted position that makes the skier susceptible to injury of the thumb when a fall occurs on an extended upper extremity.

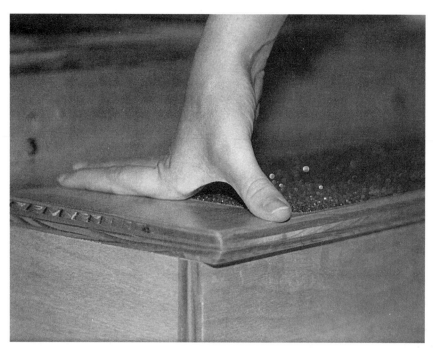

FIG. 9–7
Skier's thumb. Mechanism of injury—The fall onto the extended upper extremity will forcefully abduct the thumb, resulting in a sprain of the ulnar collateral ligament (UCL).

Clinical Presentation. The injury will follow the established grades of sprains. A grade I injury will cause pain, but there is no loss of stability of the MCP joint. A grade II lesion will cause pain, have some valgus instability, but still have a firm end point. A grade III lesion will have minimal discomfort and significant instability of the joint.[7,8]

Evaluation: Tools and Methods. The PT should take a complete history with details of the mechanism of injury. Objective measures include ROM, strength assessment, and ligamentous stress tests, which help to determine the integrity of the injured thumb. Radiographic examination is typically needed to rule out an associated fracture.[7]

Clinical Management. The level of intervention by the health-care professional depends on the intensity of the injury. The client with a grade I injury may not seek medical attention because the pain and discomfort will quickly resolve with no significant impairment. A grade II lesion is typically treated conservatively. Grade III lesions, though not common, require surgical stabilization to prevent further deformity and dysfunction. Wadsworth[7] claims that significant functional loss could occur in the client with an inadequately managed sprain of the UCL of the thumb.

If a client with a grade I UCL sprain seeks medical advice from a physician or PT, the recommended management is to provide protection and comfort. Pain control modalities, such as ice and electrical stimulation, and oral anti-inflammatory medications, may be used. As pain resolved, instructing the client in ROM exercises should help alleviate residual joint stiffness. External bracing and supports are usually not used unless the client needs to immediately participate in a potentially injurious event (e.g., return to skiing).[7]

The grade II lesion will require immobilization for a period of 2 to 4 weeks in a thumb spica cast. After removal of the cast, a removable thumb splint can be used for additional protection as strength and function returns. With removal of the fixed cast, strengthening and ROM exercises can begin. Strengthening should begin with a therapeutic putty program. ROM should be active at first with only gentle passive motion encouraged. At this stage, stability should be emphasized. Care should be taken in stretching healing ligaments. Modalities designed to relieve joint stiffness, including heat, whirlpool, or paraffin bath, may be used before exercises. If acute pain is demonstrated with active motion, the client may need to be reevaluated to rule out the presence of other pathology.[7,8]

Surgical repair of the grade III sprain will adequately stabilize the MCP of the thumb and prevent further disability. If a delay of more than 3 weeks occurs from the time of injury to the time of surgical repair, a significant risk of permanent thumb impairment may result.[9] Immediately after surgery, the hand and thumb of the client is immobilized in a thumb spica cast for 4 to 6 weeks. Upon removal of the cast, the client is fitted for a removable thumb splint that should be worn for at least an additional 6 weeks. Active motion and strengthening exercises may begin at this point. The rehabilitation team should discourage full abduction or extension (lateral) stresses on the healing thumb and encourage functional activities into opposition. ROM exercises should be performed by the client for at least 10 minutes every waking hour. Strengthening exercises with therapeutic putty are effective. If motion is severely limited, investigate the use of a dynamic, low-load splint. With the surgeon's approval, this type of splint may need to be custom made. As motion and stability of the MCP is improved, the splint may be discontinued and more aggressive strengthening exercises may be encouraged. A custom-fitted splint may be used for protection during high-risk activities.[7,8]

The expected physical therapy outcomes for managing a client with a skier's thumb include[6]:

1. Improving health-related quality of life
2. Promoting improved functional skills and return to optimal function
3. Improving safety awareness of client
4. Promoting understanding of strategies to prevent further disability

The expected time frame for achieving the outcomes for a client with a grade I injury is 4 to 6 weeks with or without medical intervention. A grade II injury, including time in the cast, should be fully healed with minimal or no disability to the client within 8 to 10 weeks. The client with the severe grade III injury will need a minimum of 12 weeks before full function is restored. More time may be needed if complications or excessive disability is noted.[7,8]

KNEE SPRAINS

Injuries to the knee ligaments include sprains of the anterior cruciate ligament (ACL), posterior cruciate ligament (PCL), medial collateral ligament (MCL), or the lateral collateral ligament (LCL). The mobility function of the knee is dependent on the inert structural stability provided by the ligaments and joint capsule as well as on the dynamic support provided by the muscles that cross the joint. Although injury to any of the ligaments is undesirable, dysfunction caused by a sprain may be overcome by overcompensating muscular strength, and dynamic stabilizing efforts to expedite to the return to the client's desired activity. Each ligament is responsible for limiting a distinct motion of the knee. The ACL ligament limits anterior translation of the tibia from under the femur as well as rotation of the tibia. The PCL limits the tibia from sliding posteriorly under the femur. In combination, the ACL and PCL limit excessive sliding during the anatomical motions of knee flexion and extension. The MCL limits valgus stresses on the knee, and the LCL limits varus stresses on the knee. In combination, the ligaments work to provide great stability for the knee while still allowing significant mobility (Fig. 9–8).[4]

Injuries to the ligaments of the knee can be devastating and may result in disability. An athlete who suffers an ACL injury may never be able to return to competition. A traumatized knee joint may develop arthritic changes over time that will eventually require a total joint **arthroplasty**. A client who sustains a knee sprain in a recreational activity may miss work as the healing process occurs. Rehabilitation for the client with a knee sprain must consider the stabilizing function of the injured ligaments while addressing the mobility of the knee joint itself. The following section will describe the management of a client with two of the more common ligamentous injuries to the knee: ACL and MCL injury.

Clinical Presentation. Damage to the ACL and MCL can occur collectively or separately. The combination injury that damages the ACL, MCL and the medial meniscus is referred to as O'*Donohue's unhappy triad*. This injury typically occurs when the client's foot is planted on the ground and a twisting motion of the knee occurs. A combination valgus force and excessive rotation of the femur on the tibia produces a force great enough to damage the ACL and the MCL, with subsequent meniscal damage caused by subluxation of the knee joint from the ligamentous instability. The client does not need to have physical contact from an opposing player. Frequently this injury occurs in isolation as the client stops and pivots on the planted extremity.[3,10]

The ACL may be damaged singularly by hyperextension of the knee beyond the joints anatomic limits. A classic example of an ACL sprain may occur when the female basketball player jumps up to rebound a ball off of the backboard and lands, hyperextending the knee. A popping sound is frequently heard, and the knee joint becomes unstable or buckles as the client falls to the floor. The MCL also can be damaged in isolation. For example, if a client is standing with complete body weight on one lower extremity and a second person falls onto the client's lateral aspect of the weight-bearing knee joint, a severe valgus force on the knee will result.

After the injury has occurred, it is likely that the client will present in the physical therapy clinic after seeing a physician, wearing a straight leg knee immobilizer. The use of a knee immobilizer after an acute ligamentous injury stablizes the knee and protects the damaged structures from further injury (Fig. 9–9).

Evaluation: Tools and Methods. A client history complete with mechanism of injury and description of the symptoms after the injury are helpful in identifying the condition. The client typically describes participating in an activity, when a sudden, audible pop was heard from the involved knee. The client may have had immediate pain that subsided or became persistent. The client may describe the onset of joint swelling after the injury as being fairly rapid (within a couple of hours). Hardaker et al.[11] reported that 77% of the examined clients with acute joint **hemarthrosis** had an accompanying ACL injury. The description of the knee "giving way" may also accompany a suspected ACL injury.[12,13] Objective measures include integumentary assessment, ROM, strength, and functional abilities of the

Arthroplasty
The reconstruction of an arthritic or diseased joint.

Hemarthrosis
The presence of blood and swelling in the joint cavity.

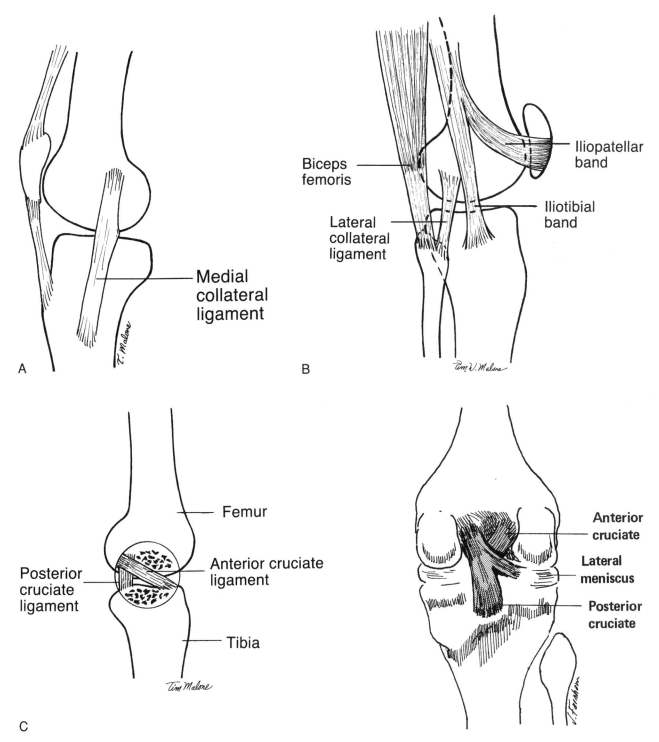

FIG. 9–8
Ligaments of the knee. The medial collateral (A) limits valgus forces on the knee joint. The lateral collateral (B) limits varus forces on the knee. The posterior cruciate and anterior cruciate ligaments (C) work in concert to provide stability of the moving knee by limiting anterior and posterior translation of the tibia. (From Norkin & Levangie, with permission.)

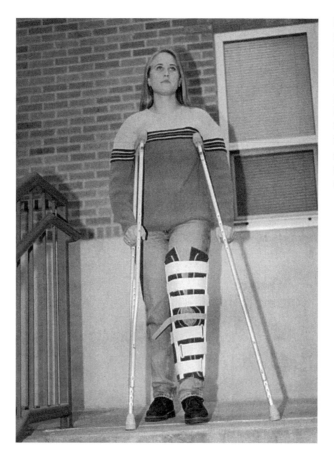

FIG. 9–9
Straight leg knee immobilizer. The use of a straight-leg knee immobilizer and an assistive device will help to prevent further damage to an acutely sprained ACL of the knee. Care should be taken during the acute and subacute stages of healing to deter the negative effects of immobilization.

knee. Special evaluation tests performed by the supervising PT to assess the integrity of knee joint structures may include[14]:

1. Lachman's test—used to assess ACL integrity
2. Anterior drawer test—used to assess ACL integrity
3. Posterior drawer test—used to assess PCL integrity
4. Pivot shift test—used to assess ACL rotatory stability
5. Valgus stress test—used to assess MCL integrity
6. Varus stress test—used to assess LCL integrity
7. McMurray's sign—used to assess meniscal integrity
8. Apley's compression and distraction test—used to differentiate between meniscal and ligamentous injury of the knee

The physician may use magnetic resonance imaging (MRI) to help confirm or reject the presence of damage to the structures within the knee. The ability of the MRI to assess the integrity of the meniscus is greater than the reliability of detecting actual ACL tears. A significant chance of false-positive results identifying an injury to the ACL. Therefore, clinical judgement and expertise should still be used as the primary assessment tool.[13]

Clinical Management. After a ligamentous knee injury, the clinical decision must be made to manage the client conservatively or surgically. The severity of the sprain and the clinical presentation of stability of the knee are major deciding factors in choosing a rehabilitation approach. Nonoperative management of a client with an MCL sprain in most cases is the first clinical option. Clients presenting with an ACL sprain can be effectively managed conservatively, if knee joint stability is not jeopardized. Clients who are not involved in strenuous activities that require jumping or direction changes may be successfully managed conservatively. Clients who present with evidence of an ACL sprain (grade I or II), but do not demonstrate joint instability or meniscal damage, are good candidates for nonoperative management. Giove et al.[15] found, in a retrospective study examining outcomes of clients that participated in rehabilitation without surgical intervention after a ligamentous knee injury, that more than half of the observed clients were able to return to their prior level of activity with only mild discomfort in the affected knee. One of the primary factors in predicting return to function was a greater-than-normal hamstring to quadriceps femoris strength ratio. Those clients who were able to increase the strength of their hamstrings found that the hamstring muscle can function as a dynamic stabilizer, assisting the torn ACL in preventing an anterior translation of the tibia from under the femur during activity (Box 9–1).[10,16]

Initial management of the acutely sprained ACL should address efforts to control the effects of inflammation and promote protection. Protection of the injured ligament is described as a brief period of immobilization and controlled weight bearing. Modalities designed to reduce joint effusion can be used. Cryotherapy, compression, elevation, and electrical stimulation are all appropriate. Functional, controlled ROM exercises, promoting knee extension and flexion, should be encouraged early to deter the adverse effects of immobilization. Figures 9–10 through 9–18 demonstrate a basic ACL rehabilitation program for the stable injury. As function improves, total body conditioning should be considered.[3,10]

Box 9–1

HAMSTRING TO QUADRICEPS FEMORIS STRENGTH RATIO IN ANTERIOR CRUCIATE LIGAMENT REHABILITATION

The role of the ACL in the knee joint is to provide stability to the moving joint. The ACL is taut in full extension and will limit hyperextension of the knee. The same ligament will also prevent the anterior translation of the tibia from under the femur during weight-bearing activities. By strengthening the hamstring muscles, which pull posteriorly on the tibia, a dynamic or active stabilization can be produced to counter the tendency of the tibia to slide anteriorly. If the quadriceps femoris muscle, which tends to pull the tibia anteriorly, is considerably stronger than the hamstrings, a muscular imbalance may result with a tendency to pull the tibia anteriorly. Normal relationships of strength between the hamstrings and the quadriceps vary, but are generally accepted as a 2:3 (hams:quads) ratio. The strength, when measured through isokinetic testing, should show quadriceps normally one-third stronger than the ipsilateral side hamstrings to achieve a balance. However, in the rehabilitation of a knee joint that has lost stability as a result of injury of the ACL, some professionals argue that the strength relationship should approach 1:1. Aggressive strengthening of the hamstrings may help to achieve the dynamic stabilization needed to replace a loss of the static stabilization from the injury to the ACL.

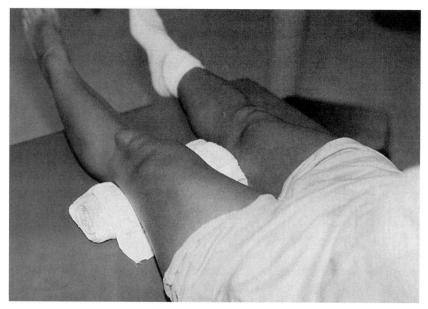

FIG. 9–10

Isometric quadriceps femoris exercises. The quad set isometric exercise produces no stress on the injured ACL, while gradually increasing the strength of the knee extensor muscles.

Rehabilitating the client with an MCL injury is frequently managed without surgery. The acute treatment rationale is similar to the management of the client with an ACL injury. Early control of inflammation and protection of the sprained area should be encouraged. Protection of the grade I or II MCL sprain should be done by placing the client in a hinged knee immobilizer with functional stops from

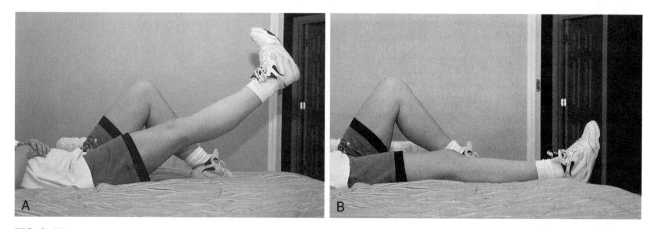

FIG. 9–11

The straight leg raise. This exercise is a combination of isometric quadriceps femoris strengthening with isotonic hip flexion. To be performed properly, the knee should be extended (terminally locked) throughout the exercise. The client should be positioned either supine with the opposite knee bent, or sitting. Start with a quad set (Fig. 9–10). After the knee is successfully locked, have the client lift the leg 12–18 in off the treatment surface (A). Some clinicians prefer the client then to hold this new position for a brief period of time, then slowly lower the leg to the starting position (B). Have the client relax between each repetition. This exercise should be performed slowly and under the control of the client.

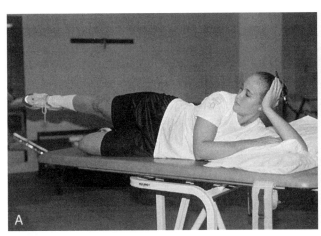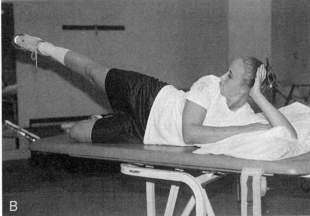

FIG. 9–12

Hip abduction. With the client positioned on the side opposite the injured lower extremity (A), the client should slowly lift the top leg, abducting the hip and keeping the knee extended (B). This exercise works to strengthen not only the hip abductors, but also the tensor fasciae latae, which inserts into the iliotibial band. The IT band crosses the knee joint laterally and can provide support to the lateral aspect of the knee.

15° to 90° of flexion. The rehabilitation team should encourage partial weight bearing with crutches during ambulation. After 3 weeks in the hinged knee brace, the client is allowed full motion of the knee. The grade III injury requires rigid immobilization at 45° with non–weight-bearing status for 3 weeks to promote healing of the damaged ligament. After the initial immobilization, the brace is unlocked, allowing motion from 0° to 90°, but limited weight bearing may be necessary for up to 3 months.[3,10]

Exercising the client with an MCL injury (grades I, II, or III) should follow the limitations of a functional brace. Early ROM exercises within the brace is desired to help deter the negative effects of immobilization. Isometric exercises of the hamstring and quads should be encouraged. When full motion is permitted, straight-leg raises in four directions, and closed-chain exercises for knee extension

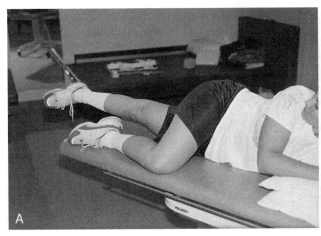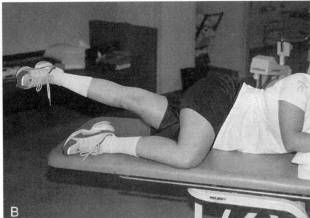

FIG. 9–13

Hip adduction. With the client positioned on the injured side and the top leg moved either anteriorly or posteriorly out of the way (A), the client should slowly lift the bottom leg, adducting the hip keeping the knee extended (B). This exercise works to strengthen the hip adductors including the gracilis, which crosses the knee joint medially.

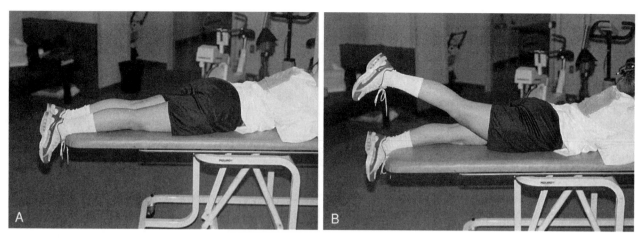

FIG. 9–14
Hip extension. With the client positioned prone (A), the client should slowly lift the involved leg, extending the hip, keeping the knee extended (B). This exercise works to strengthen the hip extensors, including the proximal hamstrings.

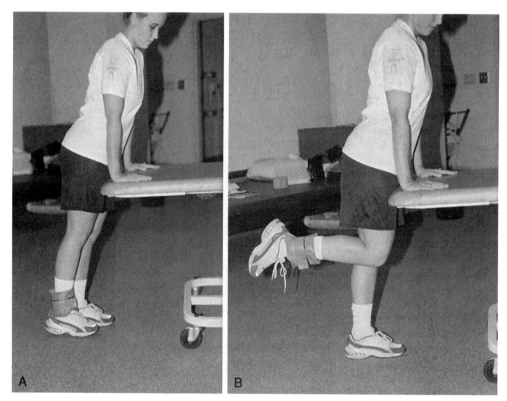

FIG. 9–15
Open-chain hamstring exercises. Standing supported at a treatment table (A), the client can actively flex the injured knee against a resistance to strengthen the hamstring muscle (B). Slow and controlled effort should be exerted by the client.

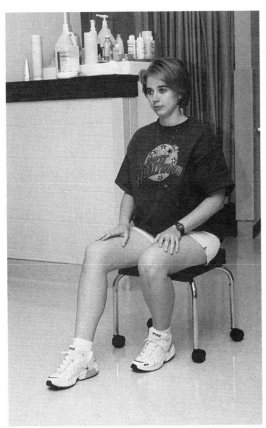

FIG. 9–16
Closed-chain hamstring exercises. To perform closed-chain strengthening exercises for the hamstring group, have the client sit on a rolling stool and pull (walk in a forward direction) the body weight across the floor.

and flexion should be performed. Stationary bikes work to facilitate increased ROM and overall conditioning. Progressive exercises should be added as tolerated by the client. After 6 weeks, the client should be ready to return to activity if full ROM is restored, no pain exists, and the strength of the leg can to tolerate necessary functional demands.[3,10]

Rehabilitation of ACL-deficient knees presents a challenge to clinicians. Loss of knee stability is a major factor that prevents the return to preinjury activity. Rehabilitation programs should focus on strengthening surrounding muscles to compensate for structural loss and prevent further joint injury. Some strengthening exercises, however, may increase stress on ACL by producing an anterior tibial displacement (ATD) force (see Fig. 9–19).[17] Displacement of the tibia produces a destructive shear force that can damage the articular surface, menisci, or joint capsule. Yack et al.[17] demonstrated that stress to the ACL is minimized when using closed-chain exercises (minisquat or parallel squat) as compared with open-chain exercises (resisted knee extension). The clients with an ACL-deficient knee had significantly greater ATD during extension from 66° to 10° in the resisted knee extension exercise as compared with the parallel squat exercise. Exercises that encourage shear forces should be avoided when rehabilitating the ACL injury.

Rehabilitating the client with a sprained ACL that demonstrates structural instability (grade II or III) is not as effective as rehabilitating the client with an injured, but structurally stable knee. Noyes et al.[18] demonstrated that through aggressive rehabilitation focusing on corrections of strength, power, endurance deficits, activity modification, and bracing, only 36% of the clients with an unstable

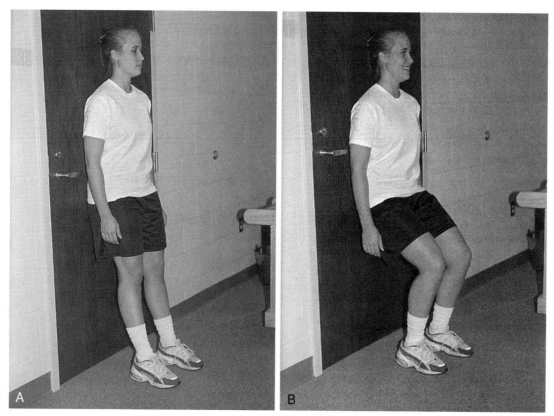

FIG. 9–17
Closed-chain quadriceps femoris exercises. Have the client stand with back against a wall or door (A). In a controlled and slow fashion, have the client lower the hips inferiorly, keeping the back against the wall, then return to the starting position (B). The client should not lower the body weight greater than 30° of flexion at the knee.

Proprioception
The awareness of posture and movement and knowledge of changes in posture and movement in relation to the body.

Kinesthesia
The ability to sense the magnitude and direction of movement in the body.

knee from an ACL injury showed significant functional improvement. Nisonson[13] reported that 60% of the clients with ACL-deficient knees treated nonsurgically, will have some type of recurrence of symptoms. The authors concluded that the modification of activity to prevent further injury or recurrence was the best predictor of success for the nonsurgically repaired unstable knee. Those individuals that did not complete rehabilitation and modify activities tended to have less successful outcomes. An unstable knee sprain that is not surgically corrected, may also put the client at risk for traumatic arthritis. ACL sprains with associated joint trauma are the leading cause of premature arthritis, accounting for up to 20% of the reported cases.[12]

Functional exercises and neurophysiological retraining, facilitating appropriate responses related to **proprioception** after a ligamentous injury, are critical in promoting return to normal function. Barrack et al.[19] found that after an ACL injury, clients had significant disturbances in **kinesthetia** noted in the lower extremity. The neurophysiological timing that sequences the recruitment of motor units is critical in developing appropriate balance, coordination, and skill. Clients with significant ligament injury or joint disruption will have a decreased ability to sense the exact position of the involved joint due in part to the disruption of the

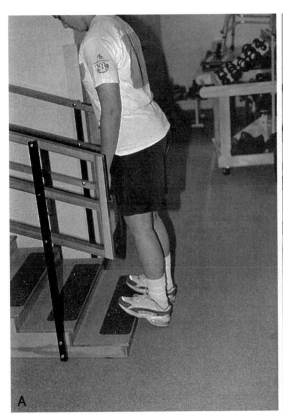
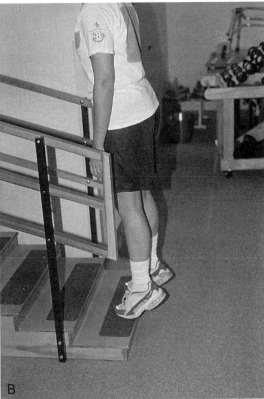

FIG. 9–18
Closed-chain plantar flexion exercises. Have the client stand on a 3–4 in step or platform with heels off the step posteriorly (A). Slowly raise and lower the body weight superiorly and return to the starting position (B). This exercise will help to strengthen the gastrocnemius muscle, which crosses the knee posteriorly, adding to the support of the knee.

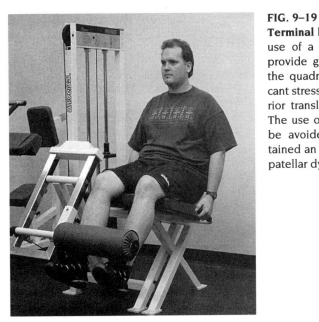

FIG. 9–19
Terminal knee extension. Although the use of a knee-extension machine can provide good resistance to strengthen the quadriceps femoris muscle, significant stress in an anterior direction (anterior translation) is placed on the ACL. The use of this type of exercise should be avoided in clients who have sustained an injury to the ACL or who have patellar dysfunctions.

Mechanoreceptors
The specialized sensory organs that receive mechanical stimuli including pressure and touch.

mechanoreceptors that are found in the ligaments and joint capsule.[20] Without appropriate and immediate positional feedback from the extremity to the central nervous system, the client is at risk for injury when sudden or unexpected events or changes in posture occur.[3]

Closed kinetic chain exercises will promote functional return. Various walking, running, and balancing drills can be incorporated into the rehabilitation of the client to facilitate proprioception. Table 9–2 describes various progressions designed to challenge the client in order to prepare him or her for a safe return to their desired activity. Figures 9–20 and 9–21 present demonstrations of proprioceptive exercises that can be easily performed in the clinical or home setting.[3]

The initial physical therapy management for the client with an unstable knee due to ACL deficiency is the same as outlined for the client with a stable knee. It is imperative that the rehabilitation team maintain open lines of communication with the orthopedic surgeon in terms of progression and expectations for return to activity. Sometimes the expectations of how rapid to progress a client are discordant among the physician, the rehabilitation team, and the client. Surgical management and rehabilitation protocols for the unstable knee are discussed later in this chapter.

Table 9–2

LOWER EXTREMITY KINESTHETIC TRAINING

Injuries to ligaments and joint capsules will decrease the ability to sense movement and postural changes in the lower extremity and the body. Exercises designed to challenge the client's proprioceptive skills and kinesthetic awareness should be included in any functional rehabilitation program when appropriate.

Walking Progression	When client can safely weight-bear on involved limb, have the client begin to:
	1. Walk first in straight lines, gradually progressing to a jog and then a run
	2. Climb stairs in a forward direction and then in a reverse direction
	3. Balance two footed on a balance board with eyes open, followed by closing of the eyes
	4. Balance one footed on a balance board with eyes open, followed by closing of the eyes
Running Progression	As skill in previous activity improves, gradually have the client add the following:
	5. Jogging in a large figure-eight pattern, progressing to smaller figure-eight patterns, gradually increasing speed to a run
	6. Sliding board activities
	7. Carioca drills (see Fig. 9–71)
	8. Plyometric exercises (including box jumps of low height, progressing to greater heights)
	9. Stopping and starting exercises such as a shuttle run or "line" drill, in which the client runs between the lines on a basketball court stopping and touching each line with his or her hands

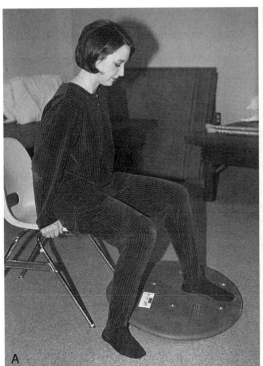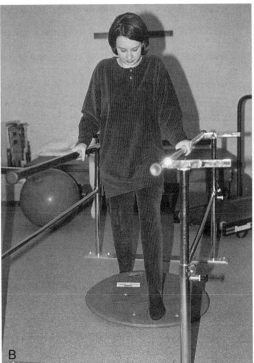

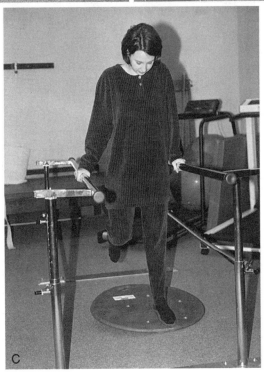

FIG. 9–20

Lower extremity proprioception exercises. The use of biomechanical ankle platform system (BAPS) board or similar device can help promote full ROM, strength, and coordination of the ankle, knee, and hip. The client can be progressively challenged while using this exercise board. First, the client can master the motion while sitting (A). Second, the client can progress to standing on the board still with body weight supported on the noninvolved limb (B). Last, the client can master the skill with all of the body weight on the injured limb (C). Challenge to the client may also occur by changing the size of the balancing sphere on the inferior surface or by adding mechanical resistance to the platform.

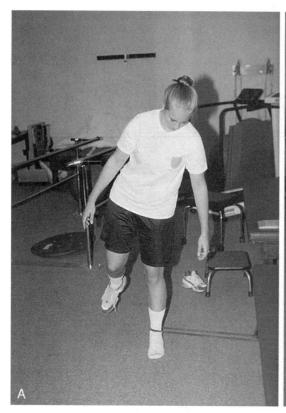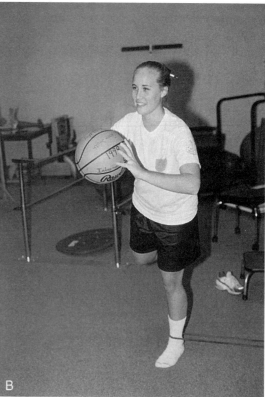

FIG. 9–21

Lower extremity proprioception exercises. When the client's pain has decreased, weight bearing and ROM are normal, and strength has improved, rehabilitation to promote normal coordination and proprioception should be addressed. One mode of exercise to improve coordination and proprioception of the lower extremity is demonstrated in this figure. Have the client stand on the involved lower extremity with a sport cord loop around the ankle and placed securely around a sturdy table. Balance on the involved lower extremity with the uninvolved limb off the ground (A). The exercise can be made more difficult by having the client close his or her eyes or by doing a functional activity, as playing catch with a ball (B).

The expected physical therapy outcomes related to the management of the client with a sprained ACL include[6]:

1. Improved health-related quality of life
2. Improved functional skills and the return of optimal function
3. Reduced risk of further disability from identified limitations
4. Improve safety awareness
5. An understanding of the risk factors that may contribute to jeopardizing health status
6. An understanding of strategies to prevent further disability

The expected time frame for achieving the outcomes for the sprained, but stable, knee should be achieved in less than 3 months. The client with a mild injury may be able to resume full activities in 4 to 6 weeks. The client with a severe sprain may need up to the full 3 months to heal. Surgical time frames for recovery are discussed later in this chapter.

ANKLE SPRAINS

The ankle joint is frequently injured during sporting activities. The ankle mortise joint is stabilized by the bony structure relationship of the distal fibula and tibia, the dome of the talus, and the ligamentous support provided by medial and lateral ligaments.[21] When the ankle is forcefully inverted or everted, damage to the supporting ligaments may occur (Fig. 9–22A). The medial ligament (the deltoid ligament) is a strong, broad ligament that limits eversion of the ankle. The lateral ligaments, including the anterior talofibular (ATF), calcaneofibular (CF), and posterior talofibular (PTF) ligaments, check inversion of the ankle. Injury of the lateral ligaments is most likely to occur as a result of an inversion sprain in combination with plantar flexion. See Figure 9–22B for an illustration of the ankle ligaments.[14,22]

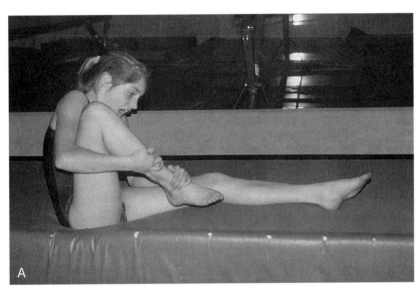

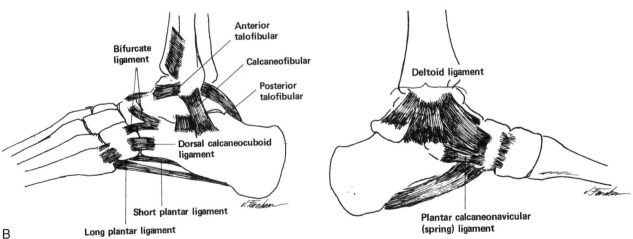

FIG. 9–22

(A) Traumatic ankle injuries. Ligamentous ankle injuries may occur as a result of forced inversion or eversion. **(B) Ligaments of the ankle.** The combination of the ATF, CF, and PTF provide for lateral ankle joint stability limiting varus forces (*left*). The strong deltoid ligament provides for medial ankle joint stability limiting valgus forces (*right*). (From Norkin & Levangie, p 385, with permission.)

The lateral ligaments can be injury graded depending on which ligament is involved. A grade I lateral ankle sprain is classified as a mild stretching with little or no tearing of the ATF. A grade II lesion results in the complete disruption of the ATF and partial tearing of the CF. Mild to moderate instability results. A grade III lesion is an unstable sprain completely disrupting the ATF and CF with some involvement of the PTF. Frequently with grade III lesions, the peroneal nerve is also damaged. Eversion deltoid sprains, occurring less frequently than inversion sprains, are more severe. Sprains of the deltoid ligament follow the same grading system as presented earlier in this chapter.[23]

Clinical Presentation

A client presenting with a mild grade I lesion will have mild swelling and tenderness over the ATF region (sinus tarsi). Generally no instability is noted with a grade I lesion. A client who has sustained a grade II lesion will have marked pain and tenderness over the injured ligaments, noted mild or moderate instability, loss of ankle and foot motion, and edema. A grade III lesion will be clinically unstable. A significant amount of swelling and loss of function will be present. The pain and tenderness may not be as severe as the grade II lesion. The presence of **ecchymosis** is almost certain 2 or 3 days after the injury has occurred.[23]

Evaluation: Tools and Methods

The evaluating PT should gather a complete history of the condition to date. Objective measures of ROM, strength, swelling, functional status, and ability to weight-bear should also be included. Palpation may help to identify tender areas and the involvement of structures. Special tests designed to identify the presence of injury to the ligaments of the ankle include (1) anterior drawer to check the integrity of the ATF ligament and (2) talar tilt inversion stress test to check the integrity of the CF ligament.[23]

Clinical Management

Conservative management of the acute lateral ankle sprain is typically effective for most clients, and physical therapy plays a critical role in that management.[23,24] An early functional management of the client with an acute lateral ankle sprain includes:

1. Protection of the injured ankle
2. Resolution of acute inflammation
3. Early ROM exercises
4. Early weight bearing

Very conservative management of the acute, stable injury would be immobilization in a cast; however, the negative effects produced from immobilization delay the full recovery of the client. Clients participating in functional rehabilitation programs compared with those given immobilization protocols have faster return to activity, fewer complications, and no long-term stability problems.[23]

Protection of the recently injured ankle is one of the first treatment concerns. Use of external supporting or protection devices in the functional management of the client with an ankle sprain is controversial regarding the effectiveness of the supporting device.[22] Taping or external bracing has been commonly used to limit

Ecchymosis
A noted skin discoloration consistent with bleeding in the tissue. The color originally will be blue to black and will change to greenish brown or yellow. Clients with dark pigmented skin will often experience darker shades in the injured tissue and the greenish brown or yellow may not be observed.

the motion of the ankle joint and to protect the joint from further injury (Fig. 9–23). Repeated injury may potentially lead to residual inflammatory symptoms and chronic instability of the ankle.[22] In active-duty soldiers, daily taping, conventional modalities, and exercise was found to be superior to the use of a gel cast, conventional modalities, and exercise.[25] Other researchers determined that some external braces significantly reduce undesired ankle motion, safely protecting the ankle joint during activity. Lofvenberg and Karrholm[22] believe that the use of semirigid bracing is effective in the management of lateral ankle sprains because of the added element of support given to the injured ankle.

Reducing the effects of acute inflammation is an immediate concern in the management of the client with an acute ankle sprain. Ice, compression, and eleva-tion have been recommended as the classic intervention for acute ankle sprains.[26,27] Ice water immersion is effective for the management of swelling after a first- or second-degree ankle sprain (Fig. 9–24).[25] The use of intermittent compres-sion pumps in combination with cryotherapy can also be an effective intervention in reducing edema (Fig. 9–25). Cote et al.[28] suggest that the preferred modality should be cryotherapy, as compared with heat or contrast bath, for all phases of ankle sprains when edema management is the goal. Michlovitz et al.[27] found that edema and pain after an acute lateral ankle sprain was reduced with the conserva-tive intervention of ice, compression, and elevation. They did not find any signifi-cant added benefit from using high-voltage pulsed stimulation (HVPS) in the conservative management of an ankle sprain. Compression is also a desired inter-vention to help mobilize fluids out of the lower leg (Fig. 9–26). Lastly, elevation is encouraged by using the positive effects of gravity to promote the reduction of edema in the injured ankle. Rucinski et al.[26] believe that elevation is the most effective modality in reducing **pitting edema** in grade I or II ankle sprains. If the lower extremity is left in a gravity-dependent position, fluid accumulation will

Pitting Edema
Pitting edema is present when the skin maintains the depression or imprint made by a compressing finger. It typically occurs distally in the extremities.

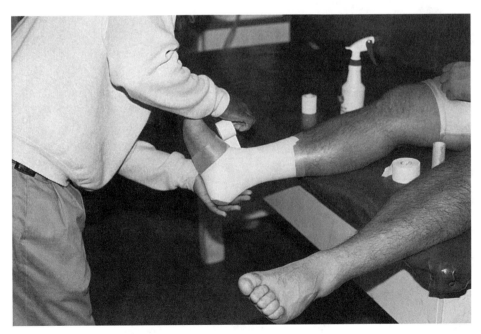

FIG. 9–23
Taping for the ankle sprain. Pictured here is one method of external support for the client who has suffered an ankle sprain.

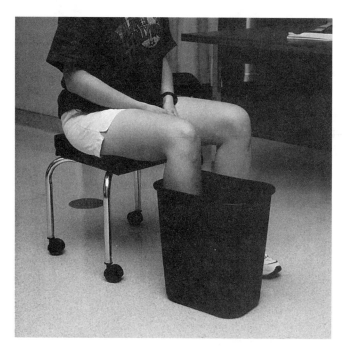

FIG. 9–24
Ice bath for ankle sprain.
An ice bath prepared in a common bucket or trash can is a very effective tool in delivering cryotherapy to the acutely sprained ankle.

occur in the lowest aspect of the extremity. If the leg is elevated above the heart, just as water rolls down a hill, fluids will be moved out of the distal aspects of the lower extremity and returned to the venous and lymphatic systems for removal from or recirculation into the body (Fig. 9–27).[23]

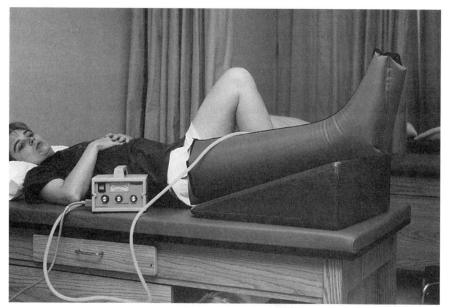

FIG. 9–25
Intermittent compression pump for ankle sprain. Compression assists with the management of acute edema after an ankle sprain. Some compression pumps work by circulating air through a sleeve, while others use cool water as the compressing medium.

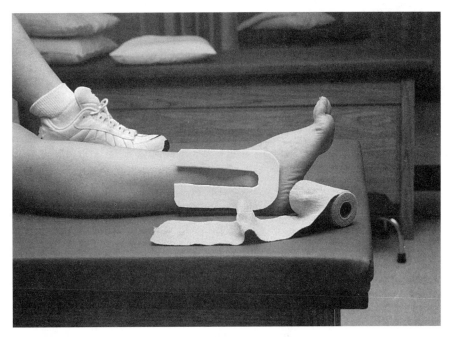

FIG. 9–26
Compression wraps for ankle sprains. The use of compression works to mobilize excessive fluids out of the injured lower extremity. Edema is a natural process of injury and inflammation, but can inhibit healing and prolong rehabilitation efforts if left unchecked. Pictured here is a lateral "horseshoe" cut from foam that is applied around the lateral malleolus and secured with an elastic wrap. The pressure from the wrap and the "horseshoe" work to move fluids proximally out of the foot. Care should be taken when applying elastic wraps to avoid constriction, adding to retention of fluids. The greatest pressure should be distally when the wrap is first applied, gradually lessening the pressure as the wrap is progressed proximally.

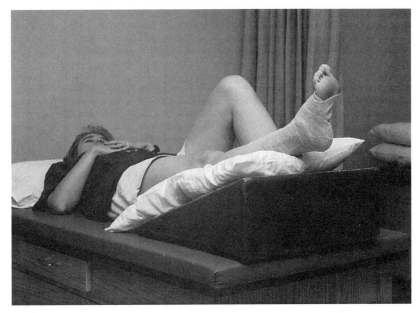

FIG. 9–27
Elevation for ankle sprains. Elevation may be the most effective means of reducing swelling in the distal lower extremity. For elevation to be effective, the injured body part should be placed above the level of the heart.

FIG. 9–28
Ankle dorsiflexion AROM. During the acute stage of the injury, AROM within the limits of pain should be encouraged. This figure demonstrates a client performing active ankle dorsiflexion.

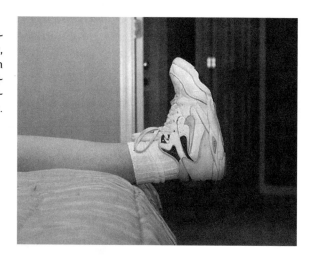

In a functional approach, early ROM is encouraged to prevent the negative effects of acute inflammation and immobilization, including edema, pain, and joint stiffness. Exercises for the sprained ankle include active range-of-motion (AROM) exercises progressing to progressive resistive exercise when tolerated by the client. AROM exercises should include ankle dorsiflexion, plantar flexion, circumduction, and toe flexion and extension (Figs. 9–28 through 9–31). When tolerated by the client, the AROM exercises can be upgraded to resistive exercises using an appropriate form of mechanical or manual resistance (Figs. 9–32 through 9–36). As tolerance to weight bearing on the injured lower extremity improves, closed-chain exercises designed to improve proprioception and coordination should be included (see Figs. 9–20 and 9–21).[3,23]

Early weight bearing is the last critical element in managing a client with an acute ankle sprain. Frequent weight bearing will result in increased proprioceptive awareness. Protection of the ankle joint early in the healing phase may be accomplished by limiting weight bearing on the affected extremity through the use of an assistive device (Fig. 9–37). A guideline for the use of assistive devices and ankle sprains includes the assessment of pain perceived by the client. If the client is able to ambulate without discomfort or gait deviations, the use of crutches is not

FIG. 9–29
Ankle plantarflexion AROM. The client in this figure is performing active ankle plantarflexion.

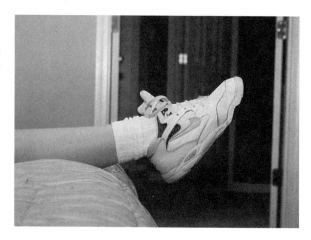

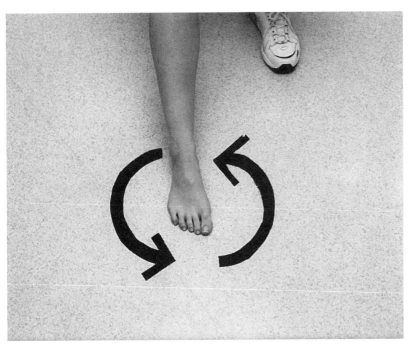

FIG. 9–30
Ankle circumduction AROM. Moving the ankle in a circular fashion will encourage all of the combination active motions of the ankle. Ankle circumduction is a combination of ankle plantarflexion, inversion, dorsiflexion, and eversion. A similar exercise is named "alphabet exercises." Instruct the client to pretend that the great toe is a pen and the task is to spell the alphabet with the great toe, foot, and ankle in letters as big as possible.

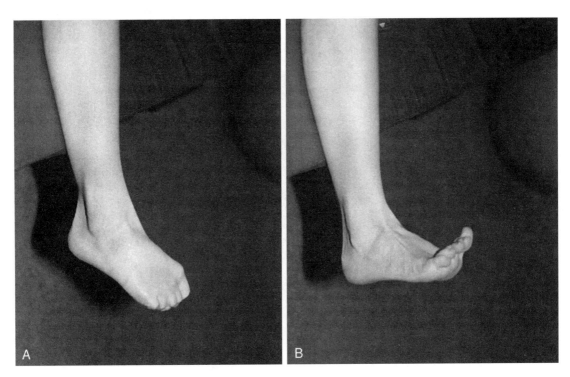

FIG. 9–31
Toe AROM. By flexing (A) and extending (B) the toes of the injured foot, the client is encouraging motion of the long toe flexors and extensors that cross the ankle joint.

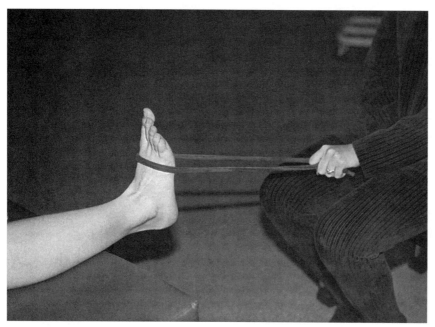

FIG. 9–32
Ankle dorsiflexion PRE. When tolerated by the client, strengthening of the muscles that cross the ankle joint should be encouraged, to reverse the effects of acute inflammation and promote the functional return of the client. The use of elastic bands is one method that applies resistance to the dorsiflexion muscles of the ankle. Other modes of resistance include ankle weights, resistive machines (see Fig. 2–11), or manual resistance.

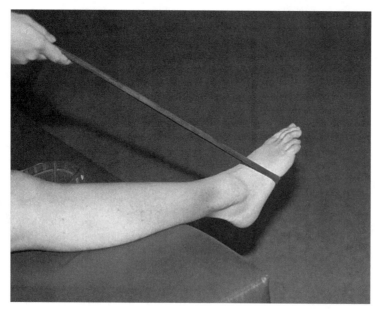

FIG. 9–33
Ankle plantar flexion PRE. Resistive plantar flexion is demonstrated with an elastic band.

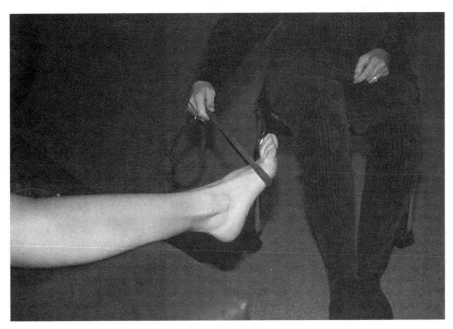

FIG. 9–34
Ankle eversion PRE. Resistive ankle eversion is demonstrated with an elastic band.

indicated. However, if the client has pain with weight bearing and an antalgic gait pattern is demonstrated, then crutches should be used.[3,23]

If the first-time injury is severe enough to be graded III, conservative immobilization is needed to allow adequate healing of the injured tissue. A functional program should not initially be pursued. A grade III lesion requires immobilization in an ankle-foot orthosis or walker boot for a period of at least

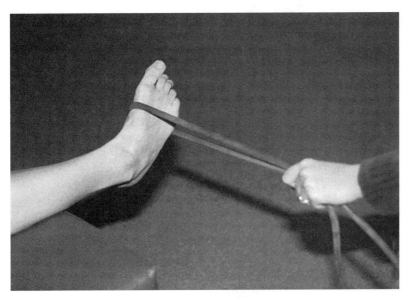

FIG. 9–35
Ankle inversion PRE. Resistive ankle inversion is demonstrated with an elastic band.

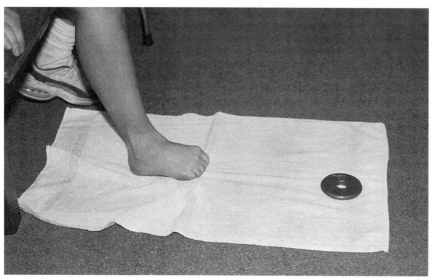

FIG. 9–36

Toe flexion PRE. Strengthening to the long toe flexors helps to provide stability of the ankle as the tendons pass posteriorly to the medial malleolus. Have the client sit with a bare foot on a long towel. Place a weight on the end of the towel farthest from the client. Ask the client to curl the towel toward herself using only her toes. Repeat the exercise several times.

FIG. 9–37

Partial weight-bearing. If the client can ambulate pain free and without gait abnormalities, the use of crutches is not necessary. If the client has pain when ambulating and gait deviations are noted, then the client should be properly fitted with crutches or another appropriate assistive device. The client should be instructed in a partial weight-bearing gait to protect the injured lower extremity body part (e.g., ankle or knee) while the body part is healing.

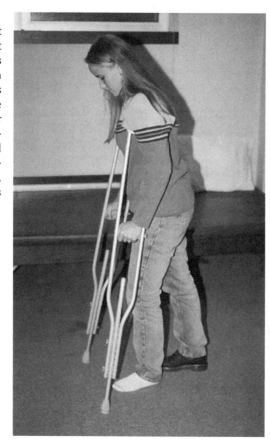

3 weeks. After the client has successfully completed the immobilization requirement, the functional rehabilitation program as outlined may begin.[24]

Clients that have chronic ankle instability from recurrent ankle sprains may be a candidate for surgery. Various stabilizing procedures are available to the surgeon. Postoperative management includes a period of immobilization and limited weight bearing. Upon removal of the immobilization cast or boot, the client will follow a similar functional rehabilitation program designed for the acute ankle sprain.[24]

The expected physical therapy outcomes for the management of a client with an ankle sprain include[6]:

1. Improved functional skills and the return of optimal function
2. Improved safety awareness of client
3. An understanding of the risk factors that may contribute to jeopardizing health status
4. An understanding of strategies to prevent further disability

For the client with a grade I or grade II injury, the expected time frame for achieving outcomes is relatively short. Most acute ankle sprains have good to excellent outcomes whether managed conservatively or operatively.[23] Scotece and Guthrie[25] reported that active soldiers that suffered a grade II ankle sprain resumed normal duties within 13 days. With grade III lesions, Meisterling[24] reported that 96% of the clients treated eventually returned to their activity of choice in an average time of 2.6 months (range 1 to 7 months). Significant factors that may deter effective rehabilitation outcomes in recurrent lateral ankle sprains included peroneal muscle weakness, tight Achilles tendon, and loss of proprioception.[24]

FOOT AND DIGIT SPRAINS

Acute and chronic foot pain is common and can be a result of sudden direct trauma; however, it is typically involved via a mechanical overuse syndrome. Foot pain in general is discussed in Chapter 10. In this chapter, a discussion of the management of acute traumatic injury to the digits of the foot is presented.

Turf Toe

A common traumatic sprain involving the digits of the foot is a condition known as "turf toe." The injury occurs to the metatarsophalangeal (MTP) joint of the great toe as a result of a hyperextension force. Resulting damage is produced to the capsule and capsular supporting ligaments on the plantar surface of the great toe. Factors contributing to hyperextension of the great toe include playing on a hard surface (e.g., artificial turf) or a flexible toe box in athletic shoes.

Clinical Presentation. The client may or may not be able to describe the mechanism of injury. A forceful hyperextension may have occurred during a competition resulting in immediate pain in the great toe. The client may notice that the pain became intense several hours after the event. Pain is usually intense and will increase with weight bearing on the injured foot. The client will typically demonstrate an antalgic gait as he or she tries to avoid placing weight onto the great toe. Motion of the great toe may be limited and the client may describe that the toe feels stiff. Extremes of the extension motion should reproduce the acute pain. The injury is graded I, II, or III depending on the severity of the ligament and capsular damage.[3,23]

Evaluation: Tools and Methods. The supervising PT should perform a comprehensive evaluation to include a complete history with mechanism of injury; objective measurements including ROM, pain assessment, amount of swelling present, presence or absence of ecchymosis, and the ability to weight-bear; and joint integrity tests. The evaluating therapist may perform ligamentous stress tests on the MTP to assess the integrity of the injured ligaments and the joint play. Often radiographic examinations are used to rule out a possible fracture.[23]

Clinical Management. Management of the client with a turf toe injury follows conservative guidelines that include protection, control of inflammation, and restoration of lost function to the involved structure. The acute grade I lesion will require modalities for pain relief, including cryotherapy. It is possible that a physician will prescribe an **anti-inflammatory drug** (NSAID) to assist in the management of acute inflammation. The use of a rigid insole and preventive taping should enable the client to quickly return to participation. A grade II lesion will require pain reduction modalities and protection as with the grade I lesion. However, if the client is not able to safely weight-bear early without pain, partial weight bearing should be encouraged. ROM exercises should be introduced to limit the effects of inflammation. The grade III lesion is potentially unstable and requires limited weight bearing. The potential for casting exists, depending on the inherent stability of the joint. Pain reduction modalities and medication are indicated for this client. After removal of the immobilization cast, ROM and strengthening exercise may be introduced. The client is able to safely return to active participation when full, pain-free motion of the great toe has been obtained.[3,23]

Modifying activities to prevent the onset of turf toe is preferable to suffering through the painful symptoms associated with the condition. Flexible shoes should be exchanged for stiff-soled or steel-plated inserts. By providing a resistance to forced hyperextension of the great toe, most turf toe injuries can be avoided.[3,23]

The expected physical therapy outcomes for managing a client with turf toe include[6]:

1. Improved functional skills and the return of optimal function
2. An understanding of strategies to prevent further disability

The expected time frame for achieving the outcomes depends on the severity of the injury. A client with a grade I injury may not miss any activity or event. With proper management, a client sustaining a grade II injury may miss as little as 1 day or as much as 2 weeks of competition. The more severe grade III injury may keep the client out of active participation from 3 to 10 weeks.[23]

 STRAINS

CLASSIFICATIONS OF STRAINS

Injury to the musculotendinous unit is called a strain. Garrett[29] claims that strains are one of the most common injuries treated in the medical profession. Strain may result from overstretching or excessive contraction forces that exceed the physiological limitations of the muscle or tendon. The severity of the injury is graded into one of three classes of injury (similar to ligamentous sprain). A first-degree strain is classified as a mild injury that results in the overstretching or

Nonsteroidal Anti-inflammatory Drug (NSAID)
A drug with an analgesic, anti-inflammatory, and antipyretic action. It is commonly used in arthritic or inflammatory conditions.

tearing of a small amount of the muscle or tendon fibers. A second-degree strain is a moderate injury that results in the tearing of half of the muscle or tendon fibers. The most severe injury is the third-degree strain, which is a complete rupturing of the musculoskeletal unit. This rupture may occur in the muscle belly, the musculotendinous junction, or the site at which the tendon inserts into the bone. If a piece of the bone pulls away at the attachment site, it is referred to as an avulsion fracture. A discussion of avulsion fractures follows later on in this chapter.[2,3]

Clinical Presentation

Grade I strains present with mild pain and discomfort during active motion. Palpation of the injured tissue may also produce some discomfort. Although pain occurs during motion, full AROM of the involved structures is still possible. Passive motion usually does not reproduce the painful symptoms. Grade II strains have extreme pain during active contraction of the involved structures. Upon palpation, a knot, depression or divot, is present over the injured tissue. Swelling may be observed, and superficial bruising will soon appear. The client will probably demonstrate protective guarding or **splinting** of the injured muscle. Grade III lesions will have marked pain during the activity that produced the injury, but the pain will quickly subside. An absolute loss of function will be observed as the client is unable to move the body part normally. Upon palpation, the ruptured tissue will often be felt as a ball that has migrated toward the intact insertion points on the bone. Passive range of motion (PROM), as in the other grades, is usually not painful.[2,3]

Splinting
A muscular spasm that protects and stabilizes an injured joint or structure. To restore normal ROM, the protective muscle spasm must be encouraged to relax.

Evaluation: Tools and Methods

The PT will perform an evaluation that consists of a complete history including mechanism of injury, if known, and course of current medical intervention. Objective measures include visual inspection, palpation, ROM, strength, and functional assessments. PROM versus AROM as a source of pain helps the therapist determine the involvement of the contractile elements. Ruling out neural tension involvement is necessary when evaluating a muscular strain. Entrapment of the nerve roots as the structures exit the spinal column can mimic signs similar to a muscular strain. For instance, a perceived hamstring injury may actually be an involvement of the neural structures from the lumbosacral plexus as opposed to muscular damage.[30]

Clinical Management

Physical therapy management for the client with a strain injury depends on the severity of the injury and the length of time between injury and treatment. Acute management for injuries of mild or moderate intensity should focus on the reduction of inflammation through appropriate modalities and medications. Early controlled motion is desired to prevent the negative effects caused by rest and immobilization. Immobilization and protection, which include limited weight bearing, may be indicated if the client is unable to ambulate safely. A gradual introduction of muscle-setting exercises should begin. If neural tension is suspected, stretching of the neural structures must be included in the rehabilitation efforts. Kornberg and Lew[30] demonstrated that conservative modalities applied directly to the hamstring muscle alone did not promote the recovery of rugby players with grade I hamstring injuries if the suspected neural involvement was not also addressed through selective stretching. Acute management of the severe grade III injury requires immobilization, and modalities to decrease inflammation. This client may be managed either conservatively through prolonged immobilization, or surgically followed by a prolonged immobilization.[2]

Treatment of a client in the subacute phase of healing should focus on the promotion of a mobile, well-healed scar. An adherent scar may deter functional return of contractile tissue. Modalities may no longer be needed as pain typically subsides. Superficial heat may be indicated before exercise if stiffness is a problem. Activities designed to promote healing and function of the scar should begin. Active and resistive exercises should be performed as tolerated. Open- or closed-chain strengthening may be used. As muscle strength and endurance improves, the client should be progressed as tolerated. Soft-tissue mobilization including myofascial release techniques or cross-friction massages may assist in making the scar functionally mobile. As the client progresses, reliance on modalities should be discouraged, and emphasis should be placed on independent exercise and return to functional activities.[2]

Chronic muscle strains may be more difficult to manage. Muscles that are continually inflamed may develop a secondary pathology, which will create a cycle of pain and reinjury. Motions or activities that promote chronic irritation and injury must be identified. The client must be educated in proper movement patterns and avoid situations that might exacerbate the condition. A full discussion of the management of the chronic pain client is presented in Chapter 10.

The expected physical therapy outcomes related to managing a client with a muscular strain include[6]:

1. Improved functional skills and the return of optimal function
2. Reduced risk of further disability from identified limitations
3. Improve safety awareness of client
4. An understanding of the risk factors that may contribute to jeopardizing health status
5. An understanding of strategies to prevent further disability

Musculoskeletal injuries heal quickly, but return to function is slower than seen in a ligamentous sprain. A muscular strain of the large muscle groups of the lower extremity (hamstrings and quadriceps femoris muscle) may take as long as 6 to 8 weeks to heal in a grade I or II injury. A client with a grade III injury may be immobilized for 6 weeks, and tissue healing may take several additional months. Athletes place great stress on their bodies, and the injured area must be strong enough to withstand the demands of the activity. Patience is necessary, both from the client and the clinician. Reinjury should be avoided.[3]

TENDINITIS

Tendinitis (inflammation of the tendons) is a condition closely related to muscular strains. Tendon irritation may come from a specific trauma or from repeated events. The management of a client with various regional tendinitis symptoms will be similar to the management described for the general strain. The rehabilitation team will focus on protection of the tendon and reduction of inflammation, followed by flexibility and strengthening exercises, scar tissue mobility, and finally, the return of function for the client. The following section presents some of the common injury scenarios that result in tendinitis.

Medial and Lateral Epicondylitis

Elbow pain is common with activities that require the use of a racket or club and even jobs that require the use of tools. Frequently the mechanism of injury is a repetitive use syndrome (e.g., caused by use of a tennis racket or hammer) that is magnified by the torque placed on the supporting structures of the wrist from the long lever (Fig. 9–38). Lateral epicondylitis, or classic tennis elbow, is described as an overuse injury resulting in a tendinitis condition primarily of the extensor carpi radialis brevis (ECRB) and extensor digitorum communis (EDC) muscles.[31] Although the short radial extensor muscles are typically involved, a severe case may involve the entire extensor mechanism.[3] An improper backhand stroke is commonly the culprit, leading to the onset of a lateral epicondylitis, but any activity that involves a repetitive use or eccentric loading of the extensor mechanism of the wrist may produce the symptoms (e.g., hammer).[32,33] Medial epicondylitis (commonly known as golfer's elbow, swimmer's elbow, or little leaguer's elbow) can result from improper mechanics during an activity placing strain on the flexor and proximal pronator muscle group and their attachment on the medial epicondyle of the elbow.[32]

Clinical Presentation. The client will describe pain in the affected elbow and forearm that is sharp and stabbing. The client may have difficulty grasping objects, making a fist, or performing active wrist extension or flexion accordingly. The condition may be acute, with the client remembering a specific incident that created the onset of discomfort, or the condition may be chronic, persisting for weeks or months without a clear mechanism of injury.

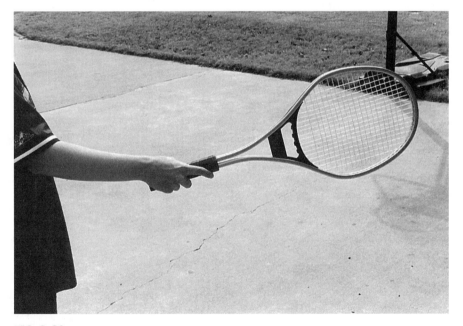

FIG. 9–38
Tennis racket and long lever arms. Holding a tennis racket creates a significantly longer resistance arm when viewing the upper extremity as a lever. The dynamic stabilizers of the wrist (flexors and extensors) have common origins above the elbow on either epicondyle. Repeated stress or resistance from the longer lever arm can produce a tendinitis of these stabilizing muscle groups.

Evaluation: Tools and Methods. A complete history should be taken including a description of the mechanism of injury and the course of treatment to date. Objective evaluation will include an assessment of motion, strength and functional abilities of the entire upper extremities (e.g., shoulder, elbow, wrist and hand). Palpation of the lateral or medical epicondyle and resisted wrist extension or flexion should reproduce the symptoms of pain.

Clinical Management. Prentice[3] claims that it is much easier to prevent an elbow epicondylitis than to treat the condition once it has occurred. Through the use of proper technique, flexibility, and conditioning, the client who participates in racket sports should be able to avoid having an irritation to either the medial or lateral epicondyle. Physician management of the condition usually involves rest, avoidance of the irritating activity, and the use of an NSAID. Resistant cases that become chronic may be treated with cortisone injections. Physical therapy management for the client with a medial or lateral epicondylitis includes[3,32,34]:

1. Acute management—pain reduction modalities
2. Subacute management—stretching of the involved musculature at both the elbow and wrist (Figs. 9–39 and 9–40)
3. Progressive resistive exercises of the involved musculature to promote both strengthening, power, and endurance (Fig. 9–41)
4. Return to function, including any modifications to activity that provokes symptoms and client education about injury prevention

In the acute stage of the injury, the goal is the reduction of inflammation. Pain reduction modalities may include iontophoresis with dexamethasone, ultrasound, phonophoresis, laser, soft-tissue mobilization, whirlpool, electrical stimulation, heat, and cold therapy.[32] Ultrasound has been recommended for the management of superficial soft-tissue inflammatory conditions such as lateral epicondylitis.[35] Forrest and Rosen[36] claim that when treating superficial conditions close to a bony prominence, a direct application technique using gel or lotion coupling agent is more effective at producing an increase in tissue temperature than the use of an indirect water immersion technique. The effects of low-intensity laser were

FIG. 9–39
Self stretching to wrist extensors. Have the client sit with the elbow of the involved limb extended. With the noninvolved hand, grasp the involved hand and digits and flex the wrist stretching the extensor muscle group. Hold for a slow count of 10–20 and repeat.

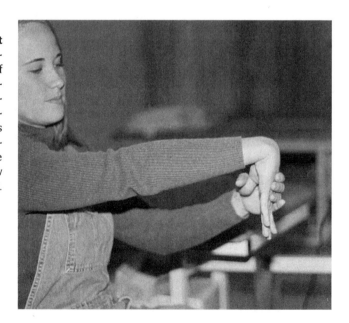

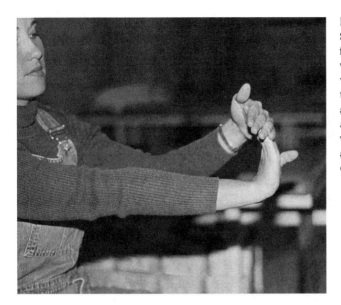

FIG. 9–40
Self-stretching to wrist flexors. Have the client sit with the elbow of the involved limb extended. With the noninvolved hand, grasp the involved hand and digits and extend the wrist stretching the flexor group. Hold for a slow count of 10–20 and repeat.

compared with those of a traditional modality in the management of lateral epicondylitis. The laser was delivered to the lateral epicondyle region at 3.5 J/cm^2 in 10-minute sessions three times a week until eight treatment sessions were completed. The comparison group received pulsed ultrasound to the treatment area at 0.35 W/cm^2 for 7-minute sessions followed by cross-friction massage for 10 minutes. Both groups showed improvement by having less pain and improved strength; however, the conventional ultrasound groups were statistically better at achieving greater reduction of pain and improvement of strength. Although the use of low-intensity lasers can be effective at reducing pain and increasing strength for clients with lateral epicondylitis compared with a placebo treatment, conventional physical therapy modalities are more effective in managing lateral epicondylitis episodes.[37,38]

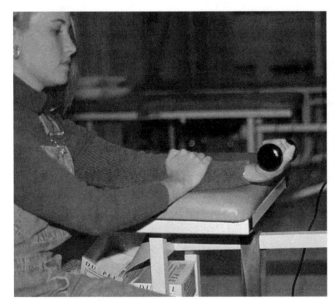

FIG. 9–41
PRE to wrist extensor muscles. Resisted wrist extension will strengthen the extensor muscle group. The focus should be on light weights with a high number of repetitions until fatigue occurs. Eccentric control is critical in developing the stabilizing function that the extensor muscle group must have to play racket sports.

Counterpressure armbands are often applied near the origin of the common extensor tendons just distal to the elbow joint to support the injury (Fig. 9–42).[3,31,39] Andrews et al.[32] stress that if the counterpressure band is used, it is not a replacement for strengthening, but simply a protective adjunctive measure. Wadsworth et al.[39] found that the use of support across the proximal attachment of the common wrist extensors provided greater strength of the wrist extensors, but not necessarily a reduction in pain associated with the lateral epicondylitis. Snyder-Mackler et al.[31] found that in healthy subjects, the Aircast tennis elbow band produced a decrease in electromyogram (EMG) activity of the EDC and ECRB proximal to the placement of the band compared with subjects using a standard band. This would suggest that the support provided by the armband may disperse forces at the common attachment site and reduce stress on the lateral epicondyle.

The expected physical therapy outcomes for managing a client with a medial or lateral epicondylitis include[6]:

1. Improved health-related quality of life
2. Improved functional skills and the return of optimal function
3. An understanding of the risk factors that may contribute to jeopardizing health status
4. An understanding of strategies to prevent further disability

The expected time frame for achieving the outcomes should be relatively short. Mild cases may show significant improvement in 2 to 3 weeks, whereas more moderate cases may need 4 to 6 weeks to fully recover. If the symptoms persist and become chronic, lasting more than 3 months, management of the condition is made significantly more difficult, and the chance for a lingering impairment increases.

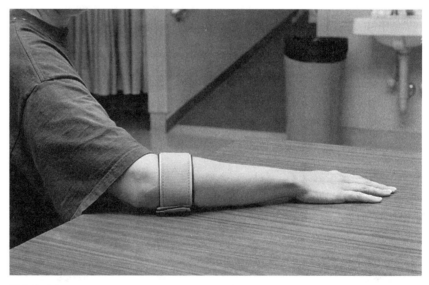

FIG. 9–42
Counter pressure arm bands. Commonly used in the management of symptoms associated with a lateral epicondylitis, the counter pressure band is positioned close to the common insertion point of the wrist extensors. Use of a counter pressure arm band should not replace strengthening and stretching (e.g., used as a crutch).

Achilles Tendinitis

Irritation of the Achilles tendon is common in runners. The tendinitis usually occurs from overuse as opposed to a specific single incident. Structurally, the gastrocnemius and the soleus muscles unite into a common tendon that inserts into the posterior superior aspect of the calcaneus. The great force demands required of the posterior calf musculotendinous group during weight-bearing or running activities in controlling the body weight may be an underlying factor in the mechanism of injury. Repeated eccentric loading will promote microtrauma in the muscle and tendon, leading to an inflammatory response. Improper foot mechanics, poor training, inadequate conditioning techniques, and tight posterior calf muscles have also been associated with the onset of an Achilles tendinitis. If the strain occurs at the musculotendinous junction of the Achilles tendon and the gastrocnemius-soleus group, the condition is known as "tennis leg."[23]

Clinical Presentation. Males account for almost 80% of the clients presenting with Achilles tendinitis. Riehl[40] claims that most of the painful symptoms associated with an Achilles tendinitis are located near the insertion on the calcaneus. A zone of pain 1 to 2 inches proximal to the bony attachment is common. Excessive pronation of the foot is a common observation in clients with Achilles tendinitis (Fig. 9–43).[40] Frequently, the client may describe a sudden change in activity as in running a greater distance or exercising at a greater intensity, without a gradual building up process. The client may also demonstrate inadequate passive dorsiflexion, demonstrating a loss of flexibility of the gastrocnemius-soleus group. Pain intensifies with weight-bearing activity, climbing

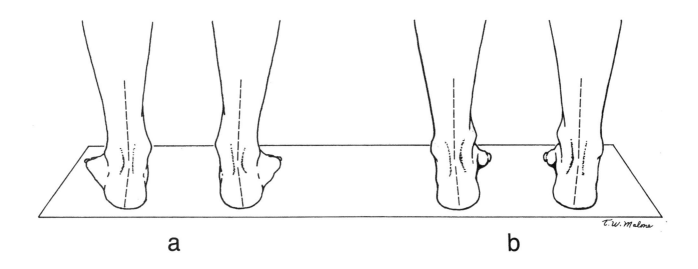

a

Calcaneovalgus

b

Calcaneovarus

FIG. 9–43
Pronation and supination of the foot. A common physical characteristic of a client with an Achilles tendinitis is excessive pronation of the foot. In the weight-bearing position, pronation of the foot is demonstrated through a combination of calcaneal valgus, plantar flexion, and forefoot adduction (A). Supination of the foot in weight bearing compromises the opposite motions of calcaneal varus, dorsiflexion, and forefoot abduction (B). (From Norkin & Levangie, p 390, with permission.)

stairs, running, or jumping. Pain decreases when activity is stopped. A palpable or audible crepitus may be present during motion.[23]

Evaluation: Tools and Methods. The evaluating PT will complete a history of the current condition and should inquire regarding the events leading up to the onset of symptoms. Objective measures should include ROM, strength and functional assessments, palpation of the posterior calf muscles and tendons, gait, and biomechanical assessment of the lower extremities. The Homans' sign may be used to determine the presence of a deep venous thrombosis, which can mimic Achilles tendinitis. The Thompson test is used to determine the integrity of the musculotendinous unit and to rule out a partial or complete tear of the gastrocnemius-soleus group.[42]

Clinical Management. The management of the client with a posterior calf irritation is dependent on the identification of the irritating event. The rehabilitation team should work to identify factors that contribute to the injury, including inadequate training habits, poor flexibility, or faulty body mechanics. Once identified, activities designed to correct the specific deficits should be incorporated. The use of proper footwear and orthotic inserts may be needed to correct faulty mechanics of the foot and ankle. A functional restoration program should initially focus on promoting healing of the injured tissue. The acute symptoms should be managed with cryotherapy, rest, and NSAIDs prescribed by the physician. Non–weight-bearing activities to maintain cardiovascular conditioning should be encouraged. This is frequently difficult with the client who is an avid runner, because the mentality of the dedicated runner is to continue to run through the pain.[40]

After the acute painful symptoms begin to resolve, the next phase of management should focus on restoring strength and flexibility, followed by a gradual return to function. Cryotherapy, ultrasound, or iontophoresis can be helpful in the reduction of inflammatory symptoms. Gentle, passive stretching of the Achilles tendon with both the knee flexed and extended should be included. The PTA should work to ensure that the stretching is occurring at the Achilles tendon by properly stabilizing the subtalar and transmetatarsal joints. Closed-chain strengthening exercises such as heel lifts work well to encourage functional eccentric use of the gastrocnemius-soleus group. The client should continue with non–weight-bearing cardiovascular exercises to prevent a loss of fitness. As strength and flexibility improves while painful symptoms resolve, a gradual running program or functional activity should be encouraged. The client should be discouraged from resuming full activities, but rather gradually increase the duration and intensity of the desired activity.[40]

The expected physical therapy outcomes for managing a client with an Achilles tendinitis include[6]:

1. Improved health-related quality of life
2. An optimal return of function
3. An understanding of the risk factors that may contribute to jeopardizing health status
4. An understanding of strategies to prevent further disability

The expected time frame for achieving outcomes is relatively slow. The Achilles tendon has a low metabolic rate, which prolongs the healing process (6 to 10 weeks). Clients who suffer from inflammation of the Achilles tendon frequently attempt to return to the activity that produced the symptoms before the injured tissue can withstand the stress associated with the activity. This potential cycle of healing and repeated trauma further delays the achievement of the expected outcomes. Asking a client not to run, if he or she is a runner, is a challenging request. The rehabilitation team should work to educate the client about activities that will exacerbate symptoms and devise alternative methods of exercise while the tendon is healing (e.g., cross-training, pool running).[23,40]

 TRAUMATIC INJURIES

CONTUSIONS

A direct blow may compress soft tissue against underlying bony tissue with a force that will produce subcutaneous bleeding. The lay term for a contusion is "bruise." The bleeding into the soft tissue may produce an external sign of a bluish-purple discoloration of the skin. Pain upon palpation may be associated with the injured area. Severe bleeding or damage to the contractile elements of the muscle as a result of direct trauma may produce pain or limited AROM. An infrequent, but potentially devastating, side effect of severe or repeated contusions is **myositis ossificans**.[43]

Myositis Ossificans
An ectopic bony formation in muscle leading to a significant functional impairment of the contractile elements.

Clinical Presentation

The quadriceps femoris muscle is a frequent location of contusions from trauma in contact sports. At the time of injury, immediate pain is often perceived by the client. Immediate discoloration is not typical, and the client will have difficulty contracting the involved muscle. The client may not seek medical attention immediately until discoloration on the anterior surface of the thigh is noted. Contusions are graded I, II, or III depending on the severity of the injury. A grade I injury is mild, with no swelling and only mild discomfort. With a grade II contusion of the quadriceps femoris muscle, the client may exhibit a noticeable antalgic gait. Muscular splinting is noted, because pain is moderate to severe. Pain will be intensified with resisted extension of the knee. The client will have a marked limitation of knee flexion and a palpable firmness over the area signifies the underlying tissue swelling. A severe grade III contusion presents with marked weakness of the muscle, severe pain, and limited motion of the knee. The client will be unable to weight-bear on the injured leg without the use of crutches.[43]

Evaluation: Tools and Methods

After the evaluating therapist completes the history of the current condition, physical observation and assessment of the injury site are indicated. Objective tools including visual inspection (which may be documented photographically), palpation, ROM, strength, circumference measurements, and functional status will be performed.

Clinical Management

Management of the acute symptoms of the contusion are the first consideration. Cryotherapy and compression are effective in limiting the bleeding within the subcutaneous tissue. A consideration during the application of cryotherapy is to place the injured body part in a position so that the adjacent muscle is in a lengthened position. If the contusion is to the anterior thigh, then the ice treatment should be applied when the knee is in flexion. This will help prevent shortening of the quadriceps femoris muscle if the swelling involves the muscular elements. Electrical stimulation is also recommended to promote acute coagulation of bleeding and reduction of edema. Muscle-setting exercises and pain-free AROM exercises should be encouraged early to lessen the effects of swelling on the muscle tissue. If gait disturbances are noted, the client should use crutches until he or she is able to ambulate normally. Treatments that increase swelling or bleeding, such as heat modalities or passive stretching, should be avoided.[43]

As acute symptoms resolve, the next rehabilitation consideration is assisting the client to return to normal function. Gradually introduce progressive strengthening exercises as limited motion improves. Functional exercises are introduced as strength improves and when motion is normal. The client is able to return to the desired activity when full, pain-free motion exists and he or she is able to participate in all functional activities without discomfort or limitation.[43]

The expected physical therapy outcomes for managing a client with a contusion include[6]:

1. An optimal return of function
2. Reduced risk of further disability from identified limitations
3. An understanding of strategies to prevent further disability

The expected time frame for achieving the outcomes is variable, depending on the severity of the injury. A client with a grade I contusion may not even seek medical attention or stop active participation in the event that produced the injury. A grade II contusion limiting knee motion may keep the client out of competition for up to 3 weeks. A grade III lesion may require up to 3 months of rehabilitation and healing time.

MENISCAL INJURIES OF THE KNEE

In the knee joint, the menisci absorb and distribute weight-bearing forces and increase the congruency and stability of the joint. The menisci are nourished passively by the synovial fluid and, when damaged, are slow to heal. Without the presence of the menisci in the knee, the potential for degenerative changes to the joint surface increases. Damage to the menisci can occur as a result of compression, distraction, or shear forces through the lower extremity. Injury frequently occurs when the knee is flexed and rotated, and injuries to the structural ligaments may occur simultaneously.[44,45]

Clinical Presentation

Meniscal injury may cause the knee joint to lock in a flexed position. This may occur as a result of damaged cartilage moving between the femoral condyles and tibial plateau, forming a wedge that limits knee motion. If the damaged tissue remains trapped within the joint, surgery will be necessary for its removal. The client will often describe the injury as a twisting motion of the knee with the feeling of an internal pop. Pain could be severe at the time of injury, but quickly subsides. Swelling is minimal unless other capsular or ligamentous injury occurred in the joint. The client can typically bear full weight on the extremity unless the knee is in a locked position.

Evaluation: Tools and Methods

The supervising PT should take a complete medical history of the client. Objective measures of skin status, palpation, ROM, strength, and functional status should be completed. Special tests used to identify a damaged meniscus of the knee include McMurray's sign and Apley's compression test.[45]

Clinical Management

Medical management for the client with a damaged meniscus usually begins with a surgical procedure. Options include the complete removal of the damaged articular disk (meniscectomy), partial meniscectomy, or a repair of the damaged tissue. Preserving as much of the tissue as possible may deter arthritic changes within the knee joint. Technological improvements in arthroscopic surgical procedures has made the repair of a damaged meniscus a routine surgical procedure. If the injury occurs in the outer third of the meniscus, where the vascular supply is substantial, surgical repair is an effective option.[46] Complication rates after arthroscopic repair are relatively low. Austin and Sherman[47] reported that complications presented in only 18% of the surgical cases, and most of those occurred with a concurrent repair of the ACL. Of the complications reported, peripheral neuropathy and arthrofibrosis were the most common. Interestingly, female clients were twice as likely to have complications as their male counterparts. If damage to the meniscus is in the inner two-thirds of the disk (poorer blood supply), then partial meniscectomy is the better option. This procedure removes only the damaged tissue leaving as much of the natural protection as possible, having the potential for successful surgical outcomes. If the damage is extensive, then a complete meniscectomy is the final option.[44]

Rehabilitation approaches will vary dramatically, depending on the nature of the surgical intervention. Clients who receive a meniscectomy will rehabilitate rapidly, whereas a repaired meniscus will significantly delay the ability to return to weight-bearing activities. Immediate concerns for the client after full or partial meniscectomy include management of postsurgical swelling and inflammation. The use of cryotherapy after arthroscopic knee surgery helps to decrease the client's dependence on pain medications and promotes early functional activities.[48] Compression also assists the reduction of edema after surgery. ROM and strengthening exercises should begin soon after surgery, as tolerated by the client. Isometric and isotonic exercises and stationary bike work are all appropriate. Progressive resistive exercises should be added when tolerated by the client. Early weight bearing is promoted through the use of partial weight bearing on crutches. Within a week to 10 days, the client should be at full weight-bearing status without the assistance of crutches. With the return of complete, pain-free ROM and strength, the client should begin functional exercises. The client should be educated about the potential for arthritic changes in the knee joint as a result of the loss of partial protection at the joint surface. The avoidance of activities that cause excessive wear and tear at the knee should be a lifelong concern.[44]

The client who successfully undergoes an arthroscopic repair of a damaged meniscus must be encouraged to be patient with the rehabilitation efforts. After surgical repair, the meniscus must be protected to ensure healing. The client will be non–weight bearing on crutches for as long as 6 weeks to avoid compressive forces. The client will also have restricted motion of the knee joint to prevent any displacement of the repaired structures. The only significant intervention during the protected phase of rehabilitation is isometric exercises of the quadriceps and hamstring groups to minimize immobilization effects. If the surgeon's protocols allow minimal active motion, then passive motion should be used to help nourish the joint structures and limit immobilization side effects to the joint capsule. Non–weight-bearing cardiovascular exercises such as an upper-extremity bike will be helpful in maintaining the fitness level of the client during this period of forced immobilization and rest.[44]

Once healing of the meniscus is deemed sufficient (4 to 6 weeks), then active rehabilitation of the client may begin. The surgeon will typically allow a gradual increase in motion through the use of a hinged knee brace with functional stops into flexion and extension. ROM and strengthening exercises should be performed within the limitations set in the brace. By the 8th to 10th week after surgery, the motion allowed in the repaired knee should be full, and the client may begin to gradually reintroduce full weight bearing during gait. Once the client is confident in bearing weight on the injured limb, motion is full, and strength is improving, the rehabilitation team should begin to introduce functional closed-chain exercises and activities. This rehabilitation process must not be rushed. The intent of the surgical repair is to save the entire meniscal element to prevent the long-term effects of the removal of the meniscus, including degenerative arthritis. The rehabilitation efforts should become aggressive only after the meniscus is well healed.[44]

The expected physical therapy outcomes for managing a client with a meniscal injury include[6]:

1. Improve health-related quality of life
2. Improved functional skills
3. An optimal return of function
4. Reduced risk of further disability from identified limitations
5. An understanding of the risk factors that may contribute to jeopardizing health status
6. An understanding of strategies to prevent further disability

The expected time frame for achieving the outcomes after a surgical intervention for the damaged meniscus depends on the type of surgery performed. Clients who have had an arthroscopic procedure (partial or full menisectomy), can return to activity in as early as 1 week to 10 days, depending on the client's tolerance and level of preinjury fitness. An average time for recovery is about 1 month. For the client who underwent a repair of the damaged meniscus, return to full activity may take as long a 4 to 6 months to ensure adequate healing of the repaired structures.

FRACTURES

A stress that exceeds the mechanical failure point of skeletal bone will produce a fracture. Active participation in sporting activities or unforseen accidents (e.g., a motor vehicle accident) can damage skeletal bones. Classifications of skeletal fractures were described in Chapter 8. Fractures are orthopedically managed through stabilization (either open or closed procedures) followed by a period of immobilization. A *boxer's fracture* is the result of excessive axial force through the closed hand that results in a fracture of the neck of the fifth metacarpal bone. A *Bennett's fracture* occurs from axial loading of the thumb that produces a fracture and a dislocation of the first carpometacarpal joint. Physical therapy intervention for the client who has suffered a fracture is often focused on the reversal of the effects of a prolonged immobilization and the restoration of normal function. The management of several common types of fractures seen in clients who participate in an active lifestyle are presented.

Crush Fractures

Severe crush injuries may involve multiple bones of the hand, including the carpal bones, producing an instability dysfunction of the hand.[49] Objects that fall onto the hand or having the hand stepped on by an opponent in a competition may produce a crushing injury to the hand.

Clinical Presentation. The client who presents to physical therapy for rehabilitation after a fracture to the metacarpal or carpal bones will typically appear after the removal of the immobilization device. The external appearance of the hand that has been crushed in a fall or from an external force may physically appear no different than any other hand; however, significant dysfunction internally both of the movement of bony relationships and of the soft-tissue structures may limit the function of the hand (Fig. 9–44). Immobilization side effects of joint stiffness, pain, and limited ROM will be common. The client may not be able to functionally close the hand or grasp objects.

Evaluation: Tools and Methods. The evaluating PT will take a complete medical history, including the onset of the fracture and the course of the current medical intervention. Objective measures include a visual inspection and documentation of the status of the skin after removal of the cast. Circumference measurements are helpful in identifying the presence of swelling or atrophy. ROM measurements of the shoulder, elbow, wrist, and digits should be completed.

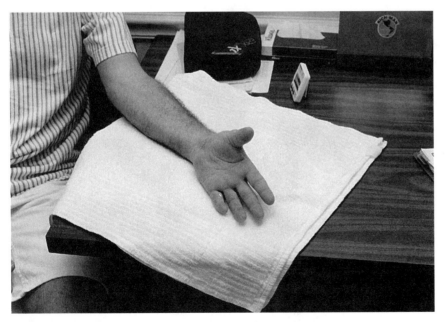

FIG. 9–44
Hand crush injury. This client's hand was crushed as a large metal box fell onto his hand, trapping the hand between a metal table and the box. Surgery was not required as the fractured first and second metacarpal bones healed well, but after 6 weeks in a cast, significant motion limitations were noted, particularly in the joints of the thumb.

Functional strength assessments of the entire upper extremity and hand should be documented. The hand-held dynamometer is one tool to assess the client's grip strength (Fig. 9–45).

Clinical Management. If the rehabilitation team has the opportunity to work with the immobilized client to prescribe home exercises, then the team should encourage as much active motion of the joints surrounding the cast as possible. The deleterious effects of immobilization have been discussed previously in this text. By performing as much active motion as possible, the client can help limit the negative effects of the necessary immobilization. Frequently with castings involving the hand, the digits remain open for motion. Active motion of the digits during immobilization works to prevent adhesion of the long finger flexors to the healing fracture (Fig. 9–46). Also, the shoulder and elbow may remain free from the cast. All available motion should be maintained while the limb is fixated in the cast.

Upon the removal of the cast, the rehabilitation team will work to restore lost function. PROM and AROM exercises will facilitate return of movement. The use of a dynamic low-load orthosis may be indicated if motion is slow in returning. Appropriate joint mobilization techniques should be prescribed to help restore normal kinematics of the involved joints. Superficial heating modalities, such as paraffin baths, work well to deliver heat to the involved hand in preparing for mobilization or stretching activities (Fig. 9–47). Whirlpools are also effective at delivering heat to the hand and have the added benefit of exercising in the water. Self-ROM exercises play a critical part in the home program in promoting improvement in the functional motion of the hand (Fig. 9–48). Strengthening exercises should focus on the restoration of a normal grip in the involved hand. Therapeutic putty of various strengths is useful for strengthening. Lastly, the client should perform coordination exercises designed to improve manual dexterity. Manipulating nuts and bolts, placing pegs in a board, and practicing writing skills are all helpful.[50]

The expected physical therapy outcomes for managing a client with a crush injury to the hand include[6]:

1. Improved health-related quality of life
2. Improved functional skills

FIG. 9–45
Hand-held dynamometer. The hand-held dynamometer is an assessment tool designed to measure grip strength. A review of the dynamometer's reliability and validity was examined in Case Study 3–1.

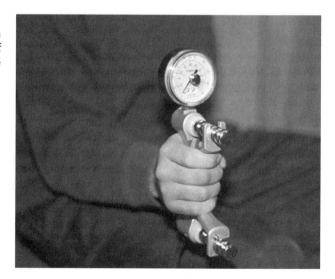

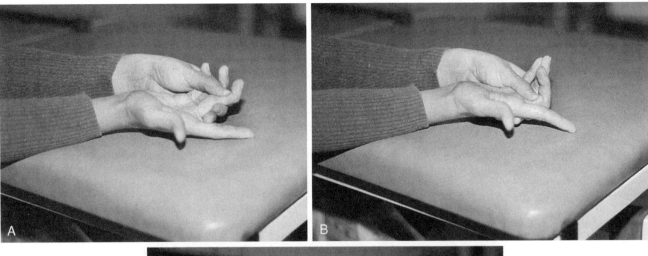

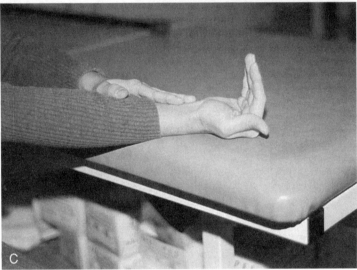

FIG. 9–46
Tendon gliding exercises. Binnell's tendon gliding exercises work to prevent the long finger flexor tendons from adhering to a fracture site. The tendons of the flexor digitorum profundus muscle are individually worked when the distal phalange is actively moved (A). Stabilizing the proximal phalange and moving the proximal interphalangeal joint will work the tendons of the flexor digitorum superficialis muscle (B). The lumbrical muscles are worked by actively performing a lumbrical grip (C). AROM should be conducted at each joint of each digit separately.

3. An optimal return of function
4. Reduced risk of further disability from identified limitations
5. Improved self-care skills and ADLs
6. An understanding of strategies to prevent further disability

The expected time frame for achieving rehabilitation outcomes after a crush injury to the hand is 3 months barring complications (e.g., reflex sympathetic dystrophy, which is discussed in Chapter 11). The restoration of the fine, coordinated movements in a functioning hand often requires longer rehabilitation efforts to achieve full recovery.

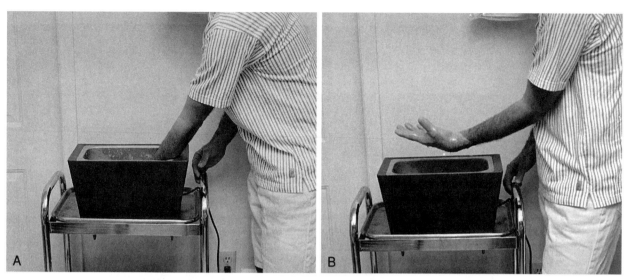

FIG. 9–47
Use of paraffin wax for hand crush injury management. Paraffin wax is an excellent medium to provide superficial heat to the hand. The injured hand is dipped into the paraffin bath (A) and after several dippings, a wax glove is produced (B). The hand is gently warmed over a 15- to 20-minute period of time in preparation for soft tissue mobilization and stretching.

Stress Fractures

A rather common injury among the athletic population is the stress fracture. It accounts for as many as 10% of all athletic injuries.[40] Repeated stress or overuse is often cited as the primary causative agent involving stress fractures. Faulty footwear and training errors have also been cited as factors that may lead to stress fractures. Commonly, the fractures occur in the lower leg involving the tibia or fibula. Tibial involvement accounts for as much as one-half of all reported stress fractures. The fibula is involved in 10% of the diagnosed cases.[51] Stress fractures of the proximal femur or femoral neck are uncommon.[52] Although the stress fracture is generally not acute in nature, the management of the injury once identified should be treated as seriously as an acute fracture.[40]

Clinical Presentation. The client may present with symptoms that are similar to a soft-tissue injury of the distal lower extremity. Symptoms include localized pain that is relieved with rest.[53] As the client continues weight-bearing activities, the pain will persist and the intensity will increase. Swelling may be present. If a client is not responding to treatment for a tendinitis or bursitis, a stress fracture should be suspected.[52]

Evaluation: Tools and Methods. Frequently, stress fractures are initially treated as other inflammatory processes that are related to overuse. Initial radiographic examination will not identify the presence of a fracture, and the injury may be diagnosed as a soft-tissue sprain or strain. If the injury does not respond to standard conservative intervention for inflammation control, then a stress fracture should be suspected. The therapist may use percussion (bone tapping) with a reflex hammer distal to the injury site if a stress fracture is suspected. The vibration created by the percussion will reproduce the symptoms. A bone scan will identify the presence or absence of a suspected stress fracture.[40,53]

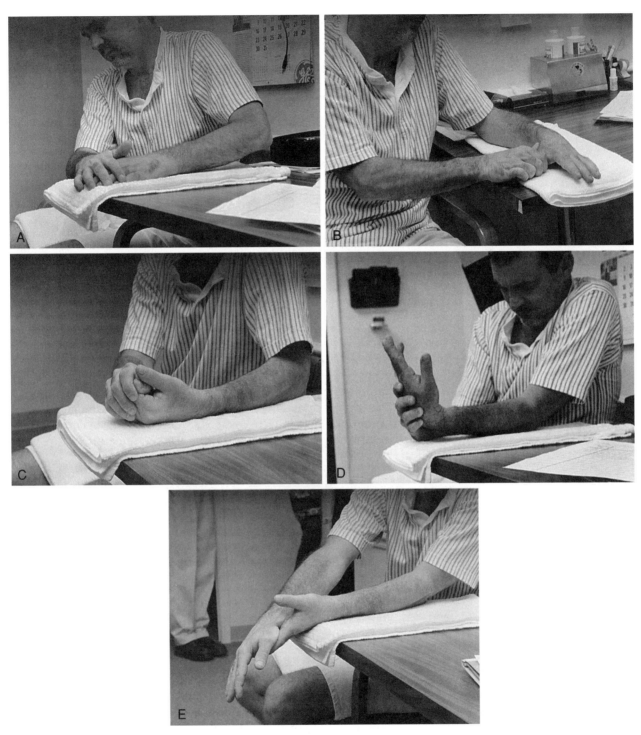

FIG. 9–48
Self ROM exercises for hand crush injury. As part of the rehabilitation for the client with a crush injury to the hand, self-stretching and ROM to the joints of the digits, hand, and wrist must be performed regularly to help restore function. Extension of the MCP joints may take the form of flattening the hand onto the treatment surface (A). Extension of the thumb and stretching the web space occurs by pulling with the opposing hand (B). Flexion of the MCP of digits 2–5 is easily performed by using the opposite hand (C). Flexion of the wrist is performed by pulling the palm of the injured hand toward the face of the client (D). Extension of the wrist is performed by stabilizing the forearm on the table and pushing the injured wrist and hand toward the floor (E).

Clinical Management. A stress fracture is indeed a fracture of the bone. This condition should be treated no more or less assiduously than any other fracture. Healing is dependent on the stability of the fracture sight, the blood supply to the area and the relief of weight-bearing stresses. The client with a confirmed stress fracture will be immobilized for a short duration (4 to 6 weeks) and be encouraged to rest and use an assistive device, as needed, to relieve weight-bearing forces.[53] Alternative methods to promote cardiovascular endurance should be encouraged that do not stress the injured bone. Pain-reducing modalities, including cryotherapy or prescribed anti-inflammatory medications, are used to help lessen the discomfort of the condition. As the pain subsides and adequate healing takes place, the client should gradually be reintroduced to the causative activity. If a biomechanical dysfunction or training error was identified as the possible cause of the stress fracture, proper client education should be conducted to develop strategies for preventing further dysfunction.[40]

The expected physical therapy outcomes for managing a client with a stress fracture include[6]:

1. An optimal return of function
2. An understanding of the risk factors that may contribute to jeopardizing health status
3. An understanding of strategies to prevent further disability

The expected time frame for achieving the outcomes for the treatment of a client with a stress fracture is relatively short. With adequate relief of weight bearing and a good blood supply, the fracture should resolve in about 6 weeks' time. The client may need activity modification, biomechanical correction, strengthening activities, and coaching in proper technique to overcome the effects of immobilization. In some cases, no intervention at all from the therapy team is needed.

Avulsion Fractures

A forceful stress that pulls the tendon and a piece of bone away from the body of the bone is called an avulsion fracture. The event can occur from a sudden traumatic force or a repeated accumulation of stress. The ischial tuberosity is a common avulsion fracture site. Cheerleaders who jump with their knee extended, producing a forceful hip flexion motion, can severely stress the origin of the three hamstring muscles at the ischial tuberosity. The tibial tuberosity is another common site of injury because forced knee flexion against a contracting quadriceps femoris muscle may pull part of the tibial tuberosity away from the tibia. Some bony avulsions are uncommon, such as avulsion at the lesser trochanter of the femur. Repeated stress from the hip flexor muscles in high-demand activities such as ballet dancing could potentially produce an avulsion of the tendon from the proximal femur.[43,53,54]

Clinical Presentation. The clinical symptoms of the client with an avulsion fracture may closely mimic those of a tendinitis, including localized pain, stiffness, crepitus, and specific pain with resisted movements of the involved musculature. An antalgic gait may be noted if the pain is significant.[40,53]

Evaluation: Tools and Methods. A history of the current condition including the mechanism of injury should be taken. Palpation of the involved structures, ROM assessment, and manual and resistive muscle testing can all be used by the PT to identify a suspected avulsion fracture. Radiographic examination will confirm or reject the suspected presence of an avulsion fracture. The avulsion fracture may be stable and nondisplaced, or it may present as a displaced bony fragment.[53]

Clinical Management. The level of surgical involvement for the management of the avulsion fracture depends on the stability of the fragments. If the avulsed fragment is unstable and displaced, the orthopedic surgeon may elect to fixate the bony separation surgically, followed by a 6-week period of immobilization. If the fracture site is deemed stable, a conservative approach is typically used by the rehabilitation team, giving the bony fragments the opportunity to heal independently.[54]

The conservative rehabilitation approach includes a period of immobilization or controlled activity, followed by a gradual return to activity. The involved body part may be physically immobilized, or the client may simply be advised to limit activity. Crutches may be used to relieve weight-bearing forces in avulsion fractures involving the tibial tuberosity and ischial tuberosity. Modalities designed to reduce inflammation are indicated, including cryotherapy, electrical stimulation, or interferential current. NSAIDs may be prescribed by the physician. Gentle stretching and ROM to prevent soft-tissue contracture of the involved structures should be included, but they should be done in the pain-free range. Stretching will also help to remodel the scar tissue along the lines of normal stress to prepare the junction between bone and tendon for activities after healing is sufficient. Modification of the stressing activity is necessary to relieve the local irritation at the point of insertion. If cardiovascular conditioning is necessary to prevent deconditioning, then an alternate, nonstressing form should be identified. Strengthening and gradual return to activity are promoted after healing of the bony fracture is assured.[40,53,54]

The expected physical therapy outcomes related to the management of a client with an avulsion fracture include[6]:

1. Improved functional skills
2. An optimal return of function
3. Reduced risk of further disability from identified limitations
4. An understanding of strategies to prevent further disability

The expected time frame for achieving the outcomes should be achieved in 3 to 4 months. Care should be taken when returning the client to competition to ensure that the healed bony junction is able to functionally withstand the tensile forces applied from the contracting muscle through the tendinous insertion.

DISLOCATION OF A JOINT

When a traumatic force produces excessive rolling in a joint, the surfaces will become discongruent and a dislocation of the joint will occur. A dislocation may occur to any of the synovial joints in the body. Pictured in Figure 9–49 is a radiographic examination of several dislocated joints. The articulating ends of the bone may spontaneously replace or reduce themselves, the client may force the bones back into place, or the joint may be manually reduced by a physician. The traumatic event will produce damage to the joint capsule and supporting ligaments, creating a state of hypermobility. If the dislocating event is repeated, the joint may become pathologically unstable and may require surgical fixation to prevent a disruption of the joint surfaces from recurring. In addition to joint capsule injury, the dislocating event may damage the articular surface or structures within the joint. This can lead to traumatic arthritic conditions in the future. The

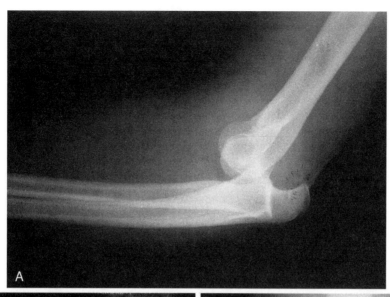

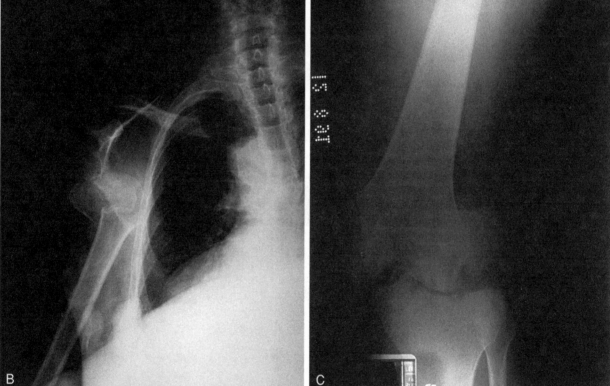

FIG. 9–49
X-rays of dislocated joints. (A) Notice the disruption of the integrity of the elbow joint. (B) An anterior dislocation of the glenohumeral joint is pictured. Notice the relative positioning between the acromial arch and the head of the humerus. (C) A traumatic dislocation of the tibiofemoral joint. Notice the displacement of the femur in relation to the tibia. Can you identify the patella? A traumatic dislocation must be successfully reduced before the restoration of function can be initiated.

management principles of treating a client who has suffered a dislocation of a joint include promoting stability of the joint, promoting normal arthrokinematics, and enabling a return to normal function.[5,49]

Shoulder Dislocation

A traumatic anterior dislocation is the most common cause of shoulder joint instability. When the shoulder is placed in a position of forced abduction and external rotation, the humeral head slides anteriorly out of the glenoid labrum. Once a dislocation of the shoulder joint has occurred, the resulting instability makes the chances of a recurrence very likely. Posterior and inferior dislocations of the glenohumeral joint also occur, but they are not as common as the traumatic anterior dislocation. After the glenohumeral joint has been dislocated, the return to function for the client is dependent on the extensiveness of the damage to the articular surfaces and the joint capsule and the residual stability of the joint itself. Common damage promoting the recurrence of an anterior shoulder dislocation is the **Bankart lesion**. A **Hill-Sachs lesion** or fractures on the humeral head may also be associated with traumatic events involving the shoulder. Clients over age 40 frequently suffer rotator cuff muscle tears (see Chapter 11).[55]

Clinical Presentation. When the client presents to physical therapy after sustaining a traumatic anterior shoulder dislocation, the involved upper extremity will most likely be secured in a sling or immobilizer. The client will have limited motion of the glenohumeral joint and may exhibit muscular guarding of the entire shoulder complex. Pain may be associated with rest or with active motion. Weakness of the shoulder muscles secondary to immobilization and pain are certain to accompany the condition.

Evaluation: Tools and Methods. The evaluating PT should complete a subjective history about the current condition. Objective measurements to be included in the examination will be visual inspection of the area, palpation, ROM, joint play, strength, and functional assessment. A special test used to identify an anterior shoulder dislocation has been named the *apprehension test*. This test is deemed positive when the client demonstrates great apprehension toward having the shoulder placed in a susceptible position for dislocation (abduction and external rotation).[42]

Clinical Management. The initial management of an acute dislocation of the shoulder is immobilization. The age of the client will determine the duration of immobilization. Younger clients under age 40 will require 4 to 6 weeks of immobilization to allow healing of the joint capsule and supporting structures. The immobilization process promotes tightening of the capsule. Clients over age 40 should require less immobilization usually lasting only until the acute pain has subsided. Immobilization for this older client population is limited in duration for prevention of an adhesive capsulitis or frozen shoulder (see Chapter 11). When the client is immobilized, active motion of the elbow, wrist, and hand should be encouraged to limit the effects of immobilization on the entire upper extremity.[5]

After the designated period of immobilization is completed, active rehabilitation can begin. AROM and PROM exercises should be performed regularly to promote normal arthrokinematics. Some clinical cases will have ROM limitations established by the referring orthopedic surgeon. These limitations should be adhered to in order to prevent the possible recurrence of a dislocation of the joint. The motions restricted are usually the extremes of movement toward the direction

Bankart Lesion
A tearing or avulsion of the anterior capsule and labrum away from the glenoid rim of the glenohumeral joint. The damage occurs as a result of a traumatic anterior dislocation and can lead to chronic instability of the shoulder.

Hill-Sachs Lesion
An indentation fracture of the humeral head as a result of an anterior shoulder dislocation. Occurs in 35–40% of first time dislocations and may jeopardize future stability of glenohumeral joint.

of dislocation. For an anterior glenohumeral dislocation, the surgeon may order the client to avoid extremes of horizontal extension and external rotation. Isometric exercises can be safely performed early in the rehabilitation efforts. Joint mobilization techniques should be performed judiciously, taking care to avoid stretching the anterior capsule of the shoulder. As active motion of the shoulder improves, strengthening of the rotator cuff muscles should be included to promote a dynamic stabilization element for the shoulder complex. Functional activities and self-care skills should be introduced as motion and strength improves. The client will be able to safely return to the desired activity when the ROM and strength of the shoulder are normal.

The expected physical therapy outcomes for the management of a client with a shoulder dislocation include[6]:

1. Improved functional skills
2. An optimal return of function
3. Reduced risk of further disability from identified limitations
4. Improved self-care skills and ADLs
5. An understanding of the risk factors that may contribute to jeopardizing health status
6. An understanding of strategies to prevent further disability

The expected time frame for achieving the outcomes for the client with a traumatic anterior shoulder dislocation is 3 to 4 months barring medical complications. The presence or absence of complicating factors will determine the success of outcomes after an anterior shoulder dislocation. Clients who suffered a dislocation but had no associated complications demonstrated successful outcomes in 80% of cases. Clients demonstrating chronic instability from the presence of a Bankart lesion or rotator cuff tear are successfully managed nonsurgically in only 12% of cases.[5]

PATELLOFEMORAL DYSFUNCTION

Dysfunction of the patella is often blamed for producing discomfort in the knee joint. Anterior knee pain is relatively common in clients with an active lifestyle; however, the mechanism producing the pain is not the same for all clients. Indeed, a wide variety of conditions that can be mechanical, traumatic, or congenital in nature may lead to similar symptoms (Table 9–3). Citing the patella as the source of all anterior knee pain is erroneous. In most cases of anterior knee pain, the surrounding dynamic structures attached to the patella or the inherent structure of the femoral groove are more likely responsible. Blaming the patella for ineffective operation is like blaming a train for not running smoothly on the train tracks if a section of the tracks is missing.[56]

A more accurate term to describe dysfunction of the patella may be knee extensor mechanism dysfunction or patellofemoral dysfunction (PFD). Davis and Prentice[44] describe that historically, every client presenting with anterior knee pain was diagnosed with chondromalacia patella (CMP). Brotzman and Head[10] state that anterior knee pain and CMP should not be used interchangeably. Chondromalacia patellae is a pathological description of articular surface changes to the posterior aspect of the patella without respect to the causal agent. A softening of the cartilage occurs in response to trauma or poor tracking mechanisms, or it may be idiopathic, which potentially leads to actual defects in the articular surfaces. This section presents the conservative management of

Table 9-3

VARIOUS PATELLOFEMORAL DYSFUNCTIONS

Many of the following conditions may produce anterior knee pain.

Mechanical Stresses	Patellar tendinitis or jumper's knee
	Prepatellar bursitis or housemaid's knee
	Osgood-Schlatter disease
	Faulty foot and lower-extremity biomechanics (including excessive foot pronation, tibial torsion, or femoral torsion)
	Inadequate flexibility (including limitations in hamstrings, gastrocnemius, and iliotibial band)
Traumatic Events	Contusions
	Patellar fractures
	Tendon rupture
	Dislocation of the patella
	Traumatic arthritis
	Chondromalacia patellae
Congenital Conditions	Lateral patellar compression syndrome
	Chronic subluxation of the patella
	Excessive Q angle
	Patella alta

---

anterior knee pain and dysfunction associated with the knee extensor mechanism, including various subcategories or conditions such as patellofemoral stress syndrome, patellofemoral pain syndrome, patellar subluxation, plica syndrome, patellar tendinitis, and chondromalacia patellae.[56]

Factors affecting the performance of the patella are many. The muscle balance between the vastus medialis and vastus lateralis of the quadriceps group, the angle of attachment of the quadriceps tendon (Q angle), and the height of the lateral wall of the femoral groove may all predispose the client to patellar dysfunction. Figure 9–50 demonstrates the dynamic activity surrounding the patella. Compressive forces on the patella can be severe at times, which may lead to dysfunction. Forces on the posterior aspect of the patella while the client is flexing the knee during stair climbing are in excess of three to four times the body weight of the client. A squatting activity may generate forces as great as seven to eight times the body weight of the client. Traumatic events, such as a lateral dislocation, may result from faulty mechanics of the extensor mechanism.[10,57]

Clinical Presentation

Many of the clients with anterior knee pain have no predisposing condition leading to the cause of the patellar pain. The pain intensity is related to activity. An increase in pain is noted when climbing or descending stairs or when moving from a sitting to standing position. Knee pain may also increase when having to sit in one position for an extended period of time (moviegoer's sign). Rest frequently relieves the discomfort. At times, the pain may be intense enough to cause the knee to give way or buckle even though no structural instability is noted. Crepitus may or may not be present.[10,44]

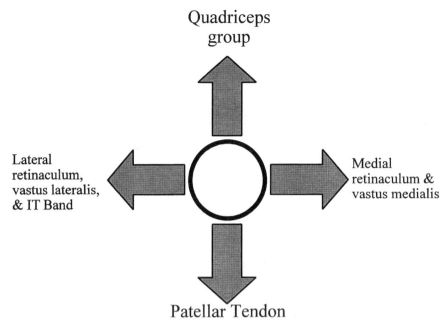

FIG. 9–50
Dynamic forces surrounding the patella.

Evaluation: Tools and Methods

Differentiating between structural misalignment and dynamic instability is an important factor leading to the management of clients with anterior knee pain. A careful history and examination should help the PT identify the true nature of the aggravating element or elements. The PT should complete an objective examination including ROM, strength, circumferential measurements, and functional assessments. A biomechanical examination of the patella is critical in implicating a cause of the anterior knee pain. Specific examination of the alignment of the patella both statically and dynamically is important. A measurement of the Q angle, which represents the angle of pull of the quadriceps group, should be taken (Fig. 9–51). The positioning of the patella may be described in accessory motion terms of gliding, tilting, and rotational components (Fig. 9–52). The position of the patella in the femoral groove can be described in relation to the height of the patella compared with the patellar tendon. Patella alta occurs when the patellar tendon is greater in length than the patella itself.[10,42,44]

The dynamic alignment or tracking of the patella may reveal excessive lateral tracking or inefficient motion within the femoral groove. An apprehension test is positive for lateral subluxation or dislocation if the client is apprehensive about the patella's being passively moved in a lateral direction. The length and strength relationships of the iliotibial band (Ober's test), gastrocnemius, and hamstring group can affect knee positioning and patellar tracking. Excessive pronation of the foot during gait will cause the tibia to internally rotate and create a lateral tracking force on the patella. Lastly, the PT should assess the functional strength of the medial and lateral dynamic patellar stabilizers. The vastus medialis oblique (VMO) muscle has an origin on the tendon of the adductor magnus and pulls the patella medially. The vastus lateralis muscle combines with the lateral retinaculum to pull the patella laterally. If the ratio of strength between these two opposing groups is unbalanced, then tracking problems may result. Clients with anterior knee pain frequently have a weaker VMO in comparison with the lateral counterpart.[10,44]

Clinical Management

Management of the client with anterior knee pain should be individually tailored to the exact aggravating mechanism. Cookbook ideas for treating knee pain, without identifying the agent of irritation, will not produce positive results, but rather lingering dysfunction. The program should be progressive (low intensity, high repetitions) without increasing symptoms, promoting proper strength, flexibility, endurance, proprioception, and the return of functional activities. Initially pain-reduction modalities (e.g., cryotherapy, electrical stimulation, iontophoresis) may be used to prepare the client for restorative exercises. Modalities that increase swelling and inflammation should be avoided. The physician may prescribe NSAIDs to help with the reduction of inflammation. Stabilizing braces, as well as supportive and corrective patellar taping techniques are good adjunctive treatments that prepare the client for exercise. These should not be used in place of exercise and rehabilitation, only as modalities to enable the client to become active.[10,44,56]

It is theorized that, despite the mechanism of onset for the symptoms of anterior knee pain, that quadriceps rehabilitation plays a substantial role in the treatment of patellar pain.[57] Strengthening protocols should be designed to address the

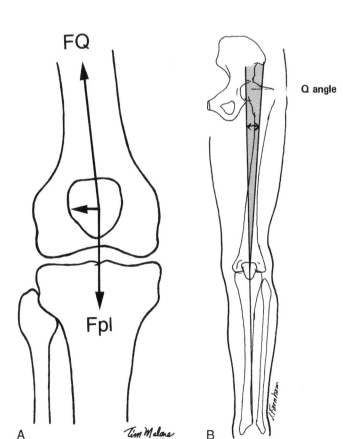

FIG. 9–51
Q-angle. The Q-angle is identified by the intersecting lines from the ASIS to the midpoint of the patella and an extended line from the tibial tubercle and the midpoint of the patella (A). The angular difference between the pull of the quadriceps (F_Q) and the pull of the patellar ligament (F_{pl}) combine to produce a slight lateral force on the patella during normal motion (B). (From Norkin & Levangie, p 371 & 372, with permission.)

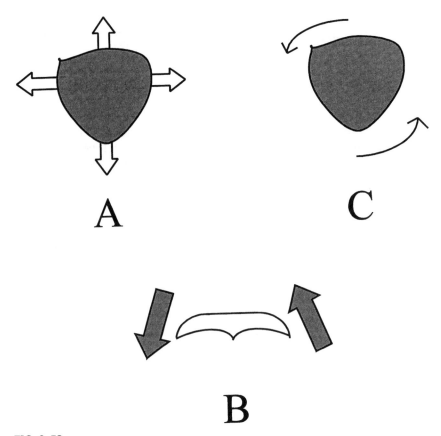

FIG. 9–52
Patellar motions. Accessory motions of the patella include gliding (A), tilting (B), and rotating (C). Gliding occurs as a result of the entire patella moving medially, laterally, superiorly, or inferiorly in the femoral groove. Tilting occurs when one pole or end of the patella moves deep while the opposite pole moves superficially. Rotating occurs as the poles or ends move in opposite directions.

balance between the VMO and the lateral dynamic structures. Isometric quad sets and straight-leg raises produce minimal posterior patellar compressive stress and have been suggested as the primary means to strengthen the knee extensor mechanism. McMullen et al.[58] investigated the difference between using static (isometric) exercise protocols and dynamic (isokinetic) exercise protocols to promote the functional improvement of the client with a diagnosis of anterior knee pain as a result of chondromalacia patellae. Compared with the control group that did not exercise, both exercise groups demonstrated a reduction in pain and improvement of strength. This should suggest that guarded strengthening activities can promote the functional recovery of the client with anterior knee pain. The authors believed that for cost-effectiveness concerns in rehabilitation (e.g., the high cost of purchasing and maintaining isokinetic equipment), isometric exercises should be considered the first choice by the rehabilitation team to manage the client with anterior knee pain.

Other strengthening protocols and tools can be used to relieve the symptoms of anterior knee pain. Biofeedback or electrical stimulation can be used as a tool to help the client isolate the VMO during exercise. Closed-chain lower-extremity exercises, hip adductor strengthening to stabilize the origin of the VMO on the adductor magnus, and short arc quads (SAQ) have all been used. Jensen and Di Fabio[59] found no significant improvement of symptoms when the quadriceps femoris of the client with patellar tendinitis was strength trained eccentrically when compared with a healthy control subject. They did, however, find a significant relationship between decreased quadriceps femoris muscle strength and greater intensity of pain. This should suggest that it is unclear which method of strengthening (i.e., isometric, concentric, or eccentric) will produce the best outcomes for clients with anterior knee pain, but it does suggest that if the exercise increases pain, strength gains will not occur.[56]

Identifying inadequate length of tissues is helpful in the rehabilitation of the client with anterior knee pain. Restricted motion from the iliotibial band, the hamstring group, and gastrocnemius muscle have all been indicated to produce excessive lateral strain on the patella.[57]

Endurance activities and functional retraining should be encouraged as symptoms decrease. When using a stationary bike, the seat should be placed as high as possible to limit the compressive forces on the patella. Stair-stepping machines work well to increase the endurance of the client, but they should be used with caution so as to not increase painful symptoms. Proprioceptive exercises can include the use of balance boards to enable the client to make a smooth transition to functional activities. When pain is resolved, a reintroduction of functional activities should be included, along with client education in strategies to prevent overuse or a recurrence of symptoms.[10,56]

The expected physical therapy outcomes related to the management of a client with anterior knee pain include[6]:

1. Improved health-related quality of life
2. An optimal return of function
3. Reduced risk of further disability from identified limitations
4. An understanding of the risk factors that may contribute to jeopardizing health status
5. An understanding of strategies to prevent further disability

The expected time frame for achieving the outcomes with conservative management of anterior knee pain as a result of a dysfunctional knee extensor mechanism ranges from 2 to 6 months. Many authors[10,44,56] believe to avoid unnecessary and irreversible surgical procedures, the client should be treated conservatively for at least 6 months before any surgical considerations. O'Neill et al.[57] believe that conservative management of anterior knee pain should be the initial treatment, even in cases of patellar subluxation or dislocation. In their study, 80% of the participants achieved satisfactory results with conservative management. If conservative management fails, then surgical intervention (such as lateral retinacular release) is recommended, but it is not guaranteed to relieve pain.[57] Cerullo et al.[60] described only poor to fair results with surgical management.

TRAUMATIC ARTHRITIS

Traumatic arthritis is the early onset of degenerative arthritic changes in a joint as a result of previous or repeated trauma. The onset of symptoms may also occur as a result of deformity, inflammatory diseases affecting the joints, and joint instabilities. Salter[49] reports that degenerative joint disease is the most common form of arthritis. Degenerative changes in the surface of the joint and joint capsule result from damage to the articular cartilage. With normal "wear and tear" after the injury, the damaged articular surface is unable to withstand the stresses placed upon it.

As athletes who sustain injuries are being managed more efficiently, allowing more athletes to play for longer periods of time, Lazenby[61] predicts that an increase in degenerative osteoarthritis will be seen.

Traumatic arthritis is not systemic in nature, but it involves only the injured joint. Weight-bearing joints are more frequently involved than non–weight-bearing joints. Pain is the most common complaint, followed by stiffness and loss of function. The pain is frequently described as a dull ache that intensifies with activity and lessens with rest. The pain may progress to a more consistent pain that does not resolve with rest. Salter[49] reports that clients will experience an increase in pain when barometric pressure changes just before the onset of a weather front.

Traumatic arthritis is a secondary form of a larger classification of symptoms known as degenerative joint disease (DJD). The complete description of the management of the client presenting with DJD will be discussed in Chapter 11. Regardless of the onset of the disease process, whether insidious or from a specific injury, the management of the condition for the client is similar.

 SURGICAL REPAIR PROCEDURES

SHOULDER OR CAPSULAR REPAIR

The shoulder complex is a complicated, interdependent dichotomy of stability and mobility. The extreme motion capabilities of the shoulder girdle provide functional positioning of the upper extremity and hand in space. However, these extreme limits of mobility make the shoulder susceptible to dislocation. The structural integrity of the shoulder complex comes from the shape of the glenoid fossae and labrum, the capsular strength, and the dynamic component of the rotator cuff muscles. If one of the supporting elements is damaged, then the overall stability of the shoulder is in jeopardy. As discussed earlier in this chapter, if the shoulder is placed in an unstable position and excessive force is transmitted through the upper extremity, a dislocation may result. Damage to the joint capsule, glenohumeral surface, labrum, and rotator cuff either individually or collectively may occur. This section addresses the repair and rehabilitation of the client with an anterior joint capsule injury after a traumatic dislocation. The rehabilitation of the client with a rotator cuff lesion is presented in Chapter 11.

Clinical Presentation

When the humeral head is traumatically forced anteriorly through the joint capsule, an avulsion or tearing of the capsule and labrum from the glenoid rim may result. The Bankart lesion causes significant anterior instability of the glenohumeral joint. These clients have poor functional outcomes when the injury is managed conservatively. The chances for repeated dislocation and the potential for the development of arthritic changes in the glenohumeral joint are significant. Surgical repair and stabilization of both the Bankart lesion and the anterior capsule constitutes the primary method of management for these clients.[5]

After surgery, the client will have the arm in an immobilizer. A surgical incision will be found anteriorly on the shoulder of the client, the incision sutured. The client will be instructed to wear the immobilizer at all times except while in therapy. After surgery, the shoulder is at great risk for damage and should be carefully handled and protected as the healing of the capsule progresses.

Evaluation: Tools and Methods

The PT should complete a standard postsurgical evaluation that includes details about the surgery, medications being used by the client, and the surgeon's rehabilitation protocols. Initially, the surgically repaired upper extremity should be objectively measured for ROM. The strength assessment and joint play of the shoulder is often deferred until healing takes place. The client should be educated about postsurgical protocols and the need for protection of the upper extremity. The client should also be made aware of the routine care of the surgical incision as well as the signs and symptoms of possible infection.

Clinical Management

The rehabilitation team will focus on the return of the client to active participation as quickly as possible without compromising the stability of the joint. The rehabilitation process can be divided into four phases:

1. Controlled motion
2. Strengthening
3. Advanced strengthening
4. Return to function

Each phase should be carefully monitored to determine that no activity is promoting excessive strain on the anterior capsule that may put the stability of the shoulder at risk.

The controlled motion phase for rehabilitation of the client after anterior capsular repair will focus on protection of the repaired joint in combination with a gradual increase in motion to limit the negative effects of immobilization. The phase will typically last for 6 weeks. The suture line should be monitored for healing, and modalities for reduction in pain and inflammation should be used. The client should wear the immobilizer at all times except when performing controlled motion exercises. Maintaining function at the elbow and hand should be encouraged by using therapeutic putty and ROM exercises. Active motion of the cervical spine should also be encouraged. Controlled motion of the shoulder should be nonstressful and kept below 90° of flexion and 60° of abduction. Passive pendulum exercises and active-assisted rope and pulley activities (see Fig. 3–3) for flexion and abduction should be encouraged. External rotation activities should be performed at the side of the body and kept within a small arc of motion less than 10°. Full external rotation and abduction will promote premature stretching of the repaired anterior capsule. Gentle isometric shoulder exercises may be introduced while the arm is immobilized to help decrease the effects of immobilization.[5,62]

After adequate healing has taken place, the client may be progressed from the controlled motion phase to the strengthening phase. The goals of this phase are progression of the client to full, pain-free motion, normal arthrokinematics of the shoulder, and improved strength and neuromuscular control. The client should be weaned from the upper-extremity immobilizer and may need a sling for protection and comfort during the transition period. The ROM restrictions should be lifted. The client should be gradually progressed to having full, pain-free motion by week 12 after surgery. Active wand exercises can be performed by the client (Figs. 9–53 through 9–55). Strengthening exercises using elastic tubing or hand-held weights may be introduced to strengthen all of the muscles of the shoulder girdle, emphasizing the scapular stabilizing muscles (Figs. 9–56 through 9–64). The PT may identify appropriate stretching and mobilization techniques to help restore normal kinematics of the repaired shoulder.[5,62]

The client is ready to begin the advanced strengthening phase when full, pain-free motion exists with no localized point tenderness in the shoulder. Strength after 12 weeks should be at a level of 70% in surgically repaired upper extremity in comparison with the nonsurgical upper extremity. The rehabilitation team will now begin to emphasize preparation for the client to improve strength, power, and endurance of the surgically repaired upper extremity. In addition to exercises performed by the client, an emphasis on speed and eccentric contractions will be encouraged in this phase. The client should increase the velocity and control of the repetitions performed during strengthening. Neuromuscular timing exercises demonstrated through proprioceptive neuromuscular facilitation patterns or other coordination activities should be included. By the end of 5 months, the client should have full motion, normal strength, and no discomfort in the shoulder.[5,62]

After the first three phases have been successfully completed by the client, the return-to-function phase may begin. The rehabilitation team will now introduce specific activities designed to prepare the client for a return to active participation. A throwing program may be designed for the gradual build-up of specific motor control for the repaired shoulder. Closed-chain activities for the upper extremity will help to promote stability and a return to function (Figs. 9–65 and 9–66). When the client can safely perform all sports-related activities with the upper extremity and the surgeon has completed a final clinical assessment of shoulder stability, the client should be ready to return to the activity of choice.[5,62]

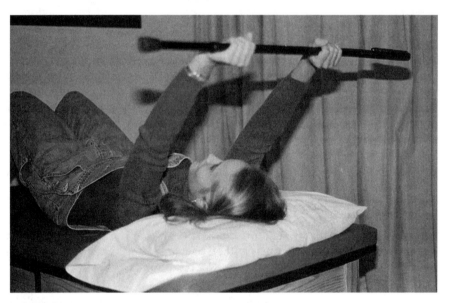

FIG. 9–53
Supine assisted shoulder flexion. A cane, broomstick, or umbrella will help the client to perform assisted range-of-motion exercises after a surgical repair to the shoulder. The motion should be smooth and controlled, performing most of the action with the noninvolved extremity. During a controlled-motion phase of rehabilitation, the client should follow range-of-motion limitations established by the rehabilitation team.

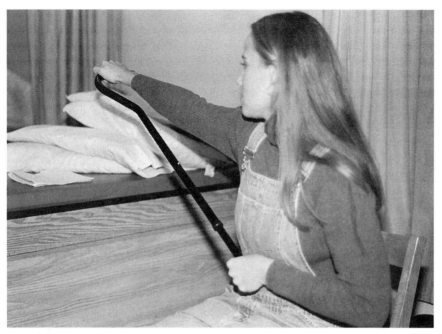

FIG. 9–54
Sitting assisted shoulder abduction. Using the cane to assist with shoulder abduction can be done from the seated position. The client should take care to remain within the established motion limitations and ensure that shoulder abduction is not substituted by side-bending the trunk.

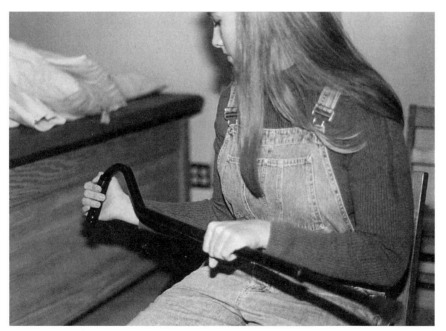

FIG. 9–55
Sitting assisted shoulder external rotation. The client can push on the cane to gently externally rotate the involved arm while in the sitting position. With the arm kept at the side of the body, small amounts of external rotation can be safely performed without overstretching the anterior capsule of the glenohumeral joint.

FIG. 9–56
Resisted shoulder flexion using elastic tubing.

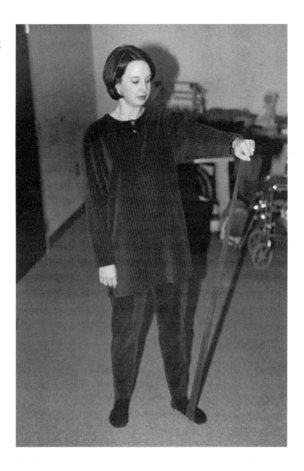

The expected physical therapy outcomes for managing a client with a shoulder ligamentous or capsular repair include[6]:

1. Stability of the repaired joint
2. Improved functional skills
3. An optimal return of function
4. Reduced risk of further disability from identified limitations
5. An understanding of the risk factors that may contribute to jeopardizing health status
6. An understanding of strategies to prevent further disability

The expected time frame for achieving the outcomes for the client after an anterior shoulder reconstruction ranges from 6 to 12 months, depending on the fitness level of the client and the intensity of the activity to which the client wishes to return. The average person in society with minimal activity demands may recover in 3 to 4 months; however, the competitive athlete may take as long as 12 months before he or she is able to return to normal competitive participation. Moreover, the client who uses the upper extremity to throw objects may take a significantly longer time in comparison with the individual who does not use the arm for throwing.

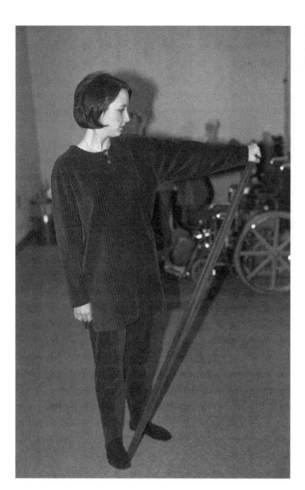

FIG. 9–57
Resisted shoulder abduction using elastic tubing.

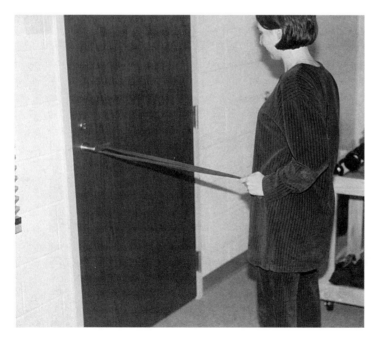

FIG. 9–58
Resisted shoulder extension using elastic tubing.

FIG. 9–59
Resisted shoulder external rotation
using elastic tubing.

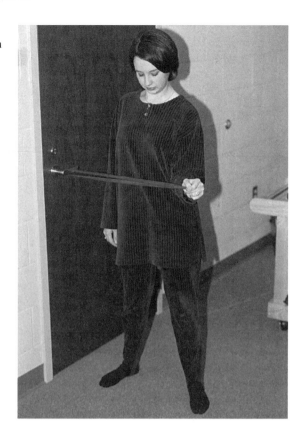

FIG. 9–60
Resisted shoulder in-
ternal rotation using
elastic tubing.

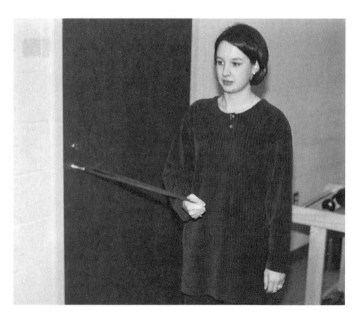

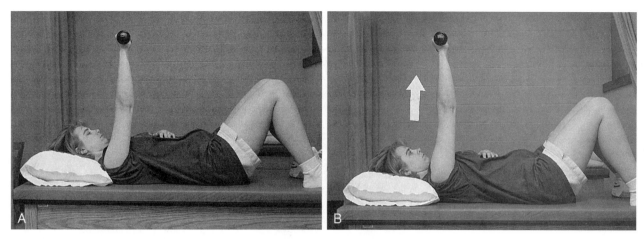

FIG. 9–61
Serratus anterior strengthening using hand weights. The motion of shoulder protraction is effective for strengthening the serratus anterior muscle. Have the client lie prone, holding the weight in the affected arm toward the ceiling (A). Keeping the elbow and wrist locked, push the arm upward (B), then slowly return to the starting point.

ANTERIOR CRUCIATE LIGAMENT

Knee instability resulting from a grade II or grade III disruption of the ACL requires surgical stabilization. The reconstructive procedures used with current technology by skilled orthopedic surgeons can promote predictable restoration of function and stability of the knee for the active client.[12]

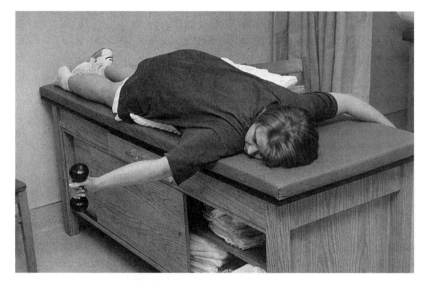

FIG. 9–62
Middle trapezius strengthening using hand weights. Repeated scapular retraction in the prone position helps to strengthen the middle portion of the trapezius muscle. Have the client lie prone with the arm extended horizontally to the side. Hold a small weight in the affected hand, with the thumb pointing upward. Instruct the client to squeeze the scapula on the side with the weight toward the opposite scapula. The client should not work to perform horizontal extension as this focuses more on the posterior deltoid muscle.

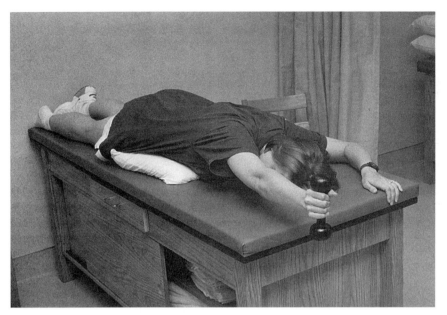

FIG. 9–63
Lower trapezius strengthening using hand weights. This strengthening position is similar to the middle trapezius, except that the arm is held 3–4 in from the ear instead of a 90-degree angle from the body. Ask the client to lift and squeeze the scapula down and in toward the spine.

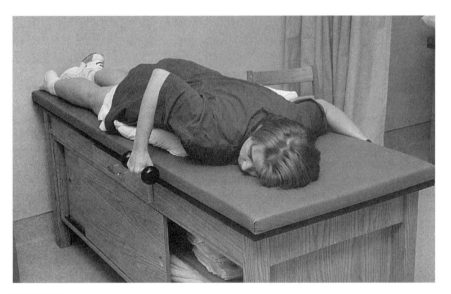

FIG. 9–64
Rhomboid strengthening using hand weights. Scapular retraction with the arm close to the side of the body will help to strengthen the rhomboid group. Have the client lie prone with a small weight in the hand on the affected side. Ask the client to lift the elbow toward the ceiling and simultaneously squeeze the scapula toward the opposite side.

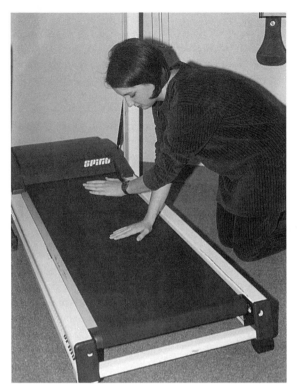

FIG. 9–65
Hand walking on treadmill. With the treadmill set on a slow speed, the client can weight-bear on the upper extremities, performing a walking pattern in a closed-chain fashion.

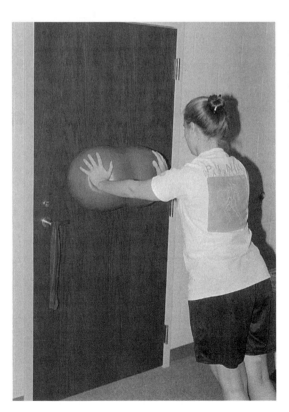

FIG. 9–66
Push-ups on therapy ball. Performing a push-up on a therapy ball challenges the dynamic stabilizers of the shoulder complex. This exercise can be started against a wall to initiate closed-chain stability and progressed to the floor as skill improves.

Autograft
The surgical process of using the client's own body tissue to replace another injured tissue.

Allograft
The surgical process of using body tissue from a donor client or cadaver to replace the injured tissue of the client.

Clinical Presentation

The **autograft** is the most common surgical reconstruction used today for repairing an ineffective ACL. The central third patellar tendon graft, or bone–patellar tendon–bone graft, is the most common of the autograft procedures (Box 9–2). Other potential graft sites include the use of tendons from the semitendinosus or the gracilis muscles, or part of the iliotibial band.[10]

The **allograft** has a much lower success rate (65% to 70%) but may be indicated if the client had a failed autograft or the donor site (patellar tendon or other tissue) is not suitable to become the graft tissue. A serious complication in using allografts is the possible transmission of diseases, including hepatitis or acquired immuno-deficiency syndrome.[10,63]

Evaluation: Tools and Methods

The PT should take a subjective history consisting of complete details of the surgical procedure, postoperative medications used by the client, and rehabilitative protocols. The client's knee will be evaluated for integumentary concerns including, skin status and surgical incision. Joint status should be objectively measured, including circumferential measurements for swelling assessment and ROM measurements. Strength of both lower limbs can be initially documented. Assessment of the client's functional status, including weight-bearing ability, gait, and transfer abilities, should be conducted.

Box 9–2

CENTRAL THIRD PATELLAR TENDON GRAFT

The surgeon will use the central-most aspect of the patellar tendon to replace the damaged ACL. A 10 mm section of the tendon will be removed with a piece of bone from the patella and a piece of bone from the tibial tuberosity still attached at both ends. The surgeon will then drill a tunnel that runs in the same anatomic direction as the client's original ACL. The tunnel will start superiorly and laterally on the femur and end inferiorly and medially on the tibia. The isolated graft is then fit into the tunnel. One end of the graft with the bone still intact is fixated to the femur, and the opposite end with the bone still intact to the tibia. The end result is the new graft functioning in a like fashion to the original ligament. The fixation devices (screws or staples) will hold the small piece of bone either to the femur or tibia and prompt a response by the body to heal the site as it would any other fracture. The small piece of bone is healed to the larger intact bone as a small isolated fracture. After a period of usually 4 to 9 months, the grafted tendon will begin to revascularize and adopt the properties and function of the old ligament. The graft, if not damaged or stretched during the rehabilitation process, will achieve the same tensile strength as the original ACL and serve as a suitable replacement for the originally damaged ligament.

Clinical Management

During the rehabilitation of a client with a surgically repaired ACL, the rehabilitation team should promote the optimal return of function. Activities should be designed to promote the restoration of full ROM, normal strength, and stability of the knee. To reintroduce the client safely to his or her preinjury lifestyle, the rehabilitation team must address the needed agility, skill, speed, and any sports-related activities. The efforts during rehabilitation should balance the need for healing and protection of the surgically repaired graft with the prevention of disuse atrophy.[10]

A variety of protocols exist for the rehabilitation of the client who has undergone ACL reconstruction. Surgeons performing the procedure will typically provide the rehabilitation team with protocols to be followed during physical therapy. Historically, a conservative immobilization approach was used that placed the surgically repaired knee in a cast for 8 weeks. The disability presented from the onset of knee **arthrosis,** and disuse atrophy was rarely overcome even by the best rehabilitative efforts. The poor outcomes from this rehabilitative approach led to the use of accelerated rehabilitation protocols, emphasizing early mobilization and activity. Despite the variations among accelerated programs, this method has become generally accepted (compared with immobilization) for rehabilitating a client after an ACL reconstruction. In general, all protocols include the following:[10]

Arthrosis
A joint disorder or dysfunction caused by trophic changes

1. Early ROM of the knee
2. Early weight bearing as tolerated
3. Inflammation and edema control
4. Avoidance of stress to graft (no open-chain extension exercises)
5. Emphasis on hamstring strength for dynamic stability
6. Proprioceptive exercises for balance and coordination
7. General strengthening and conditioning (emphasis on closed-chain exercises)
8. Cardiovascular conditioning
9. Sports-specific exercises
10. Specific criterion when the client returns to activity.

Bracing is specified in some protocols. Others stress that if graft and muscular strength is sufficient, then no external sports bracing is needed. Two basic types of braces are used after surgery: (1) rehabilitation braces and (2) functional, derotational braces (Fig. 9–67). After the ligamentous repair, the surgeon is likely to use a rehabilitation brace that covers the full length of the leg and has motion stops on the hinged knee joint. This brace is designed for acute protection, limiting some motion of the knee at the extremes of movement, while not completely immobilizing the limb. The brace is to be removed during therapy.

There is significant controversy and inconsistency in the literature, which either endorses or discourages the use of functional, derotational braces after surgical repair of the ACL. Limited evidence exists proving that the use of these sports braces limits the translation of the tibia during high-stress activities. The greatest advantage of wearing the brace comes from the clients who offer positive remarks, reporting increased confidence in the stability of the knee in the brace. Surgeons will often use the functional brace simply for that reason. The best approach is an individualized assessment of the client.[10]

Restoration of full motion is the goal of the accelerated rehabilitation protocol. The effects of immobilization on peripheral joints include adhesions, cartilage resorption and ulceration, capsular contracture, weakened ligament insertion,

FIG. 9–67
Functional ACL brace. Functional sports braces are designed to reduce the rotational effects on the knee joint during high-stress activities as well as limit the translation of the tibia from under the femur stretching the ACL. Although the researched evidence into the effectiveness of these types of braces is limited, clients often feel confident while wearing the brace. For the knee joint that is ACL deficient and unstable during activity, the use of the brace may be a necessity. Technology has produced functional sports braces that are lightweight and easily applied. The braces can be custom made to fit the client's injured knee or can be purchased at a lower price "off the shelf," in standard sizes.

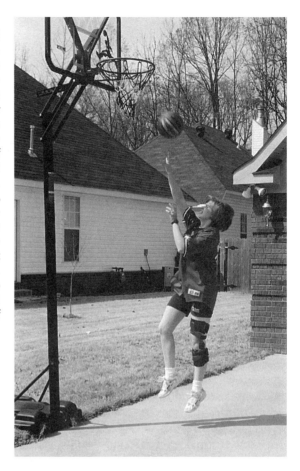

muscle atrophy, osteoporosis, and fibrofatty proliferation within the joint. Previously published studies have demonstrated benefits of using early controlled motion in reducing complications after surgery.[64,65] Fu et al.[66] suggest that achieving full terminal knee extension within the first 2 or 3 weeks is critical in the progression of the accelerated protocol. Full flexion should be gained by the eighth week after surgery.

The accelerated protocol, however, has critics who claim that the use of early controlled motion to prevent the effects of immobilization after ACL repair may jeopardize the surgical repair.[67] In the early stages of healing, the chance for mechanical disruption of the graft at the site of bony fixation is greatest in the first 3 months after surgery. Although the chances of tearing the graft itself are minimal, extreme or uncontrolled forces could potentially stretch the graft, decreasing the effective stabilization of the newly repaired joint. These concerns, however, do not seem to be supported in the professional literature. Several studies have demonstrated not only that early controlled motion is safe for the repair, but that restoring full motion after surgery helps to encourage healing and diminish postsurgical complications.[68,69,70]

To achieve full early motion of the surgically repaired knee, the rehabilitation team can use a variety of ROM exercises and stretches, but first must address the postsurgical inflammatory complications. The presence of postsurgical inflammation and pain can interfere with functional motion and rehabilitation of the repaired knee.[71] Pain and edema reduction modalities are indicated early to help manage the inflammation, including cryotherapy, elevation, and electrical stimulation. The use of continuous passive motion (CPM) after open or arthroscopically assisted ACL reconstructions may provide for less joint effusion, less postoperative stiffness, and less use of pain medications by the client and promotes terminal extension without stressing the ACL graft. McCarthy et al.[71] identified that there existed a statistical difference in the amount of pain medications used after surgery between clients using CPM and those not using CPM. Although no differences were reported in perceived pain between the two groups, the group using CPM needed less medication to achieve the same results. Rosen et al.[67] concluded that the use of CPM during the first 30 days after ACL reconstruction produced results similar to controlled supervised active motion, with no deleterious effects on stability. Full motion can also be promoted by the use of patellar mobilization techniques to assist the normal arthrokinematics of the patellofemoral joint.

In addition to achieving full active motion of the surgically repaired knee, normal strength must also be promoted. Preventing postsurgical atrophy (or neurophysiological shutdown of the quadriceps femoris) is a critical element in the accelerated program, but this goal must be accomplished without stressing the surgical graft. The greatest shear stress on the ACL is in an arc of motion from 30° of flexion to full terminal extension in an open-chain environment. Performing this arc of motion, also referred to as a SAQ is potentially the most devastating postsurgical exercise that a client could perform. Closed kinetic chain exercises, as described in previous chapters, work to promote strength gains, cocontraction, proprioception, function, and stability of the joint without increasing the shear forces on the ACL. The use of closed-chain exercises also gives the added benefit of avoiding patellar irritation, which is a common side effect in the central third patellar tendon graft surgical procedure. The greatest patellar compression force occurs from 60° to 90° of flexion and this range should be avoided when performing closed chain exercises. Wall slides, stationary cycling, and leg presses all work effectively within this safe range as closed kinetic chain exercises. Other strengthening exercises that will not place stress on the ACL include quad sets and straight-leg raises in the four directions of flexion, extension, adduction, and abduction. Care should be taken to avoid a straight-leg extensor lag while performing these exercises (see Fig. 11–31). Emphasis is placed on strengthening the hamstring muscle of the involved limb. The combined force of the hamstring group works to provide a dynamic supplement to the stability provided by the ACL.[10]

Electrical stimulation or EMG biofeedback can be used to decrease muscular atrophy as an adjunct to active contraction, but not as a replacement.[10] Postsurgically, the neurophysiological shutdown of the quadriceps femoris muscle occurs rapidly as a result of increased joint effusion. Noyes et al.[68,69] concluded that traditional postoperative rehabilitation protocols are generally ineffective in preventing the significant muscle atrophy that may occur within the first few days of surgery. Often the client needs help to "jump start" the muscle after surgery. The use of electrical stimulation can be beneficial in promoting neuromuscular retraining if performed in combination with active isometric exercises (quad sets). Delitto et al.[72] demonstrated that improved isometric strength gains in the quadriceps and hamstrings after ACL reconstruction were possible with the addition of electrical stimulation, as compared with exercise alone.

Functional progression of the client should be as tolerated. Initially, the client may be walking with the assistance of axillary crutches. A stationary bike may be the first significant overall activity the client is able to perform. As soon as the client can ambulate without gait deviations, the crutches can be discontinued. Running slowly over level surfaces in a straight line will be the next progression, followed by faster running in a straight line. Eventually, the client will participate in sports-specific activities, running, stopping, cutting, and jumping. Lephart et al.[73] demonstrated that the proprioceptive awareness in the reconstructed knee is less than that of the normal knee. The functional progression of the client should include exercises designed to challenge coordination and promote kinesthetic awareness. An example of an ACL rehabilitation protocol is presented in Table 9–4 (Figs. 9–68 through 9–71).[3,10]

The expected physical therapy outcomes for managing a client with an ACL reconstruction include[6]:

1. Improved functional skills and the optimal return of function
2. Reduced risk of further disability from identified limitations
3. Improved safety awareness of the client
4. An understanding of the risk factors that may contribute to jeopardizing health status
5. An understanding of strategies to prevent further disability

The expected time frame for achieving the outcomes varies depending on the presence of postsurgical complications and the aggressiveness of the rehabilitation team and the surgeon. Most postsurgical complications can be avoided if the client has full extension, minimal swelling, active leg control provided by the quadriceps femoris, and as much as 90° of flexion in the first 2 weeks after surgery.[10] Return to normal premorbid activity level is becoming progressively more common as only 10% to 15% of the surgical clients have severe complications, which include anterior knee pain, motion limitations, or even arthrofibrosis.[12] Shelbourne and Nitz[65] described early return to full activity in as little as 4 months if strict evaluative criteria and guidelines were met by the client. Others have described time frames of 6 to 12 months before it is completely safe to return to full activity after a surgical repair of the ACL.[3,10]

TENDON REPAIRS

Injuries to tendons can be a result of direct trauma, as in laceration with a sharp knife, or as a result of a disease process such as rheumatoid arthritis (RA). The result is a complete rupture of the tendon and a loss of function of the involved joint. A common site of tendon rupture in the client with RA is the extensor tendons of the fourth and fifth digits. To correct the deformity and dysfunction, the client must undergo a reconstructive operation. The surgeon will perform surgery to repair the tendon by attaching the damaged tendon to an adjoining group (tendon anastomosis) or by grafting a new tendon in place of the damaged tendon. Either procedure is clinically managed in the same way.[2]

Clinical Presentation

The client will most likely present to physical therapy after a period of immobilization of 4 to 6 weeks. Immobilization is necessary to allow healing of the repaired tendon without applying potentially destructive tensile stresses. The potential complications of the immobilization process include scarring and adhesion of the repaired tendons. The client will have significant atrophy and loss of function of the repaired region. Motion may be significantly limited as well.[74]

___ *Table 9–4* _____

ACCELERATED ACL REHABILITATION PROTOCOL*

Phase A: Presurgical, Postacute Injury	Client education about surgery and postsurgical protocols
	Focus on reducing acute edema and restoring normal ROM
	Restoration of normal gait
	Strengthening exercises when edema decreases and motion is normal
Phase B: Postsurgical, Initial 2 Weeks	Client in straight-leg immobilizer for protection
	CPM use from postoperative day 1 through discharge from acute care
	Cryotherapy and compression immediately after surgery
	PROM out of CPM to promote full extension and flexion to 90°
	Isometric quadriceps setting (QS) exercise (see Fig. 9–10) and straight-leg raise (see Figs. 9–11 through 9–14) when no extensor lag is present (see Fig. 11–31)
	AROM knee extension from 90° to 30° only
	Exercises performed 3×/day for first 2 wk
	Weight bearing as tolerated with crutches immediately after surgery (see Fig. 9–37)
	Prone-leg hang (see Fig. 11–30) and towel extension (see Fig. 9–68) at week 1
	Wall slides (see Fig. 9–17) and heel slides (see Fig. 11–27) at week 1
	Functional brace fit at end of week 2, progress to phase C
Phase C: Restoration of Strength (3 to 5 Weeks After Surgery)	Promote normal unassisted gait.
	Promote return to normal ADLs.
	Continue exercise program to maintain full knee extension and gradually promote full flexion (about 135°).
	Add the following strengthening exercises: toe raises (see Fig. 9–18), leg press (see Fig. 9–69), and lateral step-ups (see Fig. 2–34).
	Add conditioning exercises such as stairmaster, stationary bike, or swimming should be utilized.
Phase D: Return to Function (5 Weeks After Surgery)	Isokinetic strength evaluation with a 20° extension block at 180° and 240° per second. If strength of involved extremity is 70% of noninvolved extremity, straight-line running may begin.
	Agility drills may begin: jumping rope, lateral shuffles (see Fig. 9–70) and cariocas (see Fig. 9–71).
	Sports-specific activities may begin.
	Continuing all previous exercise and conditioning.
	Letting the response of the client and the condition of client's knee dictate progression. Any pain and edema should be addressed immediately.
	If client has gained at least 80% strength on isokinetic evaluation by week 24 and if the client is able to pass functional and agility drills, then he or she may return to active participation in sports.

Source: Adapted from Shelbourne and Nitz,[65] p 292.

*This protocol is an example of an accelerated ACL rehabilitation protocol adapted from Shelbourne and Nitz[65]. For every orthopedic surgeon who performs an ACL reconstruction, there is an equal number of postsurgical protocols. The therapy team should work in collaboration with the surgeon to construct a program specific to the individual who is recovering from surgery.

Evaluation: Tools and Methods

The evaluating therapist will perform a complete history, including details of the surgical procedure. Objective measures include a review of the integumentary system, sensory assessment to identify any deficits, ROM, strength, circumference measurements, and the functional status of the client.

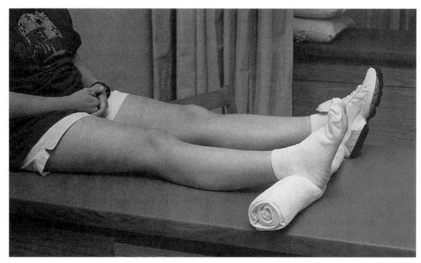

FIG. 9–68
Supine assisted knee extension. To maintain full knee extension, have the client sit long with a towel propped under the ankle of the surgical limb. Passively let gravity assist to keep the knee as straight as possible.

FIG. 9–69
Seated leg press. A closed-chain exercise that can be performed safely to strengthen the lower extremity without placing significant stress on the repaired ACL.

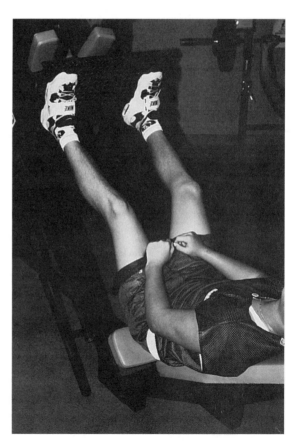

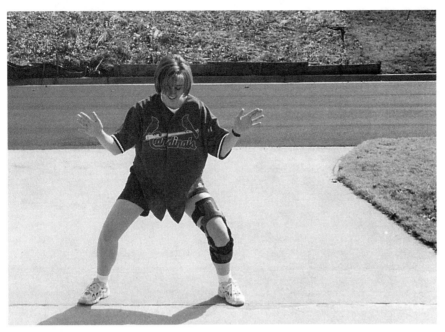

FIG. 9–70
Lateral shuffles. For a beginning agility drill, have the client slowly side step laterally going several paces in one direction and then reverse direction. As the client improves with the agility, the pace of the lateral side stepping may be increased.

Clinical Management

The gradual reversal of the effects of immobilization leading to the return of function to the client is the primary goal of the rehabilitation team. After the rigid immobilization device is removed, protective splinting may be required because of the inherent atrophy and weakness of the supporting muscle groups. AROM exercises are initiated to begin the remodeling process of the tendons and scar tissue. Initially, aggressive stretching should be avoided to prevent damaging the tendon repair. A low-load dynamic orthosis should be considered to keep a constant low-load pressure on the tissue, promoting functional realignment of the collagen fibers in the scar tissue. Gentle isometric exercises can be initiated early in the rehabilitation process. When motion and healing are sufficient, resistance may be added to the strengthening program. Client education is important in preventing future disability. Time is needed for the repair site to develop sufficient strength to withstand the great forces applied by a contracting muscle. This should be a rehabilitation consideration for appropriate return to activity.[2]

The expected physical therapy outcomes related to the management of a client with a tendon repair include [6]:

1. Improved health-related quality of life
2. Improved functional skills
3. An optimal return of function
4. Reduced risk of further disability from identified limitations
5. Improved self-care skills and ADLs

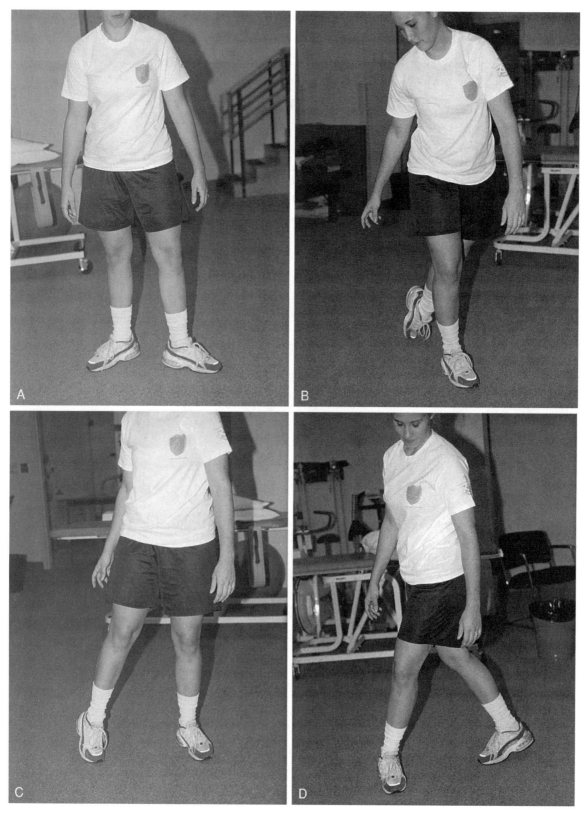

FIG. 9–71

Cariocas. This more advanced agility drill has the client moving sideways crossing one leg anteriorly over the other initially, then posteriorly on the next step. Follow the four figures (A through D), watching the progression of the clients right leg. As agility improves, increase the pace.

6. An understanding of the risk factors that may contribute to jeopardizing health status

7. An understanding of strategies to prevent further disability

The expected time frame for achieving the outcomes is 2 to 3 months after the immobilization device is no longer necessary.

 ## SUMMARY

The client with an active lifestyle may experience a variety of injuries that challenge his or her ability to return to desired activities. Ligamentous sprains, musculotendinous strains, and bony fractures caused by trauma or overuse are the most common injuries sustained by the active client. Athletes need to remain active and will wish to return to their sport as soon as possible. The rehabilitation team must balance the client's needs with the consideration of the healing process and prevention of future disability. Ligamentous sprains can be managed in an accelerated functional rehabilitation program, which will enable the client to return to participation in a relatively short amount of time. Other injuries, such as severe muscular strains, must be managed more conservatively to ensure that symptoms do not recur after treatment. Management of the orthopedic conditions in this chapter included various pain-reducing modalities, including cryotherapy, electrical stimulation, and iontophoresis. Medications commonly prescribed by the physician to decrease inflammation were discussed. ROM and strengthening exercises were addressed as methods used to limit the effects of immobilization and restore lost function. Proprioception, balance, coordination, and return-to-function exercises must be included in a rehabilitation program. These activities will facilitate the safe return to the performance of strenuous activities. Time frames related to expected outcomes for various orthopedic conditions were outlined as established by the *Guide to Physical Therapist Practice* by the American Physical Therapy Association.

 ## REFERENCES

1. Keene, JS, and Malone, TR: Ligament and muscle-tendon unit injuries. In Malone, TR, et al: Orthopedic and Sports Physical Therapy, ed 3. Mosby, St Louis, MO, 1997.
2. Kisner, C, and Colby, LA: Therapeutic Exercise: Foundations and Techniques, ed 3. FA Davis, Philadelphia, 1996.
3. Prentice, WE: Rehabilitation Techniques in Sports Medicine, ed 2. Mosby, St Louis, MO, 1994.
4. Norkin, CC, and Levangie, PK: Joint Structure and Function: A Comprehensive Analysis, ed 2. FA Davis, Philadelphia, 1992.
5. Jobe, FW, et al: Rehabilitation of the shoulder. In Brotzman, SB (ed): Clinical Orthopaedic Rehabilitation. Mosby, St Louis, MO, 1996.
6. Guide to Physical Therapist Practice. Phys Ther 77:1163, 1997.
7. Wadsworth, LT: How to manage skier's thumb. The Physician and Sports Medicine 20(3):68, 1992.
8. Calandruccio, JH, et al: Rehabilitation of the hand and wrist. In Brotzman, SB (ed): Clinical Orthopaedic Rehabilitation. Mosby, St Louis, MO, 1996.
9. Helm, RH: Hand function after injuries to the collateral ligaments of the metacarpophalangeal joint of the thumb. J Hand Surg (Br) 12(2):252, 1987.
10. Brotzman, SB, Head P: The knee. In Brotzman, SB (ed): Clinical orthopaedic rehabilitation. Mosby, St Louis, MO, 1996.
11. Hardaker, WT, Garrett, WE, and Bassett, FH: Evaluation of acute traumatic hemarthrosis of the knee joint. South Med J 83(6):640, 1990.
12. Levins, S: ACL reconstruction: The best treatment option? The Physician and Sports Medicine 20(6):150, 1992.

13. Nisonson, B: Anterior cruciate ligament injuries: Conservative vs surgical treatment. The Physician and Sports Medicine 19(5):82, 1991.
14. Hertling, D, and Kessler, RM: Management of Common Musculoskeletal Disorders: Physical Therapy Principles and Methods, ed 2. Lippincott, Philadelphia, 1990.
15. Giove, TP, et al: Non-operative treatment of the torn anterior cruciate ligament. J Bone Joint Surg Am 65:184, 1983.
16. ACL surgery and rehabilitation (special section). J Orthop Sports Phys Ther 15:256, 1992.
17. Yack HJ, et al: Comparison of closed and open kinetic chain exercise in the anterior cruciate ligament-deficient knee. Am J Sports Med 21:49, 1993.
18. Noyes, FR, et al: The symptomatic anterior cruciate-deficient knee. J Bone Joint Surg Am 65:163, 1983.
19. Barrack, RL, et al: Proprioception in the anterior cruciate ligament deficient knee. Am J Sports Med 17:1, 1989.
20. Barrett, DS, et al: Joint proprioception in normal, osteoarthritic, and replaced knees. J Bone Joint Surg Br 73:53, 1991.
21. Lane, SE: Severe ankle sprains: treatment with an ankle-foot orthoses. The Physician and Sports medicine 18(11):43, 1990.
22. Lofvenberg, R, and Karrholm, J:. The influence of an ankle orthosis on the talar and calcaneal motions in chronic lateral instability of the ankle: A stereophotogrammetric analysis. Am J Sports Med 21(2):224, 1993.
23. Brotzman, SB, and Brasel, J: Foot and ankle rehabilitation. In Brotzman, SB (ed): Clinical Orthopaedic Rehabilitation. Mosby, St Louis, MO, 1996.
24. Meisterling, RC: Recurrent lateral ankle sprains. The Physician and Sports Medicine 21(3), 1993.
25. Scotece, GG, and Guthrie, MR: Comparison of three treatment approaches for grade I and II ankle sprains in active duty soldiers. J Orthop Sports Phys Ther 15:19, 1992.
26. Rucinski, TJ, et al: The effects of intermittent compression on edema in postacute ankle sprains. J Orthop Sports Phys Ther 14:65, 1991.
27. Michlovitz, S, et al: Ice and high voltage pulse stimulation in treatment of acute lateral ankle sprains. J Orthop Sports Phys Ther 9:301, 1988.
28. Cote, DJ, et al: Comparison of three treatment procedures for minimizing ankle sprain swelling. Phys Ther 68:1072, 1988.
29. Garrett, WE: Muscle strain injuries. Am J Sports Med 24(6): S2, 1996.
30. Kornberg, C, and Lew, P: The effect of stretching neural structure on grade one hamstring injuries. J Orthop Sports Phys Ther 11:481, 1989.
31. Snyder-Mackler L, and Epler M: Effect of standard and Aircast tennis elbow bands on integrated electromyography of forearm extensor musculature proximal to the bands. Am J Sports Med 17:278, 1989.
32. Andrews, JR, et al: Elbow rehabilitation. Found in Brotzman, SB (ed): Clinical Orthopaedic Rehabilitation. Mosby, St Louis, MO, 1996.
33. Magnusson, M, and Pope, M: Epidemiology of the neck and upper extremity. In Nordin, M, et al: Musculoskeletal Disorders in the Workplace: Principles and Practice. Mosby, St. Louis, MO, 1997.
34. Harding, WG: Use and misuse of the tennis elbow strap. The Physician and Sports medicine 20(6):65, 1992.
35. Binder, A, et al: Is therapeutic ultrasound effective in treating soft tissue lesions? British Medical Journal 290:512, 1985.
36. Forrest, G, and Rosen, K: Ultrasound: effectiveness of treatments given under water. Arch Phys Med Rehabil 70:28,1989.
37. Vasseljen, O: Low-level laser versus traditional physiotherapy in the treatment of tennis elbow. Physiotherapy 78:329, 1992.
38. Vasseljen, O, et al: Low level laser versus placebo in the treatment of tennis elbow. Scand J Rehabil Med 24:37, 1992.
39. Wadsworth, CT, et al: Effect of the counterforce armband on wrist extension and grip strength and pain in subjects with tennis elbow. J Orthop Sports Phys Ther 11:192, 1989.
40. Riehl, R: Rehabilitation of the lower leg injuries. In Prentice, WE: Rehabilitation Techniques in Sports Medicine, ed 2. Mosby, St Louis, MO, 1994.
41. Clement, DB, et al: Achilles tendinitis and peritendinitis: Etiology and treatment. Am J Sports Med 12(3):179, 1984.
42. Hoppenfeld, S: Physical Examination of the Spine and Extremities. Appleton & Lange, Norwalk, CT, 1976.
43. DePalma B: Rehabilitation of hip and thigh injuries. In Prentice, WE: Rehabilitation Techniques in Sports Medicine, ed 2. Mosby, St Louis, MO, 1994.

44. Davis, M, and Prentice, WE: Knee rehabilitation. In Prentice, WE: Rehabilitation Techniques in Sports Medicine, ed 2. Mosby, St Louis, MO, 1994.

45. Wallace, LA, et al: The knee. In Malone, TR, et al: Orthopedic and Sports Physical Therapy, ed 3. Mosby, St Louis, MO, 1997.

46. Barber, FA, and Stone RG: Meniscus repair: An arthroscopic technique. J Bone Joint Surg 67Br:39, 1985.

47. Austin, KS, and Sherman, OH: Complications of arthroscopic meniscal repair. Am J Sports Med 21(6):864, 1993.

48. Lessard, LA, et al: The efficacy of cryotherapy following arthroscopic knee surgery. J Ortho Sports Phys Ther 26(1):14, 1997.

49. Salter, RB: Textbook of Disorders and Injuries of the Musculoskeletal System, Williams & Wilkins, Baltimore, 1983.

50. Lephart, S: Injuries to the hand and wrist. In Prentice, WE: Rehabilitation Techniques in Sports Medicine, ed 2. Mosby, St Louis, MO, 1994.

51. Matheson, GO, et al: Stress fractures in athletics: A study of 320 cases. Am J Sports Med 15:46, 1987.

52. Reid, DC: Prevention of hip and knee injuries in ballet dancers. Sports Med 6:295, 1988.

53. Quarrier, NF, and Wightman, AB: A ballet dancer with chronic hip pain due to a lesser trochanter bony avulsion: The challenge of a differential diagnosis. J Orthop Sports Phys Ther 28; 168, 1998.

54. Warner, WC: Rehabilitation of the pediatric patient. In Brotzman, SB (ed): Clinical Orthopaedic Rehabilitation. Mosby, St Louis, MO, 1996.

55. Cuomo, F, et al: Clinical evaluation of the neck and shoulder. In Brotzman, SB (ed): Clinical Orthopaedic Rehabilitation. Mosby, St Louis, MO, 1996.

56. Shelton, GL, and Thigpen, LK: Rehabilitation of patellofemoral dysfunction: A review of the literature. J Ortho Sports Phys Ther 14(6):243, 1991.

57. O'Neill DB, et al: Patellofemoral stress: A prospective analysis of exercise treatment in adolescents and adults. Am J Sports Med 20:151, 1992.

58. McMullen, W, et al: Static and isokinetic treatments of chondromalacia patella: A comparative investigation. J Orthop Sports Phys Ther 12:256, 1990.

59. Jensen, K, and Di Fabio, RP: Evaluation of eccentric exercises in treatment of patellar tendinitis. Phys Ther 69:211, 1989.

60. Cerullo, G, et al: Evaluation of the results of extensor mechanism reconstruction. Am J Sports Med 16:93, 1988.

61. Lazenby, T: Medical advances lead to new problem: Increase in degenerative osteoarthritis expected as athletes play longer. Pro Football Athletic Trainer. 16(1):6, 1998.

62. Thein, LA: Rehabilitation of shoulder injuries. In Prentice, WE: Rehabilitation Techniques in Sports Medicine, ed 2. Mosby, St Louis, MO, 1994.

63. Noyes, FR, et al: Bone-patellar ligament-bone and fascia lata allografts for reconstruction of the anterior cruciate ligament. J Bone Joint Surg Am 72(8):1125, 1990.

64. Ericksson, G, and Haggmark, T: Comparison of isometric muscle training and electrical stimulation supplementing isometric muscle training in the recovery after major knee ligament surgery. Am J Sports Med 7:169, 1979.

65. Shelbourne, KD, and Nitz, P: Accelerated rehabilitation after anterior cruciate ligament reconstruction. Am J Sports Med 18(3):292, 1990.

66. Fu, FH, et al: Current concepts for rehabilitation following anterior cruciate ligament reconstruction. J Orthop Sports Phys Ther 15:270, 1992.

67. Rosen MA, et al: The efficacy of continuous passive motion in the rehabilitation of anterior cruciate ligament reconstructions. Am J Sports Med 20:122, 1992.

68. Noyes, FR, and Mangine, RE: Early knee motion after open and arthroscopic anterior cruciate ligament reconstruction. Am J Sports Med 15:149, 1987.

69. Noyes, FR, et al: Intra-articular cruciate reconstruction. I. Perspective on graft strength, vascularization, and immediate motion after replacement. Clin Orthop 172:71, 1983.

70. Shelbourne, KD, et al: Arthrofibrosis in acute anterior cruciate ligament reconstruction: The effect of timing of reconstruction and rehabilitation. Am J Sports Med 19:332, 1991.

71. McCarthy, MR, et al: The effects of immediate continuous passive motion on pain during the inflammatory phase of soft tissue healing following anterior cruciate ligament reconstruction. J Orthop Sports Phys Ther 17:96, 1993.

72. Delitto, A, et al: Electrical stimulation versus voluntary exercise in strengthening thigh musculature after anterior cruciate ligament surgery. Phys Ther 68:660; 1988.

73. Lephart, SM, et al: Proprioception following ACL reconstruction. Journal of Sports Rehabilitation 1:186,1992.

74. Skoff, H: Dynamic splinting after extensor hallucis longus tendon repair: A case report. Phys Ther 68:75, 1988.

BIBLIOGRAPHY

ACL surgery and rehabilitation (special section). J Orthop Sports Phys Ther 15:256, 1992.

Andrews, JR, et al: Elbow rehabilitation. In Brotzman, SB (ed): Clinical Orthopaedic Rehabilitation. Mosby, St Louis, MO, 1996.

Austin, KS, and Sherman, OH: Complications of arthroscopic meniscal repair. Am J Sports Med 21(6):864, 1993.

Barber, FA, and Stone RG: Meniscus repair: An arthroscopic technique. J Bone Joint Surg 67B:39, 1985.

Barrack, RL, et al: Proprioception in the anterior cruciate ligament deficient knee. Am J Sports Med 17:1, 1989.

Barrett, DS, et al: Joint proprioception in normal, osteoarthritic, and replaced knees. J Bone Joint Surg Br 73:53, 1991.

Binder, A, et al: Is therapeutic ultrasound effective in treating soft tissue lesions? British Medical Journal 290:512, 1985.

Brotzman, SB, and Brasel, J: Foot and ankle rehabilitation. In Brotzman, SB (ed): Clinical Orthopaedic Rehabilitation. Mosby, St Louis, MO, 1996.

Brotzman, SB, and Head P: The knee. In Brotzman, SB (ed): Clinical Orthopaedic Rehabilitation. Mosby, St Louis, MO, 1996.

Calandruccio, JH, et al: Rehabilitation of the hand and wirst. In Brotzman, SB (ed): Clinical Orthopaedic Rehabilitation. Mosby, St Louis, MO, 1996.

Cerullo, G, et al: Evaluation of the results of extensor mechanism reconstruction. Am J Sports Med 16:93, 1988.

Clement, DB, et al: Achilles tendinitis and peritendinitis: Etiology and treatment. Am J Sports Med 12(3):179, 1984.

Cote, DJ, et al: Comparison of three treatment procedures for minimizing ankle sprain swelling. Phys Ther 68:1072, 1988.

Cuomo, F, et al: Clinical evaluation of the neck and shoulder. In Brotzman, SB (ed): Clinical Orthopaedic Rehabilitation. Mosby, St Louis, MO, 1996.

Davis, M, and Prentice, WE: Knee rehabilitation. In Prentice, WE (ed): Rehabilitation Techniques In Sports Medicine, ed 2. Mosby, St Louis, MO, 1994.

Delitto, A, et al: Electrical stimulation versus voluntary exercise in strengthening thigh musculature after anterior cruciate ligament surgery. Phys Ther 68:660; 1988.

DePalma B: Rehabilitation of hip and thigh injuries. In Prentice, WE (ed): Rehabilitation Techniques in Sports Medicine, ed 2. Mosby, St Louis, MO, 1994.

Ericksson, G, and Haggmark, T: Comparison of isometric muscle training and electrical stimulation supplementing isometric muscle training in the recovery after major knee ligament surgery. Am J Sports Med 7:169, 1979.

Forrest, G, and Rosen, K: Ultrasound: effectiveness of treatments given under water. Arch Phys Med Rehabil 70:28, 1989.

Fu, FH, et al: Current concepts for rehabilitation following anterior cruciate ligament reconstruction. J Orthop Sports Phys Ther 15:270, 1992.

Garrett, WE: Muscle strain injuries. Am J Sports Med 24(6):S2, 1996.

Giove, TP, et al: Non-operative treatment of the torn anterior cruciate ligament. J Bone Joint Surg Am 65:184, 1983.

Guide to Physical Therapist Practice. Phys Ther 77:1163, 1997.

Hardaker, WT, et al: Evaluation of acute traumatic hemarthrosis of the knee joint. South Med J 83(6):640, 1990.

Harding, WG: Use and misuse of the tennis elbow strap. The Physician and Sports Medicine 20(6):65, 1992.

Helm, RH: Hand function after injuries to the collateral ligaments of the metacarpophalangeal joint of the thumb. J Hand Surg [Br] 12(2):252, 1987.

Hertling, D, and Kessler, RM: Management of Common Musculoskeletal Disorders: Physical Therapy Principles and Methods, ed 2. Lippincott, Philadelphia, 1990.

Hoppenfeld, S: Physical Examination of the Spine and Extremities. Appleton & Lange, Norwalk, CT, 1976.

Jensen, K, and Di Fabio, RP: Evaluation of eccentric exercises in treatment of patellar tendinitis. Phys Ther 69:211, 1989.

Jobe, FW, et al: Rehabilitation of the shoulder. In Brotzman, SB (ed): Clinical Orthopaedic Rehabilitation. Mosby, St Louis, MO, 1996.

Keene, JS, and Malone, TR: Ligament and muscle-tendon unit injuries. In Malone, TR, et al (eds): Orthopedic and Sports Physical Therapy, ed 3. Mosby, St Louis, MO, 1997.

Kisner, C, and Colby, LA: Therapeutic Exercise: Foundations and Techniques, ed 3. FA Davis, Philadelphia, 1996.

Kornberg, C, and Lew, P: The effect of stretching neural structure on grade one hamstring injuries. J Orthop Sports Phys Ther 11:481, 1989.

Lane, SE: Severe ankle sprains: Treatment with an ankle-foot orthoses. The Physician and Sports Medicine 18(11):43, 1990.

Lazenby, T: Medical advances lead to new problem: Increase in degenerative osteoarthritis expected as athletes play longer. Pro Football Athletic Trainer 16(1):6, 1998.

Lephart, S: Injuries to the hand and wrist. In Prentice, WE (ed): Rehabilitation Techniques in Sports Medicine, ed 2. Mosby, St Louis, MO, 1994.

Lephart, SM, et al: Proprioception following ACL reconstruction. Journal of Sports Rehabilitation 1:186, 1992.

Lessard, LA, et al: The efficacy of cryotherapy following arthroscopic knee surgery. J Ortho Sports Phys Ther 26(1):14, 1997.

Levins, S: ACL reconstruction: The best treatment option? The Physician and Sports Medicine 20(6):150, 1992.

Lofvenberg R, and Karrholm J: The influence of an ankle orthosis on the talar and calcaneal motions in chronic lateral instability of the ankle: A stereophotogrammetric analysis. Am J Sports Med 21(2):224, 1993.

Magnusson, M, and Pope, M: Epidemiology of the neck and upper extremity. In Nordin, M, et al (eds): Musculoskeletal Disorders in the Workplace: Principles and Practice. Mosby, St Louis, MO, 1997.

Matheson, GO, et al: Stress fractures in athletics: A study of 320 cases. Am J Sports Med 15:46, 1987.

McCarthy, MR, et al: The effects of immediate continuous passive motion on pain during the inflammatory phase of soft tissue healing following anterior cruciate ligament reconstruction. J Orthop Sports Phys Ther 17:96, 1993.

McMullen, W, et al: Static and isokinetic treatments of chondromalacia patella: A comparative investigation. J Orthop Sports Phys Ther 12:256, 1990.

Meisterling, RC: Recurrent lateral ankle sprains. The Physician and Sports Medicine 21(3), 1993.

Michlovitz, S, et al: Ice and high voltage pulse stimulation in treatment of acute lateral ankle sprains. J Orthop Sports Phys Ther 9:301, 1988.

Nisonson, B: Anterior cruciate ligament injuries: Conservative vs surgical treatment. The Physician and Sports Medicine 19(5):82, 1991.

Norkin, CC, and Levangie, PK: Joint Structure and Function: A Comprehensive Analysis, ed 2. FA Davis, Philadelphia, 1992.

Noyes, FR, et al: Bone-patellar ligament-bone and fascia lata allografts for reconstruction of the anterior cruciate ligament. J Bone Joint Surg Am 72(8):1125, 1990.

Noyes, FR, et al: Intra-articular cruciate reconstruction. I. Perspective on graft strength, vascularization, and immediate motion after replacement. Clin Orthop 172:71, 1983.

Noyes, FR, and Mangine, RE: Early knee motion after open and arthroscopic anterior cruciate ligament reconstruction. Am J Sports Med 15:149, 1987.

Noyes, FR, et al: The symptomatic anterior cruciate-deficient knee. J Bone Joint Surg Am 65:163, 1983.

O'Neill DB, et al: Patellofemoral stress: A prospective analysis of exercise treatment in adolescents and adults. Am J Sports Med 20;151, 1992.

Prentice, WE: Rehabilitation Techniques in Sports Medicine, ed 2. Mosby, St Louis, MO, 1994.

Quarrier, NF, and Wightman, AB: A ballet dancer with chronic hip pain due to a lesser trochanter bony avulsion: The challenge of a differential diagnosis. J Orthop Sports Phys Ther 28;168, 1998.

Reid, DC: Prevention of hip and knee injuries in ballet dancers. Sports Med 6:295, 1988.

Riehl, R: Rehabilitation of the lower leg injuries. In Prentice, WE (ed): Rehabilitation Techniques in Sports Medicine, ed 2. Mosby, St Louis, MO, 1994.

Rosen MA, et al: The efficacy of continuous passive motion in the rehabilitation of anterior cruciate ligament reconstructions. Am J Sports Med 20;122, 1992.

Rucinski, TJ, et al: The effects of intermittent compression on edema in postacute ankle sprains. J Orthop Sports Phys Ther 14:65, 1991.

Salter, RB: Textbook of Disorders and Injuries of the Musculoskeletal System. Williams & Wilkins, Baltimore, 1983.

Scotece, GG, and Guthrie, MR: Comparison of three treatment approaches for grade I and II ankle sprains in active duty soldiers. J Orthop Sports Phys Ther 15:19, 1992.

Shelbourne, KD, and Nitz, P: Accelerated rehabilitation after anterior cruciate ligament reconstruction. Am J Sports Med 18(3):292, 1990.

Shelbourne, KD, et al: Arthrofibrosis in acute anterior cruciate ligament reconstruction: The effect of timing of reconstruction and rehabilitation. Am J Sports Med 19:332, 1991.

Shelton, GL, and Thigpen, LK: Rehabilitation of patellofemoral dysfunction: A review of the literature. J Ortho Sports Phys Ther 14(6):243, 1991.

Skoff, H: Dynamic splinting after extensor hallucis longus tendon repair: A case report. Phys Ther 68:75, 1988.

Snyder-Mackler L, and Epler M: Effect of standard and aircast tennis elbow bands on integrated electromyography of forearm extensor musculature proximal to the bands. Am J Sports Med 17;278, 1989.

Thein, LA: Rehabilitation of shoulder injuries. In Prentice, WE (ed): Rehabilitation Techniques in Sports Medicine, ed 2. Mosby, St Louis, MO, 1994.

Vasseljen, O: Low-level laser versus traditional physiotherapy in the treatment of tennis elbow. Physiotherapy 78:329, 1992.

Vasseljen, O, et al: Low level laser versus placebo in the treatment of tennis elbow. Scand J Rehabil Med 24:37, 1992.

Wadsworth, CT, et al: Effect of the counterforce armband on wrist extension and grip strength and pain in subjects with tennis elbow. J Orthop Sports Phys Ther 11:192, 1989.

Wadsworth, LT: How to manage skier's thumb. The Physician and Sports Medicine 20(3):68, 1992.

Wallace, LA, et al: The knee. In Malone, TR, et al (eds): Orthopedic and Sports Physical Therapy, ed 3. Mosby, St Louis, MO, 1997.

Warner, WC: Rehabilitation of the pediatric patient. In Brotzman, SB (ed): Clinical Orthopaedic Rehabilitation. Mosby, St Louis, MO, 1996.

Yack HJ, et al: Comparison of closed and open kinetic chain exercise in the anterior cruciate ligament-deficient knee. Am J Sports Med 21;49, 1993.

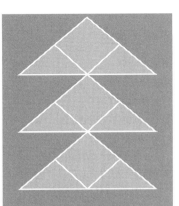

chapter 10

Clients with Repetitive Stress or Work-Related Injuries

Key Words

aneurysm
centralized
dysmenorrhea
endoscopic release
ergonomic
intermittent claudication
nonsteroidal anti-inflammatory drugs
osteomyelitis
palliative
peripheralized
spinal stenosis
spondylolisthesis
spondylolysis
spondylosis
tenosynovitis

OBJECTIVES

After completing this chapter, the PTA student will be able to:
1. Discuss the rehabilitation concerns and needs of the client with repetitive stress injuries.
2. Describe incidence, etiology, and pathophysiology of the conditions related to the industrial client presented in this chapter.
3. Identify the evaluation tools and methods used by the physical therapist to form a diagnosis, prognosis, and plan of treatment for the client conditions described in this chapter.
4. Describe the clinical management of the client conditions described in this chapter.
5. Discuss the expected physical therapy outcomes for the client conditions described in this chapter.
6. Discuss methods to identify chronic pain behavior and strategies to promote the avoidance of this behavior.

I am a great believer in luck, and I find the harder I work, the more I have of it.

Stephen Leacock

CONCERNS OF THE INDUSTRIAL WORKER: WHEN CAN I RETURN TO WORK?

Allan is a worker in the local chicken processing plant. His job is to supervise a crew of 12 employees on the floor of the plant. As part of his job duties, he must fill in on the processing line when the stationed worker needs a break. At the end of the day, he and his team are responsible for the cleaning up and the sterilizing of their area of the processing line. To complete the clean-up operation, large water-filled hoses must be lifted and used to spray down the machinery. On a Friday afternoon, the crew was getting ready to end its regularly scheduled shift. Allan felt a pulling sensation in his lower back as he and another employee were lifting the spray-down hose. Allan had to stop what he was doing and, with the help of his coworker, make his way safely to a rest station to be out of the way of the clean-up crew. After a few minutes, he was feeling better and went back to the floor. He moved slowly but was able to gingerly help the crew finish the job.

Allan drove himself home and discussed the day's events with his wife over the noise of their three young children. Allan was able to move around, but he clearly was uncomfortable. He tried to interact with his children but easily became frustrated as the pain in his back worsened. He noticed that he had difficulty getting up from the sofa and, for the most part during that evening, tried not to move. His wife suggested putting a heat pack on his back to make him feel better, which he agreed to. After a few minutes of using the moist heat, Allan noticed that his back became stiffer and his pain intensified. He took the hot pack off his back and went to the medicine cabinet to take some over-the-counter painkillers.

Sleep was not easy for Allan, but he managed. Then again, sleep was not easy in Allan's house before his injury because his youngest child was only 6-months-old. In the morning, his usual time of day to play with the kids, he had trouble getting out of bed but managed to do so. His pace throughout the weekend was slow, and he became frustrated easily because he was mad at himself for getting hurt. The only intervention that he continued was taking the medication from the medicine cabinet. Sleeping Saturday night was not much easier than the first night. By Sunday morning, the pain was not resolving, neither was it any worse.

On Monday, Allan returned to work. He tried to resume his duties on the floor but soon found himself in the employee nurse's office filling out paperwork. Soon after that, he was at the doctor's office and received an order to stay home from work for 10 days. The pain medication and muscle relaxant medication the doctor gave him did not help his back and made him feel sick to his stomach. His activity during the 10 days was minimal; he mostly lay around the house waiting for his next appointment at the doctor's office so he could be released and return to work. The time at home with the three children was not particularly restful. Allan's anxiety level increased as did his irritability. Secretly, his wife hoped for him to get better to get him out of her way in the house.

After the 10 days had elapsed, Allan was not any better and still had pain in his lower back and difficulty standing up from a chair. The doctor sent him home for another 10 days to rest. This cycle repeated twice more. On his last visit to the doctor's office, Allan was very disgruntled with the medical intervention and very frustrated over a pile of routine bills at home that he could not afford to pay because of his inability to work. He asked the doctor when he was going to be able to work. The physician replied, "I don't know. Let's send you to physical therapy."

Unfortunately, Allan's experience with the medical system is common. The institutionalization of the injured worker is prevalent, as the person moves through predescribed cycles and events, preferred providers, and management systems. Often the client is lost in the mix of paperwork and injury and appears very frustrated when he or she first arrives at the physical therapy office, potentially weeks after the onset of the condition or illness. The rehabilitation team must work to identify the needs of the client who is removed from work and integrate those needs into the recovery process. Allan is anxious for some progress and for definitive answers as to when he will be able to return to work and resume paying his bills. If this injury cycle continues, family and emotional stresses will compound the physical ailment and make managing this client even more difficult.

Work-related injuries can be sudden and traumatic as in Allan's case, or they may be a combination of small stresses that accumulate and result in major dysfunction. This chapter describes the etiologies, management, and expected outcomes of various industrial injuries related to repetitive stress.

 REPETITIVE STRESS

IMPINGEMENT, ENTRAPMENT, AND COMPRESSION SYNDROMES FROM REPETITIVE STRESS

Injuries sustained by workers on the job can place great financial hardship on both the employee and the employer. The medical sector has seen an increased client population with work-related injuries over the past 20 years, as the awareness of these injuries expands. The U.S. Bureau of Labor Statistics[1] lists that 30 cases of trauma from repetitive stress occur for every 10,000 workers in the U.S. labor force. Repetitive stress syndrome or cumulative trauma disorders (CTDs) occur when the client has sustained an injury as a result of repeatedly performing a task. If the task was performed only once, injury may not have resulted, but the cumulative effect of repeatedly performing the same task leads to dysfunction and impairment.

General types of forces that can serve as physical stressors and potentially create a repetitive stress syndrome include:

1. Repetition and force in the upper limb
2. A long duration of a single activity
3. Velocity and acceleration of machinery
4. Habitually poor posture during job performance
5. Vibration of working machines

Symptoms associated with repetitive stress include:

1. Discomfort in the effected joint or limb
2. Muscle, nerve, or joint dysfunction
3. Psychological duress from condition

As a class of injury, repetitive stress disorders can affect almost any joint in the human body. This chapter presents some of the major conditions associated with repetitive stress syndrome complete with descriptions of the client and management issues. A common underlying management premise for all disorders from repeated motion is the identification of the causal agent and modification of the situation if at all possible.[2]

Shoulder Impingement

Impingement of the shoulder can occur as the humerus elevates and traps the subacromial soft-tissue structures between the head of the humerus, the acromial arch, and the coracoacromial ligament. This injury can occur frequently in clients who use their arms for repeated overhead activity, such as lifting or throwing. Soft-tissue elements found underneath the acromial arch include the subacromial bursa and the superior aspect of the rotator cuff including the supraspinatus muscle and tendon (Fig. 10–1). The compression or impingement of these structures is a secondary problem as a result of the narrowing of the space below the acromial arch. Many factors, including structural or functional problems, can lead to irritation of the subacromial structures (Tables 10–1 and 10–2).[3,4]

The mechanism of compression is typically a fatiguing event. The rotator cuff and long head of the biceps brachii muscle work as dynamic stabilizers of the humeral head, creating a depression effect on the humeral head during elevation of the humerus. If the space between the head of the humerus and the acromion narrows from either structural deficits or dynamic instability, an impingement will result. Fatigue of the rotator cuff will lessen the dynamic stabilizing effects on the humeral head, and an excessive superior gliding may result.[3,4,5]

The prevalence of shoulder dysfunction in the workplace is common. Magnusson and Pope[6] reported that the incidence among all workers is 15% to 18% of documented industrial injuries. Women have a higher incident of shoulder dysfunction as compared with men. This is possibly related to the higher employment rate of women in occupations that require repetitive and monotonous work demands of the upper extremity. Industries cited with high incidents of shoulder dysfunction include secretarial positions, light work manufacturing and assembling, food processing, and garment industries.[6]

Clinical Presentation. The client may describe pain that is either acute or chronic in nature and can be diagnosed with various inflammatory dysfunctions, including a tendinitis or a bursitis. Pain most certainly intensifies when the humerus is forward flexed or abducted past 90°. The region around the acromial

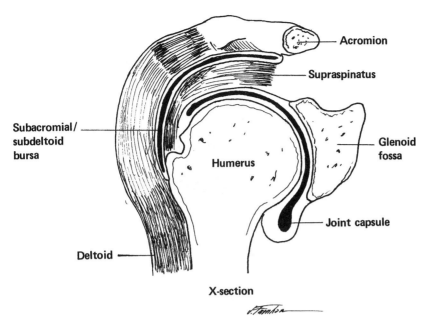

FIG. 10–1
Soft tissue located beneath the acromial arch. The small space beneath the acromial arch houses several soft tissue structures that can easily become impinged as the humerus elevates. (From Norkin & Levangie, p 221, with permission.)

arch or in the supraspinous fossae of the scapula may be tender to palpation. If the subacromial bursa is involved, an aching sensation may migrate into the lateral upper arm. Pain in the arm or neck is not uncommon. Range of motion (ROM) is usually limited by pain, but if the symptoms are persistent, joint adhesions and scarring may produce capsular motion limitations. Frequently, associated shoulder conditions of anterior instability and rotator cuff lesions are present in the client with an impingement syndrome of the shoulder.[5]

Evaluation: Tools and Methods. When the evaluating PT examines the client presenting with shoulder pain and discomfort, a complete history of the

Table 10–1

STRUCTURAL PROBLEMS THAT MAY CAUSE SUBACROMIAL IMPINGEMENT	
Structure	**Problem**
AC joint	Hypermobility
Acromion	Bony spurring
Rotator cuff	Calcium deposits in tendons
	Tendon scarring after surgical repair or from trauma
	Tears, imperfections
Humerus	Increased size of greater tuberosity

Sources: Adapted from Jobe, et al,[3] p 94; and Hertling and Kessler,[4] p 274–310.

—— *Table* 10–2 ——————————————————————

**FUNCTIONAL PROBLEMS THAT MAY CAUSE
SUBACROMIAL IMPINGEMENT**

Structure	Problem
Glenohumeral joint	Hypermobility
	Abnormal arthrokinematics (tight posterior capsule)
Rotator cuff	Paralysis of rotator cuff muscles from neurological lesion
	Tear of the muscles or tendons
	Long head of the biceps brachii grade III lesion
Scapula	Poor positioning from thoracic kyphosis
	Poor dynamic force coupling of the scapular stabilizers
	Improper glenohumeral rhythm

Sources: Adapted from Jobe, et al,[3] p 94; and Hertling and Kessler,[4] p 274–310.

current condition should be taken with a description of factors that increase and decrease symptoms, including the mechanism of injury, if known. Details of the job demands should be discovered and identified as potential causative agents. The objective examination will not only focus on the shoulder itself, but also on the entire upper extremity and cervical spine. Pain radiating from cervical dysfunctions can frequently mimic shoulder dysfunction. Objective measures of observation and palpation for muscular atrophy and misalignment should be completed. ROM, strength, deep tendon reflexes, joint stability, and functional assessments should be documented. Special tests for the shoulder include the following[7,8]:

1. ROM tests: Apley's scratch test is performed by asking the client to place one arm behind the head and the other behind the back and having the client touch opposing index fingers.
2. Impingement or provocation tests
   a. Neer impingement test is performed by forced forward flexion of the humerus.
   b. Hawkins impingement test is performed by flexing the humerus to 90° and then forcefully internally rotating the humerus.
   c. Yergason's test is designed to check the integrity of the lower portion of the tendon from the long head of the biceps brachii. The client is asked to simultaneously supinate the forearm, flex the elbow, and internally rotate the humerus against resistance with the elbow in a 90° position.
   d. Speed's test also checks the integrity of the long head of the biceps by having the client flex the arm against resistance with the elbow extended and the forearm supinated.
3. Stability tests
   a. Apprehension test is performed by placing the arm into abduction and external rotation to assess anterior joint stability.
   b. Sulcus test is performed by pulling inferiorly on the humerus and assessing the amount of downward translation of the humerus. This assesses integrity of the joint capsule.
   c. Drop arm test is used to check the integrity of the rotator cuff by having the client slowly lower the arm from full abduction to 90° of abduction.

d. "Empty can" test also assesses the integrity of the rotator cuff, particularly the supraspinatus muscle and tendon. The client is asked to empty a can with the arm abducted to 90° and horizontally flexed 30°. Resistance may produce pain or the client may not be able to hold the position.

4. Vascular and neurological tests
   a. Lhermitte's sign is described as an electrical shock that moves down the arm with cervical flexion or extension. This is indicative of cervical dysfunction, possibly a cervical **spondylosis**.

   Spondylosis
   A degenerative arthritis of the vertebrae that may cause pressure on nerve roots, resulting in radiating pain or paresthesias in the extremities.

   b. Spurling's sign occurs when pain is produced in the upper extremity when axial compression is placed on the head with concurrent extension and ipsilateral rotation. This may be indicative of nerve root compression at the cervical spine.
   c. Adson's maneuver is designed to assess for compression of the neurovascular bundle in the upper extremity and shoulder. The radial pulse is palpated as the client's shoulder is abducted to 90° with extension and external rotation and contralateral rotation of the head and neck. A diminished pulse may be indicative of neurovascular compression, as in the case of thoracic outlet syndrome.
   d. Rue's test is an assessment for **intermittent claudication** in the upper extremity. The client is asked to abduct the shoulder to 90°, flex the elbow, and rapidly flex and extend the fingers for 1 minute.

   Intermittent Claudication
   Severe pain in the extremity as a result of vascular compromise.

Clinical Management. The rehabilitation management of the client with a shoulder impingement syndrome should focus on restoring the proper rotator cuff stability, arthrokinematics, and scapulohumeral rhythm. Acute modalities designed to decrease pain and inflammation can be used. Iontophoresis, electrical stimulation, cryotherapy, and phonophoresis have all been used in the management of pain associated with shoulder impingement syndromes. Frequently, oral **nonsteroidal anti-inflammatory drugs** (NSAIDs) or injections of corticosteroids are prescribed by the physician. Early recognition of activities that increase the irritation of the shoulder should direct the client to the motions and activities that should be avoided. Part of the process of decreasing the irritation is to avoid the repeated microtrauma from the impingement process. The client may have to be instructed while at work to not lift overhead or be moved from a work station that causes the repeated impingement.[3,5]

Nonsteroidal Anti-inflammatory Drugs (NSAIDs)
Drugs that have an analgesic, anti-inflammatory, and antipyretic action. They are commonly used in arthritic or inflammatory conditions.

Exercises for shoulder impingement syndrome should work to prevent the onset of disability associated with pain and decreased activity. Pain-free ROM activities and strengthening should be encouraged early. Codman's pendulum exercises are a good early mobilization exercise (see Fig. 9–4). Isometric exercises or resistive tubing exercises can be performed safely with the arm below a 90° elevation. Motions that require the arm to be lifted above 90° should be initially avoided. Strengthening should focus on the restoration of the dynamic stabilization from the rotator cuff muscles and the dynamic stabilizers of the scapula, including the serratus anterior, rhomboid group, and middle and lower trapezius muscles (Figs. 9–59 through 9–64). As the pain and discomfort decreases, the client should be gradually progressed to a return of functional activities. The client should be educated about the factors that lead to the onset of symptoms. Strategies should be designed to prevent the onset of symptoms in the future.[5]

The expected physical therapy outcomes for managing a client with a shoulder impingement syndrome include[9]:

1. Improved functional skills and the optimal return of function

FIG. 10–2
Carpal tunnel. The structure of the proximal and distal rows of the carpal bones form an arch that, when covered by flexor retinaculum, complete a tunnel. Through this tunnel passes the tendons from the long finger flexors and the median nerve. (From Norkin & Levangie, p 274, with permission.)

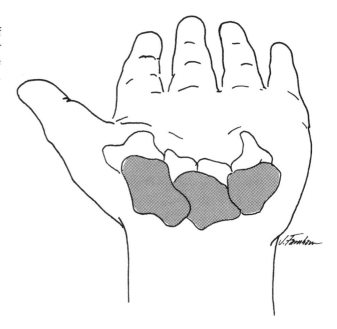

2. Reduced risk of further disability from identified limitations
3. An understanding of risk factors that may contribute to jeopardizing health status, and
4. An understanding of strategies to prevent further disability

The expected time frame for achieving physical therapy outcomes for mild impingement syndromes, including supraspinatus tendinitis or subacromial bursitis, should be in less than 6 weeks. If the offending motion or activity is not resolved or modified, the return of symptoms is likely.

Carpal Tunnel Syndrome

The anatomic space that is the carpal tunnel of the wrist houses nine flexor tendons and the median nerve covered by the transverse carpal ligament (Fig. 10–2). The physical structure is self-limiting, and any relative changes in the size or shape of the structures passing through the tunnel may affect dysfunction. Inflammation or scarring of the dynamic tendons of the flexor digitorum profundus, flexor digitorum superficialis, or the flexor pollicis longus muscles may cause damaging compression to the susceptible median nerve.[10] When compression of the median nerve from a flexor **tenosynovitis** produces symptoms in the hand, the condition is named carpal tunnel syndrome (CTS). This repetitive-use injury occurs often in clients that are performing repetitive movements or handling vibrating industrial machinery with their fingers, hands, and wrists. There is a high correlation between the incidence of CTS and the repetitive motion of the hands and wrist during work compared with sedentary, nonrepetitive jobs. The incidence of CTS is 20 cases per 1000 workers in susceptible jobs. Common examples of industrial occupations that are susceptible to compression irritation of the median nerve include garment factory workers, sawmill workers, carpenters, and food processing workers.[2,11]

Tenosynovitis
Inflammation of the tendon sheath.

Clinical Presentation. Progressive numbness and paresthesias in the areas of the hand supplied by the median nerve are characteristic signs of CTS. The median nerve supplies the radial two-thirds of the palm, the palmar surface of the first three digits, and the dorsal surface of the distal phalanges. Pain at night, weakness, and decreased functional skills of the hand may also accompany the condition. Extreme cases of median nerve compression may result in atrophy of the radial muscle of the hand with a resulting ape-hand deformity (atrophy of the thenar eminence).[10,12]

Evaluation: Tools and Methods. The history of the client should be taken by the evaluating PT, including the mechanism of injury, if known, and the date of onset. The therapist should develop a good understanding of the job demands of the client. Objectively, ROM, strength, and a functional assessment of the hand and upper extremity should be completed. Special tests that help to identify CTS include: (1) Tinel's sign (Fig. 10–3) and (2) Phalen's test (Fig. 10–4). The hand and pinch dynamometers have been used to assess the grip and pinch strength, respectively (Figs. 10–5 and 10–6). Electrodiagnostic testing including nerve conduction velocity tests may be helpful in identifying entrapment of the median nerve in the carpal tunnel.[10]

Clinical Management. Management of CTS can be either conservative or surgical in nature. Adams et al.[13] claimed that the rate of surgical management for all presented cases of CTS was 40%. Success rates of surgical decompression were marginal, because 67% returned to the same job before onset of impairment, 15% found new employment, and 18% were unemployable after a 3-year follow-up. The predictive factor related to a client's either changing jobs (15%) or not returning to work (18%) was related to being employed in a high-risk or a high-strain job. With either approach to management of CTS (surgical versus conservative), the rehabilitation team should work to relieve the aggravating factor.

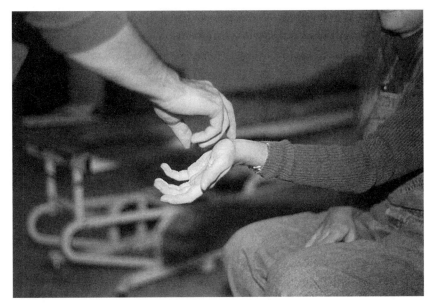

FIG. 10–3
Tinel's sign. A positive Tinel's sign occurs when tingling is elicited by gently tapping over the affected carpal tunnel. This is one special test used to identify carpal tunnel syndrome.

FIG. 10–4
Phalen's test. Compression of the median nerve occurs from forced wrist flexion. Ask the client to hold her bilateral wrists in a position of full flexion for a period of 1 minute. If the symptoms of the client are easily reproduced by this maneuver, then carpal tunnel syndrome may be suspected.

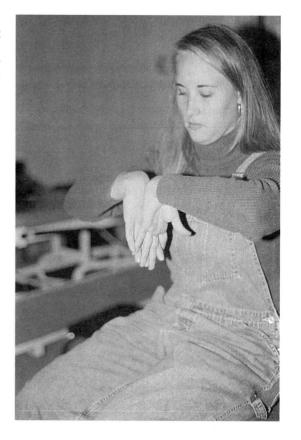

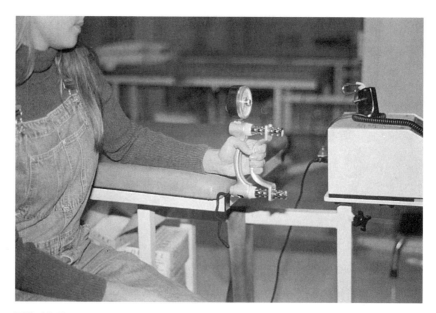

FIG. 10–5
The hand dynamometer. The client's grip strength can be assessed by squeezing the hand dynamometer. Review Case Study 3–1 for a investigation into the use of this device.

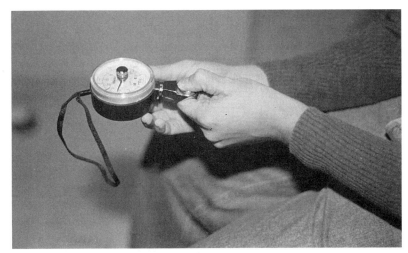

FIG. 10–6
Pinch strength. Devices such as this are able to measure the client's relative strength in the various gripping positions. See Figs. 11–43 through 11–50 for a discussion of different gripping strategies.

For mild or moderate symptoms, which account for most of the presenting cases of CTS, supporting the involved wrist and forearm in a neutral position splint for rest and protection is indicated. The client can wear the splint 24 hours a day for 2 weeks until the irritating symptoms resolve. Night splinting may continue for an additional 6 weeks if this approach is successful. The physician may prescribe NSAIDs to help reduce the inflammation and irritation of the flexor tendons passing through the carpal tunnel. Once symptoms have resolved, the client is usually released to return to work. Job modification is necessary to prevent a recurrence of the symptoms.[14]

Persistent, severe, or failed conservative management of CTS requires more aggressive measures. The physician may try direct injection of steroids into the carpal tunnel to reduce the inflammation. If the symptoms have not resolved after 6 months of therapeutic efforts, surgical release may be indicated. The orthopedic or hand surgeon may take one of two approaches to surgically relieve the pressure on the median nerve by severing the transverse carpal ligament. A carpal tunnel release (CTR) can be an open procedure that leaves a 2-inch longitudinal scar over the carpal tunnel as the surgeon severs the ligament with a scalpel. The second, less traumatic approach, is an **endoscopic release** of the same ligament. The end result of both procedures is a surgical release of the transverse carpal ligament, but the endoscopic approach may result in less scarring and a faster recovery.[14]

Physical therapy management of the client after surgery includes:

1. Encouraging full wrist and digit motion through active and passive motion exercises
2. Educating clients in caring for acute surgical incision
3. Promoting activities of daily living (ADLs) as tolerated by the client
4. Controlling edema by use of retrograde massage or custom-fitted glove
5. Managing soft tissue and scar after removal of sutures, including cross-friction massage, myofascial release, and desensitization techniques (Box 10–1).
6. Strengthening of wrist, hand, and digits via therapeutic putty or weights
7. Promoting a return to function, including self-care ADLs, manual dexterity, coordination and job performance skills
8. Modifying job structure and educating the client about risk factors leading to the potential return of symptoms

Endoscopic Release
A surgical release of tissue through a small surgical incision using an endoscope or small optical system and excision tool.

___ **Box 10–1** ___

> ### DESENSITIZATION AFTER CARPAL TUNNEL RELEASE
>
> The healed surgical incision after a CTR can be particularly sensitive and a source of great irritation to the client. Desensitization techniques can help the client to prepare the soft tissue on the palm of the hand for future work. Light pressure and tapping around the scar is usually a primary technique that encourages touching of the area. As tolerance to this approach increases, progress to deeper pressure, cross-friction massage, and rubbing various textures across the scar. Sensitivity must be normal before the rehabilitation team can effectively manage the scar. If the scarring process goes unchecked, new dysfunction from the healed scar may result.

The expected physical therapy outcomes for the management of a client after a CTR include[9]:

1. Improved health-related quality of life
2. Improved functional skills and the optimal return of function
3. Reduced risk of further disability from identified limitations
4. Improve safety awareness of client
5. An understanding of risk factors that may contribute to jeopardizing health status
6. An understanding of strategies to prevent further disability

The expected time frame for achieving the outcomes is varied. Adams et al.[13] reported an average time away from work for all clients with CTS was 4 months. The client with mild to moderate symptoms will usually return to work sooner than that average duration, and the surgical clients experience a slower return to work. Negative outcomes for the client are almost certain if the client returns to the same high-stress job without job performance modification.

de Quervain's Syndrome

de Quervain's syndrome is one of the most common repetitive-use disorders treated by hand surgeons.[10] The condition is a stenosing tenosynovitis of the abductor pollicis longus (APL) and the extensor pollicis brevis (EPB) tendons.[14] The tendons of the APL and the EPB lie deep to the extensor retinaculum and pass at an acute angle into the thumb. Various motions of the distal upper extremity can be responsible for creating stress on these tendons: (1) forearm supination and pronation, (2) wrist ulnar and radial deviation, (3) thumb abduction and extension, and (4) gripping with ulnar deviation. The original condition was described in 1895 as women who would forcefully wring out clothes would complain of pain in the radial side of their wrist and thumb. de Quervain's syndrome was then called "washerwoman's sprain."[2]

Clinical Presentation. Tenderness and pain in the region of the radial styloid process are common. Swelling may be present over the radial aspect of the dorsal part of the wrist and thumb. The client may complain that they have difficulty grasping objects in the affected hand with a power grip and that routine activities involving the thumb may be painful. In more involved cases, the pain may radiate proximally into the forearm or distally into the thumb. The client may have a loss of ROM into adduction of the thumb, and resisted extension of the metacarpophalangeal (MCP) joint may be painful. Palpation of the tendons leading to the thumb may reveal thickening and crepitus.[10,14]

Evaluation: Tools and Methods. The history of the client complete with mechanism of injury and date of onset should be taken. If the injury is work related, the therapist should inquire into the job demands of the client. Objectively, ROM, strength, and a functional assessment of the hand and upper extremity should be completed. A special test associated with de Quervain's tenosynovitis is termed *Finkelstein's test* (Fig. 10–7).

Clinical Management. Management of a client with de Quervain's syndrome generally follows conservative guidelines. Only in extreme, unmanageable cases is decompression surgery required, which involves surgically releasing the irritated sheath around the tendon. Conservatively, the client is removed from the activity that produced the condition, if easily identifiable. A thumb spica cast or custom-made orthoplast splint may be used to provide rest and support for the irritated tendons. A course of splinting may last 6 to 8 weeks or until symptoms resolve. Anti-inflammatory medications or modalities may be indicated to help promote the functional recovery of the client. NSAIDs or cortisone injections may be prescribed by the physician. The supervising therapist may form a plan of treatment using ice massage over the radial styloid process or phonophoresis with 10% hydrocortisone cream. A compressive digit wrapping with lightweight elastic tape of the thumb and wrist may be used to help reduce edema within the tendon sheaths. Active and passive exercises that do not increase pain or irritation may be included. Once pain has subsided, strengthening exercises using therapeutic putty are beneficial. A major focus of the conservative rehabilitation efforts should be modification of the repetitive forces on the client's wrist and hand. A work-site evaluation or identifying alternate methods of performing the job without causing increased stress to the client's wrist is beneficial.[14]

The expected physical therapy outcomes for managing a client with de Quervain's syndrome include[9]:

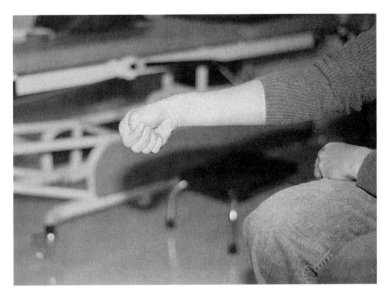

FIG. 10–7
Finklestein's test. A positive Finklestein's test occurs when pain is elicited after the client holds the thumb under flexed fingers and actively deviates the wrist to the ulnar side. This test is used to identify de Quervain's tenosynovitis.

1. Improved health-related quality of life
2. Improved functional skills and return of optimal function
3. Reduced risk of further disability from identified limitations
4. An understanding of the risk factors that may contribute to jeopardizing health status
5. An understanding of the strategies to prevent further disability

The expected time frame for achieving the outcomes for most cases is 6 to 8 weeks. Extreme cases may need surgical intervention.

Dupuytren's Contracture

The hands are a complex combination of skin, bone, tendons, ligaments, fascia, muscle, and nerves that serve the functional needs of the human upper extremity. The hand is able to forcefully grip and hold an object or lightly lift an egg without damaging the shell. This ability is in part due to the structure of the supporting elements of the hand, including the skin and fascia. The mobility of the skin over the palm of the hand is more limited than the skin covering the dorsum of the hand. The palmar aponeurosis links closely to the palmar skin and the deeper structures to provide a firm foundation for the gripping ability of the hand. Injury to the palmar surface increases the potential for scar tissue formation and decreased mobility. Thickening and contracture of the palmar fascia that limits motion of the digits is referred to as a *Dupuytren's contracture.*[15,16]

The scarring and thickening process can be caused by a specific traumatic event or a cumulative build-up of smaller events, or it may have no identifiable cause. The typical client is a male over the age 50. The adhesions can infiltrate the cords and tendons found deep within the skin on the palmar surface making it difficult for the client to extend his or her digits. The contractures are mostly noted on the ulnar side of the hand involving the fourth and fifth digits, but they may also be observed in the web space of the hand or the plantar surface of the feet. The onset is insidious and painless. A thickening of the palmar fascia develops and palpable nodules may be observed. The contracture process moves slowly, taking several years to fully develop. The MCP and interphalangeal (IP) joints are not directly involved, but they may develop a secondary capsular limitation from being in a flexed position for a prolonged period of time.[14,16]

Clinical Presentation. The client will present with a contracture of the palmar surface of the hand (Fig. 10–8).

Evaluation: Tools and Methods. The evaluation performed by the PT will consist of a history, subjective complaints, and objective measurements. Objectively, the PT will examine the ROM, strength, and functional abilities of the involved hand.

Clinical Management. If the contracture involves the fourth or fifth digit of the hand, many clients do not even seek medical attention. The primary gripping functions of the hand are performed by the first three digits (see Figs. 11–43 through 11–50 for a discussion of gripping strategies). Most clients are able to retain significant function of the hand despite the presence of a palmar contracture. Soft-tissue mobilization and remodeling interventions are generally ineffective because of the increased time factor (several years) in the development of the contracture. Dynamic splinting may be chosen as a management option; however, most clients who desire a cosmetic and functional improvement will opt for surgical release of the contracted tissue.[14]

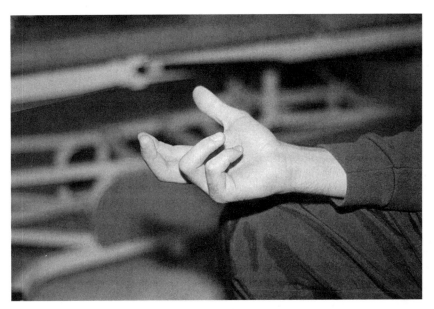

FIG. 10–8
Dupuytren's contracture. The contracture of the fascia on the palmar surface of the hand makes extension of the digits difficult.

After surgical release, the client is managed through a ROM, stretching, and education program. The client is encouraged to perform active and passive extension exercises to the digit and hands almost immediately after surgery. Passive stretching of the surgically released tissue can be performed by having the client place the hand on a flat surface (e.g., a table) and apply gentle over pressure on the dorsum of the hands and digits. A dynamic resting splint will be constructed to fit the client to keep the digits in an extended position when the client is resting or asleep. The splint will be worn for up to 6 weeks after the surgery. The client should be educated in the proper use of the dynamic splint and the correct implementation of the home exercise program.[14,16]

The expected physical therapy outcomes related to the management of a client with a Dupuytren's contracture include[9]:

1. Improved functional skills
2. An understanding of the risk factors that may contribute to jeopardizing health status
3. An understanding of the strategies to prevent further disability

The expected time frame for achieving the outcomes after surgical release of the contracted palmar fascia is 6 to 8 weeks.

Trigger Finger

The long finger flexors that drive the motion of the digits of the hand are housed inside a fibrous tendon sheath. Normally, the tendons slide smoothly through the tendon sheath just as does the cable inside the cable housing on the brakes of a bicycle. However, when inflammation occurs in the tendon sheaths as a result of overuse, the smooth flexing mechanism can turn into a rough snapping or catching of the fingers when flexed. Stenosis of the tendon sheaths leads to a condition referred to as a *trigger finger*.[14]

The etiology of a trigger finger can be blamed on a repetitive use syndrome, but the condition may develop spontaneously with no apparent mechanism of injury. Middle-aged women are the most likely clients to experience a trigger finger condition. Excessive or repeated friction inside the sheath from gripping activities of the hand may produce a thickening of the tendon or a narrowing of the tendon sheath.[16]

Clinical Presentation. The client will describe a catching or snapping of one of the digits when flexion is attempted. The trigger finger condition, as a whole, is not necessarily painful, but there may be acute discomfort with the snapping action. The digit may become locked in the flexed position because extension strength is insufficient to unlock the digit. Passively, the finger may be extended or snapped back into position. Upon palpation, nodules or knots may be felt along the irritated tendon. Often events that require forceful flexion or gripping of the hand are identified as a precursor to the onset of a trigger finger. Activities such as continuous use of heavy-duty scissors, gripping vibrating machinery, or pulling or gathering of material with the hands can cause trigger finger.

Evaluation: Tools and Methods. A history, subjective complaints, and objective measurements will be taken by the evaluating PT. Objectively, the PT will examine the ROM, strength, and functional abilities of the involved hand. The nature of the locking should be described and the causative identified.

Clinical Management. Salter[16] recommends that rest and cortisone injections are the best management for a trigger finger. These principles are still elements of the conservative approach to managing a trigger finger today. Most clients respond positively to conservative management; however, some clients that show no improvement are candidates for a surgical release of the inflamed tendon. Rest should include splinting and removal of the aggravating agent. Methods and modalities designed to reduce the inflammatory process should also be used. If the symptoms are acute, the digit should be immobilized to avoid flexion and repeated irritation within the tendon sheath. The physician may prescribe NSAIDs to reduce inflammation. The rehabilitation team should identify the stressing agent and work to eliminate that activity from the client's duties over the next several weeks. The client should be educated about the factors that may irritate the condition and activities that can be done to avoid the return of symptoms. If the conservative approach does not produce signs of improvement in 3 or 4 weeks, the physician may then resort to steroid injections.[14]

The expected physical therapy outcomes for managing a client with a trigger finger include[9]:

1. Improved health-related quality of life
2. Improved functional skills
3. An optimal return of function
4. Reduced risk of further disability from identified limitations
5. An understanding of the risk factors that may contribute to jeopardizing health status
6. An understanding of the strategies to prevent further disability

The expected time frame for achieving the outcomes is 6 to 8 weeks. If the client does not respond to conservative methods of management after 4 months and the dysfunction is deemed significant, the client may undergo a surgical release of the tendon.

Lower-Leg Compartment Syndromes

Occupational stresses and overuse rarely produce a compartmental syndrome. Overuse associated with sporting activities and secondary complications from fractures and direct trauma are more likely to be precipitating factors.[17] Compartment syndrome of the lower leg is defined as an increased pressure in the fascial compartments. The fascial sleeves in the lower leg separate the structures. If pressure is built up inside one of the closed compartments, potentially damaging compressive forces can irritate the structures housed within the compartment. There are four compartments found in the lower leg[18] :

Anterior: Structures found in the anterior compartment include the anterior tibialis muscle, deep peroneal nerve, anterior tibial artery and vein, and the extensor muscles of the toes.

Lateral: Structures found in the lateral compartment include the superficial peroneal nerve, and the peroneus longus and brevis muscles.

Superficial Posterior: Structures found in the superficial posterior compartment include the plantaris, gastrocnemius and soleus muscles.

Deep Posterior: Structures found in the deep posterior compartment include the posterior tibialis muscle, flexor muscles of the toes, peroneal artery and vein, tibial nerve, and posterior tibial artery and vein.

Clinical Presentation. Two different clinical presentations of a lower-leg compartment syndrome are applicable: acute and chronic. The client with an acute injury most likely has increased pressure in the compartments of the lower leg as a result of a direct trauma. Swelling or bleeding within the fascial compartment places acute compression on the enclosed structures. The pressure build-up potentially may exceed the viability tolerance of the peripheral nerves and may lead to irreversible nerve damage. The client may describe severe dull or sharp pain in the involved compartment, and a superficial contusion may be present. Passive stretching of the ankle will increase the symptoms. The client may describe paresthesias in the foot in the form of numbness. This is an emergency situation and the client should be taken to the emergency room for immediate decompression before permanent damage results.[18]

Chronic compartment syndrome is also referred to as exertional compartment syndrome. The symptoms present only upon exercise or exertion. This is frequently related to the increase in the muscle mass of the lower extremity during activity. During exercise, as the muscle expands in the limited space of the fascial compartments, a resulting pressure increase is noted. Pain associated with exertional compartment syndrome is usually ischemic in nature because the blood supply is slowed to the muscle. Numbness will frequently be noted as pressure compromises the function of the nerve in the involved compartment. If the deep posterior compartment is involved, then numbness may result in the plantar aspect of the foot as the tibial nerve is compressed. If the common peroneal nerve is involved, then numbness may be observed along the anterolateral surface of the lower leg and the dorsum of the foot. Frequently, this condition may mimic the symptoms of a stress fracture. With rest and the restoration of adequate circulation after exercise, the pain resolves.[18]

Evaluation: Tools and Methods. The client with an untreated acute compartment syndrome traditionally does not attend physical therapy on referral from a physician. However, in states with direct access, the potential exists that a client may appear for evaluation without first seeking medical advice from a physician. The PT, through a skillful differential diagnosis, should identify the potential of a compartment syndrome and refer the client for appropriate medical attention. Tools to help identify the presence of an acute compartment syndrome include a complete history of the onset of symptoms and objective measurements including visual inspection, palpation, sensory testing, muscle testing, circumferential measurements, and ROM assessment. Special tests that may be used include Thompson's test to assess the integrity of the plantar flexion muscle group and Homans' sign to rule out the presence of a deep venous thrombosis.[7]

Clinical Management. The client with an acute compartment syndrome is managed through an emergency fascial surgical release to relieve the pressure within the compartment. Rehabilitation after the surgical release of the fascia will follow the traditional four phases of rehabilitation: (1) controlling effects of inflammation, (2) restoring joint motion, (3) restoring muscle strength, and (4) promoting functional activities. Postsurgically, anti-inflammatory medications and modalities in conjunction with elevation of the limb and limited weight bearing are encouraged. ROM activities should begin 2 to 3 days after surgery with a gradual progression to full weight bearing. Strengthening should be considered only once the client has pain-free motion of the lower limb. At this point in time, the rehabilitation team will design a program that consists of stretching of the muscles of the lower leg, endurance activities, and gentle strengthening. A primary focus should be on promoting normal flexibility in the lower extremity. Hypertrophy of the muscles in the lower leg should be avoided after a surgical release. When the client is able, functional activities and exercises, including jogging and running, should be promoted. Client education related to the cause of the condition and methods to limit further disability should be included in the rehabilitation plan.[18]

Historically, the exertional or chronic compartment syndrome has not been successfully managed with conservative modalities. The symptoms of discomfort resolve with the cessation of activity. Conservative modalities and medications do not help the structural problem, but addressing only the current onset of symptoms. The client should be educated as to the mechanism by which the pain develops and should be encouraged to address flexibility issues related to the lower extremity as well as modification of activities that encourage symptom development. If the problem becomes persistent, a surgical release of the tissue to provide a release of pressure build-up in the compartment should be considered. Rehabilitation after a surgical release follows the same treatment plan as rehabilitation after the onset of acute compartment syndrome.[18]

The expected physical therapy outcomes for managing a client with a compartment syndrome include[9]:

1. Improved health-related quality of life
2. An optimal return of function
3. Reduced risk of further disability from identified limitations
4. An understanding of risk factors that may contribute to jeopardizing health status
5. An understanding of strategies to prevent further disability

The expected time frame for achieving the outcomes after a surgical release of the fascia is 6 to 8 weeks. Exertional compartment syndrome that is managed nonsurgically may never have a complete resolution of the symptoms unless the aggravating activity is modified or eliminated.

Shin-Splint Syndrome

A musculotendinous overuse injury affecting the anterior aspect of the lower leg is called shin-splint syndrome. Anterior shin splints are a frequent consequence of excessive eccentric loading of the anterior compartment muscles during walking or running activities. The client with shin splints will have damaging microtrauma to the muscles, tendons, or connective tissue in the anterior compartment of the lower leg. Irritation to the anterior compartment is the most common location of shin splints; however, this overuse injury may also involve the deep posterior compartment muscles. The classic factors precipitating the onset of shin splints are (1) abnormal biomechanics of the foot, (2) physical deconditioning, (3) poor flexibility, and (4) inappropriate increase in activity without a build-up of tolerance to the activity.[18]

Clinical Presentation. The client describes pain and tenderness on the anterior surface of the lower leg, along the anterolateral border of the tibia or across the anterior surface of the talocrural joint. The anterior tibialis muscle is frequently involved, and pain is demonstrated with active or resisted dorsiflexion. If the deep posterior compartment is involved, tenderness may be recognized along the medial border of the tibia, with noted involvement of the posterior tibialis muscle. Pain typically increases with activity and may decrease with rest; however, severe cases may demonstrate constant aching and pain.[18]

Evaluation: Tools and Methods. The evaluating PT should complete a history of the current condition identifying any causative agents. Objective measures will include visual inspection, palpation, ROM, flexibility, strength, sensory assessment, gait analysis, biomechanical foot, analysis, and functional assessments.

Clinical Management. As with any overuse injury, identifying the causative or aggravating agent is critical. Altering training habits, work conditions, or biomechanical foot deficiencies should all be considered in the successful long-term management of the client with lower-leg pain. The client should be educated as to the factors that may contribute to an increase or exacerbation of the symptoms. The management of the symptoms is relatively simple. It includes rest, anti-inflammatory medications, modalities, and a gradual return to activity.[18]

Debate exists over the proper modality management of clients with shin splints or overuse injuries to the lower leg. There exists limited significant data supporting or refuting the effective clinical management of shin splints. Smith et al.[19] examined the effects of four commonly used modalities in the management of pain associated with shin splints. In the use of ice massage, ultrasound, iontophoresis, or phonophoresis, their research revealed that one modality could not be statistically proved as being more effective than another in the reduction of painful symptoms. They did find, however, that all treatment groups significantly improved over the nontreatment control group, suggesting that any of the four modalities is better than no treatment.

The expected physical therapy outcomes related to the management of a client with shin splints include[9]:

1. Improved health-related quality of life
2. Improved functional skills
3. An optimal return of function
4. Reduced risk of further disability from identified limitations

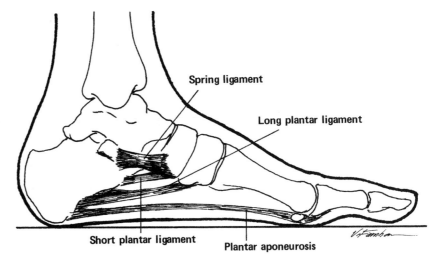

FIG. 10–9
Plantar supporting structures of the foot. The plantar fascia or aponeurosis is a major inert structural element of the plantar surface of the foot. Closely related to assist with shock absorption are the ligaments of the medial longitudinal arch. (From Norkin & Levangie, p 407, with permission.)

5. An understanding of risk factors that may contribute to jeopardizing health status
6. An understanding of strategies to prevent further disability

The expected time frame for achieving the outcomes is 4 to 8 weeks, depending on the severity of the condition. Identification and modification of the precipitating factor are needed for successful long-term management of shin splints.

Plantar Fasciitis

The plantar fascia or aponeurosis is a dense connective tissue that originates on the medial tuberosity of the calcaneus and provides for structural support and muscular origins for the foot (Fig. 10–9). With weight-bearing activities, the plantar fascia elongates to serve as a shock absorber. Differentiating the true nature of the medical diagnosis of plantar fasciitis is sometimes difficult. Hunter[20] claims that "plantar fasciitis is a catch-all term that is commonly used to describe pain in the proximal arch and heel." Pain in the posteriorinferior surface that intensifies with weight bearing is often diagnosed as an inflammation of the plantar aponeurosis. However, the origin of the aponeurosis, which is commonly the location of the pain, is also the origin for the abductor hallucis, flexor digitorum brevis, and quadratus plantae muscles. The management of this condition must address the possibility that the pain may be from either connective or muscular tissue.[21,22]

The mechanism for injury to the plantar fascia is overuse. Activities that involve running or prolonged standing can encourage repeated irritation of the structures of the plantar aspect of the foot. Associated conditions such as pes planus, pes cavus, obesity, a tight heel cord or Achilles tendon, and calcaneal valgus may cause irritation or predispose a client to developing plantar fasciitis. Spurring of the calcaneus or an osteophyte formation may or may not be associated with the onset of plantar fasciitis. Some clients present with painful symptoms, and indeed, have a formed heel spur on radiographic examination. It is also common, however, to have asymptomatic spurring of the heel due to the horizontal orientation of the spur. Further investigation is needed to confirm the absolute relationship between pain and bony spurring.[22]

Clinical Presentation. The client may complain of pain over any part of the plantar surface of the foot. The pain may be centralized in the distal aspect of the calcaneus, the medial longitudinal arch of the foot, or the central aspect of the foot. Pain is most troublesome for the client during weight-bearing activities and upon rising from bed in the morning. The pain is not sudden or acute, but rather has built up over a period of time. Frequently, there is no precipitating event or direct mechanism of injury.[22]

Evaluation: Tools and Methods. The evaluation will consist of a history including a description of the discomfort and pain. Trends in the pain are important to identify. The objective measures will include palpation of the involved structures, a biomechanical assessment of the foot, ROM, strength, and functional assessments. The physician may order radiographs or bone scans to help identify other pathologies or fractures.

Clinical Management. Hunter[20] recommends the use of soft orthotic inserts or shock-absorbing heel cups. Arch taping is often effective to help alleviate acute symptom (Fig. 10–10). Mobility exercises should address identified tight structures. The use of resting night splints may assist with the alleviation of discomfort associated with plantar fasciitis. The heel cord may be stretched using several methods (Figs. 10–11 through 10–13). The plantar fascia may be stretched by rolling the foot over a rolling pin (Figs. 10–14 and 10–15). Physicians will frequently prescribe NSAIDs and steroid injections to control the local effects of inflammation. Modification of activities that produce and increase pain is necessary. Heavy-impact activities or prolonged standing should be avoided. As symptoms resolve for the client, activity should be gradually reintroduced. If suspected biomechanical deficiencies are identified, the dysfunction should be corrected through orthotic management. Education of the client should consist of instruc-

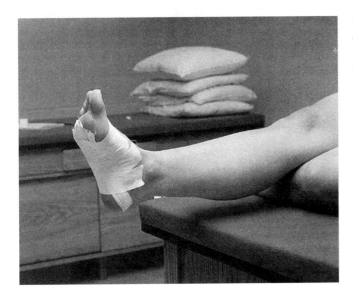

FIG. 10–10
Arch taping for plantar fasciitis. White athletic tape can be used to provide a temporary arch support to help relieve acute painful symptoms from plantar fasciitis.

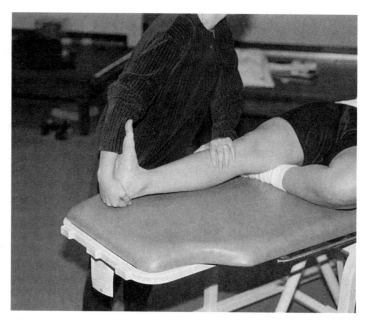

FIG. 10–11
Heel cord manual stretch. The therapist can manually stretch the heel cord by passively dorsiflexing the ankle joint while keeping the subtalar joint in a neutral position.

FIG. 10–12
Heel cord self stretch. The client can passively stretch the heel cord by leaning against a wall with the involved leg extended posteriorly, keeping the foot flat on the ground. The client should be encouraged to avoid compensating during the stretch by keeping the subtalar joint in a neutral position.

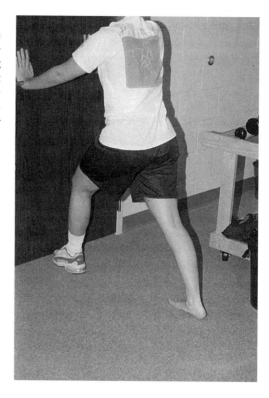

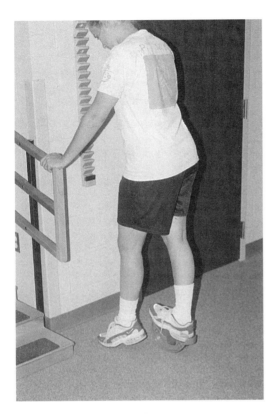

FIG. 10–13
Heel cord self-stretch with device. Mechanical devices such as the ProStretch are designed to stretch the heel cord.

tions related to the factors that contributed to the irritation of the plantar fascia. Strategies should be designed to avoid a recurrence of symptoms.[22]

The expected physical therapy outcomes for managing a client with plantar fasciitis include[9]:

1. Improved health-related quality of life
2. Improved functional skills
3. An optimal return of function

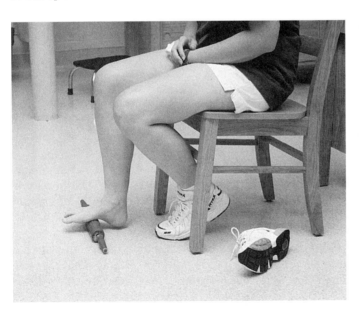

FIG. 10–14
Plantar fascia self-stretch. Using a standard kitchen rolling pin is effective in stretching the plantar structures of the foot. The client should be encouraged not to roll the pin onto the calcaneus as this may increase symptoms or irritation.

FIG. 10–15
Plantar fascia self-stretch. Windlass maneuver—by sitting with the feet flat on the floor, the client can perform the windlass effect or maneuver by keeping the foot on the floor and passively extending the toes. This will help to lengthen the plantar fascia of the foot.

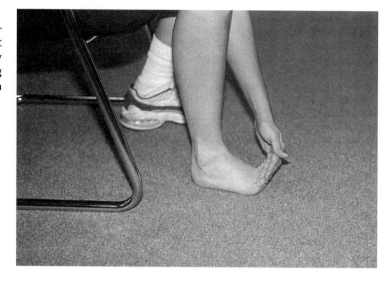

Spinal Stenosis
Constriction or narrowing of the central spinal canal or lateral intervertebral foramina.

Spondylosis
Arthritic process that involves the vertebrae of the spine.

Spondylolysis
The development of a bony defect in the lamina of the vertebrae. Most of these defects are typically found in the lumbar vertebrae.

Spondylolisthesis
A condition that results when one vertebra slips anteriorly on another. Extension activities should be judiciously avoided in clients with this condition, because spinal damage may result.

Dysmenorrhea
Pain and discomfort associated with the female menstrual cycle. Symptoms may present as painful back spasms.

Aneurysm
An abnormal widening or dilatation of an arterial wall.

Osteomyelitis
Inflammatory process involving the bone and bone marrow.

4. Reduced risk of further disability from identified limitations
5. An understanding of risk factors that may contribute to jeopardizing health status
6. An understanding of strategies to prevent further disability

The expected time frame for achieving the outcomes varies. Because of the overuse nature of this injury and the weight-bearing and shock-absorbing action of the plantar fascia, complete avoidance of repeated irritation is difficult. Because the onset of symptoms is slow, the process leads to a chronic irritation caused by chronic behaviors. The ultimate management of the symptoms is to modify the activity that is causing the irritation. Most cases should be resolved within 12 weeks.

SPINE INJURIES

Lower Back Injuries

Low back pain is the number one diagnosis treated at outpatient physical therapy clinics.[23] White and Brotzman[24] claim that 70% to 85% of all adults will experience acute back pain at some point in their lives. Back pain is commonly associated with certain conditions and events. Pregnant women have a three times greater chance of experiencing back pain during the 9 prenatal months compared to their non-pregnant counterparts. The industrial worker is more likely to experience back pain if unhappy or dissatisfied at work, if the work environment is noisy, or if there exists poor employee-employer communication. It is estimated that the societal cost of back injuries is between $20 and $50 billion dollars annually.[25]

There are many causes of low back pain, including biomechanical, traumatic, visceral, and psychogenic factors. Pain can be either acute or chronic in nature. Musculoskeletal strains, ligamentous sprains, spinal compression fractures, and herniated nucleus propulsus (HNP) are common. **Spinal stenosis, spondylosis, spondylolysis, spondylolisthesis,** and sacroiliac joint pathology may produce symptoms in the back (Fig.10–16). Hip, knee, and foot biomechanical deficits can create lower back symptoms. Internal medical conditions such as renal disease, **dysmenorrhea,** tumor, **aneurysm,** and **osteomyelitis** all may manifest externally as back dysfunction.[24]

The return-to-work outcome is a major guiding measurement when judging the effectiveness of a treatment program. Arkuszewski[26] suggested that the effectiveness of management for the client with lower back pain should be judged in relation to the client's returning to work and not going on a disability status. Other authors[27] reported as high as a 92% return-to-work rate with aggressive conservative management of clients with back injuries and dysfunction. The focus of management for the client with an acute dysfunction of the spine should include a treatment plan that enables the individual to resume normal activity and return to work as soon as possible without interventions that promote passive healing. This section discusses the management of clients with acute lower back injuries. Clients with chronic back injuries require a completely different clinical management approach, and this approach is discussed later in the chapter.

Clinical Presentation. The average age of onset for acute low back pain is 30 years, with the greatest occurrence of injury around age 50. Pain can be described as either **centralized** or **peripheralized**. The pain can be dull or sharp, constant or intermittent. Most clients will be able to describe the event that led up to or precipitated the onset of acute symptoms. The client may have difficulty in standing, sitting, or weight bearing. Gait dysfunctions (e.g., decreased trunk rotation, slow cadence, and decreased stride length) are common with acute back injuries. Transitional movements from sit to stand or from supine to sit may be difficult. With acute back discomfort, the client is frequently able to find a position that helps to relieve the symptoms.

Centralized
Pain is said to be centralized if the symptoms remain in the region of the spine.

Peripheralized
Pain is said to be peripheralized if the symptoms radiate into one or both of the extremities.

Evaluation: Tools and Methods. The PT will perform an extensive evaluation that will identify the source of the discomfort. A history will help reveal precipitating factors and the mechanism of injury, if known. The active range of motion of the spine will be assessed, as should the segmental mobility of the involved vertebrae. Posture examinations will reveal appropriate alignment of structures and noted skeletal deviations. The therapist will frequently perform a holistic evaluation, looking not only at the injured area, but also associated areas

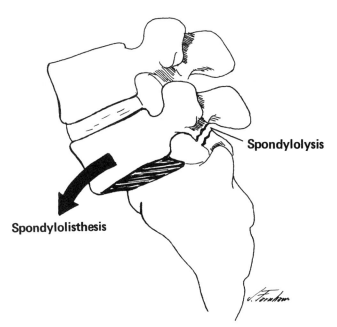

Spondylolysis

Spondylolisthesis

FIG. 10–16
Spondylosis, spondylolysis, and spondylolisthesis. These three words have created great confusion in many students due to the similarities in the word construction and the similarities of the involved body region. Spondylosis is an arthritic process affecting the vertebrae. Spondylolysis is a defect occurring in the lamina of the vertebrae. Spondylolisthesis is an actual forward slippage of one vertebra over another. (From Norkin & Levangie, p 164, with permission.)

and structures that may be potential sources of pain. Nerve root integrity, manual muscle testing, reflex testing, and a complete sensory examination may be included. Palpation of the involved structures and simple observation of the client's movements are helpful. There exist many special tests associated with the lumbar spine, and manual therapists are currently adding more diagnostic tools and movements as this text is being written. One of the classic special tests associated with back pain is the passive straight-leg raise (SLR) test. The SLR test is positive when pain in the back and limited motion of the hip is noted as the examiner passively flexes the hip while keeping the knee extended with the client in a supine position. This may be indicative of disk or sciatic nerve involvement. A second common special test is the pelvic obliquity or alignment examination. By examining the relative heights of the anterosuperior iliac spine (ASIS) and posterosuperior iliac spine (PSIS) of the pelvis, the therapist is able to identify potential rotations or shifts in the sacroiliac joint that may produce pain.

Clinical Management. The management goals for the client with an acute low back injury are the same as those for any other musculoskeletal dysfunction. The management goals include:

1. Alleviating or modifying the painful symptoms
2. Promoting healing
3. Restoring normal motion and arthrokinematics
4. Promoting adequate strength and stability of the spinal muscles
5. Encouraging appropriate functional activities in order to prepare the client to return to work or the prior level of function
6. Providing education in an attempt to minimize future episodes of back pain[24]

The classic intervention for acute back injury is bedrest. The physician may often prescribe muscle relaxant medication and pain-killing or analgesic medication. Studies by various authors have all concluded that bedrest not only is ineffective in the management of acute back pain, but also promotes a slower return-to-work rate. Clients given 7 days of bedrest after an acute back injury return to work an average of 60% greater or longer than comparable clients not given prolonged bedrest. Cardiovascular deconditioning, muscle atrophy, bone loss, and hypercalcemia leading to the formation of kidney and bladder stones may all accompany bedrest.[24]

Passive modalities have often been an integral treatment for lower back injuries. To the credit of the researchers in the allied health professions, the former reliance on passive modalities (e.g., moist heat, ultrasound, massage) as the primary treatment plan for clients with low back pain has greatly decreased. Acute management of an injury should be designed to reduce the negative effects of inflammation. Cryotherapy and electrical stimulation are some of the more effective modalities at the disposal of the rehabilitation team and should be used for the acute back injury the same as they would be used for an acute knee or ankle injury. Reimbursement in the physical therapy profession for passive modalities has come under criticism. Third-party payers are becoming less likely to support the use of passive treatments only in the management of low back (or any) injuries. Modalities should be carefully chosen primarily to achieve an established goal. With acute management of lower back injuries, the primary goal is to reduce pain and inflammation. Modalities should be chosen to achieve those goals, not simply used as **palliative** treatments.

A variety of literature is presented prescribing management of the client with a back injury, but there is little consensus among authors.[28] Various exercise

Palliative
A treatment that relieves or alleviates pain without curing it.

protocols have been described ranging from no activity to protocols including isometric exercises, dynamic concentric and eccentric programs, dynamic stabilization protocols, and extension and flexion exercises. McKenzie[29] reported that 98% of the clients experiencing pain for less than 4 weeks had excellent outcomes if their pain was controlled initially through exercise. Manniche et al.[30] demonstrated that clients with chronic low back pain responded positively to intense dynamic exercise programs. Clients regularly performing more than 100 repetitions of dynamic trunk and extremity exercises had improved conditions 74% of the time, whereas the placebo group performing the same dynamic exercises, yet only doing 20 repetitions, had improvement ratings in 42% of the cases. The control group, which did no exercises, demonstrated improvement only 18% of the time. Hansen et al.[31] suggested that treatment approaches to clients with back injuries vary depending on the gender and activity level of the client. Male clients tended to respond better to traditional physical therapy (isometric exercises), whereas female clients responded better with intensive dynamic back exercises. Those clients that performed moderate to hard work responded better to traditional physical therapy, whereas those clients with sedentary or light work demands had a greater success rate with dynamic exercise programs. Kellett et al.[32] demonstrated that over a 1½-year period, workers who regularly exercised lost less time from work due to back pain when compared with a control group over the same period.

Manual therapy has appeared frequently in the literature for the management of lower back pain. Janda[33] examined the use of manual therapy (including mobilization of joint restrictions, and addressing length and strength imbalances of the spine, pelvis, and extremities) and found that 91% of the clients over an 8-year period demonstrated improvement and 75% were able to return to their normal activities. The authors concluded that motivation to improve and adherence to the exercise programs were critical factors that determined the success of the treatment. Kinalski et al.[34] also found manual means to be effective at reducing back pain. Compared with passive modality sessions, the average length of treatment time was less for the client receiving manual therapy. Overall, both groups improved, but the passive modality group required a greater amount of time to achieve the same results. Patijn and Durink[35] believed that the use of manual interventions for musculoskeletal problems results in lower rates of absenteeism among injured employees. Arkuszewski[26] found that the average number of treatments was less for therapists applying a manual therapy approach compared with a control group, and that clients treated with manual therapy returned to their previous work at a rate of 60%, whereas the control group returned to their previous job only 36% of the time.

Various exercise protocols have been described for the management of clients with acute low back dysfunction. Boxes 10–2 through 10–4 describe the treatment approach by Robin McKenzie (Figs. 10–17 through 10–29).[24,36] Box 10–5 presents the classic Williams flexion exercises (Figs. 10–30 through 10–33),[12,24] Lastly, Box 10–6 discusses the dynamic lumbar stabilization protocols (Figs. 10–34 through 10–47).[12,24] Many other approaches to the management of spinal dysfunction exist. Manual therapists will balance spinal dysfunction with mobilization and repeated exercise to promote functional gains. Functional and return-to-work activities for the management of clients with lower back dysfunction are presented later in the chapter. A common premise that should flow through any treatment approach used is the avoidance of peripheralizing or radicular symptoms. If an exercise produces pain that radiates into the lower extremity, then it should be avoided. Frequently, pain may initially increase in the lumbar area itself, but as long as pain or numbness does not move into the lower extremity, this is acceptable. Pain increases in the lumbar spine are usually mechanical in nature, whereas radiating symptoms are usually a result of a neurological compression or involvement and thus should be avoided.[29] This chapter is not a comprehensive overview of every

Box 10–2

MCKENZIE'S TREAT YOUR OWN NECK OR BACK:

Robin McKenzie, a New Zealand physiotherapist, developed a comprehensive evaluation and management approach to neck and back pain centered on the empowerment of the client to manage his or her own pain. Two small booklets in the "Treat Your Own" series were produced for client education purposes and summarize the treatment approach for back or neck pain. Incorrectly associated with only a method of extension exercises, the McKenzie approach is a comprehensive approach designed to systematically evaluate and treat back and neck dysfunction. Relevant to the management concepts for the neck or back is the concept of centralization versus peripheralization. As the client improves, pain should centralize, or move to the neck or back. If the pain is moving into either the upper or lower extremity, the treatment approach is aggravating the condition. Repeated exercise motions, activities, and rest patterns should be chosen with respect to promoting centralization of the pain and avoiding peripheralization of the symptoms. Pain is classified by three syndromes or conditions: (1) dysfunction, or adaptive shortening or changes unable to handle stresses; (2) disorders of posture or symptoms associated from poor postural alignment; or (3) derangement, or an involvement of the disk, creating neurological symptoms.

McKenzie believes that most back problems are a result of being in a flexed posture for too long throughout the day. Sitting at a desk, standing with a slumped posture, or driving a car all promote a flattening of the lumbar lordosis, and forward head. Very little, if any time is spent throughout the day correcting this flexed posture of the lower back or cervical spine. Six lumbar exercises (see Figs. 10–17 through 10–22) and seven cervical exercises (see Figs. 10–23 through 10–29) are described as tools to centralize pain and discomfort. The exercises performed repetitively should encourage a centralization of the discomfort. McKenzie found that extension movements worked best when followed by lateral movements. Rarely did flexion movements produce a centralization in the pain. The rehabilitation team should address posture and factors leading to postural deficits and work to improve client awareness and understanding of methods to prevent the return of symptoms.

McKenzie describes a client empowerment process that should be used for clients who demonstrate acute neck (see Box 10–3) or lower back (see Box 10–4) symptoms. Advantages of the McKenzie approach include empowerment of the client to help himself or herself and positive results with acute management of back or neck pain. Disadvantages of the McKenzie approach include (1) the client must desire to be an active participant, (2) the results with chronic pain clients are poor, and (3) the therapist must be able to effectively prescribe appropriate movements.

Box 10–3

TREATING ACUTE NECK SYMPTOMS

Empowering the client is to educate him or her regarding the negative effects that most activities have on posture. Sitting, reading, and computer work all create stress, placing the head and neck in a forward position. If acute pain occurs, the client should do the following:

1. Avoid quick, rolling motions.
2. Avoid positions that reproduce or aggravate the pain.
3. Acute modalities, such as ice, will aid the client at home to reduce pain.
4. Do not put the neck into greater flexion while sleeping by using excessive pillows.
5. Promote good cervical alignment while resting by using a towel or cervical roll.
6. Begin exercises as pain decreases. Avoid peripheralizing the symptoms.

Box 10–4

TREATING ACUTE LOWER BACK SYMPTOMS

A client with acute lower back symptoms can be educated to take the following steps to help limit or minimize his or her discomfort.

1. Immediately find a comfortable position. Usually this is prone. Acute modalities, such as cryotherapy, work well to limit pain.
2. Use proper body mechanics if lying in a bed to preserve lumbar lordosis. Use a towel roll that is fastened around the waist to achieve this goal.
3. When pain decreases, begin prone exercise progression (prone, prone on elbows, and prone press-ups) in attempt to centralize any discomfort.
4. If pain is greater on one side and not centralizing, move hips away from the painful side, and repeat prone progression.
5. Rest as much as possible in a properly supported position.
6. Avoid forward flexion for 3 to 4 days.
7. As pain resolves, return to normal activities, being aware of proper posture at all times.

approach to the management of spinal injuries, but rather an introduction to some of the more common methodologies. The PTA should be effective at implementing techniques described in the plan of treatment by the supervising PT. A comprehensive review of the spine and spinal mechanics is beyond the scope of this text and is indeed the focus of many well-written, current books.

Surgery should be reserved for clients who cannot be managed satisfactorily by an aggressive rehabilitation program. Saal and Saal[27] reported that 90% of the clients examined with a disk herniation and radicular symptoms had good or excellent results with an aggressive active rehabilitation program. Surgical approaches that have been traditionally used for the management of lower back pain include laminectomies, lumbar fusions, and diskectomies. Indications for

Text continued on page 366

Box 10–5

WILLIAMS FLEXION EXERCISES

Originally described in the 1930s, these exercises were designed to (1) increase the space of the intervertebral foramina and open the facet joints, (2) strengthen the abdominal muscles as a spinal stabilizer, and (3) stretch the hip flexors, hamstrings, and back extensors. Although original results as described by Dr. Williams were positive, certain flexion activities of the spine can place significant increased pressure on the intervertebral disk and should be avoided in clients with a suspected disk lesion. Figures 10–21, 10–22, and 10–30 through 10–33 demonstrate the Williams flexion protocol.

Box 10–6

DYNAMIC LUMBAR STABILIZATION PROTOCOLS[24]

The research that is presented in support of early mobility of the client with an acute back dysfunction promotes the concept that no matter the severity of the pain as perceived by the client, each individual should be able to do some activity to promote a return to function. Those individuals in whom early mobility is promoted not only tend to have shorter periods of disability, but also tend to manage discomfort more readily. Dynamic stabilization programs were developed along the premise that the spine is a dynamic element supported by muscles and ligaments. Clients could be taught to stabilize the injury by increased neuromuscular control. The root of any management program for the spine is education about the function of the spine and the proper body mechanics associated with lifting and moving objects.

The management of the client with an acute back dysfunction using dynamic stabilization exercises should focus on strengthening the dynamic stabilizers of the spine (the abdominal muscles) to sufficiently cocontract during functional activities to protect and support the spine. All activities and exercises should begin from a pain-free neutral position. Various limb exercises are added as the client gains abdominal motor control and strength in one posture. Eventually, the postures are made progressively more challenging in attempts to carry over strength gains into functional activities. The phases of progression in a dynamic stabilization program include (1) addressing flexibility issues (see Figs. 10–34 through 10–36), (2) addressing spinal mobility issues (see Figs. 10–20 through 10–22), and (3) performing progressive stabilization exercise training (see Figs. 10–37 through 10–47).

Advantages of the dynamic stabilization program include active exercise, postural control, and return to functional activities. Critics of the program believe that the spine is a dynamic element, and encouraging bracing or muscle splinting may limit normal arthrokinematic movement of the spine. The client should also be trained in rotational movements. Functional activities, while keeping the spine in a neutral position, do not guarantee that injury will be prevented.

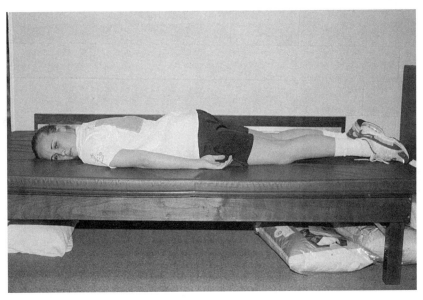

FIG. 10–17
Prone lying. Lying in the prone position is an exercise to help reduce stress on the lumbar spine and encourage relaxation. Often acute painful symptoms in the lumbar spine are increased with sitting. Encourage the client to lay prone and relax for 4–6 minutes. Have the client focus on taking deep breaths.

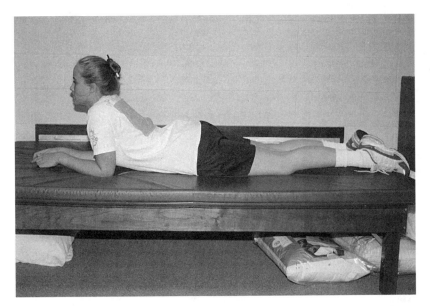

FIG. 10–18
Prone on elbows. Increasing the lumbar lordosis should be slow and gentle. Have the client place the arms under the trunk and lift up to the elbows position holding for a few minutes. Pain may intensify in the lumbar region, but this is appropriate and will subside. If pain radiates into the lower extremity, stop the exercise and notify the supervising physical therapist.

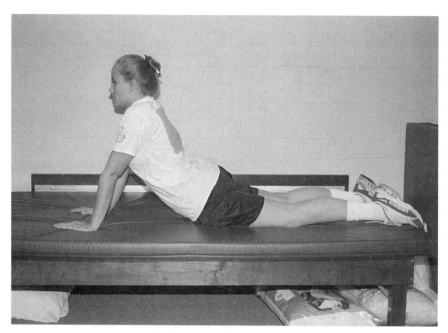

FIG. 10–19
Prone press-ups. Have the client extend the trunk by extending the elbows. The hips, pelvis and legs should remain relaxed and in contact with the surface. The movement should be slow and controlled, holding at the end range for a second or two, then return to the starting position. If pain increases centrally, do not force, but also do not stop. If the pain peripheralizes, stop the exercise and contact the supervising physical therapist.

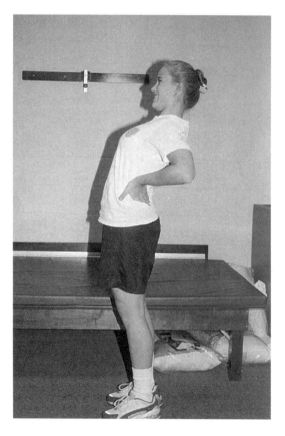

FIG. 10–20
Extension in standing. The lumbar lordosis can be promoted by extending the trunk in standing. This is a particularly good exercise for someone who sits flexed for long periods of time. Have the client place hands on the posterior aspect of hips and extend the trunk as far as possible. Hold for a second or two, then return to the starting position.

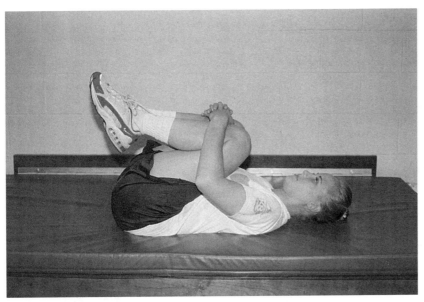

FIG. 10–21
Flexion in supine position. A classic exercise in William's flexion exercises, is also promoted by McKenzie if it works to centralize the pain and discomfort. Have the client pull both knees to the chest and hold for 1–2 seconds. McKenzie believes that all flexion exercises should be followed by a session of prone lying to restore normal a lordotic posture.

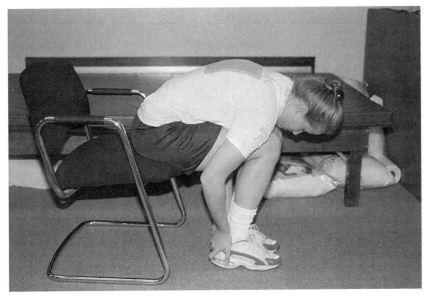

FIG. 10–22
Flexion in sitting. Forward flexion of the lumbar spine can help restore normal motion and should be used if pain is centralized or eliminated. McKenzie feels that after a flexion exercise is performed by the client, a prone press-up should be done to help restore the normal lumbar lordosis.

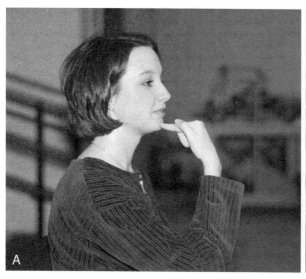
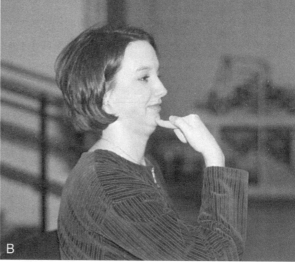

FIG. 10-23
Cervical retraction. Retracting the head and cervical spine is the result of pulling the head backward. Have the client place the index finger on the chin (A) and pull the head and chin directly posterior (B). The finger is used for feedback in keeping the head level. No rotation of the head should occur. The finger should move directly backwards keeping eyes level with the horizon. Hold the position for several seconds and relax. This will help to reduce the negative effects of a forward head posture.

FIG. 10-24
Cervical extension in sitting. Have the client gently tilt the head posteriorly as if looking toward the sky. Hold each extension exercise for several seconds and return to the starting point. The exercise can be varied by gently rotating the head a little to the right or left once the head is extended. Any pain should centralize in the cervical spine. If pain increases in the arm, stop the exercise and contact the supervising physical therapist.

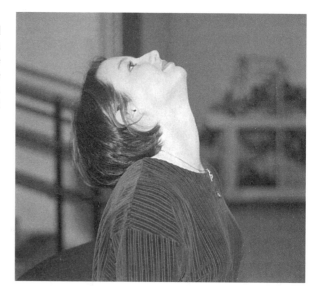

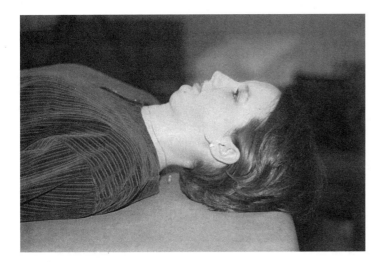

FIG. 10–25
Cervical retraction in supine position. A variation of the sitting cervical retraction exercise can be performed supine for those clients with extreme discomfort or who are unable to maintain good cervical alignment when performing the retraction. Have the client try to flatten the neck against the surface on which he or she is lying. Hold for a few counts and relax.

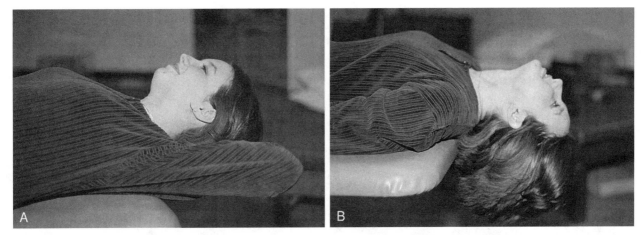

FIG. 10–26
Cervical extension in supine. Extension may be encouraged by hanging the head off the bed. Support the head in neutral with one hand (A) and gently lower the cervical spine into extension (B). Once maximum extension is achieved, gentle rotation may be performed by slowly moving the nose to the left and right about 1 in. Do not actively lift the head, but passively lift using the hand. Do not encourage the client to raise to sitting until resting for a few moments. Avoid any use of a pillow, as this promotes cervical flexion.

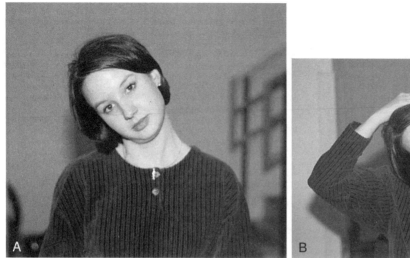
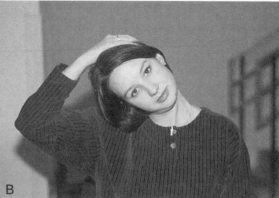

FIG. 10–27
Cervical side bending. A lateral side bend can help elongate the upper trapezius muscle (A). Gentle over-pressure may assist this exercise (B). If this exercise causes increased pain in the arm, stop and contact the supervising physical therapist.

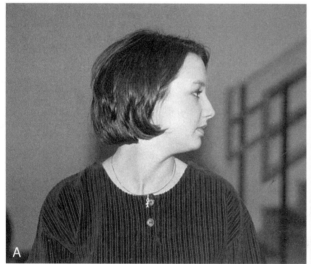
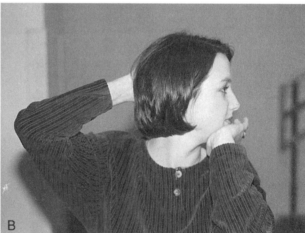

FIG. 10–28
Cervical rotation. Have the client look to the left or right, maintaining good cervical alignment (A). Over-pressure can help to lengthen tight structures (B).

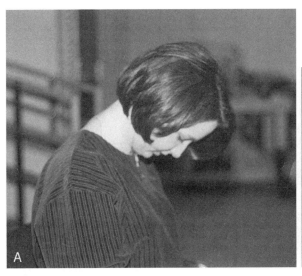
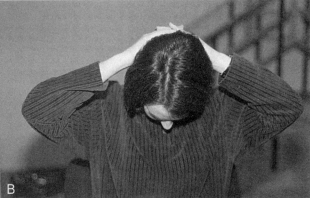

FIG. 10–29
Cervical flexion in sitting. Drop the head forward, gradually stretching all of the posterior structures of the neck (A). The weight of the hand can be added as a gentle over-pressure (B). No pulling from the hand is required. Flexion activities should be followed by cervical retraction and extension. This exercise is particularly helpful for tension headaches.

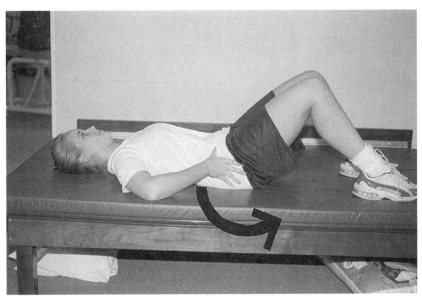

FIG. 10–30
Posterior pelvic tilt. Have the client lie in the hook-lying position and place the fingertips on each respective ASIS. Ask the client to gently rotate the pelvis posteriorly as if trying to flatten the back onto the treatment surface (arrow). Hold for several counts and relax.

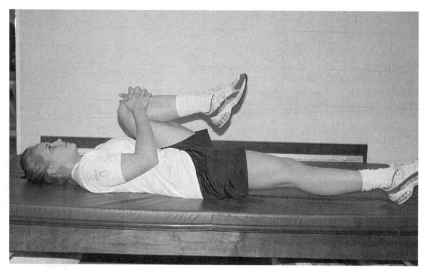

FIG. 10–31
Single knee to chest. The single knee to chest can help to stretch the hip flexors on the extended leg. Have the client hold one knee to the chest while keeping the opposite knee extended. The double knee to chest exercise is used to elongate the lower back extensor muscles.

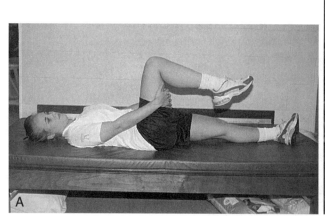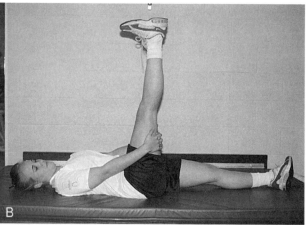

FIG. 10–32
Hamstring stretch. Have the client support the leg to be stretched by grasping the posterior aspect of the thigh (A). Ask the client to actively extend the knee to stretch the hamstring muscle group, keeping the hip in 90 degrees of flexion (B). Hold for a slow count of 20–30 and relax.

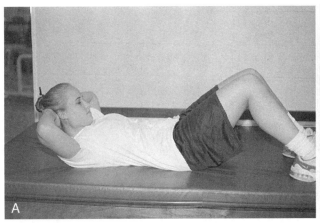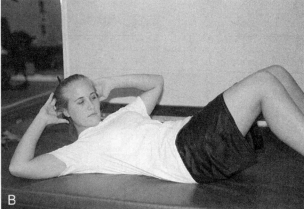

FIG. 10–33

Abdominal crunch. The client can support the head and neck with his or her hands and gently lift the head and shoulders off the supporting surface (A). The client should be encouraged not to hold his or her breath and to perform the repetitions slowly and in a controlled fashion. The exercise can be varied by rotating the trunk to the left or right (B). Strengthening the abdominal muscles is a critical aspect for the client with any back injury as the abdominal muscles are the only anterior dynamic supporting element of the spine.

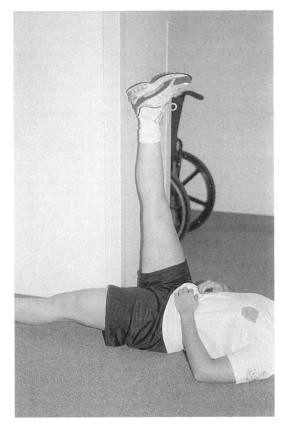

FIG. 10–34

Hamstring stretch against a wall. A loss of flexibility of the hamstring group can place the pelvis in a posterior rotation, placing stress on the lumbar spine. Stretching can be done by propping the leg up against a wall and hold for durations greater than 30 seconds. Care should be taken not to produce discomfort in the lumbar spine.

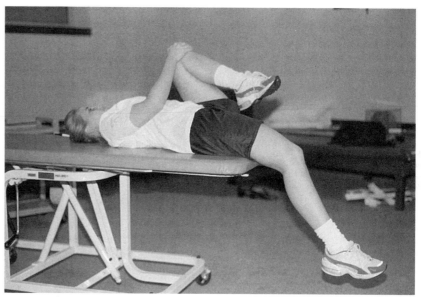

FIG. 10–35
Hip flexor stretch. Tight hip flexor muscles can place an anterior rotational stress on the pelvis causing lumbar spine discomfort. The Thomas position is a method to promote stretching of the hip flexor group.

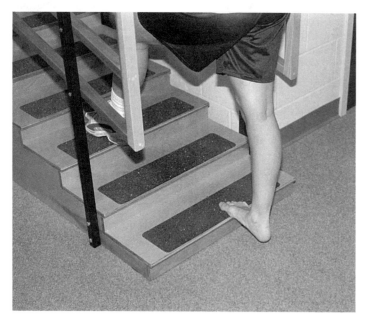

FIG. 10–36
Heel cord stretch. Tight heel cords can limit dorsiflexion of the ankle during gait and create undue stress on the closed kinematic chain. Previous methods to stretch the heel cord have been presented earlier in this chapter (see Figs. 10–11 through 10–13). Another method to promote stretching of the heel cord is to have the client hang the heel off a step. This method helps to keep the spine of the client in a neutral position.

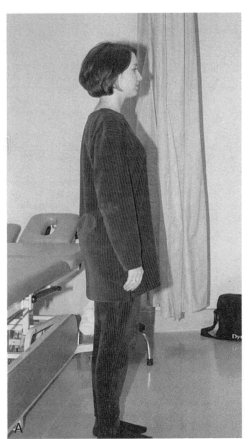

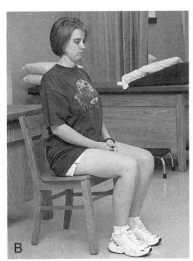
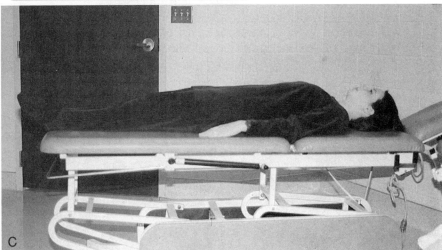

FIG. 10–37
Neutral spine. Finding the point where the spine is pain free and in a neutral position is key to all dynamic stabilization exercises. The client will learn to find this point by anteriorly or posteriorly rotating the pelvis in different postures (A, B, and C). Once this neutral pelvic position is learned, it should be maintained throughout the progressive sequences of the dynamic stabilization program.

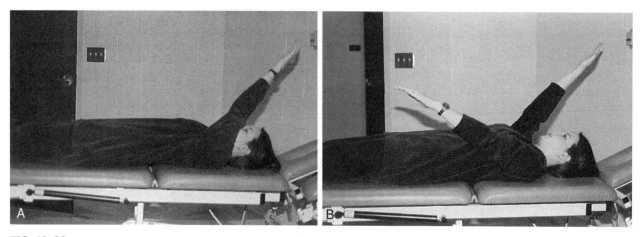

FIG. 10–38
Neutral spine with arm movement. Once the client has learned to maintain the neutral spine, dynamic activities can be added such as lifting one arm (A), followed by alternating arms (B).

back surgery should include acute neurological dysfunction with signs of muscular weakness and paresthesias. The surgical procedures will often relieve the potentially devastating neurological symptoms but may frequently leave the lower back pain unresolved.

The expected physical therapy outcomes for the management of a client with low back pain include[9]:

1. Improved health-related quality of life
2. Improved functional skills
3. An optimal return of function
4. Reduced risk of further disability from identified limitations
5. Improved self-care skills and ADLs
6. An understanding of risk factors that may contribute to jeopardizing health status
7. An understanding of strategies to prevent further disability

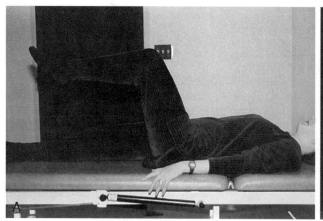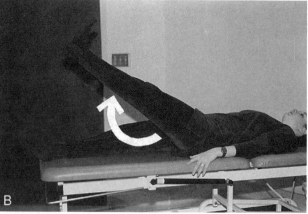

FIG. 10–39
Neutral spine with leg movement. Lower extremity movements are more challenging to the stabilization efforts of the client. A single bent leg lift (A) can be followed by extending the unsupported leg (B).

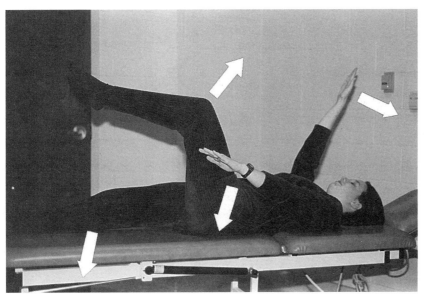

FIG. 10–40
Neutral spine with arm and leg movement. Once easier movement patterns are learned keeping the spine in a neutral position, then the therapist can instruct the client to combine both upper and lower extremity movement (arrows).

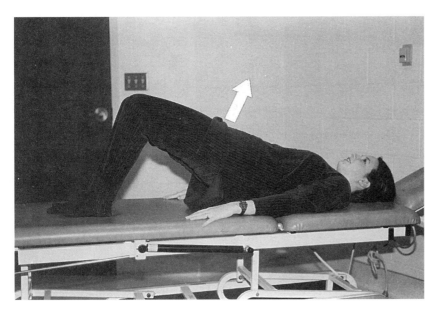

FIG. 10–41
Bridging. Bridging is an advanced exercise that will promote lower extremity motion while challenging the ability of the client to maintain a neutral pelvis (arrow). Exercises should be slow and controlled with progressively increased repetitions.

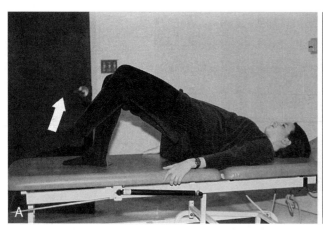
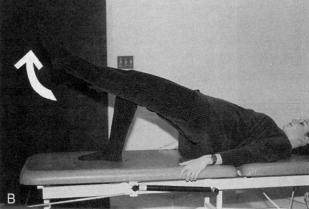

FIG. 10–42
Dead bug lift. An advanced bridge exercise has the client maintain the bridge position and then slowly unload one of the lower extremities (A). Once this is mastered, the client can perform a leg thrust (B) from the dead bug position. If the client is unable to maintain a neutral spine during the dynamic activity, a less challenging form of exercise should be encouraged.

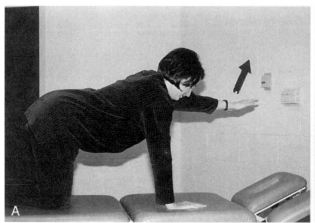
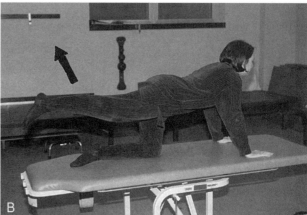

FIG. 10–43
All-fours position. The quadrupled or all-fours position is an advanced exercise. Once the neutral pelvis is maintained, the client can dynamically lift an arm (A) or a leg (B).

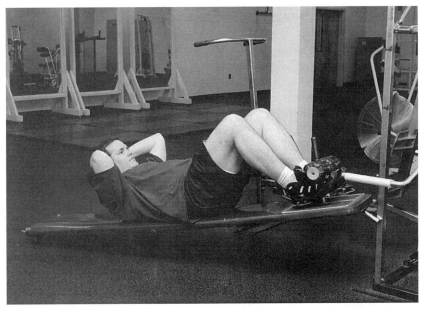

FIG. 10–44
Abdominal crunches. Abdominal strengthening may be advanced to using crunches as pictured in Fig. 10–33, and progressed to using slant boards.

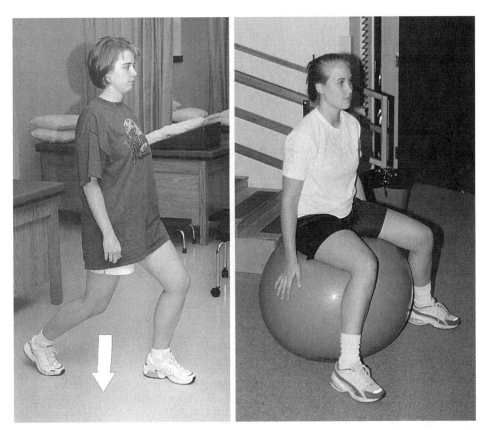

FIG. 10–45
Postural challenges. Once the client has progressed through the challenges designed by the rehabilitation team maintaining a neutral pelvis, advanced postural challenging exercises should be incorporated. The lunge (A) and the therapy ball (B) are significantly advanced exercises.

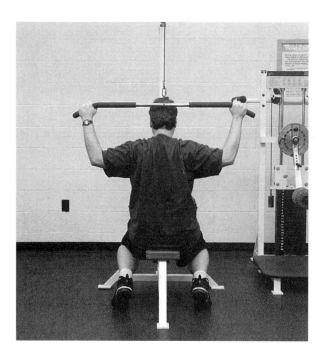

FIG. 10–46
Upper body exercise. General upper body strengthening can be encouraged as the client improves. With each repetition, the client should focus on the main purpose of stabilizing the spine in a neutral position. The latissimus pull down is pictured here.

The expected time frame for achieving the outcomes for an acute low back injury is 6 to 8 weeks. Of all acute back injuries, 80% to 90% respond positively in this short period regardless of the management approach or protocols. Interestingly, White and Brotzman[24] claim the return-to-work rate is relatively low for the client who has retained an attorney or in the presence of threatened litigation.

Cervical Injuries

Clients with cervical injuries can present from various postural or traumatic events. One of the most commonly treated neck injuries in physical therapy is pain and

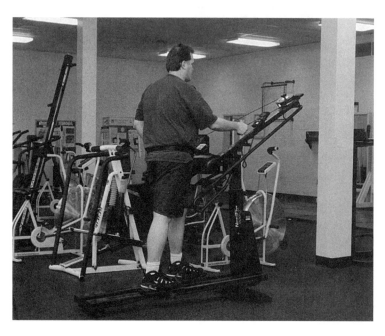

FIG. 10–47
Aerobic exercise. A return to function is not complete without an aerobic program. Any mode can be safely utilized if the client is able to maintain a neutral spine during the activity. Ski simulation machines gained great popularity as an aerobic tool that dynamically moves all extremities.

dysfunction associated with a motor vehicle accident (MVA). In a whiplash injury, the client's head and neck are forcefully flexed followed by a forceful hyperextension. The term "whiplash" is not, however, descriptive of the structures involved or the extent of the disability. From a whiplash injury, a muscular strain or ligamentous sprain may result, if not a combination of both. In either case, proper assessment and identification of the involved structures are critical for proper management of the dysfunction.

The cervical spine is designed to support and provide mobility for the head. Combination motion of the head and cervical spine allow approximately a 180° arc of movement from side to side and from top to bottom. In comparison with the lumbar vertebrae, the cervical vertebrae are smaller and do not have the major weight-bearing capacity of their lumbar counterparts. Strong ligaments, long muscles, and structural alignment play a pivotal role in maintaining the head in an upright posture. Faulty postural mechanics or a traumatic event can lead to injury of any of these dynamic or static elements. Cervical pain from faulty postural mechanics is nearly as common as pain associated with traumatic injury.[37]

Clinical Presentation. Pain and dysfunction in the cervical spine can be related to pain and dysfunction in the upper extremity. Entrapment of the spinal nerve roots of the brachial plexus may create symptoms (e.g., pain, numbness, muscular weakness) that radiate into the shoulder or distal extremity. Treating peripheral symptoms without managing the central problem or dysfunction is generally ineffective. Cervical pain may be centralized in the neck without radiating symptoms. The pain may be present in the neck and shoulder. Clients may describe pain in the cervical region and discomfort in the distal extremity. The upper-extremity discomfort may be greater than the actual cervical discomfort. Neurological signs of weakness and paresthesias may accompany the cervical pain. Pain may be either acute or chronic.[38]

Evaluation: Tools and Methods. An examination by the PT should focus on a problem-oriented history. The client should try to identify factors or events that have created the current medical condition. The client should also describe how the dysfunction is limiting his or her ability to perform routine activities and job performance duties. The nature of the pain should be described as clearly as possible, particularly which activities cause symptoms to improve or worsen. Objective measures will include a postural evaluation, palpation, ROM, strength assessment, neurological screen, and functional assessment. The evaluating PT may use some of the cervical tests mentioned in the shoulder impingement section (e.g., Lhermitte's sign, Spurling's sign, Adson's maneuver, Rue's test). Other measures include axial loading and distraction as well as individual vertebra provocation tests.[7,38]

Clinical Management. The management of the client with an acute cervical injury will focus on:

- Minimizing painful symptoms
- Reducing inflammatory symptoms
- Restoring normal motion and arthrokinematics
- Improving strength and stability
- Promoting the return to functional activities
- Educating the client on injury prevention and future recurrence

Acute management of painful symptoms is often treated with NSAIDs as prescribed by the physician. Muscle relaxant and narcotic analgesics may also be used. The use of immobilization devices to successfully manage an acute cervical soft-tissue injury is controversial. Borchgrevink et al.[39] demonstrated that in two comparison groups, the clients that were encouraged to resume normal activity after suffering a cervical injury in an MVA performed significantly better on six follow-up examinations than those clients who were encouraged to limit activity and wear a soft cervical collar.

Passive modalities designed to reduce the complications of acute inflammation should be encouraged. Cryotherapy and electrical stimulation are helpful in reducing pain. As an adjunctive treatment to conventional physical therapy, the use of a helium-neon (He-Ne) laser may also be an effective means for reducing pain associated with cervical trigger points and muscle spasm.[40] Cervical traction, if prescribed in the plan of treatment, works to perform distraction of the cervical facet joints and may help to alleviate acute painful symptoms. Positioning using cervical pillows or towel rolls may assist the client in finding a comfortable resting position (Fig. 10–48).[38]

Exercises to promote ROM, strengthening, and postural awareness should be added to the progression of the client's treatment as acute pain and discomfort subside. Active range-of-motion exercises and self stretching exercises are

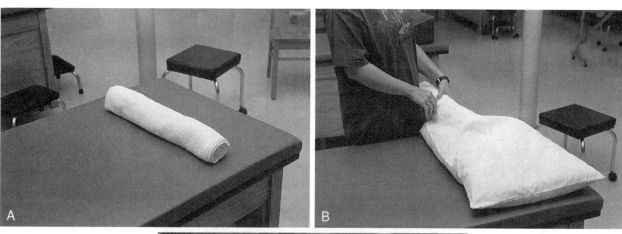

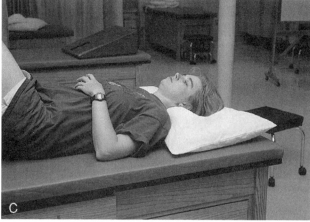

FIG. 10–48
Cervical support in supine. Various pillows are designed to support the neck in the supine position. Avoiding extremes of flexion should be encouraged. The use of a simple towel roll (A) strategically placed in the pillow case (B) can effectively support the cervical spine for the client when sleeping (C).

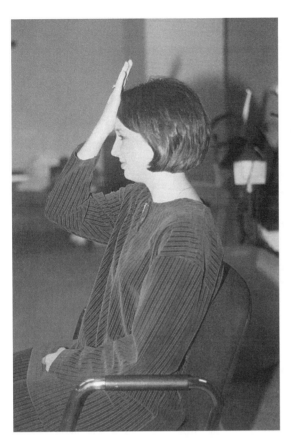

FIG. 10–49
Isometric cervical flexion. The client can perform resisted cervical isometric flexion by resisting at the forehead. Movement should not be encouraged. The client is asked to perform a maximal isometric contraction by gradually increasing the anterior resistance followed by gradually decreasing the resistance. Proper posture should be encouraged at all times. The client may begin these exercises in the supine position, and as strength improves, advance to sitting or standing.

beneficial in helping to restore lost motion (see Box 10–4).[41] Isometric exercises help to promote holding and stability of the cervical spine. These exercises can be started in the supine position to help keep good cervical alignment and gradually progressed to a sitting position, as tolerated by the client (Figs. 10–49 through 10–52). Functional activities of the cervical spine should include postural awareness exercises and education. If the client performs activities that challenge

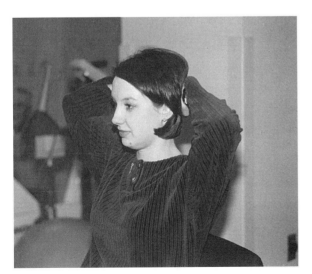

FIG. 10–50
Isometric cervical extension. The hands placed behind the head are effective in resisting the extension motion of the cervical spine. In supine, the table or mat serves as the resistance.

FIG. 10–51
Isometric cervical rotation. Have the client resist rotation by placing the hand against the temple, rotating toward the side on which the pressure is being applied. Again, as with all isometric exercises, movement should not be encouraged, but rather a graded increase and decrease of resistance.

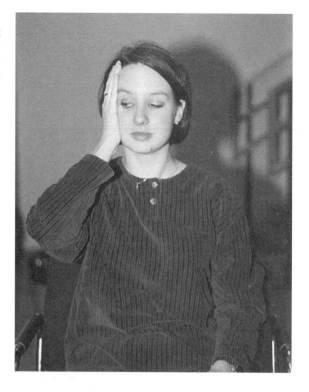

posture throughout the day, endurance and strength training of the upper arms and back should be considered. Strategies should be discussed to prevent the recurrence of symptoms.

The expected physical therapy outcomes related to managing a client with cervical dysfunction include[9]:

1. Improved health-related quality of life
2. Improved functional skills

FIG. 10–52
Isometric cervical side bend. Side bending can be resisted by placing the hand above the ear.

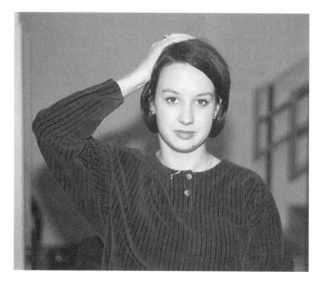

3. An optimal return of function
4. Reduced risk of further disability from identified limitations
5. Improved self-care skills and ADLs
6. An understanding of risk factors that may contribute to jeopardizing health status
7. An understanding of strategies to prevent further disability

The expected time frame for achieving outcomes for clients with cervical injuries is similar to lower back injuries. DeRosa and Porterfield[38] claim that "most cases of spinal pain have a favorable prognosis and a natural tendency toward spontaneous resolution." Clients generally respond positively in 6 to 8 weeks. If the dysfunction was a result of faulty posture or biomechanics, promoting an understanding of strategies to prevent the onset of symptoms in the future is important.

INDUSTRIAL REHABILITATION

The concept of industrial rehabilitation has taken many identities, names, and protocols over the past 20 years. Work hardening, industrial medicine, functional restoration programs, chronic pain management, and multidisciplinary pain teams have all been used to describe some aspect of the process for enabling a client to return to work after sustaining an injury. The basis of an industrial rehabilitation program is the care and prevention of the injured worker. Elements of a comprehensive industrial rehabilitation program should include:

1. A job **ergonomic** analysis to determine the suitability of and mechanical stresses on an individual performing a job
2. A functional capacity evaluation of the client to assess the individual's ability to perform certain jobs
3. Procedures for the immediate first aid and acute care of an injured worker
4. Procedures for ensuring the care of the injured worker promoting a return to work
5. Process for measuring outcomes and effectiveness of program.

Ergonomic
The science concerned with the fitting of a job to an individual's anatomic, physiological, and psychological characteristics to enhance performance and reduce the chance of injury.

Ergonomic Analysis

A specialized aspect of the rehabilitation team is the involvement in the prevention of injuries and disabilities. The traditional medical model for physical therapy professionals has been the management of the client after an injury has occurred. As health-care costs have increased and the need to reduce expenditures through the prevention of costly injuries has been emphasized, the rehabilitation team has become involved in the analysis of the workplace. An ergonomic analysis performed by a skilled team will help to identify components of a workplace that may potentially lead to injury or disability for the client working at that particular job or station. Assessing the use of machinery and its effects on the worker's posture and motion are critical. Normal measures designed to identify potentially excessive stresses can be applied to various elements of an individual's job performance. The evaluating team will make suggestions related to altering methods of job performance and designing tools to help the individual better perform the expected duties. McElligott et al.[42] concluded that improvements in job design and on-site rehabilitation can produce a financial savings to employers by reducing the number of industrial injuries.

Functional Capacity Evaluation

A branch of the ergonomic analysis related to the workstation is the screening of the individual who is working at the station. Elements of some machinery cannot be changed for various physical or financial reasons and thus physical and psychomotor characteristics of the individual who must work at the station are identified. These essential job performance functions should be related to the fundamental nature of the job performance and be nondiscriminatory. Any person who is able to meet the individual characteristics should be eligible for the position.

Before or after an injury, the rehabilitation team may perform a comprehensive functional capacity evaluation for the worker. This evaluation is designed to measure the individual's functional abilities to perform a certain job. Critical factors or essential job functions for a specific job can be used for a comparison to deem whether the client is able to safely participate in the desired job. Elements of the functional capacity evaluation may include all or some of the following:

1. ROM assessment
2. Strength assessment (either through manual muscle testing or isokinetic testing)
3. Functional tests
   a. Lifting assessment
   b. Carrying assessment
   c. Dexterity and small-object manipulation assessment
4. Aerobic capacity and overall conditioning

Acute Care of the Injured Worker

The initial management of the injured worker does not typically involve the physical therapy team, unless a PT is employed by the actual industry. Traditionally, an occupational health nurse is available for immediate care of minor injuries sustained by the employee. In the case of severe injuries, the nurse will contact the appropriate emergency medical system. The injured worker will be seen by a physician either in an emergency room or at a clinic approved by the company. The occupational health nurse will attempt to limit unnecessary trips to the emergency room by making appropriate, less costly referrals to a local physician. Emergency room bills are traditionally a large expense for most medical insurance programs. By controlling visits, the cost of health care is contained. The physician will examine the injured worker and make appropriate medical recommendations. The physical therapy team may now become involved with the injured client if the condition warrants intervention. Management of conditions described in this chapter are then pursued accordingly to ensure the return of the client to work.

Deconditioning Syndrome

The conditioning of an injured worker is critical to the successful return of the client to the previous level of work skills. Mayer et al.[43] demonstrated that an intensive functional retraining program focusing on overall body conditioning of the client was successful. Choosing clients who had not improved with conventional or surgical intervention, the program consisted of education, exercise for fitness, work simulation, repetitive motions, and psychological counseling. The program participants were obligated for 3 successive weeks for 58 hours per week.

The return to work rate was 82%. For those workers who failed to return to work after the conditioning program, inadequate strength for the performance of job duties was most frequently cited. This research suggests that the medical processes used after a client is injured may lead to the physical deconditioning of the client, which further extends the functional disability and inability to return to work. Mayer et al. concluded that back education alone was ineffective in ensuring that a client would return to work. A program of intensive physical reconditioning will help promote a functional atmosphere that limits the effects of deconditioning after injury, and enables the worker to safely return to their job.

Work Conditioning Functional Restoration Program

From the onset, in order to prevent excessive disability caused by industrial injury or accident, the client should be encouraged to participate actively in a functional restoration or work conditioning program. Hazard et al.[44] found a positive return-to-work success rate for clients that actively participated in a functional restoration program. After 1 year of observing the performance of the graduates of the restoration program, 81% were employed, compared with only a 40% employment rate for those who did not complete the program. Lindstrom et al.[45] concluded that low back pain clients who were encouraged to be active had less time off from work and returned to work faster than a control group of clients who were not encouraged to be active. Reilly et al.[46] reported that with a supervised, structured restoration program, the chances that a client with low back pain will be compliant with the exercise program increase. Regular weekly participation in a conditioning program can improve aerobic fitness and conditioning as well as produce a decrease in subjective pain reports.[46]

Critics dispute the efficacy and cost-effectiveness of placing a client in an aggressive functional restoration program, citing that no significant benefits are gained compared with the cost that is incurred.[47] Bendix et al.[48] in a comparison study of three different approaches to management of clients with chronic low back pain, demonstrated that the results of functional restoration programs were superior to those of either simple back education or psychological counseling. A significant human as well as economical benefit was gained by the participants in the intensive, multidisciplinary functional restoration program.

The multidisciplinary team approach in returning a client to work is comprised of various health-care fields. The physician often directs the medical management. The psychologist is involved to assist with cognitive behaviors and attitudes. The physical therapy team participates in the physical conditioning, job simulation, and client education. Sometimes an exercise physiologist is incorporated into the team to manage the fitness of the individual. A case manager is the director and coordinator of the team effort. Elements of the functional restoration program include all of the following[43]:

1. Baseline evaluation through the functional capacity evaluation (FCE)
2. Psychosocioeconomic assessment
3. Physical reconditioning of identified deficits from FCE
4. Job simulation
5. Client education on fitness and ergonomics
6. Cognitive and behavior modification to avoid pain behaviors
7. Outcome assessment

The physical reconditioning of the injured worker is considered after any acute management of the injury has been resolved. Cardiovascular conditioning may take many forms. Walking on a treadmill is one type of activity that will help improve cardiovascular conditioning and prevent the onset of a deconditioning syndrome (Fig. 10–53). Stationary bikes, upper-extremity ergometers, or stair machines may also be used. The program should focus on identified strength or flexibility deficits found in the FCE. The client should be given the exercise program and encouraged to actively control the rehabilitation, as though he or she were actually at work performing job duties. Passive treatments and modalities are not usually involved at this level of care. If passive techniques are therapeutically required elements of the plan (e.g., ice pack or stretching performed by the therapist), the client should be shown how to apply the techniques independently. The treatment is then appropriately dispensed by the client when needed. This is part of the empowerment process related to industrial rehabilitation.

Job simulation activities should be encouraged during the participation in a functional restoration program. The rehabilitation team should identify the key elements of the client's job duties and incorporate them into the designed activities. If the client must stand for 8 hours a day, all therapeutic activities performed should be done in a standing position. If the client must manipulate small objects with the hands, then small objects should be provided to the client to manipulate repetitively. Rest breaks from rehabilitation should be designed in accordance with the client's work environment. Some facilities actually incorporate the use of time clocks to have the client "punch" in and out for therapy. Every activity should have a purpose and be designed to promote return to work.

Injury Prevention and Client Education. Education is a critical element in any restoration program. The client must demonstrate knowledge about the injury and the events that precipitated the injury. Strategies to prevent further disability or a return of symptoms should be pursued. Sikorski[49] reported that after a 1-year

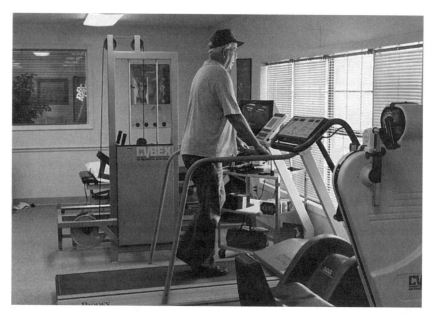

FIG. 10–53
Treadmill for back injury management. Despite the back injury, activity at a tolerable level should be promoted to prevent the onset of disuse atrophy. A treadmill is one mode of exercise to accomplish this goal.

follow up of 142 clients with mechanical low back pain, the clients reported that the most beneficial aspect of the medical intervention was education on posture and body mechanics. Klaber et al.[50] believed that client education was critical in lessening long-term disability associated with back pain. When comparing clients who received a regular back school program, there was a significant decrease in functional disability compared with a group that only exercised. Although the exercise group improved by having reduced painful symptoms, this group tended to revert to their pre-exercise condition over a period of 16 weeks. Leboeuf-Yde and Kyvik,[51] after their investigation of the onset of back pain and dysfunction in the adult population, believed that educational efforts for the prevention of back injuries should be focused on the adolescent individual. If body mechanics, prevention techniques, and awareness of disability associated with back injury are instilled in the youthful population, the net effect would be an overall decreasing of back injury in the adult population.

Measuring Outcomes. Demonstrating positive outcomes for the functional restoration program will ensure that industries will rely on the service provided by the rehabilitation team. As discussed previously, reducing long-term financial obligations for the industry by preventing costly medical claims will help the overall well-being of the client. Weir et al.[52] supported the cost-effectiveness of multidisciplinary pain management teams. These researchers found that clients who used the services of the chronic pain treatment centers relied less frequently on other health services (emergency room visits), thereby reducing the total cost for the health-care providers. Programs that actively work to promote physical recovery for the injured worker should gather data related to length of treatment, associated costs, disability, and return-to-work status. These outcomes are observed by the insurance industry and are important cost-effectiveness points of discussion.[43]

CHRONIC PAIN

Pain is frequently the reason why clients seek medical intervention. The onset of chronic pain can have significant financial, personal, and societal implications.[53] Chronic pain and its implications is one of the most costly health problems in America. Estimates provided by the National Institutes of Health approach $50 billion dollars of annual health-care expenses including direct medical expenses, lost income, lost productivity, compensation payments, and legal bills.[54] Chronic low back pain affects about 15% of the adults in the United States. Five million of these clients have some partial functional disability from the pain, and another 2 million have severe impairments that prevent them from working. Low back pain accounts for 93 million workdays lost every year and costs over $5 billion in health care.[54]

Avoiding Chronic Pain Behavior

Clients with chronic pain can be not only difficult to manage, but also resistant to treatment.[53,55] The perception of persistent pain often leads the client to seek health advice from multiple practitioners with various therapeutic interventions. Description of the characteristics of the average client with chronic pain that participated in one study included a 48-year-old with low back pain, leg pain, six past hospitalizations, two surgical operations, and numerous failed conservative treatment interventions. The average client had been unemployed for 2 years, had a history of medication abuse, and was currently receiving workers' compensation.[55] Another report described that over half of the clients using services at a chronic pain clinic have poor psychosocial adjustment to the condition.[52] The prognosis for employment of a client with a long history of lower back pain is poor.[44]

Burry and Gravis[56] demonstrated that men involved in heavy labor occupations had a higher incidence of back injury claims compared with those in white-collar jobs. Lifting (55%) was by far the most common mechanism of injury. Interestingly, up to 70% of the claimants had a history of back pain and dysfunction. Regarding medical intervention, the study demonstrated that claimants cited positive results from rest and painkillers and gave low ratings to exercise. The positive aspect of the study is that 82% of the claimants returned to work within 4 weeks regardless of treatment intervention.

Distinguishing between types of pain is relevant for clinical treatment of clients with chronic pain conditions. During intervention, and with a long history of the presence of pain, the client may not be able to differentiate successfully between acute or chronic symptoms. Acute pain is usually temporary with a rapid onset and usually a rapid resolution. The presence of acute pain is a warning signal from the body that the client has done something that is potentially injurious to the body. In comparison, chronic pain has been persistent for a long period of time (usually measured in months or years). The nature of the pain may be continuous as is the case for a client with a chronic lower back ache, or intermittent in the case of the client with chronic migraine headaches. Typically, there is no reason for the pain to remain persistent, and medical intervention has not alleviated the painful condition.[53]

Once pain has been resistant to resolve and lasts for many months or even years, chronic pain behavior may result. The client may establish a predictable "memory" pattern of the chronic pain or develop "pain talk" patterns. Pain memory is retained as patterns of pain, and pain responses are ingrained into the neural patterns of the client. A similar touch, feeling, or stressful condition will trigger a painful response even though the actual current stimulus was not sufficient to produce acute pain. The client may have emotional responses to the presence of the chronic pain including anger and depression. Attention of the client is frequently focused on the presence of the pain, and the client frequently engages others in discussions about his or her pain. Associated symptoms include loss of appetite, constipation, and sleep disturbances. The symptoms may be enhanced as a result of social dysfunctions encouraged by the chronic pain, including disruption of the family unit or social network. Identifying the presence of behaviors associated with chronic pain and incorporating plans to address the psychological and emotional needs of the client are critical in effectively managing the presence of chronic pain.[53]

Management emphasis to avoid chronic pain behavior should be to empower the client. Active participation of the client in the rehabilitation efforts is critical. Passive treatments and modalities encourage dependence. Teaching a client to control his or her own pain grants freedom and self-reliance.[53] Flor et al.[57] concluded that chronic pain clients treated with a multidisciplinary approach tended to improve and return to work at a greater rate than clients treated only by one health-care discipline. In a separate study, Stieg et al.[58] concluded that properly trained multidisciplinary rehabilitation teams can provide an effective means for reducing the long-term financial implications of the client with chronic pain. A third study by Guck et al.[59] also demonstrated that the participants in a multidisciplinary chronic pain center had positive outcomes in 60% of the cases, whereas the control group had no successful outcomes. In the present atmosphere of cost containment in health care, effective programs demonstrating measurable and predicable outcomes for clients are desirable.

The PTA should be an integral part of the rehabilitation team, helping to empower the client. Pain that persists and does not resolve should not be continually rewarded by applying palliative modalities. The assistant should be aware that the client may develop dependent behaviors that do not promote the functional return to active participation in society. If these behaviors are observed, the supervising PT should be consulted, and strategies to decrease dependent behavior should be considered.

Disability Syndrome

A disability syndrome is produced when there exists little or no incentive for the client to improve. Workers' compensation laws were originally designed to protect the rights of the injured worker but have evolved into an institution of expectations and delays. The worker expects to receive compensation for a sustained injury. As the level of injury severity increases, so does the expectation of financial compensation. Claims may take years to resolve, and the severity of the injury must be observed during the delays in litigation or there is a lower level of financial gain. If disability checks are regularly received while the employee is away from work, then there is less financial incentive to return to work. The rehabilitation team must be aware that in cases involving chronic pain and litigation settlements, a balance exists between psychological pain and disability and physical pain and disability. Sometimes, the correction of the painful dysfunction is beyond the scope of the physical care that the physical therapy team can provide.[60]

 SUMMARY

The client who suffers injury and disability related to the performance of job duties presents with unique physical and psychosocioeconomic problems. The nature of being injured presents stress, but the addition of missing work related to the injury coupled with financial obligations compounds an already difficult situation. Many work-related injuries are related to overuse or a cumulative trauma disorder. Dysfunction can result from standing for an excessive time, from repeatedly manipulating an object such as a screw driver, or from reaching over head. The back is a site of frequent injury, and management of back dysfunction puts an excessive strain on the medical and insurance industries. Management of acute musculoskeletal dysfunction should focus on combating the effects of inflammation, restoring normal motion, improving strength, and returning the client to a functional level for return to work. Modalities and techniques that are passive in nature encourage dependent behavior and may promote disability behaviors. Acute pain that is unresolved may develop into a chronic pain condition. Chronic pain is not necessarily physical in nature: A psychosocial component must be considered in the management of the client with chronic pain. Industrial rehabilitation is a comprehensive treatment approach designed for the prevention of injury and the care of industrial clients. The FCE is designed to identify the current abilities of the client related to functional activities. The ergonomic job analysis is the evaluation of the workstation as it relates to the human element. Education and a multidisciplinary approach to care for the industrial client is critical in preventing a recurrence of symptoms. The medical system of management of the injured worker often establishes a deconditioning of the client because time-off from work creates a decreased tolerance of the employee to sustain regular job demands. Time frames related to expected outcomes for various orthopedic conditions were outlined as established by the *Guide to Physical Therapist Practice* by the American Physical Therapy Association.

REFERENCES

1. Bureau of Labor Statistics Data. US Department of Labor, Washington, DC, 1998 [http://stats.bls.gov:80/datahome.htm].
2. Armstrong, TJ, and Martin, BJ: Adverse effects of repetitive loading and segmental vibration. In Nordin, M, et al (eds): Musculoskeletal Disorders in the Workplace: Principles and Practice. Mosby, St Louis, MO, 1997.
3. Jobe, FW, et al: Rehabilitation of the shoulder. In Brotzman, SB (ed): Clinical Orthopaedic Rehabilitation. Mosby, St Louis, MO, 1996.
4. Hertling, D, and Kessler, RM: Management of Common Musculoskeletal Disorders: Physical Therapy Principles and Methods, ed 2. Lippincott, Philadelphia, 1990.
5. Marks, PH, FU, FH: Treatment of shoulder disorders. In Nordin, M, et al (eds): Musculoskeletal Disorders in the Workplace: Principles and Practice. Mosby, St. Louis, MO, 1997.
6. Magnusson, M, and Pope, M: Epidemiology of the neck and upper extremity. In Nordin, M, et al (eds): Musculoskeletal Disorders in the Workplace: Principles and Practice. Mosby, St Louis, MO, 1997.
7. Hoppenfeld, S: Physical Examination of the Spine and Extremities. Appleton & Lange, Norwalk, CT, 1976.
8. Cuomo, F, et al: Clinical evaluation of the neck and shoulder. In Nordin, M, et al (eds): Musculoskeletal Disorders in the Workplace: Principles and Practice. Mosby, St Louis, MO, 1997.
9. Guide to Physical Therapist Practice. Phys Ther 77:1163, 1997.
10. Anderson, M, and Tichenor, CJ: A patient with de Quervain's tenosynovitis: A case report using an Australian approach to manual therapy. Phys Ther 74:314, 1994.
11. Rempel, D, and Punnett, L: Epidemiology of wrist and hand disorders. In Nordin, M, et al (eds): Musculoskeletal Disorders in the Workplace: Principles and Practice. Mosby, St Louis, MO, 1997.
12. Kisner, C, and Colby, LA: Therapeutic Exercise: Foundations and Techniques, ed 3. FA Davis, Philadelphia, 1996.
13. Adams, ML, et al: Outcome of carpal tunnel surgery in Washington State worker's compensation. Am J Ind Med 25, 527, 1994.
14. Calandruccio, JH, et al: Rehabilitation of the hand and wrist. In Brotzman, SB (ed): Clinical Orthopaedic Rehabilitation. Mosby, St Louis, MO, 1996.
15. Bednar, MS: Clinical evaluation of the wrist and hand. In Nordin, M, et al (eds): Musculoskeletal Disorders in the Workplace: Principles and Practice. Mosby, St Louis, MO, 1997.
16. Salter, RB: Textbook of Disorders and Injuries of the Musculoskeletal System: Williams & Wilkins, Baltimore, 1983.
17. Zetterberg, C: Epidemiology of the lower extremity. In Nordin, M, et al (eds): Musculoskeletal Disorders in the Workplace: Principles and Practice. Mosby, St Louis, MO, 1997.
18. Riehl, R: Rehabilitation of the lower leg injuries. In Prentice, WE (ed): Rehabilitation Techniques in Sports Medicine. 2nd ed. Mosby, St Louis, MO, 1994.
19. Smith W, et al: Comparative study using four modalities in shinsplint treatment. J Orthop Sports Phys Ther 8:77, 1986.
20. Hunter, S: Rehabilitation of foot injuries. In Prentice, WE (ed): Rehabilitation Techniques in Sports Medicine, ed 2. Mosby, St Louis, MO, 1994.
21. McPhoil, TG: The foot and ankle. In Malone, et al (eds): Orthopedic and Sports Physical Therapy, ed 3. Mosby, St Louis, MO, 1997.
22. Brotzman, SB, and Brasel, J: Foot and ankle rehabilitation. In Brotzman, SB (ed): Clinical Orthopaedic Rehabilitation. Mosby, St Louis, MO, 1996.
23. Jette, AM, and Davis, KD: A comparison of hospital-based and private outpatient physical therapy practices. Phys Ther 71:366, 1991.
24. White, AH, and Brotzman, SB: Low back disorders. In Brotzman, SB (ed): Clinical Orthopaedic Rehabilitation. Mosby, St Louis, MO, 1996.
25. Bigos, SJ, et al: Treatment of the acutely injured worker. In Nordin, M, et al (eds): Musculoskeletal Disorders in the Workplace: Principles and Practice. Mosby, St Louis, MO, 1997.

26. Arkuszewski, Z: The efficacy of manual treatment in low back pain: A clinical trial. Journal of Manual Medicine 2:68, 1986.

27. Saal, JA, and Saal, JS: Nonoperative treatment of herniated lumbar intervertebral disc with radiculopathy: An outcome study. Spine 14:431, 1989.

28. Batte, MC, et al: Managing low back pain: Attitudes and treatment preferences of physical therapists. Phys Ther 74:219, 1994.

29. McKenzie, RA: The Lumbar Spine: Mechanical Diagnosis and Therapy. Orthopedic Physical Therapy Products, Minneapolis, MN, 1981.

30. Manniche, C, et al: Intense dynamic back exercises for chronic low back pain: A clinical trial. Pain 47:53, 1991.

31. Hansen, FR, et al: Intensive, dynamic back-muscle exercises, conventional physiotherapy, or placebo-control treatment of low-back pain. Spine 18:98, 1993.

32. Kellett KM, et al: Effects of an exercise program on sick leave due to back pain. Phys Ther 71:283, 1991.

33. Janda, V: Treatment of chronic back pain. Journal of Manual Medicine 6:166, 1992.

34. Kinalski, R, et al: The comparison of the results of manual therapy versus physiotherapy methods used in treatment of patients with low back pain syndromes. Journal of Manual Medicine 4:44, 1989.

35. Patijn, J, and Durinck, JR: Effects of manual medicine on absenteeism. Journal of Manual Medicine 6:49, 1991.

36. McKenzie, R: Treat Your Own Back, ed 5. Orthopedic Physical Therapy Products, Minneapolis, MN, 1992.

37. Norkin, CC, and Levangie, PK: Joint Structure and Function: A Comprehensive Analysis, ed 2. FA Davis, Philadelphia, 1992.

38. DeRosa, C, and Porterfield, JA: The spine. In Malone, TR, et al (eds): Orthopedic and Sports Physical Therapy, ed 3. Mosby, St Louis, MO, 1997.

39. Borchgrevink, GE, et al: Acute treatment of whiplash neck sprain injuries: A randomized trial of treatment during the first 14 days after a car accident. Spine 23:25, 1998.

40. Snyder-Mackler, L, et al: Effects of helium-neon laser irradiation on skin resistance and pain in patients with trigger points in the neck or back. Phys Ther 69:336, 1989.

41. McKenzie, R: Treat Your Own Neck. Orthopedic Physical Therapy Products, Minneapolis, MN, 1992.

42. McElligott, J, et al: Low back injury in industry: The value of a recovery program. Conn Med 53:711, 1989.

43. Mayer, TG, et al: A prospective short-term study of chronic low back pain patients utilizing novel objective functional measurement. Pain 25:53, 1986.

44. Hazard, RG, et al: Functional restoration with behavioral support: A one-year prospective study of patients with chronic low-back pain. Spine 14:157, 1989.

45. Lindstrom, I, et al: The effect of graded activity on patients with subacute low back pain: A randomized prospective clinical study with an operant-conditioning behavioral approach. Phys Ther 72:279, 1992.

46. Reilly, K, et al: Differences between a supervised and independent strength and conditioning program with chronic low back syndromes. J Occup Med 31:547, 1989.

47. Sturgis, ET, et al: Pain center follow-up study of treated and untreated patients. Arch Phys Med Rehabil 65:301, 1984.

48. Bendix, AF, et al: Comparison of three intensive programs for chronic low back patients: A prospective, randomized, observer-blind study with 1-year follow-up. Scand J Rehabil Med 29:81, 1997.

49. Sikorski, JM: A rationalized approach to physiotherapy for low-back pain. Spine 10:571, 1985.

50. Klaber Moffet, JA, et al: A controlled, prospective study to evaluate the effectiveness of back school in the relief of chronic low back pain. Spine 11:120, 1986.

51. Leboeuf-Yde, C, and Kyvik, KO: At what age does low back pain become a common problem? A study of 29,424 individuals aged 12–41 years. Spine 23:228, 1998.

52. Weir, R, et al: A profile of users of specialty pain clinic services: Predictors of use and cost estimates. J Clin Epidemiol 45:1399, 1992.

53. Simon, JM: A multidisciplinary approach to chronic pain. Rehabilitation Nursing 14:23, 1989.

54. Chronic Pain: Hope through Research. US Department of Health and Human Services National Institutes of Health, November 1989, publication 90-2406 [http://www.nih.gov/health/chip/ninds/cronpain/chronpna.htm].

55. Swanson, DW, et al: Program for managing chronic pain, I: program description and characteristics of patients. Mayo Clin Proc 51:401, 1976.

56. Burry, HC, and Gravis, V: Compensated back injury in New Zealand. New Zealand Medical Journal 101:542, 1988.

57. Flor, H, et al: Efficacy of multidisciplinary pain treatment centers: A meta-analytic review. Pain 49:221, 1992.

58. Stieg, RL, et al: Cost benefits of interdisciplinary chronic pain treatment. Clin J Pain 1:189, 1985.
59. Guck, TP, et al: Multidisciplinary pain center follow-up study: Evaluation with a no-treatment control group. Pain 21; 295, 1985.
60. Mayer, TG: Rehabilitation of the worker with chronic low back pain. In Nordin, M, et al (eds): Musculoskeletal Disorders in the Workplace: Principles and Practice. Mosby, St Louis, MO, 1997.

BIBLIOGRAPHY

Adams, ML, et al: Outcome of carpal tunnel surgery in Washington State worker's compensation. Am J Ind Med 25, 527, 1994.

Anderson, M, and Tichenor, CJ: A patient with de Quervain's tenosynovitis: A case report using an Australian approach to manual therapy. Phys Ther 74:314, 1994.

Arkuszewski, Z: The efficacy of manual treatment in low back pain: A clinical trial. Journal of Manual Medicine 2:68, 1986.

Armstrong, TJ, and Martin, BJ: Adverse effects of repetitive loading and segmental vibration. In Nordin, M, et al (eds): Musculoskeletal Disorders in the Workplace: Principles and Practice. Mosby, St Louis, MO, 1997.

Batte, MC, et al: Managing low back pain: Attitudes and treatment preferences of physical therapists. Phys Ther 74:219, 1994.

Bednar, MS: Clinical evaluation of the wrist and hand. In Nordin, M, et al (eds): Musculoskeletal Disorders in the Workplace: Principles and Practice. Mosby, St Louis, MO, 1997.

Bendix, AF, et al Comparison of three intensive programs for chronic low back patients: A prospective, randomized, observer-blind study with 1-year follow-up. Scand J Rehabil Med 29:81, 1997.

Bigos, SJ, et al: Treatment of the acutely injured worker. In Nordin, M, et al (eds): Musculoskeletal Disorders in the Workplace: Principles and Practice. Mosby, St Louis, MO, 1997.

Borchgrevink, GE, et al: Acute treatment of whiplash neck sprain injuries: A randomized trial of treatment during the first 14 days after a car accident. Spine 23:25, 1998.

Brotzman, SB, and Brasel, J: Foot and ankle rehabilitation. In Brotzman, SB (ed): Clinical Orthopaedic Rehabilitation. Mosby, St Louis, MO, 1996.

Bureau of Labor Statistics Data. US Department of Labor, Washington, DC, 1998 [http://stats.bls.gov:80/datahome.htm].

Burry, HC, and Gravis, V: Compensated back injury in New Zealand. New Zealand Medical Journal 101:542, 1988.

Calandruccio, JH, et al: Rehabilitation of the hand and wrist. In Brotzman, SB (ed): Clinical Orthopaedic Rehabilitation. Mosby, St Louis, MO, 1996.

Chronic Pain: Hope through Research. US Dept of Health and Human Services, National Institutes of Health, Washington, DC, November 1989, publication 90-2406 [http://www.nih.gov/health/chip/ninds/cronpain/chronpna.htm].

Cuomo, F, et al: Clinical evaluation of the neck and shoulder. In Nordin, M, et al: Musculoskeletal Disorders in the Workplace: Principles and Practice. Mosby, St Louis, MO, 1997.

DeRosa, C, and Porterfield, JA: The spine. In Malone, TR, et al: Orthopedic and Sports Physical Therapy, ed 3. Mosby, St. Louis, MO, 1997.

Flor, H, et al: Efficacy of multidisciplinary pain treatment centers: A meta-analytic review. Pain 49:221, 1992.

Guck, TP, et al: Multidisciplinary pain center follow-up study: Evaluation with a no-treatment control group. Pain 21; 295, 1985.

Guide to Physical Therapist Practice. Phys Ther 77:1163, 1997.

Hansen, FR, et al: Intensive, dynamic back-muscle exercises, conventional physiotherapy, or placebo-control treatment of low-back pain. Spine 18:98, 1993.

Hazard, RG, et al: Functional restoration with behavioral support: A one-year prospective study of patients with chronic low-back pain. Spine 14:157, 1989.

Hertling, D, and Kessler, RM: Management of Common Musculoskeletal Disorders: Physical Therapy Principles and Methods, ed 2. Lippincott, Philadelphia, PA, 1990.

Hoppenfeld, S: Physical Examination of the Spine and Extremities. Appleton & Lange, Norwalk, CT, 1976.

Hunter, S: Rehabilitation of foot injuries. In Prentice, WE (ed): Rehabilitation Techniques in Sports Medicine, ed 2. Mosby, St Louis, MO, 1994.

Janda, V, Treatment of chronic back pain. Journal of Manual Medicine 6:166, 1992.

Jette, AM, and Davis, KD: A comparison of hospital-based and private outpatient physical therapy practices. Phys Ther 71:366, 1991.

Jobe, FW, et al: Rehabilitation of the shoulder. In Brotzman, SB (ed): Clinical Orthopaedic Rehabilitation. Mosby, St Louis, MO, 1996.

Kellett, KM, et al: Effects of an exercise program on sick leave due to back pain. Phys Ther 72:283, 1991.

Kinalski, R, et al: The comparison of the results of manual therapy versus physiotherapy methods used in treatment of patients with low back pain syndromes. Journal of Manual Medicine 4:44, 1989.

Kisner, C, and Colby, LA: Therapeutic Exercise: Foundations and Techniques, ed 3. FA Davis, Philadelphia, 1996.

Klaber Moffet, JA, et al: A controlled, prospective study to evaluate the effectiveness of back school in the relief of chronic low back pain. Spine 11:120, 1986.

Leboeuf-Yde, C, and Kyvik, KO: At what age does low back pain become a common problem? A study of 29,424 individuals aged 12–41 years. Spine 23:228, 1998.

Lindstrom, I, et al: The effect of graded activity on patients with subacute low back pain: A randomized prospective clinical study with an operant-conditioning behavioral approach. Phys Ther 72:279, 1992.

Magnusson, M, and Pope, M: Epidemiology of the neck and upper extremity. In Nordin, M, et al (eds): Musculoskeletal Disorders in the Workplace: Principles and Practice. Mosby, St Louis, MO, 1997.

Manniche, C, et al: Intense dynamic back exercises for chronic low back pain: A clinical trial. Pain 47:53, 1991.

Marks, PH, FU, FH: Treatment of shoulder disorders. In Nordin, M, et al (eds): Musculoskeletal Disorders in the Workplace: Principles and Practice. Mosby, St Louis, MO, 1997.

Mayer, TG, et al: A prospective short-term study of chronic low back pain patients utilizing novel objective functional measurement. Pain 25:53, 1986.

McElligott, J, et al: Low back injury in industry: The value of a recovery program. Conn Med 53:711, 1989.

McKenzie, RA: The Lumbar Spine: Mechanical Diagnosis and Therapy. Spinal Publications, New Zealand, 1981.

McKenzie, R: Treat Your Own Back, ed 5. Spinal Publications, New Zealand, 1992.

McKenzie, R: Treat Your Own Neck. Spinal Publications, New Zealand, 1992.

McPhoil, TG: The foot and ankle. In Malone, TR, et al (eds): Orthopedic and Sports Physical Therapy, ed 3. Mosby, St Louis, MO, 1997.

Norkin, CC, and Levangie, PK: Joint Structure and Function: A Comprehensive Analysis, ed 2. FA Davis, Philadelphia, 1992.

Patijn, J, and Durinck, JR: Effects of manual medicine on absenteeism. Journal of Manual Medicine. 6:49, 1991.

Reilly, K, et al: Differences between a supervised and independent strength and conditioning program with chronic low back syndromes. J Occup Med 31:547, 1989.

Rempel, D, and Punnett, L: Epidemiology of wrist and hand disorders. In Nordin, M, et al (eds): Musculoskeletal Disorders in the Workplace: Principles and Practice. Mosby, St Louis, MO, 1997.

Riehl, R: Rehabilitation of the lower leg injuries. In Prentice, WE (ed): Rehabilitation Techniques in Sports Medicine, ed 2. Mosby, St. Louis, MO, 1994.

Saal, JA, and Saal, JS: Nonoperative treatment of herniated lumbar intervertebral disc with radiculopathy: An outcome study. Spine 14:431, 1989.

Salter, RB: Textbook of Disorders and Injuries of the Musculoskeletal System. Williams & Wilkins, Baltimore, 1983.

Sikorski, JM: A rationalized approach to physiotherapy for low-back pain. Spine 10:571, 1985.

Simon, JM: A multidisciplinary approach to chronic pain. Rehabilitation Nursing 14:23, 1989.

Smith W, et al: Comparative study using four modalities in shinsplint treatment. J Orthop Sports Phys Ther 8;77, 1986.

Snyder-Mackler, L, et al: Effects of helium-neon laser irradiation on skin resistance and pain in patients with trigger points in the neck or back. Phys Ther 69:336, 1989.

Stieg RL, et al: Cost benefits of interdisciplinary chronic pain treatment. Clin J Pain 1:189, 1985.

Sturgis, ET, et al: Pain center follow-up study of treated and untreated patients. Arch Phys Med Rehabil 65:301, 1984.

Swanson, DW, et al: Program for managing chronic pain. I. Program description and characteristics of patients. Mayo Clin Proc 51:401, 1976.

Weir, R, et al: A profile of users of specialty pain clinic services: Predictors of use and cost estimates. J Clin Epidemiol 45:1399, 1992.

White, AH, and Brotzman, SB: Low back disorders. In Brotzman, SB (ed): Clinical Orthopaedic Rehabilitation. Mosby, St Louis, MO. 1996.

Zetterberg, C: Epidemiology of the lower extremity. In Nordin, M, et al (eds): Musculoskeletal Disorders in the Workplace: Principles and Practice. Mosby, St Louis, MO, 1997.

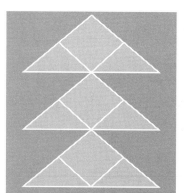

Geriatric Clients

OBJECTIVES

After completing this chapter, the PTA student will be able to:

1. Discuss the rehabilitation concerns and needs of the geriatric client.
2. Relate the factors and conditions necessary to maintain balance.
3. Describe the incidence, etiology, and pathophysiology of the conditions presented in this chapter related to the geriatric client.
4. Identify the evaluation tools and methods used by the PT to form a diagnosis, prognosis, and plan of treatment for the client conditions described in this chapter.
5. Describe the clinical management of the client conditions described in this chapter.
6. Discuss the expected physical therapy outcomes for the client conditions described in this chapter.

Key Words

abductor wedge
allodynia
arthroplasty
avascular necrosis
crepitus
extrinsic risk factors
hyperhidrosis
intrinsic risk factors
nociceptors
open reduction and internal fixation
osteophytes
perturbation
synergy

Successful aging is a combination of good life-style and behavioral habits, including exercise, diet, and socioeconomic well-being.[1]

Carole B. Lewis and Jennifer M. Bottomley
Geriatric Physical Therapy: A Clinical Approach

CONCERNS OF THE GERIATRIC CLIENT: HOW DO I PREVENT A LOSS OF FUNCTION?

THE COMMUNITY-DWELLING CLIENT

Falls are a common problem for those geriatric clients living in the community. Koch et al.[2] claims that the "elderly persons in the community . . . constitute a majority of persons at risk for falls and immobility." For persons over age 65, falls occur in one-third of the population. Of the clients that sustain a fall, half cannot get up without assistance, and 1 of 10 suffers some type of serious injury. Fear of falling is reported by one of every four community-dwelling, geriatric clients.[2,3] Falling at home is a frequent cause of injury to the geriatric client. For clients over age 75, 70% of all emergency room visits are directly related to falls. Of all emergency room admissions by the geriatric client, 4 of 10 will result in an extended hospital admission. The average fall-related hospital stay for geriatric clients is 12 days. Narrow spaces and doors, throw rugs and furniture, electric cords, and small animals may all present potential environmental hazards for the geriatric client. Internal factors related to visual disturbances or decreased flexibility can also precipitate a fall for the geriatric client. Preventing a loss of function as the geriatric client ages is a major concern of both the client and the health-care industry. If a client is hospitalized because of a fall-related injury, one of every two clients will never return to his or her home but will be discharged to some form of long-term institutional care.[4,5]

The concerns of the community-dwelling client center on the loss of function. Intrinsic or extrinsic risk factors may limit the individual's ability to live independently and force a sudden lifestyle change. Falling will usually be a critical first indicator that signals the decline in function of the geriatric client. Many of the factors that precipitate falling are correctable and should be addressed by the health-care team. Safely navigating a walker in a limited area is one such example (Fig. 11–1). When readying clients to return home, the rehabilitation team should prepare the individual for task-specific activities that will be encountered in the home setting. Too often, the client is rehabilitated in the accessible environment of the physical therapy gymnasium. Unique challenges presented by uneven surfaces, low furniture, pets, or carpeted floors are not encountered or practiced. It should not be assumed that because a client can safely maneuver a walker in a hospital room, the same ability would carry over to the home environment.

For a client to be a safe community dweller, he or she must demonstrate the ability to walk functional distances in the home and in the community. Fatigue or poor endurance from cardiovascular diseases may limit an individual's ability to walk safely through a grocery store. Frequently, **extrinsic risk factors** such as uneven surfaces, unrepaired sidewalks, or stairs are encountered as the client journeys through the community. As the clients begins to limit activities because of perceived or real limitations and fears, the deconditioning cycle will begin to consume the client. If the client does not venture out of the home for fear of falling, muscle atrophy and endurance losses will occur. The client should be encouraged to stay as active as possible to prevent the onset of any functional loss. Chandler et al.[6] scientifically investigated the functional improvements associated with strengthening the lower extremities of the community-dwelling client. Using the simple intervention tool of elastic tubing, strength gains of up to 16% were noted in the clients who exercised regularly over a 10-week period. Strength gains were noted in the hip extensor and abductor, knee extensor and flexor, and the ankle plantar and dorsiflexor muscle groups. The control group actually demonstrated a

Extrinsic Risk Factors
Those characteristics related to environmental conditions that may predispose the client to an injury.

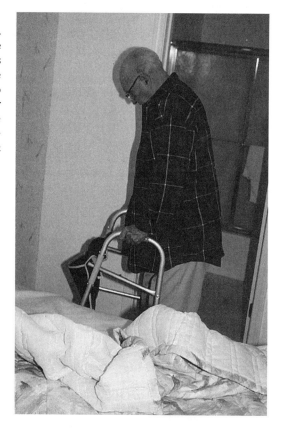

FIG. 11–1

Narrow ambulation spaces at home. The homes of most geriatric clients are not well suited for the space demands of medical equipment and assistive devices. Working with the client to navigate safely in crowded areas or modifying the environment should be a primary concern for the rehabilitation team when preparing a geriatric client for returning to home.

decrease of strength in the same muscle groups of up to 3% during the same period. Functional gains were noted by the clients who demonstrated improved mobility skills, an increase in gait velocities, and an increased perceptual awareness in avoiding falls.

Innovative programs are being implemented targeted at empowering the geriatric client to take an active role in managing the aging process and preventing disability. A Seattle senior center–based self-management and disability prevention program focused on health, maintaining function, and appropriate health-care utilization in community-dwelling geriatric clients. A 1-year follow-up investigation identified that participants in the study had perceived a decrease in disability, actually spent fewer days in the hospital as compared with the control group, and demonstrated increased physical activity.[7] Preventing the onset of disability and the loss of function in most geriatric clients can be a simple process. Education of the geriatric population in issues related to prevention should be delivered by the physical therapy professionals. The end result could be less of a strain on the health-care system by limiting the number of problems related to preventable declines in function in this population.

THE NURSING HOME CLIENT

As previously discussed, institutionalization of the geriatric client who has suffered a fall-related injury is quite common. In Western societies, the quality of life issues related to nursing home care is not generally viewed in a positive light. The average client living in a nursing home was described by Joseph and Boult[8] as being 83.5-years-old and predominantly female (69%). Nursing home clients demonstrated a high prevalence of dementia (83.5%) and functional disabilities (87.2%) that affected the performance of two or more activities of daily living (ADLs). Even though placement in a long-term nursing facility is often needed, these clients should be viewed with no less dignity and respect than any other client being treated with an orthopedic condition. Frequently, intervention from the rehabilitation team can improve the quality of life for the client living in the nursing home.

Engle et al.[9] developed a model of needs and concerns of the client living in a nursing home based on interviews with actual clients. Rather than focusing on dying (even with the terminally ill client), the goal of the health-care team for the client living in a nursing home should be to improve the quality of living in the following ways:

1. Improving the quality of day-to-day living
2. Promoting adequate pain relief for debilitating conditions
3. Promoting sufficient chewing and swallowing
4. Incorporating desired participation in religious activities
5. Providing respectful and prompt care

Residents of the nursing homes in this study validated these components of health-care intervention as the most important factors leading to an increased quality of life.

Falls, with subsequent fall-related injuries, can be a leading cause of disability in the nursing home client. Of all the documented incidents related to nursing home residents, falls are the largest category.[10] A fracture of some sort will occur in 5% of the cases when a client falls to the ground.[11] Other injuries that are typical include contusions, sprains, strains, abrasions, or head injuries. Kiely et al.[12] examined risk factors predicting fall susceptibility. A 1-year follow-up study

Intrinsic Risk Factors
Those characteristics related to
the individual that may
predispose the client to an
injury.

examining 18,855 residents of nursing homes in the state of Washington produced a list of **intrinsic risk factors** that may lead to falls by a nursing home resident:

1. Previous history of falling
2. Wandering behavior demonstrated by the client, or a psychiatric diagnosis
3. Use of a cane or walker by the client
4. A recent, noted decline of ADL performance
5. Age of the client greater than 87 years
6. Unsteady gait demonstrated by the client
7. Ability to transfer independently
8. Inability of the client to follow directions, or impaired memory and judgement
9. Altered proprioception demonstrated by the client
10. Use of sedative medication by the client
11. Independence with wheelchair propulsion
12. Male gender

The strongest fall-predicting factor identified was a history of falls. If a client had previously fallen, the chance of a recurrent fall was three times greater than if a client had never demonstrated a history of falling. Mion et al.[10] examined falls in a long-term rehabilitation setting and summarized that although overall, only 37% of the total number of clients experienced a fall, that particular percentage of clients constituted nearly three-fourths of all the documented falls. The client is most likely to fall in his or her own room, from a wheelchair on the evening shift within the first 2 weeks of being admitted to the facility. This may be related to orientation to new surroundings, or complications from new medications or surgery, which may alter cognitive perceptions or proprioception. Screening elements to prevent disability from injuries sustained in a fall should include a thorough history of previous falls by the client from a reliable source.[10] Screenings and fall prevention programs should include the following elements:

1. Assessing risk factors
2. Assessing the staffing and availability of client assistance when clients are up in wheelchairs
3. Increasing the number of visual observations of clients while out of bed
4. Ensuring that the client is able to use a call or buzzer system
5. Collecting, monitoring, and assessing data related to falls in the facility
6. Removing potentially dangerous environmental barriers
7. Periodically reassessing the client for changes in status

CONCERNS OF BALANCE IN THE GERIATRIC CLIENT

Once believed to be a natural part of aging, loss of balance in the geriatric client is now identified as a cumulative effect of multiple impairments.[2,3,13] Many of these impairments are easily identifiable and correctable, which would greatly benefit the geriatric client in preventing falls from a loss of balance. The prevention of falls from balance disturbances should be a team effort. It is true that physical impairments may potentially cause loss of balance; however, medical conditions (e.g., postural hypotension, visual, or hearing impairment) or medications (e.g., sedatives) also may add to the risk of falling.[2]

Gait is the ultimate functional task relative to good balance. The dynamic principle of balance is to keep the center of mass (COM) within the base of support (BOS). When the COM moves outside of the BOS, the individual is unstable and will fall toward the direction in which the COM was displaced. Gait is no more than the ability to continually "lose your balance" and regain stability before falling. As the COM is continually displaced in a desired direction, the individual becomes a complex combination of dynamic and static elements collaborating to allow locomotion. When factors decrease the ability of the individual to sense appropriate balance reactions, the potential to fall is increased. Pathology often leads to a breakdown of the coordinated systems needed to maintain balance.

Balance maintenance is a complex, dynamic combination of predetermined events. Normal balance is the coordinated efforts of sensory input, integration by the central nervous system, and musculoskeletal action in either the standing or sitting position.[14] Normal postural sway is described as an inverted pendulum swinging as much as 12° in an anteroposterior (AP) direction and up to 16° from side to side (Fig. 11–2).[14] Variations and motion within the span of dynamic stability for posture maintenance are expected and should be smooth and rhythmic. If the COM is forced outside the BOS, the body has exceeded the limits of stability and some response is necessary, or a fall will result. Challenges to the displacement of the COM outside the BOS can be addressed in a reactive manner from appropriate neurophysiological feedback. Challenges to the displacement of the COM outside of the BOS may also be proactive from anticipated actions or feed-forward input.[15] Two basic methods or strategies of muscular **synergy** exist for

Synergy
A cooperative, coordinated effort of two or more muscles in the body designed to accomplish a predetermined task.

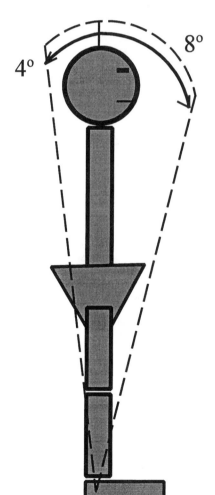

FIG. 11–2
Normal postural sway. The normal upright posture of the human is described as an inverted pendulum swaying as much as 4 degrees posteriorly and 8 degrees anteriorly. If the sway exceeds these normal parameters, some mechanism or strategy is needed to maintain the center of mass over the base of support and prevent a loss of balance.

the client to effectively manage balance challenges to prevent falling: (1) fixed support mechanisms and (2) change in support mechanisms. For a visual comparison of balance strategies, see Figure 11–3.

Fixed support mechanisms are synergistic movement patterns designed to readjust the COM over the BOS without unloading the lower extremities. Two different strategies are ingrained into the central nervous system as responses for a loss of balance: (1) ankle synergy and (2) hip synergy. The ankle synergy pattern is activated in response to small, slow postural sways and challenges. A larger base of support on a firm surface and the ability to sense the base of support are prerequisites for an adequate ankle synergy response to prevent a loss of balance. It is not a voluntary movement, but a postural reflex designed to keep the COM over the BOS. If a force on the fixed segment is in the posterior direction, then a backward **perturbation** occurs. The postural challenge is a reaction to control an anterior sway of the body. This is visualized by picturing the perturbation direction as if a rug was being pulled from beneath the client in that direction. The gastrocnemius-soleus, hamstring, and paraspinal groups work synergistically to

Perturbation
The state of disturbance or change in a direction.

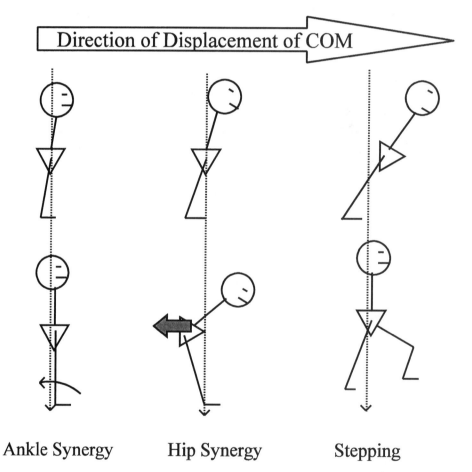

Direction of Displacement of COM

Ankle Synergy   Hip Synergy   Stepping

FIG. 11–3
Comparison of balancing strategies. As the challenge to the displacement of the center of mass increases in an anterior direction, different strategies for maintaining balance are progressively used. This figure represents, on the left, strategies to control small challenges (ankle synergy) and progresses toward the right to strategies that control large displacements of the center of mass (stepping).

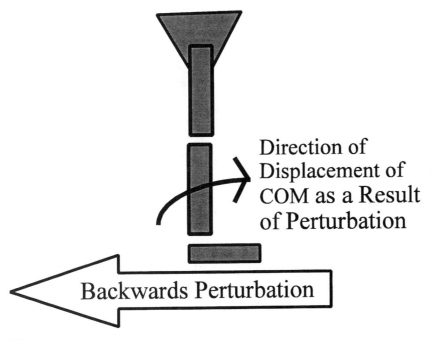

Direction of
Displacement of
COM as a Result
of Perturbation

Backwards Perturbation

FIG. 11–4
Ankle synergy with backward perturbation. Challenges to posture are described in terms of the direction of the displacement or perturbation. Imagine standing on a carpet and someone pulling the rug from underneath you. The direction that the carpet is moving is the direction of the perturbation with the opposite direction resulting in the displacement of the COM from outside the BOS. The gastrocnemius muscle will work to limit the anterior translation of the tibia, preventing the COM from leaving the BOS. The hamstring group and paraspinal group also work to limit the anterior displacement.

pull the tibia and the body posteriorly back over the talus, stopping the anterior motion. This helps to offset the backward perturbation (Fig. 11–4). If the postural challenging force is in an anterior direction or a forward perturbation, the client loses his or her posture in a posterior direction. The dorsiflexors, quadriceps femoris group, and abdominal muscles contract to pull the tibia and body anteriorly on top of the talus to control the COM in a distal to proximal fashion (Fig. 11–5). Once balance mechanisms are incorporated into the adult, the ankle synergy is a major component in preventing falls and maintaining balance within the normal framework of the postural sway. The ankle synergy can be compromised as a result of decreased flexibility, decreased strength, neural timing, and central nervous system processing. Often, geriatric clients are found to have a decreased reliance on or decreased ability to elicit the ankle synergy in controlling upright postural sway.[14]

The second fixed mechanism is the hip flexion or extension synergy pattern. These patterns are designed for larger amplitude challenges and faster displacements of the center of mass. The hip synergy patterns are also activated when the base of support is relatively small or the surface is not firm. A backwards perturbation results in an excessive, sudden anterior displacement of the COM. The abdominal and hip flexor muscles rapidly activate to move the buttocks posteriorly in a proximal to distal fashion. This rapid movement posteriorly of the pelvic region helps to offset the anterior displacement of the COM (see Fig.

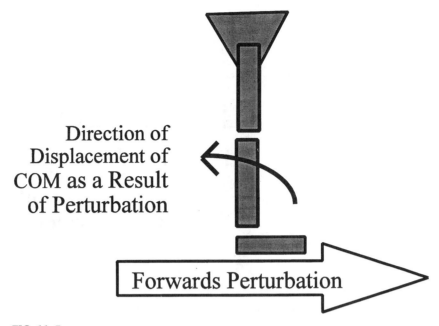

Direction of
Displacement of
COM as a Result
of Perturbation

Forwards Perturbation

FIG. 11–5
Ankle synergy with forward perturbation. If the perturbation is in a forward direction, the displacement of the COM is in the posterior direction. The anterior tibialis, quadriceps femoris, and abdominal muscles will react to pull the body anteriorly over the feet.

11–6A). The reverse hip reaction works to control excessive or sudden movements of the COM in a posterior direction (anterior perturbation). The hamstring muscle group and the paraspinal muscles (hip extension synergy) work together to thrust the pelvis anteriorly to prevent a fall in a posterior direction (see Fig. 11–6B). This response to the displacement of the COM can be limited by decreased flexibility and strength of the hips and spine, decreased nervous system processing time, and depressed sensory inputs (vestibular system).[14]

Change in support mechanisms are used for larger, more dramatic displacements of the COM. Stepping (stumbling) and grabbing (reaching) mechanisms can be used to maintain the client in an upward posture. If the COM is displaced sufficiently in an anterior direction, the client must take a step, lengthening the BOS to keep an upright posture. This is the normal mechanism of walking and running. Grabbing strategies are also utilized when a client feels that by reaching for an object added support will be provided (e.g., chair, wall, table). Often gait assistive devices are "reached for" or "grabbed" to assist with balance to prevent a fall. While the inclusion of upper extremity motion is a critical element in the complex processes of maintaining upright posture, there exists a danger in promoting a reliance on grabbing strategies in the client that is prone to falling. First, the client may not be able to reach the object to increase the base of support fast enough to prevent a fall. Second, the client may not possess adequate stabilizing strength in the upper extremities to provide support, and thus, may fall. Lastly, the displacement of the upper extremity to "reach" for support may actually encourage a greater shift of the COM outside of the BOS and precipitate a fall.[1,13]

Changes across the life span can predispose a geriatric client to falling. Some

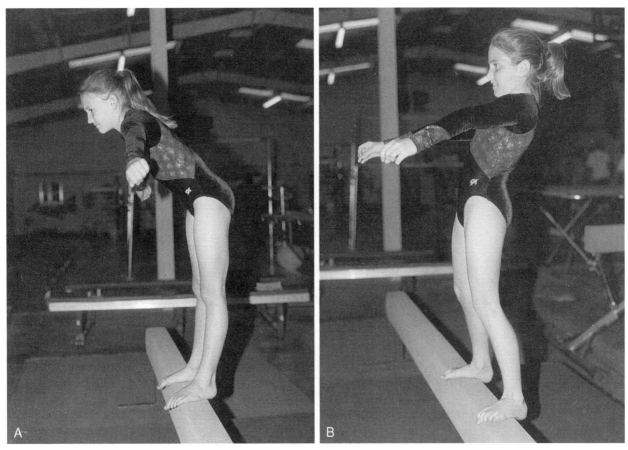

FIG. 11–6
Hip synergy. Watching a gymnast on a balance beam will help clarify the use of hip strategies. To stay on the balance beam (a narrow 4-inch base), the gymnast will rapidly respond to anterior or posterior displacements of the center of mass by moving the pelvis posteriorly or anteriorly, respectively. (A) The gymnast reacts by moving her COM posteriorly (hip and trunk flexion) as she feels her balance being lost in an anterior direction. (B) The gymnast reacts by moving her pelvis anteriorly (paraspinal and hamstring muscles) as she senses her balance being displaced posteriorly.

geriatric clients lose the ability to respond adequately to slow or sudden displacement of the COM. The normal postural sway increases slightly as aging progresses. Notably, clients who have a history of falls have greater postural sway parameters compared with those who do not have this history. Some critics argue that changes in normal postural sway are not a normal aspect of aging, but are indeed a result of pathology.[16] Muscle recruitment timing and magnitude deficits alter normal distal-to-proximal recruitment of muscles, making the ankle synergy ineffective. The client's altered direction of recruitment (proximal to distal) encourages hip synergies to activate before ankle responses, potentially displacing the COM excessively in the opposite direction and resulting in a fall. Sensory perception changes (e.g., proprioception, visual, hearing, vestibular) can all limit the input to the balance maintenance system. A delay of nerve conduction in geriatric clients may also curtail the response time of protective synergies and strategies. Flexibility and strength can also play a role in limiting the effectiveness of appropriate strategies. Woollacott[16] observed that more than half of the falls in their study were related to clients with some sort of central nervous system pathology. Singly, or in various combinations, these elements may make the geriatric client more susceptible to falling. As much as 25% of all falls may be related to poor balance and dysfunctional gait patterns.[4,16]

Therapeutic intervention to alter or improve identified deficits in postural control is multifaceted. The postural control mechanism consists of many interdependent areas (Fig. 11–7). Improvements in one facet will not necessarily prevent a client from ever losing his or her balance. Each influencing component must be carefully examined and deficits identified. Strategies to overcome or modify the identified deficits should be incorporated, if feasible, into the rehabilitation plan.[17] Educational sessions that include information on the influences that the environment or medications may have on posture should be regularly conducted with the client until the knowledge becomes second nature. Exercises designed to build strength are often performed at slow velocities, whereas those designed to improve balance response should be conducted at faster speeds and in task-specific postures. The client should practice repeatedly changing postures from sitting to standing, from supine to sitting, and from various heights and surfaces. Any gains in balance should be dedicated to maintaining the center of gravity within the BOS.[6] A variety of challenges should be presented in gait-training programs, including ambulating over a variety of surfaces, distances, and textures. Challenges should be presented during ambulation as often as challenges are introduced to static or quiet standing. Winstein[18] concluded that although static standing posture abilities can be improved through exercise, the static gains do not carry over into balance improvements during locomotion or dynamic activities. Multifaceted exercise programs designed to improve balance

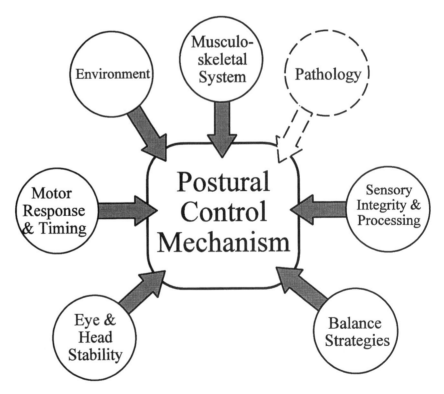

FIG.11–7
The Postural Control System.

and mobility in community-dwelling geriatric clients are effective in preventing falls.[3,13] Regular participation in structured exercise regimens are also predictive of decreasing falls among community-dwelling geriatric clients.[4]

Multifaceted exercise programs designed to improve balance are individualized programs based on a comprehensive evaluation identifying specific impairments and risk factors. Balance gains in one environment or task should not be considered inclusive of all tasks or situations. Balance is specific to the task at hand performed by the client. Keshner[15] concludes, "it is tempting to believe that we can teach a specific pattern of movement that will resolve all of the postural problems presented to our [clients]. The key to success in developing balance, however, is to develop adaptable and flexible strategies that will meet the multiple demands presented in a complex environment."

Balance, as briefly described in this section, can be inappropriately labeled as a predetermined concrete series of events. Instead balance should be viewed by the clinician as a dynamic, flexible process that is responsive to the specific condition or task.[15,17] Balance deficits can be successfully addressed, prevented, altered, and improved by the rehabilitation team. Woollacott[16] stressed that "data support[s] the hypothesis that aging does not have to lead to a decline in function within the postural control system. On the contrary, if one is able to sustain a lifestyle that minimizes pathology, balance control may remain normal into old age."

 ## CONDITIONS AND IMPAIRMENTS AFFECTING THE GERIATRIC CLIENT

OSTEOPOROSIS

Osteoporosis is the process by which a bone becomes mechanically unstable and susceptible to fracture because of a loss of bone mass. Low bone mineral density (BMD) has been associated with an increased risk of sustaining a fracture in clients with osteoporosis.[19] In the United States, 25 million people are diagnosed with osteoporosis or have low BMD, placing them at great risk for disability.[20] Outside of the normal effects of aging, osteoporosis demonstrates excessive loss of bone. Typically involving the hip, the distal arm, and the spinal vertebrae, the end results of osteoporosis is a bone that is unable to absorb mechanical forces, resulting in disruption or fracture of the tissue.[21] The development of osteoporosis can be related to the activity level of the client, some of whom can present with significant functional impairments.[22] Other risk factors leading to a loss of bone density have been well documented in many published studies (Table 11–1). Osteoporosis can also be related to other conditions or pathologies (Table 11–2).[20]

Disability associated with osteoporosis in Western societies is common.[23] One-third of American women over age 65 will sustain a fracture of the spine, and one-fifth will sustain a fracture of the hip. Nationally, 7 of 10 fractures in clients over age 45 are related to osteoporosis.[20] Up to as many of as one-fourth of the clients sustaining a hip fracture as a result of osteoporosis will need long-term institutional care after the injury. A client with a distal radius bone density less than the average bone density for her age group is likely to fracture her distal wrist at a rate six times greater than someone with normal bone density. Likewise, a client demonstrating a significant loss of bone density in the femoral neck has a seven times greater risk of fracturing the hip in a fall compared with a person of similar age and normal bone density.[11] The annual cost to the health-care sector

___ Table 11–1 ___

RISK FACTORS ACROSS THE LIFE SPAN LEADING TO OSTEOPOROSIS	
All ages	1. Low calcium intake
	2. Low estrogen state (postmenopause)
	3. Inactivity, immobility, and lack of weight-bearing exercise
Children and young adults	1. Corticosteroid use
	2. Early onset of menopause
	3. Delayed puberty
	4. Malnutrition
	5. Amenorrhea
	6. Abuse of alcohol
Male clients	1. Aging (over 70-years-old)
	2. Hypogonadism
	3. Abuse of alcohol

___ Table 11–2 ___

ONSET OF OSTEOPOROSIS FROM A SECONDARY PATHOLOGY OR CONDITION	
Medications and medical treatments	1. Steroids (such as prednisone)
	2. Anticoagulants (such as heparin and warfarin [Coumadin])
	3. Thyroid hormone
	4. Radiation treatments
Genetic conditions	1. Osteogenesis imperfecta
	2. Marfan's syndrome
	3. Turner's syndrome
	4. Klinefelter's syndrome
Other pathologies and conditions	1. Grave's disease
	2. Hyperparathyroidism and hyperthyroidism
	3. Cushing's syndrome
	4. Chronic renal failure
	5. Malnutrition
	6. Diabetes
	7. Immobility associated with spinal cord injury (either congenital or acquired)
	8. Rheumatoid arthritis
	9. Cancer
	10. Alcoholism

for the treatment of osteoporosis exceeds $13 billion, with 70% of those dollars used for managing hip fractures alone.[11,20,24]

The development of osteoporosis varies dramatically depending on the race and gender of the client. African-American women develop osteoporosis significantly less often than any other ethnic or racial group. Asian women have a low incidence of hip fractures as a result of osteoporosis, but have an equal prevalence of spinal fractures when compared with white women. Latino women have a greater incidence of osteoporosis compared with African-American women, but still significantly less than white women. Typically, men do not demonstrate the onset of osteoporosis until much later in life. By age 75, one-third of men are affected by changes in BMD. Although women experience fractures of the hip three times more often than their male counterparts, the death rate 1 year after a hip fracture is 26% greater in men than women.[20]

Clinical Presentation

Clients with osteoporosis are usually seen in the physical therapy setting not for the osteoporosis condition itself, but for disabilities associated with the onset of bone loss. Fractures of the hip, wrist, proximal humerus, and spine are the typical conditions that will direct the client to the services of physical therapy professionals. The typical client will be a postmenopausal white woman. Visual inspection may reveal a kyphotic posture with a forward head. Apparent deformities, however, need not always be present. When the client has a kyphotic posture, a dull, lingering back ache commonly is observed.[23] The client may describe difficulty sleeping, fatigue, and loss of motion in the upper extremities and the cervical spine. Osteoporosis and repeated fractures to the spine may produce a loss in height for the client. The client with severe deformity of the spine will experience the greatest morbidity and loss of function including the inability to sleep, dress, and effectively use the upper extremities.[25]

Historically, clients with osteoporosis have not been addressed or treated until symptoms or disability presents. With the changing face of health care and reimbursement structures, it is necessary to address the treatment and prevention of osteoporosis in the population as a whole. Osteoporosis directly and indirectly accounts for more than 320,000 annual hospital admissions of women over age 45 for management of various conditions. If the rehabilitation team is able to limit disability in the enrolled population as a whole by prevention of costly disabilities, the long-term financial savings for the health-care sector and the improvement of the quality of life for the clients served will be tremendous.[20]

Evaluation: Tools and Methods

Evaluating the client with osteoporosis should entail a comprehensive documentation of risk factors and medical history. Functional assessments related to balance, mobility, and risk of falling should be carefully performed. Complete sensory evaluations (e.g., vision, vestibular, somatosensory) may reveal subtle risk factors that could lead to falling or future disability. Motor and flexibility assessments should be related to functional abilities. A self-perception scale of functional performance is helpful in identifying limitations perceived by the client.

Clinical Management

Sinaki and Grubbs[23] believe that the best management of the problems associated with osteoporosis is prevention in susceptible populations. Munnings[24] believes that a few lifestyle changes can make a significant difference in maintaining bone density versus succumbing to the effects of osteoporosis. Tresolini et al.[20] suggest that promoting the health of the bone should be ongoing across the life span and not when the symptoms are observed. A balanced triad of management to prevent osteoporosis in postmenopausal women includes: (1) nutrition rich in calcium, (2) exercise beyond normal ADLs, and (3) hormonal supplements (estrogen). Table 11–3 presents a life-span approach to the prevention of osteo-porosis.[20]

Nutrition as a whole can have a positive or negative influence on BMD. Practicing good nutritional habits should be a consistent behavior across the life span, not a sudden change for immediate results. Calcium in the diet plays a large role in the maintenance of bone density, but it should not be considered the only necessary element. Many marketing ploys display vitamins and supplements rich in calcium as a primary means in preventing disability from osteoporosis. These claims are mostly marketing hype and have little founded evidence in successful outcomes. Calcium is found in such foods as dairy products, salmon, broccoli, and tofu. Vitamin D and citric acid are also necessary for the uptake of calcium. If these components are not present in the body, the calcium will not be adequately absorbed into the system for use by the body. Vitamin D can be obtained from drinking milk that is fortified with vitamin D; eating eggs, cheese, butter, liver; or spending time in the sun (about 10 minutes daily is sufficient). Homebound clients, who are not regularly exposed to the sun, should be encouraged to get vitamin D through other dietary means. Citric acid is commonly found in most fruits. Supplements should be considered only if the client is not obtaining the adequate vitamins and minerals from a routine diet.[20]

Foods that limit calcium uptake and simple malnutrition both have a negative effect on BMD. Foods and dietary substances such as wheat bran, caffeine, alcohol, and sodium all block the uptake of calcium into the system. Eating to prevent a loss of bone mass should include avoiding these types of foods. Poor nutrition, as seen in populations in underdeveloped countries or young females with anorexic and bulimic behaviors, can significantly alter the ability of the body to develop strong and healthy bones. These changes and patterns may be irreversible. Eating for healthy bones should be practiced across the life span, not simply in old age.[20]

Part of the management of osteoporosis is exercise. A general increase in activity, although it can promote an improved quality of life for the client, may not directly promote a specific increase in the density of long bones, which are susceptible to fracture. Exercises must be designed with a specific weight-bearing and stress-producing component. The identified exercises must be at an intensity greater than routine ADLs and performed on a regular basis. Water activities, though beneficial for some painful conditions, lessen the effects of gravity reducing the stress on bone. Direct weight-bearing stress and resistance related to Wolff's law direct the balance of bone growth. Ayalon et al.[26] demonstrated that through total body exercises and exercises designed specifically to load suspect bones, an increase in bone density was noted after 1 year of participation by the study group. The control group demonstrated a continual decline in bone density. Some studies have shown that in postmenopausal women, as much as 1% of the bone density is lost for each calendar year of life.[20] Chow, et al,[22] found that aerobic capacity and bone density were improved in two different exercise groups of postmenopausal women after one year of exercise when compared to a non exercise control group. They found no significant difference gains between the group that only exercised aerobically and the group that exercised aerobically and with progressive resistive exercises. The control group in this study did demontrate a loss of bone density over the same one year period of time which suggests that any type of exercise is better in preventing osteoporosis than no exercise at all. Nelson et al.[27] found that high-intensity strength-training exercises were effective in preserving bone density along with improving muscle mass, strength, and balance in postmenopausal women. In this study, high-intensity

Table 11–3

LIFE-SPAN APPROACH TO THE PREVENTION OF OSTEOPOROSIS

Client Population	Exercise	Nutrition	Special Considerations
Pediatric	Encourage various weight-bearing activities.	Well-balanced diet	If unable to eat dairy products, consider alternative means of ensuring calcium and vitamin D intake.
Premenopausal adult	Encourage weight-bearing activity, resistive exercises, and postural exercises.	Well-balanced diet	Activity is critical. Avoid behaviors that promote osteoporosis.
Postmenopausal adult	Encourage weight-bearing activity, resistive exercises, postural exercises, and flexibility exercises.	Well-balanced Supplements if needed	Hormonal replacement therapy.
Geriatric without signs of osteoporosis	Encourage weight-bearing activities, resistive exercises, and postural exercises. Stress fall prevention.	Well-balanced diet Supplements if needed	Perform fall prevention assessment and routine medical exam.
Geriatric with signs of osteoporosis	Encourage weight-bearing activities (as tolerated). Postural and resistive exercises should be performed only with direct supervision. Stress fall prevention.	Well-balanced diet Supplements if needed	Perform fall prevention assessment and routine medical exam.

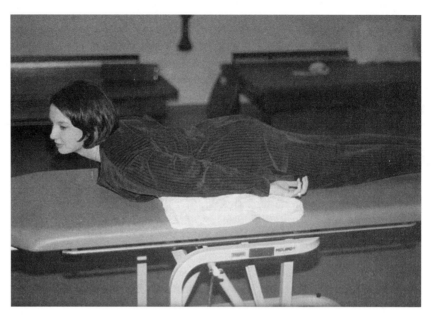

FIG. 11–8
Isometric back extension exercises for osteoporosis. The client assumes a prone position, with a pillow placed comfortably under the abdomen. With the arms at the sides of the client, the client slowly extends the spine, retracts the scapulas, and lifts the head. Movement from the floor is not excessive, but a rather small distance. The client holds the position for five counts then slowly returns to the original position. Have the client repeat exercise 15 times.

isotonic weight lifting was performed twice per week for 52 weeks. Muscle groups targeted included the hip, knee, back, and shoulder extensors as well as the abdominal muscles using a hydraulic resistance machine for three sets of eight repetitions. The intensity level was at 80% of the established 1 rep max (1 rep max = the amount of weight that is able to be lifted by the client one time) with a new 1 rep max established every 4 weeks. Nelson et al. concluded that even though some pharmacological and nutritional management methods for clients with osteoporosis are effective in limiting the loss of bone, strength training promotes these same benefits with the added benefits of strength gains, improved balance, and muscle mass. Therefore "strength training in postmenopausal women . . . has the clinical potential to prevent osteoporotic fractures by simultaneously influencing multiple risk factors."[27]

With respect to the improvement of osteoporosis in the spine of the geriatric client, varying results have been published as to which exercise is most effective. Sinaki and Mikkelsen[28] believe that although exercise in general is encouraged for the client with osteoporosis, not all exercises are helpful, and indeed some can be harmful. When examining the effects on the spinal column using flexion or extension exercises, a significant difference was found identifying extension exercises as the safer exercise to prevent the advancement of spinal deformity, wedging, or fracture. Over a 1½-year study of women with osteoporosis, an overall progression rate of spinal deformity was noted (44%). However, the group that performed flexion exercises demonstrated increased spinal wedging or compression fractures in 89% of the cases, whereas those clients performing extension exercises demonstrated deformity in only 16% of the cases. This research evidence may suggest that extension or isometric exercises may be the most appropriate form of spinal exercises to prevent the progression of deformities from osteoporosis.[23,28]

When performing back extension exercises, care should be taken not to overstress the spine or extend any deformity or discomfort. Sinaki and Grubbs[23] found that none of the women with osteoporosis who volunteered to participate in the extension exercise investigation deteriorated by performing a home program, and several with long-standing back discomfort actually reported a reduction in symptoms. Back extension isometric exercises and hip extension exercises were included in the home program for postmenopausal women with osteoporosis (Figs. 11–8 and 11–9). The McKenzie method of promoting extension described in Chapter 10 may be helpful in preventing the onset of kyphotic posture deformities. Table 11–4 presents an overall summary of exercise principles related to the client with osteoporosis.

The most susceptible population for disability associated with osteoporosis is the postmenopausal woman. This is due, in part, to the decline of the hormone estrogen. Estrogen is needed for the development and maintenance of bone density. The onset of menopause brings a decline in the production of estrogen and a resultant imbalance of bone deposits and resorption. Increased bone resorption is noted particularly in trabecular bone. This is one reason for the involvement of the vertebral bodies, which are composed of mostly trabecular bone. It has been documented that from ages 50 to 80 in women, bone density

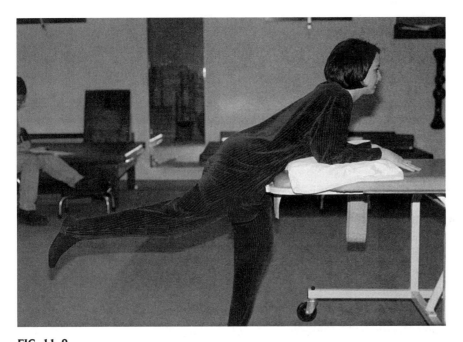

FIG. 11–9
Hip extension exercises for osteoporosis. This exercise is also referred to as a "mule kick." With the trunk and spine supported by the plinth or bed, have the client extend one hip, keeping the knee bent. Care should be taken not to move the spine excessively, creating either an increased or a reduced lumbar lordosis. Have the client isometrically hold the hip extension for 5 seconds and slowly return to the starting position. Repeat the exercise 15 times. This exercise and the isometric back extension exercise were described by Sinaki and Grubbs to be an effective intervention for osteoporosis management if performed regularly by the client four times per week.

Table 11–4

EXERCISE PRINCIPLES FOR THE CLIENT WITH OSTEOPOROSIS

1. **Specificity of exercise:** Bone density gains will only be realized in body parts that are exercised.
2. **Overload principle:** Bone density gains will only occur if the bone is progressively overloaded. Great care should be taken with overloading bones demonstrating osteoporosis because of the increased risk of pathological fracture.
3. **Reversibility principle:** If exercise stops, gains in bone density will be reversed.
4. **Some exercise is better than none:** If the client is physically unable to perform strenuous exercises, then non–weight-bearing activities are better than not exercising at all.
5. **Avoid long-duration activities:** Activities that are low load, high repetition performed for more than 5 hr/wk may not enhance bone density. Excessive exercise may lead to amenorrhea and should be avoided.
6. **High loads, low reps:** The most effective form of resistance training is greater loads with fewer repetitions.
7. **Eat, eat, eat:** Adequate nutrition through a well-balanced diet is critical. Unhealthy eating coupled with the use of supplements will not prevent the onset of osteoporosis.
8. **Avoid activities that produce deformities:** Forward flexion exercises of the spine may increase kyphotic deformities related to osteoporosis. Falls should be preventable if possible.

---

lessens by almost 30%. Hormonal replacement therapies have been incorporated into the treatment parameters for osteoporosis because of this significant increased risk of bone loss in this population. The benefits and risks of replacing deficient estrogen in the postmenopausal woman should be a discussion between the client and physician. However, estrogen replacement therapies are ineffective if not accompanied by proper nutrition and exercise.[20]

Osteoporosis can have an impact on the psychological and social well-being of the client. In the United States and many other cultures, the simple mention of the word "osteoporosis" often strikes fear and anxiety in many women. Images of disability, pain, and loss of function are commonly associated with the word osteoporosis within the lay community. The prevention of disability and fractures related to osteoporosis can often produce anxiety in those clients afflicted with the condition. Depression can accompany anxiety if not addressed by the rehabilitation team. Despite the best preventative efforts, fractures may still occur, giving the client a sense of failure. The cycle of chronic pain, disability, and depression may begin to alter the self-esteem of the client. Physical appearance in Western societies is associated with self-esteem, and with the acquisition of a kyphotic posture, the client may feel awkward and sensitive about appearance. Frequently, women stricken with this disease find that clothing no longer fits, preventing them from wearing their usual clothing. If left unattended by the rehabilitation team, this cycle of disability, depression, and loss of function may inhibit attempts to promote successful outcomes and treatment.[20,29]

The expected physical therapy outcomes for managing a client with osteoporosis include[30]:

1. Improved health-related quality of life
2. Improved functional skills
3. An optimal return of function
4. Reduced risk of further disability from identified limitations
5. Improved safety awareness
6. Improved self-care skills and ADLs
7. An understanding of risk factors that may contribute to jeopardizing health status
8. An understanding of strategies to prevent further disability

The expected time frame for achieving the outcomes is variable and ongoing. The management of osteoporosis should truly be a life-span approach. Short-duration changes in behavior are an ineffective means of dealing with disability associated with osteoporosis. Women over age 40 can be proactive in limiting the debilitating effects of the disease. Simple home exercise programs (in combination with proper nutrition and hormonal replacement therapy after menopause) can improve posture and back strength as well as promote the emotional well-being of the client.[23]

FRACTURES

As discussed in the sections related to falls and osteoporosis, a fracture is the end result of both conditions. Collectively or separately, falling and osteoporosis lead to an excessive number of hospitalizations for broken bones in the geriatric population. Disability related to fractures in the geriatric population is one of the major health epidemics facing managed care. Risk factors associated with fractures in geriatric clients can be either intrinsic or extrinsic in nature.[4,31] Intrinsic risk factors include:

1. Demographics of the client (age, sex, height, and race)
2. Relevant medical history (history of maternal hip fracture, medications) and presence of pathology (cancer)
3. Nutritional status
4. Activity level and functional status (inability to rise from a chair without using arms, loss of flexibility, or use of an assistive device for gait)
5. Cognitive status
6. Visual status (poor depth perception, contrast sensitivity)
7. BMD (osteoporosis)
8. Weight gain since age 25

Geriatric clients who sustain fractures to their extremities are at risk for developing neuropsychological problems immediately after the injury.[32,33] However, Jelicic et al[34] describes that no decline in cognitive function was observed in clients two months after the fracture had occurred. This probably suggests that impaired cognitive behavior that is observed in the geriatric client after an extremity fracture is often a result of factors related to the hospitalization process. Stress, anxiety, sleep disturbances, and medications either singly or collectively may be responsible for the high occurrence of cognitive dysfunction in the geriatric client after sustaining a long bone fracture.

Shoulder Fractures

Fractures of the proximal humerus are common and are typically a result of falling. The fall can be a result of intrinsic or extrinsic factors, but the end result is the

Open Reduction and Internal Rotation (ORIF)
An open surgical procedure designed to reduce the bony deformity and stabilize the fractured components. Various screws, pins, and plates can be used in the stabilizing procedure.

broken bone. Slightly more nondisplaced fractures occur compared with displaced proximal humeral fractures. The orthopedic surgeon will evaluate the stability of the fracture and either perform an **open reduction and internal fixation** (ORIF) on an unstable fracture or simply immobilize the stable fracture (Fig. 11–10). A total joint replacement may also be considered by the orthopedic surgeon (this is addressed in the arthroplasties section of this chapter). At times, the fracture is severe enough that a surgical option is not considered, because there potentially is not enough healthy or sturdy bone to reconstruct. These clients are managed conservatively and will eventually heal, but they lose significant motion and function of the involved shoulder.

Clinical Presentation. The client may present as soon as 1 week after injury. If being treated in the acute care facility, the client will potentially begin rehabilitation in functional skills on the first or second day after the injury. The injured upper extremity will be immobilized in either an over-the-neck sling or a shoulder immobilizer that is secured to the trunk. Noted bruising and edema may encompass the shoulder girdle. If swelling is a problem, gravity may force extracelluar fluid into the distal upper extremity and hand, causing motion dysfunctions there. Pain will be significant, and the client may have difficulty breathing deeply, turning in bed, or coming to a seated position. Once the client has moved through the transitional movement from supine to standing, the client is usually comfortable enough to perform ambulation (i.e., barring other complicating factors, including hypotension, other injuries sustained in the fall, or preexisting conditions).

Evaluation: Tools and Methods. A comprehensive evaluation including a subjective history and onset of the current disability should be taken. The evaluating therapist should perform a visual inspection of the injured or surgically

FIG. 11–10
Proximal humeral fracture. Pictured is a postoperative X-ray of a client who received an ORIF to stabilize a proximal humeral fracture. This client suffered the fracture in a fall.

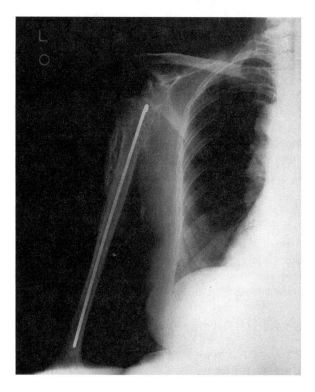

repaired area, documenting integumentary status. Range of motion (ROM) and strength assessment of the neck, ipsilateral elbow, and hand as well as the contralateral entire upper extremity should be completed. Many therapists will delay assessment of motion and strength of the fractured shoulder until a more substantial amount of healing has taken place. Gait, functional skills, posture, pain, and balance assessments should also be documented.

Clinical Management. Fractures are typically managed through immobilization, casting, or surgical reduction and fixation.[20] The use of a weighted cast is sometimes an option for management of the proximal humeral fracture. The cast is placed on the distal humerus and proximal forearm, immobilizing the elbow and, at times, the wrist. With the elbow immobilized in 90° of flexion and the entire upper extremity placed in a sling, a distraction of the proximal humerus results. The weight of the cast acts similarly to an orthopedic traction appliance attached to a client's bed. This method can be effective at reducing the bony fracture, but the potential of losing motion in the associated joints of the upper extremity is significant.[1]

When deemed appropriate by the orthopedic surgeon, gentle motion of the shoulder should begin. Often as early as the first week, the client may begin Codman's pendulum exercises to prevent the onset of restricted motion of the shoulder and the remainder of the upper extremity. Performing early motion near a fracture site appears to be encouraging an established fracture contraindication. This, however, is an exception to the rule, because the benefits are deemed to outweigh the risks of performing the motion. If the geriatric client's shoulder is immobilized for a significant length of time, the likelihood of experiencing associated complications increases (e.g., adhesive capsulitis, reflex sympathetic dystrophy). Gentle, controlled motion will promote long-term function and a short-term reduction in pain, swelling, and irritation. The therapist should be aware of the nature of the fracture and ensure that the application of early motion is not so aggressive as to jeopardize the stability of the fracture site. Active motion also can be encouraged by performing shoulder shrugs or circles as well as active motion for the elbow and hand. Passive motion and stretching may disrupt the integrity of the healing fracture and should not be performed until sufficient healing has occurred.[1]

Addressing self-care and functional skills early in the rehabilitation process is necessary. Frequently, teaching the client how to safely eat, dress, write, and perform other self-care skills is needed to encourage early independence. If the client has injured the dominant hand, temporary retraining emphasizing the nondominant hand may be necessary for some tasks.[1]

Overall activity will help limit the disability associated with the onset of the fracture. The client should be encouraged to ambulate and perform self-care as much as possible. Gait skills should be addressed early in the rehabilitation efforts to prevent the onset of disuse atrophy. If complicating factors are present, such as balance deficits or associated fractures, these must be concurrently addressed. Working with the client who sustained a proximal humeral fracture and a femoral neck fracture, with a non–weight-bearing (NWB) status on either the upper or lower extremity is quite a mobility challenge for the rehabilitation team and the client.

Strengthening exercises will be incorporated into the treatment plan after some healing has occurred. Usually by the third week after the injury, the client should be doing gentle resisted isometric or setting exercises to the shoulder girdle muscles. Active motion of the shoulder can begin, with pain used as a guideline.

Great emphasis should be placed on early and proper motion of the scapula. The injury and subsequent immobilization frequently interrupts the normal scapulo-humeral rhythm, which allows full motion of the shoulder complex. The client should be encouraged to perform quality movements of the shoulder rather than multiple movements performed poorly. The quality versus quantity issue is relevant because quantity will not ensure good quality. If the motion is repeatedly performed incorrectly, the client will adapt to the incorrect movement pattern in accomplishing shoulder movement. Correcting unsatisfactory movement patterns when further into the rehabilitation process is often difficult. Encourage good quality over sheer quantity in performing all exercises.[1]

The fracture should be healed by the eighth week. Factors that may delay healing for the client include poor nutrition, presence of osteoporosis, and reinjury to healing tissue. If adequate healing has taken place and motion limitations are still a significant problem, appropriate joint mobilization and stretching may become a part of the treatment plan. Great care should be taken when performing joint mobilization on a geriatric client with a proximal humeral fracture due to not only the recently healed fracture, but also to the potential presence of osteoporosis. As active motion is improved, a continual reexamination of proper scapular movement should be included. The client should be gradually challenged with functional activities using the healed upper extremity.[1]

The physical therapy expected outcomes[30] include:

1. Improved health-related quality of life
2. Improved functional skills
3. Improved self-care skills and ADLs
4. An understanding of strategies to prevent further disability

The expected time frame for achieving outcomes is 3 to 6 months. Barring complications, the humerus will heal in the expected time frame of 8 weeks, but function of the shoulder may slowly follow physiological healing. These clients often will not regain full, normal motion of the shoulder, but they should aspire to being fully functional when using the upper extremity.

Elbow Fractures

Injuries to the elbow may involve soft tissue, bony tissue, or nervous tissue. Typically, the elbow sustains injury as a result of direct trauma, as when falling. Injury may produce a dislocation of the elbow joint, but typically some sort of fracture to the distal humerus, proximal ulna, or radius is the result. One-third of all elbow fractures involve the radial head.[1,35]

Clinical Presentation. After the orthopedic surgeon manages the case, the client will be immobilized. Traditionally, the client begins physical therapy upon removal of the immobilization device. Initially, a significant loss of elbow and forearm motion is common. Typically, a significant amount of pain is associated with elbow fractures.[1] A paralysis of the hand may result from a compromise of the blood flow if the fracture disrupted the brachial artery. A Volkmann contracture is described as muscular atrophy from a circulatory compromise. A vascular compromise should be considered if the client demonstrates the following signs[35]:

1. Severe forearm pain
2. Painful and limited finger movement
3. Prominent veins, purple discoloration of the hand
4. Initial paresthesia soon followed by anesthesia in the hand

5. Loss of radial pulse followed by a loss of capillary refill
6. Pallor and paralysis in the hand

Evaluation: Tools and Methods. The evaluation performed by the PT may include a subjective history of the injury and pain. Objective measures include upper-extremity ROM, strength, and sensory assessments. Integumentary status should be evaluated, including the integrity of the circulatory system. Functional measures of the hand should be initially documented for future comparison to assess progress and the effectiveness of the intervention program.

Clinical Management. Extemity fractures are traditionally managed through casting, with some cases needing surgical reduction and fixation.[20] Radial head fractures in the geriatric client are often managed by ORIF, and certain cases require a surgical excision of the radial head.[1] Immobilization after surgery in a hinged brace or cast is common, lasting 3 to 4 weeks. If the client has access to a therapist while immobilized, education should be provided regarding (1) ROM exercises, (2) swelling reduction, and (3) signs of circulatory compromise. If the hand and shoulder are free to move, then active motion at these adjacent joints should be encouraged to limit concurrent dysfunction. If swelling is observed distally, this should be managed with elevation, cryotherapy, and potentially compression. Persistent edema will cause great discomfort and may lead to conditions such as reflex sympathetic dystrophy (see later discussion). Circulatory compromise signs should be reported immediately to the physician for management.[35]

When the cast is removed, active motion exercises of the elbow should begin. Passive stretching and mobilization should be performed with great care and only at the direction of the supervising PT. Early isometric exercises can be done to encourage strengthening. As motion improves, strengthening using progressive techniques should be introduced. Motions emphasized include elbow flexion and extension followed by forearm supination and pronation. Practicing and relearning functional activities should begin as soon as tolerated by the client.[34] Functional limitations that may present after a fractured elbow include difficulty turning a door knob, feeding oneself, going from sit to stand with the assistance of the upper extremities and carrying objects.[35,36]

According to the Preferred Practice Patterns,[30] the expected physical therapy outcomes related to the management of a client with an elbow fracture include:

1. Improved health-related quality of life
2. Improved functional skills
3. Improved self-care skills and ADLs
4. An understanding of strategies to prevent further disability

The expected time frame for achieving the outcomes is 3 to 4 months.

Wrist

The wrist and hand constitute the final or terminal functional link for the entire upper extremity. The role of the shoulder and elbow is to place the hand strategically so that a desired function may be adequately performed. When injury occurs to the wrist or hand, a significant functional deficit occurs for the geriatric client. More than 90% of all fractures involving the wrist result from a fall.[11] A Colles fracture results from a fall on an extended arm with the wrist in an extended position (Fig. 11–11).

FIG. 11–11

X-ray of a client with a distal radial fracture.
Notice the deformity of the distal radius as the fractured elements are dorsally displaced. A Colles fracture will result in a "dinner fork" deformity. If the distal fractured elements are displaced anteriorly, the fracture is named Smith's.

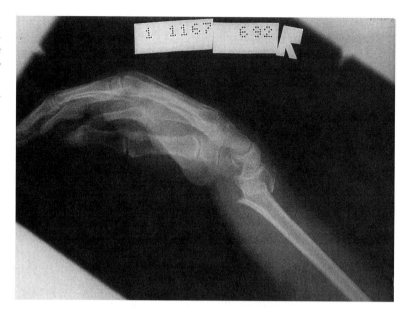

Clinical Presentation. The average client presenting with a fractured wrist is between ages 50 and 65. The frequency of fractures involving the wrist does not increase after age 65, as a plateau effect is demonstrated.[11] Nevitt and Cummings[11] believe that the plateau effect is a result of clients over age 65 tending not to have effective protective mechanisms in the upper extremities due to declining strength. Protective responses, such as extending an arm during the process of falling, may increase the likelihood that a client may sustain a fracture of the wrist. When the geriatric client attends physical therapy, it is usually after a short period of immobilization. A noted deformity may be present after the healing process has completed: the wrist is dorsally displaced, and the distal extremity resembles a dinner fork.

Evaluation: Tools and Methods. The evaluation performed will contain a subjective history of the current condition and status of pain. Objective measures should be taken in regard to the ROM, strength, and sensation of the wrist and hand. Functional assessments for gripping and self-care skills are likely to be completed. Integumentary assessment for the integrity of the skin and the presence of edema should also be completed.

Clinical Management. Most distal wrist fractures are managed through a closed reduction, followed by a period of immobilization in a cast or splint. Some cases require surgical fixation.[20] The rehabilitation team may have the opportunity to work with the client while the wrist is immobilized to establish an effective home program routine. The client should focus on edema reduction while in the cast. This can be accomplished by elevation and active motion of nonimmobilized joints. The rehabilitation team should ensure that the client actively moves all of the digits to prevent the long finger tendons from adhering to the fracture site during the healing process. Sometimes, dynamic splinting is added to the cast to ensure that motion of the digits is preserved. The cast may be removed in 2 to 4 weeks and replaced with a rigid splint.[34,37]

When healing is deemed sufficient by the orthopedic surgeon (between 4 and 6 weeks), active rehabilitation may begin. Upon the removal of the cast, pain and edema will need to be controlled. Topical modalities such as heat or cold as well as electrical stimulation may be needed. Active range of motion (AROM) exercises and mobilization of the wrist and carpal bones may begin to improve the client's motion. Passive range of motion (PROM) and stretching can be performed within the pain tolerance of the client. Early in the rehabilitation program, isometric gripping exercises, such as squeezing a tennis ball or therapeutic putty, are beneficial. If needed, functional electrical stimulation may be used to assist with strengthening of the wrist and digit muscles. By the sixth to eighth week after the injury, complete healing of the fractured wrist should occur. At this time, the client's wrist should be assessed to begin more aggressive stretching and strengthening if appropriate.[1] Clients with surgically managed wrists will follow the same rehabilitation guidelines upon direction of the surgeon.[37]

In the geriatric population, distal wrist fractures are associated with significant morbidity and loss of function. The fractured wrist may result in chronic pain, traumatic arthritis, and neuropathies. The onset of post-traumatic arthritis can lead to debilitating pain in the client. Knirk and Jupiter[38] reported that as many as 90% of clients experiencing a distal radius fracture will develop traumatic arthritis. Reflex sympathetic dystrophy (RSD) is a condition that frequently is associated with distal wrist fractures. Early awareness of the signs and symptoms of RSD are helpful in managing the condition (see later discussion).[20,37]

The expected physical therapy outcomes for managing clients with wrist fractures include[30]:

1. Improved functional skills
2. Reduced risk of further disability from identified limitations
3. Improved safety awareness of the client
4. Improved self-care skills and ADLs
5. An understanding of strategies to prevent further disability

The expected time frame for achieving all of these outcomes is 3 to 6 months. After 6 months, half of all geriatric clients with a Colles fracture subjectively report only fair outcomes. However, the morbidity and loss of function does not produce significant dependence on others. Despite the loss of function, less than 1% of the clients report having to rely on others to compensate for the disability.[20,39]

Pelvic

A pelvic fracture sustained by a geriatric client is usually due to a fall. When seen in younger clients, pelvic fractures are usually a result of high-energy impact events, such as motor vehicle accidents. A pelvic fracture is also associated with other multiple injuries because of the violent nature of the fracturing force. The mortality rate for clients with a pelvic fracture is as high as 20%.[40]

Pelvic fractures can occur to any combination of the pelvic bones, resulting in either a stable or unstable fracture. The union of the two ilia, ischia, pubes, and the sacrum form a pelvic ring when viewed superiorly (Fig. 11–12). If trauma results in a fracture to any of the bones of the pelvis, the stability of the fracture is judged by the integrity of the pelvic ring. If the fracture disrupts the pelvic ring, the client will not be able to bear weight on his or her lower extremities without jeopardizing the stability of the fracture site. Pelvic instability is described either as a rotational instability or a vertical instability. A type A pelvic fracture is stable both vertically and rotationally. A type B pelvic fracture is vertically stable, but rotationally unstable. A type C pelvic fracture is both vertically and rotationally unstable. If the fracture is unstable, surgical fixation is required to prevent further damage and morbidity to the geriatric client.[40]

FIG. 11–12
Pelvic ring. The weight-bearing unit formed by the two innominate bones and the sacrum is a supportive ring. If a fracture disrupts the ring, the weight-bearing ability of the pelvis becomes unstable and surgery is required.

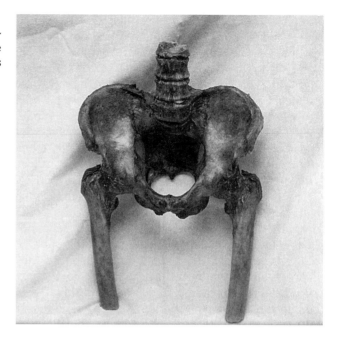

Clinical Presentation. The client with a pelvic fracture will be seen in the acute care setting for conservative management either after a stable pelvic fracture or after surgical fixation for an unstable pelvic fracture. Pain and discomfort are significant for these clients. Transitional movements are difficult and painful to perform. Most clients prefer to remain in bed, reluctant to move. This behavior can lead to respiratory or circulatory compromise. In a client who is medically stable, often a difficult aspect of treatment is the attempt to convince the client of the importance of getting up and out of bed, despite the pain.

Evaluation: Tools and Methods. In the acute care facility, the evaluation will focus on the functional abilities of the client. Subjective pain reports are documented as well as a description of the events leading up to the fracture of the pelvis. Objectively, ROM and strength measures may be taken, but pain may significantly limit the validity of the data. Sensory and balance assessments should be documented. The functional status of the client should be assessed including bed mobility, rolling, coming to a seated position, and gait skills.

Clinical Management. Stable pelvic ring fractures are managed conservatively without surgery. In the acute care setting, these clients are encouraged to get out of bed as quickly as possible to prevent the onset of secondary conditions associated with bedrest (e.g., pneumonia, kidney stones, and disuse atrophy). During the first week of rehabilitation, the client is allowed to bear weight as tolerated (WBAT) on the lower extremities using a walker. Treatment should focus on functional activities of bed mobility, transfers, and gait training. The client is most likely using pain medications that could affect balance and sensory feedback, so gait training should be performed with this in mind. By the second week after the injury, the rehabilitation team may begin gentle strengthening exercises. Isometric exercises are usually tolerated well early in the strengthening program. Closed-chain strengthening is often preferred to open-chain strengthening by the client due to comfort. Open-chain exercises (e.g., a straight-leg raise) can place a long-lever arm force on the pelvis that may produce discomfort. A particular emphasis on the hip abductor muscles should be addressed, because this muscle group is a major dynamic stabilizer of the pelvis during gait. By the fourth to sixth week, the client should be full weight bearing (FWB) and should be able to return to most activities as tolerated. When no gait deviations are noted and sufficient healing of the pelvis has occurred, the client may discard the assistive device (unless otherwise needed for other conditions).[40]

If the fracture produces an instability of the pelvic ring, surgical fixation is necessary. These clients will have a limited weight-bearing program for as much as 3 months after surgery.[40] Clients with a type B rotational instability are limited to touch toe weight bearing (TTWB) on the involved side for at least 6 weeks. Strict adherence to this guideline is needed to prevent jeopardizing the surgical repair. Isometric exercises to the hip are safe during the first 6 weeks, but no open-chain activities that stress the pelvis should be performed. If the client is able to safely walk using a TTWB pattern, gait training should be conducted. Functional concerns related to safe transferring and bed mobility should be addressed. This client will probably need a wheelchair for some mobility during this period, so wheelchair management education should be performed. Partial weight bearing (PWB) may begin as early as 6 weeks if healing is adequate. At this time, closed-chain strengthening exercises may be added to the program. Functional activities should be updated to accommodate the increased weight-bearing status. FWB is probably not likely until 12 weeks have passed. At that time, more aggressive strengthening and a full return to activities may begin.[40]

Fractures that are vertically and rotationally unstable (type C) have significantly delayed weight-bearing limitations. The client may not begin any weight bearing until the sixth week after surgery, so the first 6 weeks of rehabilitation should focus on independent wheelchair mobility. The primary focus should be functional activities of transferring in and out of bed to the wheelchair. Isometric exercises can be safely performed to help decrease disuse atrophy. A walker may be used to assist with transfers from the wheelchair to the commode or to stand at the side of the bed. Walking any significant distance should be discouraged. At 6 weeks, if sufficient healing has taken place, the client may begin PWB and gradually increase his or her ambulation skills. Closed-chain exercises may be tolerated at this point in the rehabilitation of the client. At 12 weeks, more aggressive ambulation and strengthening may begin if the surgeon feels adequate healing has taken place.[40]

The expected physical therapy outcomes when managing a client with a pelvic fracture include[30]:

1. Improved functional skills
2. An optimal return of function
3. Improved safety awareness of the client
4. Improved self-care skills and ADLs
5. An understanding of risk factors that may contribute to jeopardizing health status

The expected time frame for achieving the outcomes is 6 to 8 weeks in the conservatively managed client. The client with a stable pelvic fracture should progress well without severe complications, with pain as the major limiting factor. As the fracture heals, the pain should subside. The expected time frame for achieving the outcomes is 4 to 6 months for the client who was surgically managed. The significant delay in FWB abilities after surgery prevent a speedy recovery for this client.

Hip

The most common acute orthopedic condition affecting the geriatric population is the hip fracture.[1] Nevitt and Cummings[11] reported that almost 90% of all hip fractures occur as a result of falling. The average client presenting with a hip fracture is about 60-years-old, but the frequency of hip involvement increases exponentially with age.[11] White women are more likely to sustain a hip fracture than any other racial subgroup.[41] If the client is younger than 50, then the client is two times more likely to be male than female. However, if the client is 70-years-old, then the odds reverse for a 2:1 female to male ratio. This suggests the significant physiological and lifestyle changes that occur with the aging population.

If the client falls and physically impacts the ground near or directly on the hip joint, the chances of sustaining a fracture are substantially increased.[11] In general, falls that are to the side, backward, or straight down increase the chance that the hip joint will be the initial point of impact. Sixty-six percent of sustained hip fractures occur from a fall to the side. Interestingly, if the client falls and is able to break the fall on an extended upper extremity, the chances of sustaining a hip fracture are decreased (but the chances for fracturing the wrist are increased). If the client is able to land on the soft-tissue area of the buttock as opposed to the lateral aspect of the hip joint, the chances for fracture are less. The hardness of the surface (e.g., a concrete compared with a grassy surface) landed upon also has a direct impact on the prevalence of hip fractures.[11,42]

Mortality rates as high as 23% within the first year after suffering a hip fracture have been documented.[31] Some estimates have reported a death every 10 minutes nationwide from complications associated with a hip fracture.[1]

Clinical Presentation. The geriatric client usually sustains a proximal hip fracture in one of two areas. Forty-nine percent of all hip fractures are trochanteric,

FIG. 11–13
X-ray of a client with a proximal femur fracture. Notice the deformity altering the normal angle of inclination between the femoral shaft and neck. The external appearance of this client's limb was shortened and externally rotated compared to the noninvolved limb.

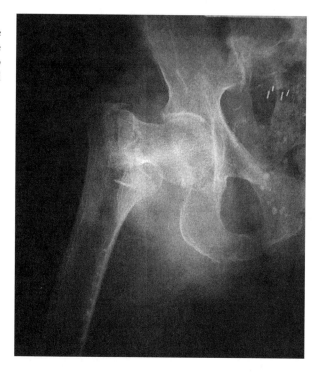

and 47% involve the femoral neck.[43] The neck and intertrochanteric region of the femur have a higher concentration of cancellous bone as opposed to the more dense cortical bone. There tends to be a decreased vascular supply to this area as well. Figure 11–13 represents a radiographic examination of a client who has sustained a fracture of the proximal femur.

The client is traditionally seen after surgery in the acute care setting for initial rehabilitation. Staples or sutures will secure the client's lateral incision. A protective, absorbent dressing and possibly a surgical drain exiting the incision may be in place. Some facilities use postsurgical prophylactic measures to prevent the formation of a deep venous thrombosis (DVT), including intermittent compression pumps, compression stockings, and/or elevation of the lower extremity.

Evaluation: Tools and Methods. The evaluating PT will complete a comprehensive evaluation of the client and establish a plan of treatment. Sometimes, the evaluation is based on standardized measurement tools. These standardized assessment tools have common scoring systems and are used to assess the function of the client by the rehabilitation team (Box 11–1). The plan of treatment may be established according to specific protocols from either the physician or the facility. At the minimum, the evaluation should contain a history of the current condition and status of pain. Objectively, the evaluation should assess the skin and sensory integrity, ROM, strength, and balance assessments. Functional activities (e.g., bed mobility, transfers, gait skills) should be judged.

Clinical Management. Most hip fractures are surgically reduced and fixated (ORIF).[20] Figure 11–14 presents a surgically reduced and stabilized proximal hip fracture. Lewis and Bottomley[1] stress the importance of early mobility and weight bearing on the involved limb as soon as medically appropriate. This will promote a return to normal gait, balance, and proprioception and enhance the healing of the bone. Russell and Palmieri[40] stress the importance of early activity after a hip surgery by claiming:

> It is important that once stabilization is obtained, these patients begin to get up, sit in a chair, and ambulate frequently, since many are borderline ambulators before injury. Early mobilization also helps to minimize the complications of prolonged bed rest.

Hip fractures are usually managed following established guidelines and protocols of the facility or surgeon (Table 11–5). Weight-bearing parameters should be observed to promote the integrity of the surgical repair. The surgeon will determine the weight-bearing parameters depending on the type of fixation used and the integrity of the bone. Weight-bearing guidelines include NWB, TTWB, PWB, WBAT, or FWB. All gait and transfer training skills should be conducted within the established weight-bearing restrictions.

Bed mobility concerns should be addressed by the rehabilitation team with the client who has sustained a hip fracture. The client must be taught how to successfully manage bed coverings and transition from supine to sitting before the client can safely consider ambulating (Fig. 11–15). Ankle pumps are a prophylactic exercise designed to deter the postsurgical complications of edema and pooling of blood in the distal lower extremity (Fig. 11–16). Excessive blood pooling or decreased venous flow can lead to an active DVT. Most movements and activities in the lower extremities are contraindicated in the presence of an active DVT. Activity may dislodge the blood clot, causing it to become a pulmonary embolus, which can cause severe respiratory compromise or sudden death.

Box 11–1

STANDARDIZED ASSESSMENT FORMS

Many medical facilities are using standardized evaluation tools based on a numerical rating system with multidisciplinary input. The Functional Independence Measure (FIM[SM]), Tenetti Balance Test, Barthel Index, or Peabody Developmental Motor Scales are examples of standard assessment tools. These tools are helpful in assessing outcomes, as data are compiled into easily tracked numbers and categories. A limitation of the standardized tool is that it may not be individualized enough to accurately measure and reflect the needs or improvement of the specific client. Below is a simulated example of a standardized tool that the PT may use to assess a client:

Scoring		admission	goal	week 1	week 2	week 3	week 4	discharge
7. Completely independent 6. Modified independent using a device 5. Supervised 4. Minimal assistance 3. Moderate assistance 2. Maximal assistance 1. Dependent								
	Transfer: Bed to chair							
	Transfer: Sit to stand							
	Transfer: Toilet							
	Transfer: Tub or shower							
	Gait:							
	Wheelchair skills:							
	Stairs:							

Avascular Necrosis
Death of the bone due to an insufficient blood supply.

Chronic pain after a hip fracture may occur. Strategies to avoid the onset of chronic pain are biomechanical in nature. Hip abductor strengthening helps to promote stability of the pelvis during locomotion, limiting excessive stress and strain on the lower back, pelvis, and lower extremity. Carefully evaluating the respective leg lengths after a hip surgery will also reduce mechanical wear and tear on the client. If a leg-length discrepancy is present after surgery, appropriate shoe lifts or orthotic devices should be used. **Avascular necrosis** is a complicating factor that can mimic chronic pain after a hip fracture. If the blood supply is disrupted to the head of the femur after a proximal hip fracture, then irreparable joint damage may result. If avascular necrosis is detected, the client will undergo a total hip reconstruction to correct the problem.[20,44]

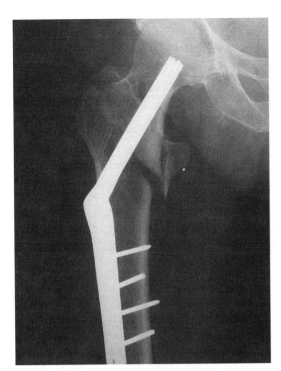

FIG. 11–14
A common orthopedic procedure is the open reduction and internal fixation (ORIF) of a proximal hip fracture. The orthopedic surgeon uses a combination of nails, pins, and screws to reduce the fracture and promote stability.

Table 11–5

HIP FRACTURE REHABILITATION PROTOCOL	
Time Frame	**Activities**
Day 1	Perform isometric quad, hamstring, and gluteals exercises. Perform ankle pumps. Perform AAROM: heel slides, hip abductions, adduction, SLR. Provide bed mobility training. Issue home exercise program and discuss rehabilitation plan.
Day 2	Review exercises from previous day. Provide bed mobility training. Begin gait skills from side of bed following WB status.
Day 3–7	Continue exercise program, increase AAROM to AROM as tolerated. Add hip flexor stretch (Thomas stretch). Promote independence with transfer skills. Increase gait tolerance. Enhance standing balance skills and weight shifts. Perform home evaluation and assistive device assessment.
Day 8–21	Establish discharge parameters. Increase gait independence: advanced assistive device (allowed by WB guidelines). Increase standing balance activities. Incorporate standing AROM exercises: flexion, abduction, extension, adduction and toe raises (if allowed by WB guidelines).
Discharge	Client is independent in all bed mobility. Client is able to ambulate 100 ft in hall independently with appropriate assistive device. Client is independent with appropriate bathroom transfers.

AAROM = active assistive range of motion; SLR = straight-leg raising; WB = weight bearing.

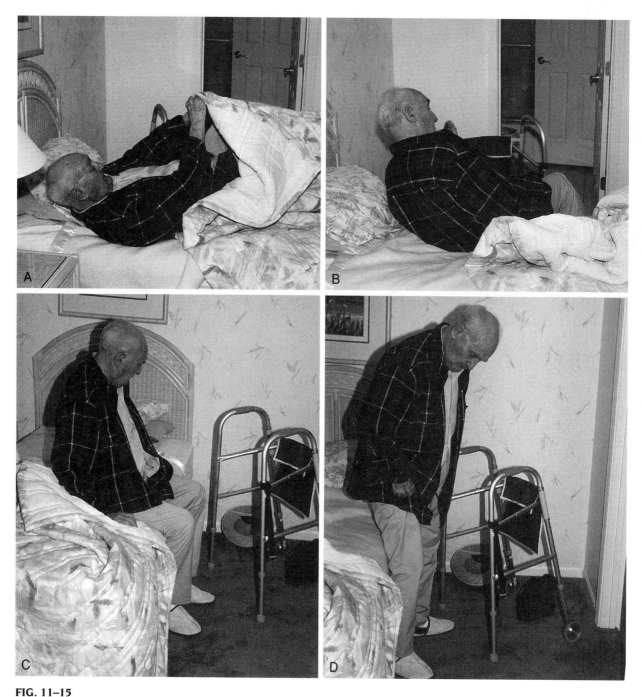

FIG. 11–15

Bed mobility concerns after a hip fracture. The client who has suffered a hip fracture and subsequent surgical repair must be taught how to safely transition from a supine to a sitting position in order to prepare for gait activities. Managing the bed covers is often not easy, but is a necessary first step (A). Next, a semi–log roll to the side of the bed in combination with swinging the feet and lowering legs off of the bed provides momentum to gain a sitting position (B). Sitting at the side of the bed is necessary for a short time to allow acclimation to an upright posture. If the client moves too quickly to a standing position, dizziness may result (C). Finally, the client should be ready to transfer from sitting to a standing position (D).

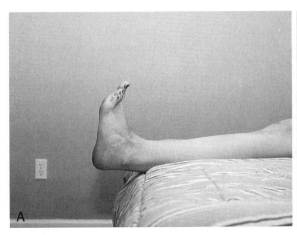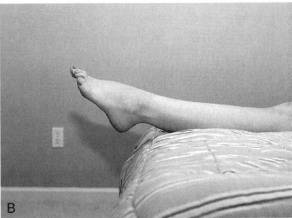

FIG. 11–16
Ankle pumps. AROM of the ankle including dorsiflexion (A) and alternating plantarflexion (B) will help to reduce to postsurgical effects of long bone surgery, including hip fractures, hip replacements, and total knee replacements.

The expected physical therapy outcomes for managing a client with a proximal hip fracture include[30]:

1. An optimal return of function
2. Reduced risk of further disability from identified limitations
3. Improve safety awareness of the client
4. Improved self-care skills and ADLs
5. An understanding of risk factors that may contribute to jeopardizing health status

The expected time frame for achieving the outcome is 6 to 8 weeks, barring medical complications.

Ankle

Fractures of the ankle are less common in the geriatric population than fractures of the hip, spine, or distal wrist. When they occur, however, significant disability may result, limiting gait and transferring abilities. The integrity of the ankle mortise joint is maintained by the interosseous membrane between the tibia and fibula as well as the medial and lateral malleolar ligaments. If a fracture is sustained and the supporting elements of the joint are destroyed, the client will need a surgical reduction to stabilize the fracture site. If a fracture is present, but the ankle joint remains stable, then conservative immobilization should be adequate to provide for adequate healing of the damaged bones.[45]

Clinical Presentation. Typically, the geriatric client who enters physical therapy with a fractured ankle has already been immobilized for 6 weeks. The acute care rehabilitation team may have had the opportunity to work with the client when the cast was applied for gait training and a simple home exercise program. When the cast or immobilization device is removed, the client will have noted loss of ROM and strength. Residual swelling and pain may be present with movement, but the chief complaint is usually stiffness in the joint.

Evaluation: Tools and Methods. A physical therapy evaluation will cover the subjective history of the client, including the mechanism of injury with current medical treatments or medications. ROM, strength, and sensory assessments should be included in the objective data. Balance and functional concerns can also be addressed. The integrity of the skin and circulation should be monitored.

Clinical Management. Distal lower-extremity fractures can be managed conservatively through casting, or surgically if the severity of the fracture dictates invasive procedures.[20] Nondisplaced, stable fractures with an intact ankle mortise joint can be immobilized in a cast or in a walking, removable boot. If the fracture is displaced or the stability of the ankle mortise joint is questionable, then an ORIF is required. The ability to bear weight on the injured extremity is dictated by the orthopedic surgeon. Some surgeons will promote early weight bearing for a stable fracture in a cast, but others believe that conservative TTWB is needed for surgically repaired fractures. The rehabilitation team should follow the guidelines of the surgeon, encouraging the most appropriate functional locomotion possible for the client within the restrictions.[45]

When the client is removed from the immobilization device (usually after 6 weeks), active rehabilitation may begin. The focus of rehabilitation should be restoring normal joint arthrokinematics, increasing strength, and facilitating proprioception of the injured ankle. ROM activities and joint mobilization will help restore normal motion. Strengthening can be undertaken by progressive resistive exercises, including elastic tubing and ankle weights. Closed-chain exercises will help restore strength as well as proprioception in the injured extremity. The rehabilitation team should work to identify gait and balance dysfunctions that may lead to future problems for the client. Some clients are simply sent home and told to move their ankle without the benefits of a full rehabilitation program. Significant long-term morbidity can result from a loss of motion and strength in the ankle. The client may be more susceptible to falls from inadequate strength or balance reactions. The client may also be predisposed to traumatic arthritis and chronic pain.

The expected physical therapy outcomes for managing a geriatric client with a fractured ankle include[30]:

1. An optimal return of function
2. Improved safety awareness of the client
3. Improved self-care skills and ADLs
4. An understanding of risk factors that may contribute to jeopardizing health status
5. An understanding of strategies to prevent further disability

The expected time frame for achieving the outcomes 8 to 12 weeks from the time of injury.

Spinal

Vertebral fractures in geriatric populations account for more than 5 million restricted activity days in clients over age 45.[20] Fractures of the spine associated with osteoporosis are small and persistent, resulting in kyphotic or hyperkyphotic deformities in the client. The fractures typically affect the anterior portion of the vertebral body, resulting in compression or collapse of the anterior structure of the vertebrae. The cumulative effect of the spinal fractures is a loss in axial height of the client.

Clinical Presentation. Pain is the most common and limiting factor associated with spinal compression fractures. Osteoporosis produces no physical pain, but fractures associated with the outcomes of osteoporosis are extremely painful and debilitating. The periosteum of the bone contains an abundance of **nociceptors**. The client with a spinal compression fracture presents with substantial pain. One subtype of spinal fracture is "silent" during the development of osteoporosis and prevents identification of the condition for many years. Most fractures related to the spine and osteoporosis will produce extreme discomfort and disability.[46]

Nociceptors
Pain receptors in the peripheral nervous system.

Pain associated with a spinal fracture will limit most of the client's functional abilities. Difficulty will be demonstrated during mobility tasks, such as getting out of bed, rolling, bending, or standing up from a chair. Frequently, the client will demonstrate nausea and a loss of appetite due to the severity of the pain. The inability to remain active because of the pain will lead to the added complication of immobility, including muscle atrophy, kidney stones, respiratory compromise, decreased circulation, and depressed cardiovascular efficiency. Side effects of pain medication can produce constipation, further increasing the client's discomfort.[20]

Evaluation: Tools and Methods. The PT will evaluate the client focusing on function and disability. A comprehensive history may reveal elements or risk factors related to osteoporosis and the history of the current medical condition. Subjective pain measures are often documented on pictures or as a numerical scale. Objective measures for ROM, strength, posture, gait, sensation, functional mobility, and risk for fall should be documented.

Clinical Management. The resolution of pain associated with spinal compression fractures is largely dependent on the ability of the client to adequately heal. The presence of other pathology, poor nutrition, and medications may limit the healing process and delay a full recovery. Most spinal compression fractures are managed conservatively without surgical intervention. Surgery is required only when neurological symptoms or spinal instability is suspected. The client is traditionally placed into a hyperextension type trunk orthosis that limits flexion.[20]

Activities designed to limit pain and promote mobility should be encouraged. Conservative modalities that reduce pain and encourage the relaxation of painful muscle guarding should be used. Controlled mobility should be promoted early to prevent the onset of disuse atrophy and bone loss. Frequently, pain-reducing medications are prescribed by the physician with instructions to rest. A fine line between activity and rest should be identified. The client should always use pain as a guideline and should avoid any activity that increases painful symptoms.[20]

The client should be educated to avoid forward flexion of the trunk so as to avoid extending the deformity. Assistive devices (reaching sticks) and strategies (energy conservation) to complete household activities should be investigated by the rehabilitation team and used by the client. Postural awareness should be encouraged when the client is sitting or lying down, when performing transitional movements, and when walking. The rehabilitation team should educate the client on how to properly transfer into and out of a car, reducing the risk of injury.[20]

Even in the more acute phase of pain in the spinal compression fracture, some exercising is tolerated and may indeed help reduce pain. As pain subsides from spinal compression fractures, an exercise program designed to improve strength, posture, and endurance should begin. Aggressive exercises should be discouraged, as well as postures (flexion) that would encourage deformity of the spine. Spinal extension exercises, both isotonic and isometric, should be used.

Deep-breathing exercises help enhance pulmonary function, preventing potential respiratory conditions. Relaxation exercises are frequently helpful in reducing muscle guarding and pain. Closed-chain activities, for example the wall slide or partial squat, combine several elements into one comprehensive exercise, including postural awareness, strengthening of the lower extremities, balance, coordination, and promoting client confidence in weight bearing.[20]

Clients with spinal compression fractures have the potential for continued disability associated with repeated fractures of the spine. At times, the pain appears chronic, but in reality, it is a continuous cycle of new pain presenting with new compression fractures as the old fracture heals and resolves. If the condition progresses to a chronic state, it is more likely a result of deconditioning and faulty posture rather than a single compression fracture. Exercise is a critical element in the management of chronic pain. Identifying faulty posture and corrective treatment plans should be incorporated. Cardiovascular conditioning and weight bearing can both be accomplished through a regular walking program. If the client is unable to tolerate walking on dry land, pool therapies should be considered as an exercise alternative. However, the PTA should understand that water exercise does not promote an increase in bone mass.

The expected physical therapy outcomes for managing a client with spinal compression fractures include[30]:

1. Improved health-related quality of life
2. Improved functional skills
3. Reduced risk of further disability from identified limitations
4. Improved safety awareness of the client
5. Improved self-care skills and ADLs
6. An understanding of risk factors that may contribute to jeopardizing health status
7. An understanding of strategies to prevent further disability

The expected time frame for achieving all outlined outcomes, barring any complicating condition, should be 8 weeks. In the presence of a positive healing environment, the vertebrae should heal and the pain will resolve. The onset of spinal fractures associated with osteoporosis does not immediately signal a greater onset of mortality, but if the deformity and persistence of fractures extends for more than 1 year, the survival rate declines rapidly for each continued year of life. The increase in the mortality rate for these clients with each passing year is not fully associated with the osteoporosis or the fracture, but with concurrent morbid conditions, including compromised lung capacity, pneumonia, and other fractures.[20]

DEGENERATIVE JOINT DISEASE

Degenerative joint disease (DJD) is the most common arthritic disorder involving one or more joints in the human body. Lewis and Bottomley[1] claim that "the most prevalent orthopedic condition is osteoarthritis." Characteristics of the disease include local deterioration of the articular cartilage that is progressive in nature. Inflammation of the synovial lining of the joint accompanies the degenerative changes. Many synonyms for DJD exist, including osteoarthritis, osteoarthrosis, and degenerative arthritis. Degenerative changes are more common in women than men. In the client population older than 60, 40% of the female population demonstrates degenerative changes in one or more joints, whereas 20% of the male population has osteoarthritis detected on x-ray examinations. The radiographic confirmation of osteoarthritis is demonstrated by a narrowing of the normal joint space. Zetterberg[47] reported that with the inclusion of **osteophytes**, around 12% of the U.S. population may be afflicted with degenerative joint disease. For those clients who reach age 75, as much as 70% may exhibit some signs of osteoarthritis. The knee is the most commonly involved joint, followed by the hip joint.[1,44]

Osteoarthritis can be classified into two distinct populations: primary osteoarthritis is a result of many potential etiologies, whereas secondary osteoarthritis or traumatic arthritis is a result of a known disease or traumatic event. Etiologies of primary osteoarthritis may include premature aging, genetic predisposition, or be unknown. Racial influence is significant in cases of primary osteoarthritis. Incident rates per 100,000 people demonstrated that people of Asian decent had a rate of 1.5, Hispanic 5.1, African-American 8.3, and white 29.4. Activity in the heavy work industry was a correlation factor for men, whereas obesity had a positive correlation for women. Men who work as farmers, construction workers, or firefighters have a higher incidence of degenerative changes in the hip joint. Obesity and sporting activity will increase the risk of developing osteoarthritis in the knee joint.[47]

Secondary DJD is frequently the residual effect of a traumatic event. Secondary DJD is frequently referred to as traumatic arthritis. Direct trauma to the joint surface may produce a lesion that eventually becomes arthritic in nature. Congenital abnormalities, joint infections, long bone deformities, and joint instability may predispose a client to demonstrating arthritic changes later in life. Traditionally, osteoarthritis is unilateral in nature and involves weight-bearing joints.[44]

The client with DJD of the hip or knee will complain of a general aching sensation in the hip that worsens with weight bearing. Associated conditions (e.g., bursitis, tensor fascia lata tendinitis) must be ruled out when the hip is involved. Patellofemoral dysfunction should be ruled out when the knee is involved. In the knee, the articular cartilage will be progressively worn away. The knee joint capsule will thicken and osteophytes may form. Proprioception is diminished as the degeneration progresses in the weight-bearing joints. Frequently on radiographic examination, the normal joint space in either the hip or knee is significantly narrowed (Fig. 11–17A).

The management of either onset of DJD to any joint is identical. Controlling pain and inflammation is accomplished through rest, modified activities, conservative modalities, and nonsteroidal anti-inflammatory drugs. Strengthening and flexibility exercises for the diseased joint should be promoted to alleviate pain and promote functional abilities. Clients with DJD of the hip frequently have strength deficits in the hip abductor and extensor muscles.[1] Contrary to some opinions, the inert structures of the joint (cartilage and ligaments) are not the major shock-absorbing structures. Indeed, the dynamic elements (muscles) surrounding the joint account for as much as 80% of the shock absorption of forces through a weight-bearing joint. With this fact in mind, the rehabilitation team should work to control the weight-bearing forces by increasing the strength of the muscles surrounding the joint. In the hip, the extensors and abductors are important, whereas in the knee, the strengthening efforts should focus on quadriceps and hamstring groups. Because of the progressive nature of the disease, including the continued wear and tear process through everyday activities, complete destruction of the articular cartilage will eventually result. In that circumstance, a joint replacement or **arthroplasty** should be considered.[1,44]

Osteophytes
A bony outgrowth from normal bone structures.

Arthroplasty
The surgical reconstruction of a diseased joint surface.

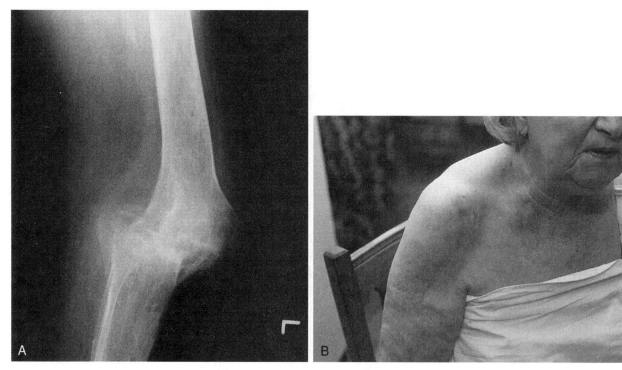

FIG. 11–17
Degenerative joint disease. (A) The knee is the most common joint affected by degenerative arthritis. Pictured is an X-ray of a left knee (lateral view) demonstrating degenerative changes. Notice the decreased joint space and shifting of the femur anteriorly on the tibia. (B) Healed surgical incision after a total shoulder replacement. This client had a total shoulder replacement approximately 1 year before this photo was taken.

ARTHROPLASTIES

Total Shoulder Replacement

Osteoarthritis of the shoulder is rare, exhibited in only 2% of geriatric shoulder dysfunction. Most of the presenting symptoms are a result of traumatic pathology, including joint instability or dislocation, but may include severe rheumatoid arthritis as well. The client who demonstrates signs and symptoms of degenerative changes in the glenohumeral joint has a constant dull ache, **crepitus,** weakness, and difficulty sleeping. A hard end-feel may be observed with passive movement of the shoulder joint. A joint replacement for the shoulder is warranted if arthritic symptoms severely limit ADLs, or following a fracture of the proximal humerus that has not sufficiently healed.[1]

Clinical Presentation. The client with a total shoulder replacement enters physical therapy very soon after the surgery for rehabilitation. An over-the-neck sling or immobilizer will hold the surgically repaired shoulder close to the client's trunk. The involved arm will be significantly weak and nonfunctional, leaving the client only one upper extremity to perform most, if not all, self-care activities. See Figure 11–17B for a healed incision after a total shoulder replacement.

Evaluation: Tools and Methods. The evaluation will consist of a subjective history and description of pain. Objective measures will included current ROM and sensory status. Strength evaluation of the surgically repaired shoulder is often

Crepitus
A clicking or crackling sound heard or palpated during the movement of a joint.

deferred until later in the rehabilitation program. The PT will evaluate the cervical region and the opposite extremity to assess the readiness of the client for one-handed activities. Gait, balance, and posture may be addressed.

Clinical Management. Client rehabilitation efforts are divided into two categories, depending on the presence of secondary soft-tissue compromise. Those clients with good rotator cuff and scapular stabilizer muscles have a better opportunity to gain significant functional abilities and are treated a bit more aggressively. Those clients with dysfunctional or poor rotator cuff muscles are treated more conservatively with lower expectations for significant functional gains.[48]

Rehabilitating the client with an intact rotator cuff and a total shoulder arthroplasty will begin the first day after surgery. The client should be instructed in AROM exercises of the elbow, wrist, and hand. Education and practice of one-handed activities should be incorporated early into the rehabilitation efforts. On the second or third day after surgery, motion activities of the shoulder should begin. Capsular restrictions or adhesive capsulitis should be prevented and early motion encouraged. Passive activities to stimulate ROM include (1) CPM, (2) manual or self-PROM, (3) pendulum exercises, and (4) rope and pulley (at week 2). Early strengthening efforts should focus on the prevention of rotator cuff muscle atrophy. Isometric shoulder exercises can be performed with the arm at the side of the body. Modalities such as ice and electrical stimulation can be used for pain control if needed. At the minimum, exercises should be performed daily. A complete home program should be developed for the client early, with home participation occurring between clinical visits.[48]

By the fourth week after surgery, more aggressive activities can begin. The client should be using a rope and pulley and performing wand exercises, gradually increasing motion of the shoulder. Joint mobilization can be added to reduce the motion limitations of the shoulder. AROM exercises should begin in the seated or standing position, with the client moving into flexion, abduction, and extension. The client should focus on quality movements, moving the arm from the side of the body up in a short arc about 45°. The client should not be encouraged to see how far the extremity can be move, but rather how *well* it can be moved. Elastic tubing exercises can begin with the arm at the side to strengthen the rotator cuff muscles. Emphasis on the scapular stabilizers and restoring normal scapulohumeral rhythm should begin.[48]

The expected outcome or return for the client with a total shoulder replacement and an intact rotator cuff is functional use of the upper extremity. Normal, full ROM and strength are not the ultimate goals. Shoulder flexion and abduction to 160° and internal and external rotation to 75° should be achieved. Shoulder strength should be about 60% of the opposite extremity, with good scapular control. The focus at this point is on self-care and functional skills. The client should continue a level of activity and exercise with the shoulder indefinitely, even after initial goals have been achieved. Home exercise programs maintaining ROM should help to prevent a loss of function in the surgically repaired joint (Fig. 11–18). Functional activities each day should gradually challenge the client to reach for greater heights, both figuratively and literally (Fig. 11–19).[48]

The client who undergoes a total shoulder replacement and has poor integrity of the rotator cuff has a poorer prognosis for functional recovery. The rehabilitation efforts follow the same guidelines previously discussed, except the client progresses at a much slower rate. Expectations for recovery should include a pain-free, partially functioning shoulder. Clients who achieve 120° of shoulder

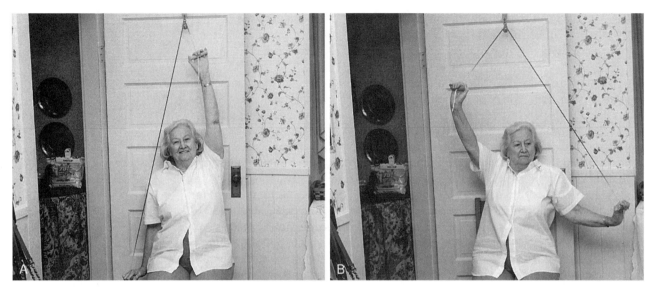

FIG. 11–18
Home exercise program after a total shoulder replacement. Over-the-door pulleys can be performed routinely by the client at home (A, B). Initially, the tool can help increase range of motion after surgery, but the pulleys progress to a maintenance tool, preventing the loss of motion in the shoulder.

flexion and 45° of external and internal rotation should be considered as having a successful outcome. Strength within the limited motion should be 50% to 60% of the opposite side. Even with a conservative approach, a focus on continued exercise and a gradual increase in function should be a lifelong attitude.[48]

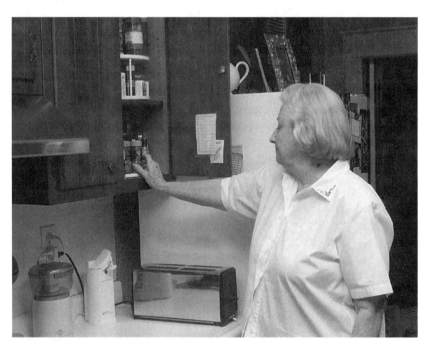

FIG. 11–19
Functional activities after a total shoulder replacement. Reaching into a cabinet is an activity that combines range of motion with function. The client can judge functional progress by the height that can be reached.

The expected physical therapy outcomes related to managing a client after receiving a total shoulder replacement include[30]:

1. Improved health-related quality of life
2. Improved functional skills
3. Improved self-care skills and ADLs

The expected time frame for achieving the outcomes is 6 to 12 months. Normal expectations should be discussed early in the client's rehabilitation, because the joint replacement will not give the client the shoulder of a 20-year-old athlete. The differences between functional expectations and normal expectations should be made clear and fully understood.

Digit Replacements

Deformities of the digits can severely impact the ability of a client to perform self-care skills (Fig. 11–20). Pain from diseased joints may also hinder the functional abilities of the client. Joint arthroplasties can be performed on the interphalangeal (IP) and the metacarpophalangeal (MCP) joints of the fingers and thumbs to correct deformity and reduce pain (Fig. 11–21). A combination of bony reconstruction and soft tissue correction may improve the functional abilities of the diseased hand.[37]

Clinical Presentation. Clients who undergo joint arthroplasty surgery of the digits are mainly those individuals with rheumatoid arthritis (RA) or osteoarthritis. Various deformities are associated with the digits of the hand. The client with RA will exhibit significant tissue proliferation, swelling, pain, loss of motion, and warmth in the involved joints of the hand. Muscle imbalances, tendon ruptures, capsular weakening, and bony erosion may contribute to the deformity process in the RA client as well. The fingers of the client will be viewed as deviating toward the ulnar border of the hand. This medial deviation of the proximal phalanx at the MCP joint is referred to as an *ulnar drift*. A swan-neck deformity is observed in the client who has proximal interphalangeal (PIP) hyperextension and DIP flexion. A boutonniére deformity results when the PIP is flexed and the distal interphalangeal (DIP) extended. Functionally, the client's ability to grasp and hold objects will be diminished. There may be difficulty performing simple self-care activities such as combing the hair, buttoning a shirt, or brushing teeth.[35,37]

Evaluation: Tools and Methods. The PT performing the evaluation will complete a thorough history of the client's condition complete with documentation of the functional abilities of the client. Individual ROM measurements of the digits, hands, and upper extremity will be assessed. Strength measurements of the

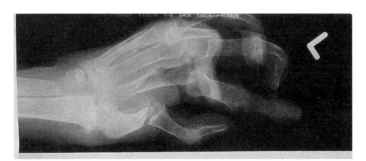

FIG. 11–20
Digit deformity of the hand. This is an X-ray of a severely deformed arthritic hand. Notice the marked angulations and overlapping of the digits. This client has great difficulty and pain associated with the performance of activities of daily living because of the arthritic changes.

FIG. 11–21
Interphalangeal joint replacement of the hand.
Pictured is an X-ray of a proximal interphalangeal (PIP) joint replacement of the third digit on the left hand. Joint replacements of the IP joints can be used to restore function by correcting deformity or by reducing pain.

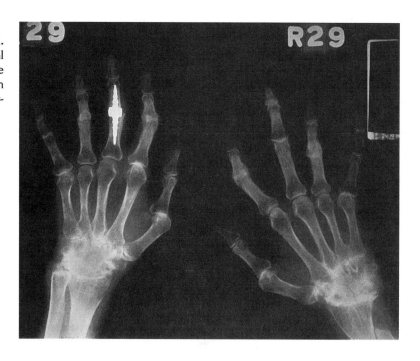

hand may be deferred for functional assessments, because pure strength measurements may not be indicative of the client's ability to perform certain tasks. Gait, sensory, posture, and balance assessments may also be included.

Clinical Management. Rehabilitation after a joint replacement for the IP or MCP joints of the hand varies depending on the surgeon's protocols and preferences. Frequently, these clients are treated by hand rehabilitation specialists who have extensive background knowledge and experience. General parameters may include splinting for support of the involved structures, gentle early ROM, and strengthening at 6 weeks after surgery. If concurrent soft-tissue reconstruction to the tendons was performed, motion may be delayed for several weeks until sufficient healing has occurred. The splinting mechanisms can be either a resting splint or dynamic splint to assist with the gradual elongation of the soft-tissue structures. These splints are custom made using various forms of moldable plastics, rubber bands, fishing line, Velcro, hooks, and glue. The prevention of contracture after surgery is an early concern. ROM activities are performed on all nonimmobilized joints and may be passively performed to the surgical joint if approved by the surgeon. Strengthening will not begin until the sixth week (possibly the eighth week) and may be performed by using therapeutic putty, rubber bands, and various gripping tools.[37]

The expected physical therapy outcomes related to managing a client with joint replacements of the digits include[30]:

1. Improved health-related quality of life
2. Improved functional skills
3. Reduced risk of further disability from identified limitations
4. Improved self care skills and ADLs
5. An understanding of risk factors that may contribute to jeopardizing health status
6. An understanding of strategies to prevent further disability

The expected time frame for achieving the outcomes is 6 months. The client may have to continue a regular intensive home program of ROM, strengthening, and splinting to maintain gains achieved in the original rehabilitation program.

Total Hip Replacement

The hip replacement surgery is a common procedure treated in orthopedic rehabilitation centers across the country. A prosthesis takes the place of the natural components of the proximal femur and acetabulum (Fig. 11–22). A total hip replacement or hip arthroplasty can be performed by an orthopedic surgeon for clients with a hip fracture, severe osteoarthritis or RA, or bone cancer. Hip replacements are also performed in cases of severe, uncontrollable pain or previous surgical replacement failures.

Clinical Presentation. The client will often be seen in the acute care setting 1 or 2 days after the surgery has been completed. The client will have a longitudinal surgical incision over the anterior, lateral, or posterolateral aspect of the involved hip. Staples frequently hold the incision intact with a protective absorbent dressing covering the area. The client may be positioned in an **abductor wedge** that is securely placed between the lower extremities of the client to prevent the prosthesis from dislocating during movements in bed or during transfers (Fig. 11–23).

Evaluation: Tools and Methods. The physical therapy evaluation will address the current functional status of the client. Transfer ability, gait skills, balance, and posture will be assessed. Some evaluating therapists defer a ROM and strength assessment of the surgical hip until later in the rehabilitation program. An assessment of the client's cognitive abilities to follow established protocols that prevent prosthetic dislocation is sometimes necessary. An evaluation of the integumentary status, including skin integrity surrounding the surgical incision, should be conducted.

Abductor Wedge
A large, triangle-shaped foam pillow that has straps on each side to secure the apparatus to each lower extremity of the client. Used after a total hip replacement to prevent the client from crossing his or her legs in bed and to hold the surgical hip in a slightly abducted position.

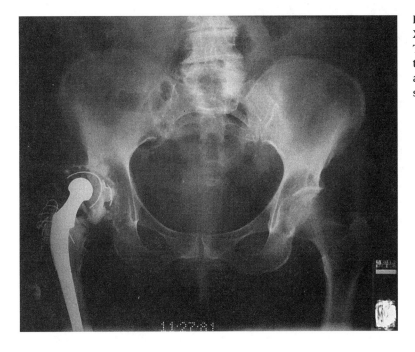

FIG. 11–22
X-ray of a client with a total hip replacement. The femoral prosthesis performs the function of the neck and head of the femur, whereas the acetabular prosthesis provides a smooth, stable surface.

FIG. 11–23
Dislocation of a total hip replacement. Pictured is an X-ray of a hip replacement that has become dislocated. Notice the positioning of the head of the prosthesis superior to the acetabulum. Dislocations of hip arthroplasties may occur as a result of excessive hip motion produced when the client crosses his or her legs, puts on a pair of shoes, or rolls over in bed. Hip replacement range-of-motion precautions should be followed as a guide to minimize the risk of dislocation.

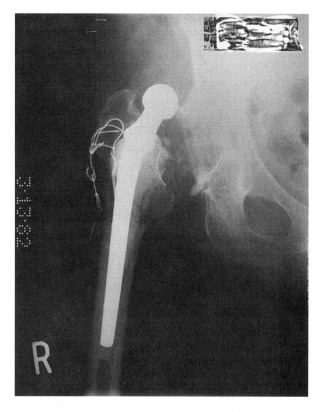

Clinical Management. Clients with total hip replacements are almost exclusively managed according to a specific protocol established by a physician. The operating surgeon either will dictate the parameters of rehabilitation after the client has successfully completed surgery or will have an established protocol in place to be followed at the facility. The protocols will also vary depending on the type of fixation used for the hip replacement (cemented versus cementless) and the surgical approach used (anterior vs. posterior).[49]

Weight-bearing protocols will differ depending on the type of fixation used. Surgeons who opt for a cemented approach will use a type of bone cement to hold the prosthetic components in place. The cement used will reach maximal strength in about 15 minutes after it is set in the operating room. With this type of fixation, the client will be allowed WBAT using a walker immediately after surgery. Cementless fixation occurs as a result of pressing the prosthesis into the available bone. The ultimate fixation comes as the bone grows into the components of the prosthesis. The stability of the noncemented hip replacement does not come for several weeks after surgery until new bone growth is implanted into the prosthesis. Surgeons, to prevent slipping of the prosthesis, will restrict weight bearing to TTWB or PWB with a walker for up to 6 to 12 weeks. Maximal stability of the noncemented hip is probably not achieved, however, until 6 months after surgery.[49]

Other variations in protocols after a total hip replacement center on the NWB forces allowed on the hip. Some protocols will prohibit straight-leg raises because of the excessive torques placed on the hip joint and the fear of loosening the femoral prosthesis. Excessive hip rotation forces that occur while moving from sit to stand are discouraged as well. The client should be encouraged to use his or her arms as much as possible to help lift his or her body out of a chair and reduce the stress on the hip joint. Excessive rotational forces that occur from a Trendelenburg gait should also be avoided. The use of assistive devices to correct any gait deviation should be incorporated until the client is able to ambulate without deviations (this may take many months or even years).[49]

One chief concern for the long-term integrity of the implanted hip prosthesis is the prevention of a dislocating episode (see Fig. 11–23). After a total hip replacement, some clients will experience the femoral prosthesis (ball) dislocating from the acetabular component (socket). Many speculative conditions can predispose a client to a dislocation including:

1. Excessive movement in certain combination patterns, causing instability
   a. Anterior surgical approach (susceptible to anterior dislocation): relative hip position of extension, adduction, and external rotation
   b. Posterior surgical approach (suspectible to posterior dislocation): relative hip position of flexion, adduction, and internal rotation
2. Poor client compliance with postsurgical precautions
3. Inadequate surgical alignment of prosthetic components

No conclusive data exist on predicting a dislocating episode, but general evidence indicates that most episodes of dislocation occur soon after the surgery, rather than later in the healing and rehabilitation process. This situation may be related to the amount of soft-tissue healing that has occurred. Some clients will be required to maintain the motion limitations on the repaired hip for up to 6 months, whereas others are required to continue total hip replacement precautions throughout life, as follows[1]:

• Do not lie on the surgical side.
• Do not cross legs.
• Do not remove pillow from between legs while in bed.
• Do not sit in low chairs.
• Do not sit on a regular toilet seat.
• Do not bend over to pick up *anything*!
• Do not sit up in bed and reach to pull up covers.
• Do not stand up from the back of a chair (slide to the front).
• Do not bring your knees to your chest.
• Keep legs apart when sitting.

Critical rehabilitation management areas include safe transfers, progression of the weight-bearing abilities, strengthening of the hip muscles (in particular the abductors), balance activities, self-care skills, and proper education on the maintenance of the surgically replaced hip. Initial rehabilitation efforts should focus on the functional mobility of the client executing safe transfers while not jeopardizing the integrity of the hip replacement. Despite the trauma of the surgery and the immediate need for rest after a surgery, the rehabilitation team must promote early mobility to prevent the onset of DVT. The risk for development of DVT is greatest in the first 3 weeks after surgery. Gait activities should follow the weight-bearing prescription of the surgeon. Isometric hip and knee exercises (quads, hamstrings, gluteals, and abductors) as well as ankle-pumping exercises should begin immediately. AROM hip exercises may be performed early or later in the rehabilitation program, depending on the protocols of the physician. The hip abductor muscles have been described as the most critical element for strengthening after a total hip replacement surgery in preventing gait deviations. Avoiding a postsurgical hip flexion contracture can be accomplished by performing a Thomas stretch. With the client lying supine, have the client pull the uninvolved leg toward the chest and then press the surgical leg into the mattress of the bed. Standing balance activities and lower-extremity ROM should be incorporated into the rehabilitation program as soon as tolerated by the client. The use of the abductor wedge while the client is in bed usually lasts for 6 weeks.

The physical therapy expected outcomes for managing a client with a total hip replacement include[30]:

1. An optimal return of function
2. Reduced risk of further disability from identified limitations
3. Improved safety awareness of client
4. Improved self-care skills and ADLs
5. An understanding of risk factors that may contribute to jeopardizing health status
6. An understanding of strategies to prevent further disability

The expected time frame for achieving the outcomes is 6 to 12 weeks. The client may be discharged from the acute care setting to a long-term care facility, long-term rehabilitation unit, or directly to home with the home health services. Clients with total hip replacement surgeries generally have successful outcomes. Johnsson et al.[50] suggested that it is critical for the rehabilitation team to help the client with concerns of progressing with assistive devices and performing functional skills well beyond the acute phase of rehabilitation. As the client improves related to ROM, strength, and balance, new methods and strategies are needed to safely accomplish functional tasks at home.

Total Knee Replacement

Not unlike a total hip replacement surgery, the total knee replacement (TKR) is a successful surgical procedure. Clients with severe arthritic deformity, pain, or weight-bearing dysfunctions are candidates for a knee arthroplasty. Unlike the hip replacement, the knee replacement is significantly more prone to infection, and the rehabilitation team should be keenly aware of and educate the client about the signs of infection after surgery. The TKR tends to cause significantly greater discomfort for the client. The rehabilitation team should work to educate the client early in the rehabilitation process on the issues of moderate to severe pain and the need to progress through severe discomfort.[1,49]

Clinical Presentation. The client with a TKR will most likely present in the acute care setting with a protective dressing covering the recent surgical incision. Staples or sutures will secure the longitudinal incision that spans the anterior or anterolateral surface of the knee. Pain medicine will probably be used by the client for control of the postsurgical discomfort and a full-length lower-extremity compression stocking may be applied to prevent the onset of DVT. The client may have a straight-leg immobilizer to be used during gait for protection of the knee and assistance in maintaining terminal extension. The immobilizer is also useful in preserving terminal extension of the knee if the client sleeps with the device in place. After the surgical incision is healed, the knee of the client will look similar to Figure 11–24. A radiographic examination of a total knee arthroplasty is pictured in Figure 11–25.

Evaluation: Tools and Methods. The evaluation performed by the PT may follow a functional outcome form used by the facility. It should contain a subjective

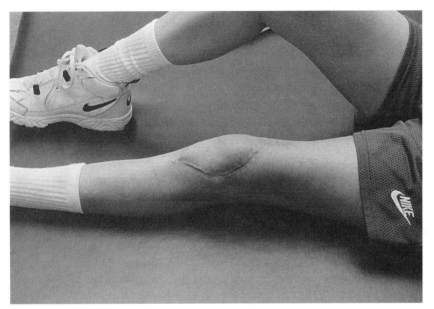

FIG. 11–24
Healed incision of a TKR. The surgical incision used by the orthopedic surgeon
may be longitudinal in an anterior fashion, or anterolateral as pictured here.

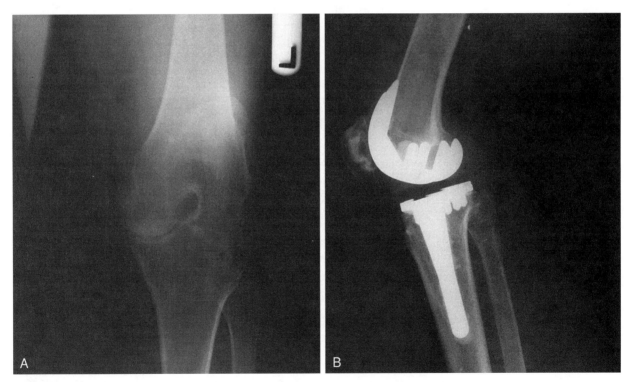

FIG. 11–25
X-Ray of a client with a total knee replacement. Pain and degenerative changes are indications for joint replacement.
An arthritic knee (A). Notice the narrowing of the joint space and the uneven articulating surfaces. Notice the placement
of the distal femur prosthesis that resurfaces the femoral condyles and the proximal tibial prosthesis that acts as the
receptacle for the new femoral condyles (B).

history, including a description of pain and discomfort. Objectively, ROM measurements of the surgical and nonsurgical knee and lower extremity should be documented. Strength, sensory, and balance assessments may also be documented. Functional skills including bed mobility skills, transfer skills, and gait skills will be included.

Clinical Management. Protocols are frequently used in the rehabilitation of the client with a knee arthroplasty. Common to all protocols is the need for early, aggressive motion. If the ROM is not restored early during the healing phases of the soft tissue, long-term dysfunction may result. If significant motion limitation is present after surgery, the surgeon may opt for a manipulation under anesthesia to forcefully gain greater motion. Because of the effects of healing of the soft tissue, most surgeons prefer to perform a manipulation closer to the surgery date than farther from the date. If significant healing has taken place and a manipulation is performed, greater force to sever adhesions is needed and may result in postmanipulation complications. This procedure is potentially more painful than the original operation.[49]

The client should be instructed initially in ankle-pumping exercises to help promote venous return in the distal lower extremity (see Fig. 11–16). This simple active ROM exercise of the ankle helps to facilitate circulation, reduce edema, and deter the risk of the onset of DVT. The incidence of DVT in post-TKR clients is 10% or greater.[49]

Pain control is important in the initiation of rehabilitation after TKR surgery. Significant pain can be a detriment to exercise, walking, or performing the necessary activities that will assist in the return to optimal functioning. Delaying in beginning ROM activities due to pain may allow the repaired knee to heal in a shortened or contracted position. Angulo and Colwell[51] concluded that the use of transcutaneous electrical stimulation is indicated for the reduction of postopera-

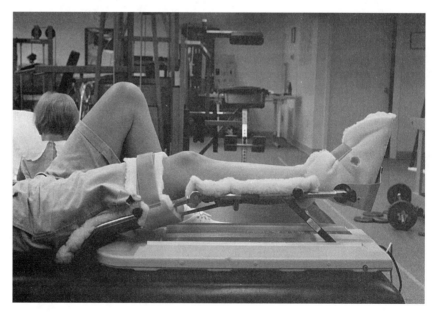

FIG. 11–26
Utilizing continuous passive motion (CPM) after a TKR can help reduce the length of stay in the hospital as well as postsurgical complications. Review Chapter 5 for full details on the clinical utilization of CPM.

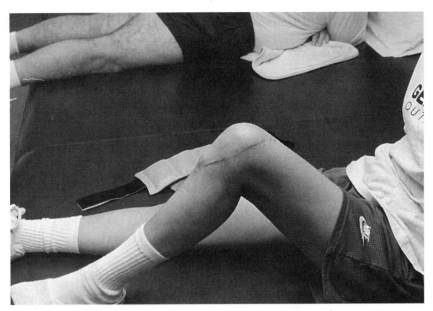

FIG. 11–27
Heel slides. Knee flexion can be promoted by having the client long sit on a therapy mat and actively slide the heel toward the buttock. When a good stretch of the soft tissue is achieved, have the client hold the position allowing elongation to occur. Many repetitions of this exercise are needed.

tive pain. Cryotherapy has been frequently used in various forms to help alleviate postsurgical pain and swelling. Physicians rely heavily on pain-killing narcotics to block pain perception. The PTA will soon discover that lower pain levels in the client will result in more productive treatment sessions.

Continuous passive motion has been widely used postsurgically for the client who undergoes TKR surgery (Fig. 11–26). Gose[52] in a retrospective study indicated that the use of CPM reduced the length of stay and the number of postoperative complications in clients who received a TKR as compared with those clients who received a TKR without CPM. Gose did not find, however, a significant difference in the ROM of the two comparative groups. Some studies have shown that aggressive early CPM use may increase the incidence of wound complications.[49]

Exercises to promote the functional return of the client after TKR surgery should address restoring ROM, strength, balance, and coordination in the affected limb. Promoting maximal knee flexion and extension of the knee is a slow process, but is necessary in regaining functional use of the knee. If the client cannot flex the knee past 90°, then there will be difficulty getting in and out of cars, sitting in a movie theater, or climbing stairs. If the client cannot obtain full extension, then significant gait deviations will result, potentially leading to excessive wear and tear on the opposite extremity or the spine. Heel slides (Fig. 11–27) and sitting knee flexion (Fig. 11–28) will help promote gains in flexion. AROM or PROM exercises can be used to help facilitate knee extension. Active or electrically assisted quad sets can help promote terminal knee extension. Passive techniques include using the opposite extremity to help stretch the knee (Fig. 11–29) or allowing gravity to passively extend the knee (Fig. 11–30). The use of mobilization techniques, either sustained or oscillatory, can significantly benefit the improvement of motion.

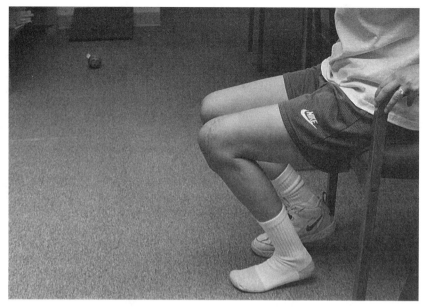

FIG. 11–28
Sitting knee flexion. The client may also achieve knee flexion by sitting in a stable chair and gradually pulling the involved limb under the chair. The opposite extremity may assist the pulling process.

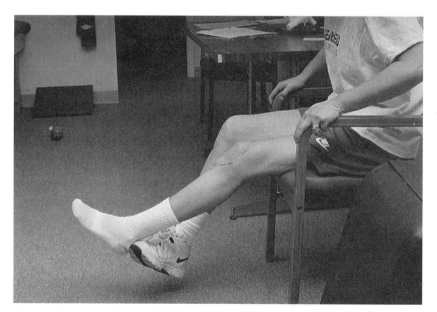

FIG. 11–29
Self-assisted passive knee extension. In the sitting position, the client can use the opposite extremity to help terminally extend the knee. When a good stretching sensation is perceived, the client should hold the stretch to allow for elongation of the soft tissue structures.

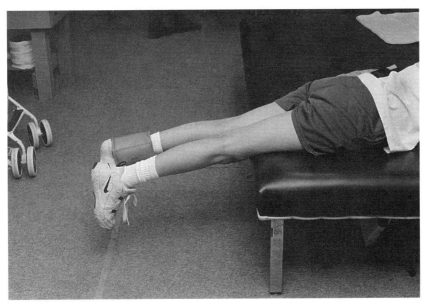

FIG. 11–30
Gravity-assisted passive knee extension. Prone leg hangs will use the effects of gravity to help extend the knee passively. Ensure that the patella is free from compression from the table, to avoid irritation. The client may lie in this position for up to 20 minutes as tolerated to help promote plastic elongation of the structures. The addition of ankle weights should be considered if tolerated by the client.

Techniques should focus on the mobility of both the tibiofemoral joint and the patellofemoral joint. Review specific mobilization techniques in Chapter 7.

Strengthening exercises should include the restoration of strength to the knee and adjacent joints of the lower extremity as well as the promotion of functional endurance. After total joint surgery to the knee, strength of the quadriceps femoris is critical in promoting safety during gait activities and transfers. If the knee extensor musculature is physically unable to maintain the knee in an extended position when weight bearing, there is a greater risk of falling (Fig. 11–31). Exercises that strengthen the quadriceps femoris muscle include isometric quad sets, straight-leg raises, mechanically resisted large arc quads (Figs. 11–32 and 11–33), or closed-chain exercises (Figs. 11–34 and 11–35). Strengthening the abductors of the hip helps promote stability of the pelvis during gait activities (Fig. 11–36). Addressing the strength of the hamstrings will help promote muscular balance around the knee joint (Fig. 11–37). Balance and coordination concerns can be addressed through closed-chain exercises that strengthen the entire lower extremity and facilitate the proper neuromuscular timing of the involved dynamic elements (see Figs. 11–35 and 11–38).

The physical therapy expected outcomes[29] to manage the client with a TKR include:

1. An optimal return of function
2. Reduced risk of further disability from identified limitations
3. Improved safety awareness of client
4. Improved self-care skills and ADLs
5. An understanding of risk factors that may contribute to jeopardizing health status

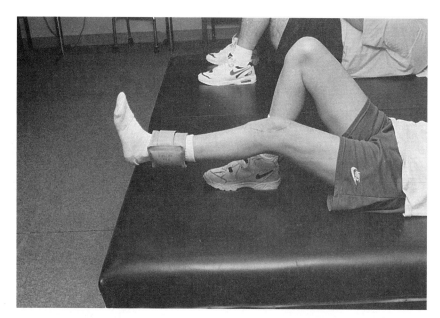

FIG. 11–31

Knee extensor mechanism lag. Pictured here is a client who has recently undergone a total knee replacement on her left side due to arthritic changes in the knee joint. As she lifts the leg against resistance, a noticeable lag or inability to maintain terminal knee extension is noted. This client's lag was measured at 25°. Some controversy exists over whether to have this client perform straight leg raises in the presence of an extensor lag. Critics believe that if the quadriceps femoris muscle is repeatedly exercised, encouraging a lag, then the muscle will adapt (specificity of exercise) to this position as normal. A better approach to strengthening may be keeping the client in a terminal position, performing isometric exercises or reducing the resistance to the point at which the client can actively maintain terminal knee extension while performing the exercise.

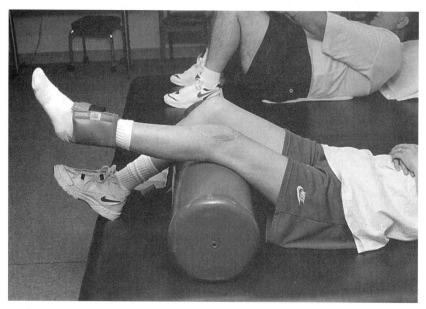

FIG. 11–32

Large arc quads (LAQ) with ankle weights. Placing the involved knee over a bolster will assist the client in moving the knee joint through a large ROM. Emphasis should be placed on the client's achieving terminal extension of the knee at the end of motion.

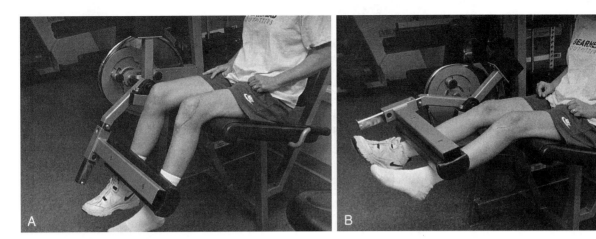

FIG. 11–33
Large arc quads (LAQ) with knee extension machine. Sitting knee extension machines (A) can also provide for a large arc of motion for knee extension (B). Care should be taken as with LAQ with ankle weights, that terminal knee extension is achieved and patellar irritation avoided.

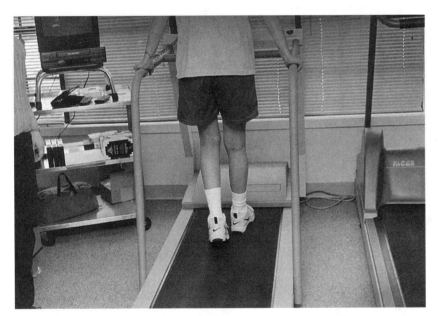

FIG. 11–34
Closed-chain lower extremity. Treadmill—This client is performing a closed chain exercise for the lower extremity as she is walking backward on this treadmill (this is a reversible treadmill). The two-dimensional picture does not fully illustrate the amount of work the quadriceps femoris of this client is performing.

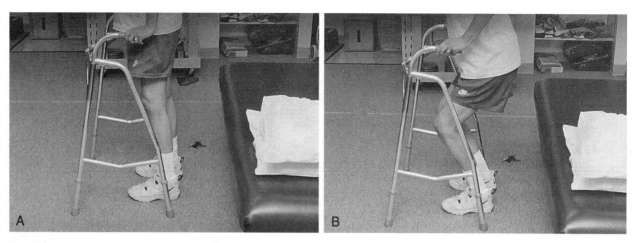

FIG. 11-35
Closed-chain lower extremity. Squats—The client can use a walker as an assistive tool (A) in order to perform standing closed chain squats for the lower extremity (B).

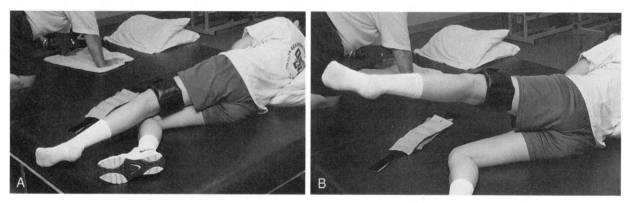

FIG. 11-36
Resisted hip abduction. The gluteus medius muscle is a primary stabilizer of the pelvis during locomotion. Strengthening hip abduction is important for promoting stability during gait. The ankle weight can be placed proximally (A) on the thigh for the client to perform hip abduction (B). If the same weight is moved distally, the force needed to move the limb is increased.

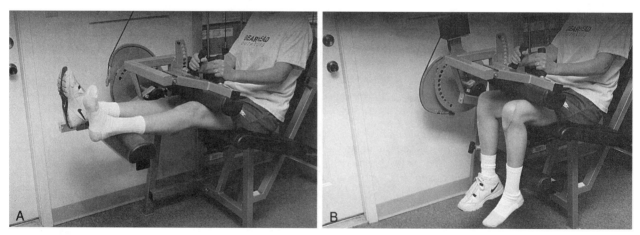

FIG. 11-37
Resisted knee flexion. A sitting knee flexion machine (A) can provide adequate resistance for the hamstring group (B).

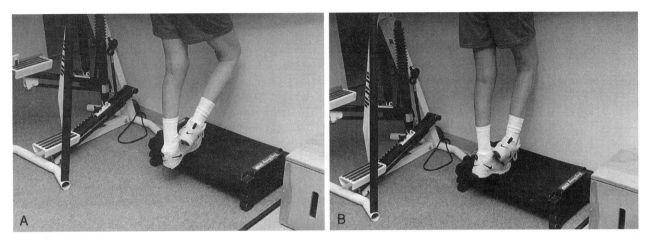

FIG. 11–38
Closed-chain lower extremity. Toe Raises—This client is standing on the edge of an aerobic step (A) and repeatedly raises and lowers her body weight on the involved leg (B).

The expected time frame for achieving the outcomes is 3 to 6 months. Most clients should achieve functional motion in the surgical knee (about 110° of flexion), but not significantly much more.

FUNCTIONAL IMPAIRMENTS

Rotator Cuff Tears

The blending into a common cuff of the supraspinatus, infraspinatus, subscapularis, and teres minor tendons forms the dynamic stabilizer for the glenohumeral joint. A rotator cuff tear is one of the two most common shoulder pathologies seen in the geriatric population (the other is bursitis and will be discussed later in this chapter). The etiology of the rotator cuff dysfunction in the geriatric population is usually insidious without a specific traumatic event. A gradual eroding of the cuff from osteophytes or from abnormal arthrokinematics are potential precursors to a rotator cuff tear. Traumatic incidents are possible, but they are more common in younger, more active populations. The classic client with a rotator cuff tear is a baseball pitcher; however, many clients across the life span can develop the same pathology. Functional deficits in the rotator cuff will cause improper arthrokinematics and decreased stability of the humeral head. The client may be more susceptible to impingement problems if excessive superior gliding in the glenohumeral joint is a result. Conservative management of small tears and dysfunctions is possible. Surgical repairs of the rotator cuff are necessary when the dysfunction is significant and when the pain is intolerable.[1]

Clinical Presentation. One of the most frequent complaints from individuals in geriatric population with rotator cuff pathologies is the inability to sleep. Crepitus or clicking in the shoulder joint may occur if the lesion has begun scarring or the joint capsule is fibrotic. Weakness of the rotator cuff muscles will be measurable, and atrophy may be observed. Abnormal movement and arthrokinematics may be noted as the client tries to lift the arm to the front (flexion) or side (abduction). The client may elevate the scapula in an unsuccessful attempt to gain more ROM. With traumatic, grade III lesions, the client will be unable to lift the arm from the side of the body because the humeral head cannot be stabilized in the glenoid fossa.[1]

When the client is first seen in the physical therapy setting after the rotator cuff has been surgically repaired, the affected arm will most likely be protected in an over-the-shoulder sling. At this point in the rehabilitation efforts, the shoulder of the client is functionally weak and the client is unable to lift the arm or protect it from further injury. Staples or sutures most likely are present holding the superior surgical incision secure (Fig. 11–39).

Evaluation: Tools and Methods. The evaluating PT will take a complete history including details of the operation, if available. Following surgery, if physician protocols are to be part of the rehabilitation program, then a copy of the protocol sheet should be incorporated into the plan of treatment. Initial ROM measurements of the repaired shoulder should be documented, as well as assessments of pain and swelling. An initial status of the surgical incision should be thoroughly recorded. The presence of staples or sutures, as well as drainage amount, color, and odor, should be noted. Strength and functional assessments of the shoulder are frequently deferred until later in the rehabilitation process. However, the comprehensive evaluation will include the cervical, elbow, and hand regions to document a baseline of strength and movement. Care and periodic reassessment should help identify the onset of secondary complications after rotator cuff repair or injury, such as RSD or adhesive capsulitis.

Clinical Management. Conservative management for the torn rotator cuff is symptomatic. Pain and inflammation should be controlled through modalities and medications prescribed by the physician. ROM activities that avoid painful arcs of

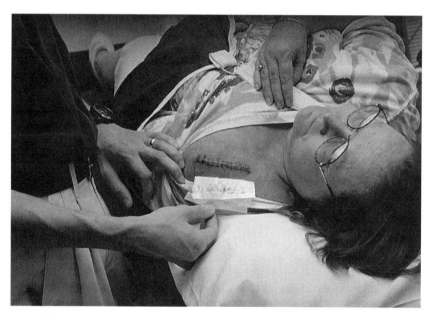

FIG. 11–39
Rotator cuff repair incision. The incision for most rotator cuff repairs is made superiorly and secured with staples. A protective dressing covers the incision to protect the healing tissue from the irritation of clothing and the possibility of infection. Drainage from the site could stain clothing as well.

motion should be included. As the pain reduces over time, a gradual strengthening program designed to promote the integrity of the rotator cuff should be undertaken. Elastic tubing or small hand weights and isometric protocols are adequate for the resistance exercises. Functional activities should be developed as strength and motion improve. The geriatric client with a torn rotator cuff may never achieve full motion and normal strength, but should indeed be functional with the upper extremity. For this very reason, a significant portion of minor rotator cuffs in geriatric clients are managed conservatively.[1]

After a surgical repair of the dysfunctional rotator cuff, adherence to established physician protocols is required. Acute discomfort after the surgery may be alleviated with the use of topical modalities designed to reduce pain and inflammation. A period of PROM typically precedes any AROM exercises. Wand exercises, self-ROM, or over-the-door pulleys are effective tools in accomplishing passive motion. Strengthening is frequently limited to isometric exercises with the arm in the sling or at the client's until active motion is allowed. The delivery of superficial heat before ROM and mobilization activities may help relax the client and reduce discomfort (Fig. 11–40). Gentle PROM exercises can accompany gentle grade I or II oscillations or grade I sustained mobilization techniques to promote an increase in motion (Fig. 11–41). Great care should be taken to promote the restoration of normal joint arthrokinematics and the avoidance of injury to the recently repaired structures.[35]

As the protocol dictates, AROM and strengthening are permitted. PROM gains will quickly exceed AROM gains in most surgically repaired rotator cuffs. At times, the client may become frustrated because he or she cannot (or must not) actively move the arm. This is to be expected and is not out of the ordinary. Gradual strengthening will eventually lead to independent control of the repaired

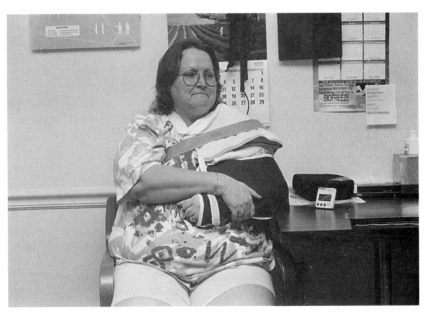

FIG. 11–40
Superficial heat applied to the client with a rotator cuff repair. A moist cervical heat pack can be secured superiorly on the client's shoulder to deliver superficial heat on a surgically repaired rotator cuff. Sometimes the weight of a larger moist heat pack may not be tolerated by the client.

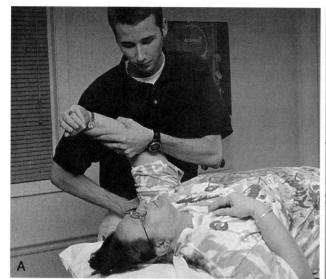
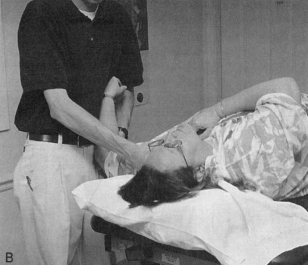
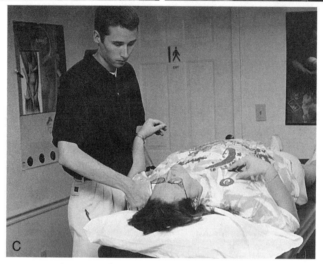

FIG. 11–41

ROM after a rotator cuff repair. With the client positioned supine, the therapist can easily access the repaired shoulder to perform ROM exercises. Shoulder flexion (A), abduction (B), and external rotation (C) are performed in the early stages of rehabilitation without forcing the extremes of ROM or causing pain. External rotation is best performed initially with the arm at the side of the client to avoid potential impingement of the greater tuberosity under the acromial arch when the arm is abducted to 90°. The therapist should firmly and securely manage the weight of the extremity because the client will not yet have adequate strength to support the arm. Be sure to encourage the client to relax if the desired motion is passive.

extremity. At that time, functional activities should be included to stimulate the mechanoreceptors and proprioceptors found throughout the arm. The client should not be encouraged to rush through the rehabilitation process, but to have patience.

The expected physical therapy outcomes for managing a client with a rotator cuff repair include[30]:

1. An optimal return of function
2. Improved self-care skills and ADLs
3. An understanding of strategies to prevent further disability

The expected time frame for achieving the outcomes after a rotator cuff surgical repair is 6 to 12 months.

Adhesive Capsulitis

Also known as a "frozen shoulder," geriatric clients are prone to develop capsular limitations of the shoulder after a traumatic incident or sometimes for no particular reason. Adhesive capsulitis can complicate primary conditions as in a rotator cuff injury or repair, which will cause significant functional limitations of the shoulder and upper extremity.[1] Ultimately, the dysfunctional joint capsule leads to abnormal arthrokinematics of the glenohumeral joint, preventing smooth and effective movement.

Clinical Presentation. A frozen shoulder may be either primary or secondary, depending on the precipitating factor. A primary frozen shoulder is of unknown etiology. A secondary frozen shoulder is the result of a known pathology, such as a fracture or a rotator cuff injury. Typically, the dominant extremity of the client is involved. The classic periods that can be identified by the client when looking back on the condition include (1) painful or freezing phase, (2) stiffening or frozen phase, and (3) thawing phase.

The *freezing phase* of a frozen shoulder may last 2 to 9 months. The pain in the shoulder is gradual and diffuse, with no noticeable loss of motion. The client has a subtle loss of glenohumeral motion and discomfort and also tends to avoid using the extremity. The *frozen phase* may last 4 to 12 months, causing motion restrictions but very little pain. The classic characteristic of a frozen shoulder is capsular tightness. The loss of motion is a result of an inflammatory process that causes the joint capsule to adhere to the anatomic neck of the humerus. The capsule may even adhere to itself in the redundant inferior axillary fold. As the condition progresses, a loss in joint space and accessory motion is noted. External rotation and abduction movements of the shoulder are significantly limited, followed by decreased flexion and internal rotation. The client may assume a protracted scapular posture, demonstrating concurrent muscle atrophy of the deltoid, rotator cuff, biceps, or triceps muscles. Tenderness can be palpated along the anterior joint capsule of the involved shoulder. In the *thawing phase*, no clear definition exists as very few consistent characteristics are clinically present. The time frame for return to function is variable. Some clients may regain full motion, while others retain a significant disability.[1,48]

Evaluation: Tools and Methods. The evaluation for a client with an adhesive capsulitis will contain a medical history and subjective reports of the condition, including the level and quality of pain and perceived functional limitations. Objective measures include assessment of ROM, strength, joint play, and posture.

Clinical Management. Effectively managing a client with a frozen shoulder depends on the early identification of the adherent condition. If it is several years before the geriatric client seeks medical attention, then it is unlikely that significant amounts of motion will be regained. Early intervention is essential. The onset of the condition is insidious, and thus the client may not notice the inability to fully reach overhead. This activity is not a regular part of every elderly client's day. When the client notices that he or she cannot reach into the top cabinet (about 130° off flexion), that is usually when medical attention is sought. By that time, however, almost one-third of the glenohumeral motion has been lost.

The ultimate goal for the rehabilitation of a frozen shoulder is to improve functional mobility of the shoulder. This is typically accomplished through joint mobilization techniques that stretch the joint capsule and restore normal arthrokinematics. Topical modalities such as heat, ultrasound, or cold may be used as preparatory agents for mobilization and stretching. Ice should be used for intense pain reduction, but only if tolerated by the client. Appropriate joint mobilization techniques should be performed according to the plan of treatment to facilitate gains in the direction of joint limitations. As motion improves, AROM exercises and strengthening should supplement the treatment. Isometric exercises can progress to resistive activities, as tolerated by the client. Great care should be taken to avoid any painful motion that may promote reflexive tightening of the shoulder girdle muscles and soft tissue. Frequently, postural exercises for correction of deficits are helpful in the ultimate management of a client with a frozen shoulder.[35,48]

If the client fails to progress, further investigation is necessary. The client may have sustained an associated fracture, rotator cuff tear, or pathological condition that was not initially identified. Manipulations under anesthesia or surgical intervention may be considered for cases resistant to conservative stretching and mobilization.[48]

The expected physical therapy outcomes related to the management of a client with adhesive capsulitis include[30]:

1. Improved health-related quality of life
2. Improved functional skills
3. Reduced risk of further disability from identified limitations
4. Improved self-care skills and activities of daily living
5. An understanding of risk factors that may contribute to jeopardizing health status
6. An understanding of strategies to prevent further disability

The expected time frame for achieving the outcome is 3 to 6 months after the condition has been identified. The cumulative amount of time from the onset of the condition may last as long as 2 years if there was a significant delay in seeking medical attention.

Reflex Sympathetic Dystrophy

Reflex sympathetic dystrophy syndrome is an excessive or abnormal response of the sympathetic nervous system following an injury. RSD is a disorder that affects as many as 5% of injured clients, usually following a trauma to the face, neck, or extremities. It is not specific to the geriatric population, but can occur across the life span. Most commonly, RSD is observed in the upper extremity following a neck, shoulder, elbow, or wrist injury. There is no direct relationship between the severity of an injury and the onset of symptoms associated with RSD. Despite the intense discomfort associated with the symptoms of RSD, immediate, early detection is often delayed. Stralka[53] reports that the average client does not seek medical attention for the painful symptoms for 10 days. Further prolonging the diagnosis of this painful condition is the fact that medical professionals often misdiagnose the symptoms for those of another condition.

There are many synonymous terms associated with reflex sympathetic dystrophy. Some authors even believe that RSD is a generic term for more specific conditions.[53] *Sudeck's atrophy, shoulder-hand syndrome, post-traumatic pain syndrome, algodystrophy,* and *major and minor causalgia* are terms that have been associated with

RSD. Current debate continues to separate symptom deviations between neurogenic and vascular pain. This section presents RSD as one overall painful condition causing significant impairment to afflicted clients.[35,53]

Clinical Presentation. The signs and symptoms of RSD form a self-perpetuating circle (Fig. 11–42). Common complaints and problems associated with RSD include:

1. Diffuse or burning pain
2. Hypersensitive skin
3. **Allodynia**
4. Peripheral edema
5. **Hyperhidrosis**
6. Vasomotor instability
7. Increased bone resorption
8. Depressed motor function
9. Integumentary dystrophic changes (including shiny skin and loss of normal skin wrinkles)

Allodynia
Pain perceived by the client from a stimulus that would not otherwise cause a painful response.

Hyperhidrosis
Sweating more than would be expected for the environmental conditions.

The onset of symptoms is highly variable and unpredictable. RSD can manifest in clients after an inflammatory process, surgery, immobilization for fractures, superficial burns, and traumatic injuries. The client may develop symptoms from common orthopedic conditions, such as sprains, dislocations, fractures and amputations. The symptoms are grouped into three general stages of the disease process. Some clients exhibit only a few symptoms presented above, whereas others manifest with almost all of the symptoms listed. The most prevailing clinical observation is perceived pain by the client that is disproportionate to the severity of the actual injury. Table 11–6 presents the general clinical course of RSD.

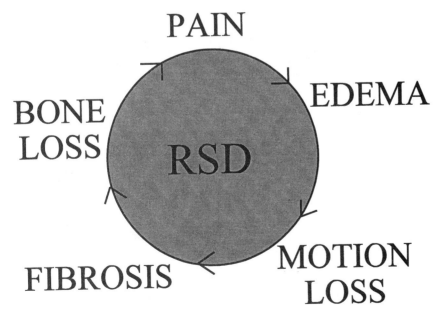

FIG. 11–42
Cycle of pain associated with RSD.

Table 11–6

CLINICAL COURSE OF REFLEX SYMPATHETIC DYSTROPHY

Phase 1: Acute Stage (onset can be immediate or delayed)	Edema that is soft and pliable Acute, intense pain Hyperasthesias Loss of ROM in affected part Spasms of associated muscles Hyperthermia
Phase 1: Late Signs (onset 3–6 wk after start of phase 1)	Cold, clammy, and cyanotic skin Osteoporosis (Sudeck's atrophy) Hair and nail changes Hyperhidrosis
Phase 2: Dystrophy Stage (onset anywhere from 2–6 mo after phase 1)	Pain lessens Edema that is tough and firm Loss of skin wrinkles Shiny skin Hyperesthesias Joint stiffness Hyperhidrosis Muscular atrophy Hair and nail changes
Phase 3: Atrophy Stage (onset anywhere from 6–12 mo after phase 1)	Pain continues to lessen Diffuse muscular and bony atrophy Fascial thickening Joint ankylosis Cool, glossy skin

Evaluation: Tools and Methods. Identifying a client with RSD is key to the successful treatment of the client. Frequently the rehabilitation team may be working with a client for a primary injury and should be aware of an onset of hypersensitivity that is disproportionate to the injury being treated. If RSD is suspected by the PTA, then the supervising PT should be contacted immediately. Management of the client with RSD is achieved through an interdisciplinary pain management center including a physician, anesthesiologist, psychologist, and therapist. The evaluating team must not only be skilled in the treatment of the condition, but must also be compassionate with regard to the extreme pain and discomfort the client has experienced. When the PT evaluates the client specifically for RSD, a detailed description of the pain and precipitating factors should be identified. Objective measures of ROM, edema, sensation, and integumentary status should be documented. Also, for proper management, the therapist should identify elements or activities that exacerbate the vasomotor tone or make the symptoms worse. By focusing on elements that relax the vasomotor tone or decrease the symptoms, a starting point for treatment can be found.[53]

Clinical Management. An understanding of the pain cycle that accompanies the signs and symptoms of RSD is central to the management of the client. The extreme perceived pain results in the avoidance of movement. The self-imposed immobilization causes stiffness and edema. The immobilization also leads to disuse atrophy of the muscles and decreases the ability of fluids to move through the extremity. Edema increases, creating fibrotic adhesions in the muscles and joints. Osteoporosis may soon enter the clinical picture, completing the painful cycle leading back to increased pain and discomfort. Breaking the pain cycle is critical to the successful management of the client with RSD. The effective management of RSD does not center on resolving one of these components, but on bringing about a gradual decrease in all the components of the pain cycle. If the rehabilitation team is successful in reducing only one component, a brief reduction in symptoms may result, but the symptoms are likely to return.[53]

Initial management of the client with RSD should focus on pain reduction, edema control, and improving ROM. The starting point frequently begins with interventions that do not increase the symptoms, gradually expanding treatment. It is difficult to follow a specific protocol for clients with RSD, because each case is extremely individualized. What works for one client may be an exacerbating factor for another. The general medical approach to management of the pain is trying various medications to depress the excessive sympathetic response of the client. Analgesics, corticosteroids, NSAIDs, antidepressants, anticonvulsants, and nerve blocks have all been used. TENS has been indicated because of the relatively low amount of side effects of long-term use. Desensitization techniques, such as rubbing and tapping different textures on the skin or using a fluidotherapy machine, may be of benefit to help decrease hypersensitivity. Superficial modalities do not seem to be beneficial in reducing pain and may increase the hypersensitivity to touch. Edema control may be managed through the use of compression pumps, gloves, elevation, retrograde massage, and possibly high-volt galvanic stimulation. Motion concerns can be managed through CPM, dynamic splinting, and AROM exercises. Weight-bearing exercises on the involved extremity seem to be helpful in promoting ROM as well as bone integrity. Other areas to address in the management of the client with RSD include stress management and the return to functional activities.[53]

The expected physical therapy outcomes related to the management of a client with RSD include[30]:

1. Improved health-related quality of life
2. Improved functional skills
3. Reduced risk of further disability from identified limitations
4. Improved self-care skills and ADLs
5. An understanding of strategies to prevent further disability

The expected time frame for achieving the outcomes is highly variable. The duration of the pain is not related to any measurable severity of the initial injury. Symptoms associated with RSD last up to 6 months in 75% of the cases. The remaining cases may have pain and discomfort for longer than 1 year. The best management approach is the early detection and prevention of the symptoms.[53]

Hand Deformities

Hand deformities that will limit the functional abilities of the geriatric client are common. According to Lewis and Bottomley,[1] the three most common pathologies leading to deformities of the hand in the geriatric client are (1) RA, (2) DJD, and (3) Dupuytren's contractures (see Chapter 10). In the RA process, the synovial lining of the joint becomes diseased and weakened. The degenerative overuse process associated with DJD is more common than RA and usually involves the IP joints of the digits and the carpometacarpal joint of the thumb.

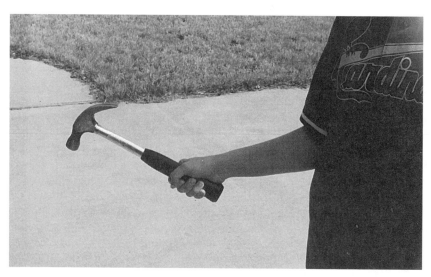

FIG. 11–43
Power grip, cylindrical. Power grips are used for forceful actions of the upper extremity, such as lifting or moving objects. The power grips are mostly isometric, fingers being flexed against the palm of the hand. The thumb is used to conform to the shape of the object and to add power and support to the grip. Pictured here is a cylindrical grip used to hold objects, such as a hammer.

Clinical Presentation. The client with RA may have classic deformities of ulnar drift of the digits, boutonniére, or swan-neck deformities. Joint stiffness, particularly in the morning, and pain are also common complaints by the client. Clients with DJD of the digits will have significant pain, swelling, and weakness associated with the condition.

The hand serves as the manipulative tool of the client's environment. Through a variety of power and precision gripping patterns (Figs. 11–43 through 11–50), the client is able to interact with the environment. To perform adequate precision

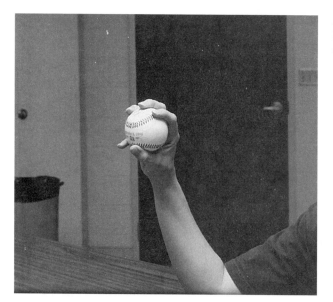

FIG. 11–44
Power grip, spherical. The power spherical grip is used for grasping objects such as a baseball.

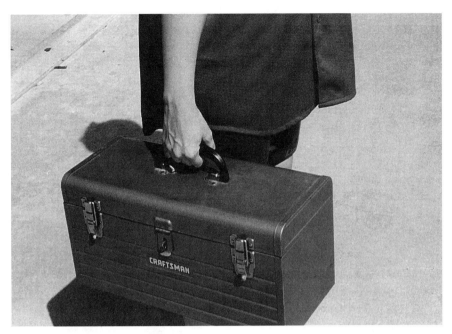

FIG. 11–45
Power grip, hook. The power hook grip is used for carrying a tool box.

grips, the thumb and first two fingers of the client must be fully functional. Successful power grips are performed by using the same digits as the precision grips, but with the addition of the last two fingers as power supplementors.[35]

Evaluation: Tools and Methods. Measuring grip strength using a hand dynamometer has been a traditional method to assess hand strength (see Figs.

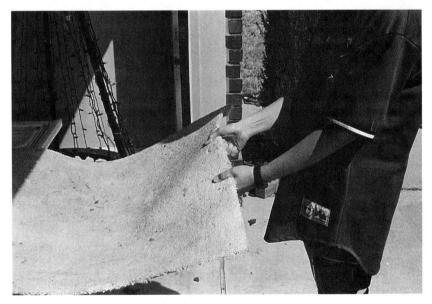

FIG. 11–46
Power grip, lateral prehension. Carpet layers promote the use of the lateral prehension grip to pull the carpet tight. The object is secured forcefully between the thumb and the lateral aspect of the hand.

FIG. 11–47
Precision grip, pad to pad. Precision grips almost exclusively use the thumb, index and middle finger to manipulate objects. The palm of the hand is not used, and the muscle contractions are mainly fine, graded isotonic contractions. Sensory feedback from the hand is critical for skillful manipulation of an object. Pictured here is a pad-to-pad grip, which is the type used when picking up a pencil.

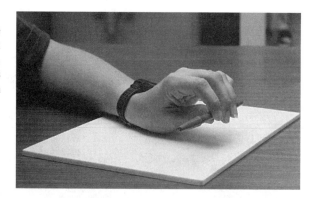

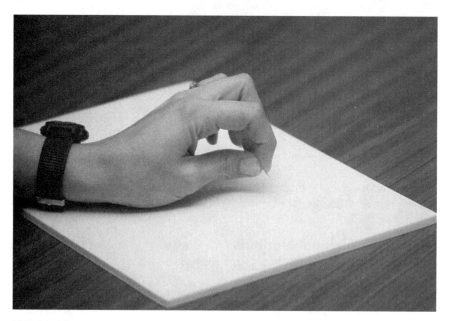

FIG. 11–48
Precision grip, tip to tip. A tip-to-tip precision grip is frequently used when a client sews.

FIG. 11–49
Precision grip, pad to side. The pad-to-side grip is used for skilled actions, such as throwing a dart.

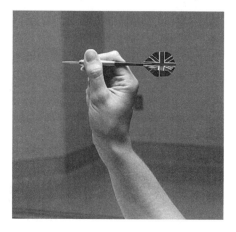

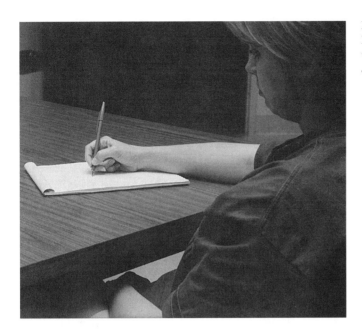

FIG. 11–50
Precision grip, three-point chuck. This precision grip is used when holding a pen or pencil to write (also referred to as a tripod grip or three-jaw chuck).

10–5 and 10–6). However, numerous studies have demonstrated that the geriatric client's grip strength can be influenced by various elements, including mental status and balance. Grip strength should be judiciously used as an assessment of function in the geriatric client.[1,54] Other tools to document the status of the client include ROM and functional measurements. The direct strength measured on a dynamometer can be used to judge individual progress, but should not be correlated to direct function of the hand. Some clients with significant hand deformities and weakness are indeed quite functional.

Clinical Management. The client with RA or DJD should be managed symptomatically. Intervention by the rehabilitation team will not reverse the condition, but decreased symptoms and functional improvement can be realistic goals. ROM exercises and topical heat modalities (whirlpool, fluidotherapy, paraffin bath) will help to alleviate stiffness of the joints. Some clients, during periods of exacerbation, find that the usually helpful heating agents may become irritating. If superficial heat benefits the client, methods should be investigated for the client to independently deliver the modality at home. There are many small home paraffin units or table fluidotherapy units available on the market today. Splinting and joint protection are critical so as to not advance the deformity or cause injury to the diseased hand. Some clients can use night splints to help limit the deformity, whereas others will have custom-made splints designed for support of their body part. Strategies should be discussed early for the efficient management of routine activities at home. By identifying less stressful methods of opening jars, dressing, or playing cards, the client can maintain a full, active lifestyle. Durable medical equipment catalogs have extensive supplies of various tools designed to make the small activities of life a bit easier. If the impairment of the hand and digits is significant and the client is no longer able to perform self-care skills adequately, then a joint replacement might be considered.[1,35]

The physical therapy expected outcomes to manage a client with RA include[30]:

1. Improved functional skills
2. Reduced risk of further disability from identified limitations

3. Improved self-care skills and ADLs
4. An understanding of strategies to prevent further disability

The expected time frame for achieving the outcomes is 4 to 6 weeks. The client should be educated in a comprehensive home exercise program for the lifelong management of the symptoms associated with the deformities.

Toe and Foot Deformities

Deformities of the foot are seldom causes of great mortality in the geriatric population, but are frequent sources of great morbidity and disability. Clients with pain and dysfunctional feet experience pain and discomfort with weight-bearing activities affecting almost every aspect of life. One survey reports as many as 30% of community-dwelling geriatric clients complaining of discomfort in their feet.[55] Many of the foot problems experienced by the geriatric population are due to poorly fitting or inadequate supporting footwear.

Clinical Presentation. Common problems include calluses, corns, and toe deformities. *Calluses* form from excessive friction resulting in a build-up of skin over the irritated area (typically found on the sole of the foot). *Corns* are built-up areas of skin typically on the bony areas of the digits as a result of friction. Corns can be particularly painful if excessive pressure is applied from footwear. *Toe deformities* can be clawlike or even overlapping. Often these are a result of narrow toe boxes (front of shoe) that the client has worn throughout life. Hallux valgus is a lateral deviation of the great toe with a medial deviation of the first metatarsal. Pes cavus is an excessively high medial longitudinal arch of the foot. Pes planus is an inadequate medial longitudinal arch of the foot that gives the appearance of a flatfoot.[35]

Evaluation: Tools and Methods. The evaluating therapist should consider a holistic evaluation when addressing the geriatric foot. Integumentary assessments of the skin could reveal potential for skin breakdown due to diminished circulation or diabetes. The PT will evaluate the integrity of the skin, dryness, and the presence of calluses. ROM, strength, and sensory evaluations should be completed. A particular assessment of vibratory and position senses should be conducted as part of the overall balance assessment of the client. The footwear of the client should be assessed for the potential of causing excessive friction areas, leading to blisters or calluses. To assess the integrity of the arches of the foot, the evaluating PT may have the client step into a small tub of water and then onto the floor. The outline of the foot can then be assessed. A client with a high arch (pes cavus) will have a narrow footprint with no water contacting the ground in the area of the medial arch. The client with a flat arch (pes planus) will have a wide foot print as the medial longitudinal arch actually contacts the ground. The evaluating therapist may also perform a gait assessment and determine the dynamic relationships of the bones of the foot.

Clinical Management. Toe and foot deformities can usually be successfully managed conservatively. Anti-inflammatory modalities can be directed at the hallux valgus conditions that are painful. Ultrasound, whirlpool, and iontophoresis have all been used to lessen the discomfort associated with the stretching of the medial joint capsule of the great toe. Joint mobilization and strengthening exercises for the intrinsic and extrinsic muscles of the foot and toes may be beneficial. Splinting or orthotic management (e.g., the use of toe spreaders) is often helpful in correcting toe deformities such as overlapping toes. Shoe inserts benefit the client with arch dysfunctions or a painful heel. Client education about proper footwear that gives adequate arch support and does not restrict the toes is important.

The expected physical therapy outcomes related to managing a client with toe and foot deformities include[30]:

1. Improved health-related quality of life
2. Reduce risk of further disability from identified limitations
3. An understanding of risk factors that may contribute to jeopardizing health status
4. An understanding of strategies to prevent further disability

The expected time frame for achieving the outcomes is 4 to 6 weeks. Painful deformities of the foot and toes are usually well managed by decreasing the inflammation and empowering the client to prevent the recurrence of symptoms through the use of proper footwear and compliance with a home exercise program.

Bursitis

Hip Bursitis. Greater trochanteric bursitis is a common problem affecting not only geriatric clients, but younger populations as well.[56] In the lower extremity, roughly 18 bursal sacs surround the hip joint and 10 protect the knee joint.[47] The most common bursitis is caused by friction as the iliotibial band rubs over the greater trochanteric bursa.[57]

Clinical Presentation. Sharp pain over the greater trochanteric region is a chief complaint with associated aching in the lateral aspect of the same lower extremity.[56] The pain and intensity will typically increase with weight-bearing activities and is alleviated with rest.

Evaluation: Tools and Methods. Palpation of the suspected area is one of the chief assessment tools available to the PT. The palpation examination may produce pain and tenderness or may reveal the presence of crepitus.[56] The comprehensive evaluation will include a description of the pain and a history of events leading up to the current condition. Objective tests include ROM, strength, sensory, and balance assessments. A postural and gait examination may identify structural deficits that may promote the painful condition.

Clinical Management. Management of the symptoms associated with greater trochanteric bursitis include stretching of the iliotibial band (Fig. 11–51), strengthening of the abductors and extensors of the hip, modalities designed to decrease the effects of inflammation (short-wave diathermy, ultrasound, and iontophoresis), and modifying activities that reproduce symptoms. Frequently the physician will use NSAIDs and, occasionally, may use corticosteroid injections for pain relief.[56]

The expected outcomes to manage the client with a greater trochanteric bursitis include[30]:

1. Improved health-related quality of life
2. An optimal return of function
3. An understanding of strategies to prevent further disability

The expected time frame for achieving the outcomes is 4 to 6 weeks. The client should be given an effective home program designed to prevent the recurrence of

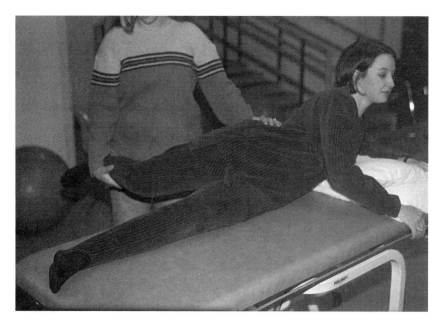

FIG. 11–51
Stretching of the iliotibial (IT) band. To stretch a tight IT band, place the client in a side-lying position with the affected side up and the therapist standing behind the client. Stabilize the client with the right hand at the hip posteriorly to prevent rotation or sliding off of the plinth. Support under the knee with the left hand, keeping the knee in 90° of flexion. To stretch, extend the hip and then use gentle adduction, allowing the knee to drop down behind the client off of the plinth. Care should be taken not to irritate an inflamed bursa at the hip.

symptoms, including flexibility and strengthening exercises as well as modification of aggravating behaviors.

Shoulder Bursitis. One of the more common shoulder dysfunctions seen in the geriatric population is symptoms associated with bursitis, which are more prevalent than osteoarthritis involving the shoulder.[1]

Clinical Presentation. Signs and symptoms include tenderness in the area of the inflamed bursa and pain with movement. Pain can be elicited with palpation distal to the acromial arch along the superior aspect of the humeral head. Pain may also be provoked by passively abducting the arm past 90°. The client will frequently note that with rest, the symptoms decrease. Frequently, the client can describe that there was a recent episode of overuse through increased activity of the irritated upper extremity.[1]

Evaluation: Tools and Methods. The evaluating therapist should take a comprehensive history to identify any precipitating factors that may lead to the onset of pain and disability. Subjective measures include a description of the pain, noting aggravating and alleviating conditions. Objective measures include palpation, ROM, strength, sensory, and functional assessments of the upper extremity and cervical spine. A positive impingement test may reproduce symptoms.

Clinical Management. Conservative management of the subacromial bursitis is generally effective. Pain-reducing modalities including ice, heat, iontophoresis, or ultrasound can be used. Frequently the physician will prescribe NSAIDs and, occasionally, corticosteroid injections for pain relief. Activities and motions that reproduce the pain should be avoided. Isometric exercises with the arm at the side of the body in a pain-free position should begin immediately or when tolerated to avoid the onset of disuse atrophy. ROM and strengthening exercises can progress in a pain-free range, avoiding the painful arcs of motion (i.e., exercising above and below this region). As the client demonstrates a significant reduction in pain and an increase in strength, a gradual return to functional activities should be promoted. The client should be educated on the factors that led to the onset of painful symptoms, and strategies should be developed to avoid a recurrence of symptoms in the future.[1]

The physical therapy expected outcomes to manage the client with a subacromial bursitis include[30]:

1. An optimal return of function
2. Reduced risk of further disability from identified limitations
3. Improved self-care skills and ADLs
4. An understanding of risk factors that may contribute to jeopardizing health status

The expected time frame for achieving these outcomes is 4 to 6 weeks. Acute bursitis conditions will easily resolve if repeated irritation to the soft tissue is avoided.

POOL THERAPIES

Pool therapies are the final presentation in this text for the PTA. Water as a modality for healing is one of the oldest and most frequently used agents in the profession of physical therapy. Hydrotherapy can be used to deliver heat or cold to an affected body part or to cleanse an open wound. Total body or limb immersion can also be used as an exercise tool to promote improvements in ROM, strength, and endurance. Pool therapies can provide an environment of comfort for severely arthritic clients or promote increased independence for the client with paralysis. Water can be used as a motivator for exercise and can promote desired facilitation or inhibition of neurologically impaired clients. The unique physical properties of water add or limit this medium as an exercise modality.

Many health professionals have advocated the use of pool therapies as a successful tool in the management of various conditions; however, evidence of the efficiency of such programs is limited.[58] Vogtle et al.[58] described that a group of individuals examined who participated in pool therapy demonstrated improved ROM and decreased pain, while experiencing a pleasurable social experience. Improvements related to strength and cardiovascular endurance from pool therapies were demonstrated by Danneskiold-Samsoe et al.[59] in clients with RA without producing adverse effects. The strength of the study group improved over that of the control group, but their overall strength was still significantly weaker when compared with that of normal, healthy individuals.

The physical benefits of exercising in water include the following considerations. Buoyancy is the physical property of water that supports the body when immersed. Weight relief is promoted as the effects of gravity are decreased. Muscle contractions when submerged in the water are purely concentric in nature. Ease of movement is granted as the client can slowly move in the water, controlling any painful segment. Through the support of the water, or the use of floatation devices, a low-resistance environment in which to move a body part can be achieved. Easy handling by the therapist is also provided in the pool. The therapist can work on gait skills of the client when submerged, working to correct deviations. The therapist also can easily support the weight of the body through the use of life jackets or floatation devices, helping to reduce the stress of dry land activities. Movement pattern education for weak muscles is promoted in the water environment. The client can move the body part with graded resistance and great support in the desired pattern, whereas if on dry land, the effects of gravity would prevent the same weak muscle from lifting the body part. A client with a Trendelenburg gait on dry land due to a weak gluteus medius muscle can actually have a normal gait pattern when submerged.

Pool group therapy improves socialization, motivation, and cost-effectiveness.[60] When performed as a class, pool therapies promote peer support, competition, and comradery. Geriatric pool programs in community centers encourage activity and participation. The exercise atmosphere can be supportive both emotionally and physically. Dry land exercise may be painful, thus decreasing compliance. If the client is able to exercise pain-free in the water, the program is likely to be continued. The effectiveness of the program from a cost perspective may be justified when performed in groups, because the more clients involved in one session, the less the overall cost. One therapist would be able to work with certain clients, whereas others would be individually exercising.

Orthopedic clients who have traditionally been managed with aquatic therapy include clients with DJD, RA, chronic musculoskeletal pain, work-related injuries, and orthopedic surgical clients. Therapeutic goals of pool therapy include[61]:

1. Improved ROM
2. Normalized tone
3. Strength gains
4. Relieved weight bearing and decreasing joint compression
5. Decreased pain
6. Improved cardiovascular endurance
7. Return to functional activities

Therapeutic activities that can be performed in the water include any activity that may be painful or difficult to perform on dry land. A client may work on progressive sitting from a supine position in the shallow end of the water or on steps that enter the pool. The client can simulate the transition from sit to stand, demonstrating less compressive forces on the lower extremity. If the client has difficulty weight bearing because of pain, progressive standing and weight bearing can be performed by shifting weight onto either lower extremity as well as increasing tolerance to standing. Gait training in the pool can help promote a normal pain-free gait cycle while increasing endurance and distance. Gait that is painful on dry land may be performed more readily in the pool, improving the client's tolerance and confidence.[62]

Range of motion can be promoted in the water as the buoyancy effect can assist with gentle ROM exercises. When standing with the water level to the client's shoulder, the arm can be placed at the side, and the effects of the water can assist the arm to the surface through the available ROM. The client can work horizontal to the surface of the water in a gentle motion pattern, or from the surface of the water down to the side of the body in a sagittal or frontal pattern.

Contraindications and precautions for pool therapy include severe cardiopulmonary dysfunction, open wounds, active infectious disease, immunodeficiency, and hypertension. Some health-related precautions may prevent clients who demonstrate urinary or bowel incontinence from actively participating in pool therapy programs. The client who is significantly fearful of water may not benefit from an aquatic program.

Client compliance will significantly improve if the medium allows very little or no pain during the exercise. Arthritic clients who have severe pain with weight bearing will find a reduction in pain associated with weight bearing as the water helps to reduce joint compression. As discussed in the section on osteoporosis, the major detriment to exercising in water for clients with osteoporosis is the very thing that makes exercising in water attractive for clients with painful orthopedic conditions: the reduction of the stress on the body. To prevent a loss of bone, hydrotherapy may not be the best exercise choice. The freedom of movement can also increase confidence in performing the difficult activity, but may not carry over to performing the same activity on dry land. However, if the alternative is not to exercise at all, then hydrotherapy is beneficial for the geriatric client and should be encouraged.

 SUMMARY

The geriatric client has unique needs related to the prevention of a loss of function. Osteoporosis, or the loss of bone density, is a common occurrence in the geriatric population that affects white women more than any other group. Risk factors associated with the onset of osteoporosis are well documented and center on the triad of exercise, nutrition, and hormone replacement as a lifelong approach to preventing the onset of this debilitating condition. Falls are one of the leading causes of morbidity and mortality in the geriatric population. The mechanics of a fall are important factors in predicting the injury. If the client falls onto an extended upper extremity, the chance of fracturing the wrist is increased. If the client falls and lands near the hip, the chance of a hip fracture is increased. If the client is able to break the fall by landing on something soft or grabbing an object, the risk of fracture is lessened but soft-tissue injury is more likely. Bone density will also play a critical role in whether a client sustains a fracture. Activities and programs designed to educate the client about preventing falls and maintaining bone density should be encouraged.

Many orthopedic conditions will limit the functional abilities of the geriatric population. Fractures are usually a result of a falling incident or the onset of osteoporosis and will account for most of the therapeutic treatment from the rehabilitation team working with the geriatric population. DJD is a gradual erosion of the bony surfaces compromising the integrity of the synovial joint. Degenerative changes can be seen in any joint, but such changes commonly affect weight-bearing joints and are not symmetrical in nature. If joint destruction is severe and the discomfort unmanageable, then a joint replacement or arthroplasty may be considered. Common sites of joint replacements are the hip and knee; less common sites are the shoulder, digits of the hand, and elbow. Other functional impairments described include rotator cuff tears, the frozen shoulder, RSD, and hand and foot deformities.

The rehabilitation team can effectively manage the geriatric client with a functional limitation by implementing an established plan of treatment. General management guidelines include controlling pain and inflammation, restoring functional ROM and strength, educating the client in the prevention of a recurrence of symptoms, and assisting the client with concerns over how to perform functional tasks safely when at home. Balance deficits can be addressed through a variety of management techniques, including flexibility, strengthening, neuromuscular timing, and development of appropriate balancing strategies.

Pool therapies are effective for motivating the geriatric population to exercise. Benefits may include ROM, increased strength, socialization, and confidence.

Indications and contraindications were discussed. The pool provides a positive atmosphere for clients with debilitating pain because it allows them to exercise in a pain-free environment by relieving the normal weight-bearing forces on the body. A negative consequence of the relief of weight-bearing forces in a water environment is the limited ability to prevent bone loss.

 # REFERENCES

1. Lewis, CB, and Bottemley, JM: Geriatric Physical Therapy: A Clinical Approach. Appleton & Lange, Norwalk, CT, 1994.
2. Koch, M, et al: An impairment and disability assessment and treatment protocol for community-living elderly persons. Phys Ther 74:286, 1994.
3. Nevitt, MC, et al: Risk factors for injurious falls: A prospective study. J Gerontol 46:M164, 1991.
4. Shumway-Cook, A, et al: The effect of multidimensional exercises on balance, mobility, and fall risk in the community-dwelling older adults. Phys Ther 77:46, 1997.
5. Patla, AE, et al: Identification of age-related changes in the balance-control system. In Duncan, PW (ed): Balance: Proceedings of the APTA Forum. APTA, Washington, D.C., 1990.
6. Chandler, JM, et al: Is lower extremity strength gain associated with improvement in physical performance and disability in frail, community-dwelling elders? Arch Phys Med Rehabil 79:24, 1998.
7. Leveille, SG, et al: Preventing disability and managing chronic illness in frail older adults: A randomized trial of a community-based partnership with primary care. J Am Geriatr Soc 46(10):1191, 1998. Available at [http://www.amgeriatrics.com/].
8. Joseph, A, and Boult, C: Managed primary care of nursing home residents. J Am Geriatr Soc 46(9):1152, 1998. Available at [http://www.amgeriatrics.com/].
9. Engle, VF, et al: The experience of living-dying in a nursing home: self-reports of black and white older adults. J Am Geriatr Soc 46(9):1091, 1998. Available at [http://www.amgeriatrics.com/].
10. Mion, LC, et al: Falls in the rehabilitation setting: Incidence and characteristics. Rehabilitation Nursing 14:17, 1989.
11. Nevitt, MC, and Cummings, SR: Type of fall and risk of hip and wrist fractures: The study of osteoporotic fractures. J Am Geriatr Soc 41:1126, 1993.
12. Kiely, DK, et al: Identifying nursing home residents at risk for falling. J Am Geriatr Soc 46(5):551, 1998. Available at [http://www.amgeriatrics.com/].
13. Tenetti, ME, et al: Risk factors for falls among elderly persons living in the community. N Engl J Med 319:1701, 1988.
14. Nashner, LM: Sensory, neuromuscular, and biomechanical contributions to human balance. In Duncan, PW (ed): Balance: Proceedings of the APTA Forum. APTA, Washington, D.C., 1990.
15. Keshner, EA: Reflex, voluntary and mechanical processes in postural stabilization. In Duncan, PW (ed): Balance: Proceedings of the APTA Forum. APTA, Washington, D.C., 1990.
16. Woollacott, M: Postural control mechanisms in the young and old. In Duncan, PW (ed): Balance: Proceedings of the APTA Forum. APTA, Washington, D.C., 1990.
17. Horak, FB, and Shumway-Cook, A: Clinical implications of posture control research. In Duncan, PW (ed): Balance: Proceedings of the APTA Forum. APTA, Washington, D.C., 1990.
18. Winstein, CJ: Balance retraining: does it transfer? In Duncan, PW (ed): Balance: Proceedings of the APTA Forum. APTA, Washington, D.C., 1990.
19. Grisso, JA, et al: Risk factors for falls as a cause of hip fracture in women. N Engl J Med 324:1326, 1991.
20. Tresolini, CP, et al (eds): Working with Patients to Prevent, Treat and Manage Osteoporosis: A Curriculum Guide for the Health Professions, ed 2. National Fund for Medical Education, San Francisco, CA, 1998.
21. Aisenbrey, JA: Exercise in the prevention and management of osteoporosis. Phys Ther 67:1100, 1987.
22. Chow, R, et al: Effect of two randomised exercise programmes on bone mass of healthy postmenopausal women. BMJ 295:1441, 1987.
23. Sinaki, M, Grubbs, NC: Back strengthening exercises: Quantitative evaluation of their efficacy for women aged 40 to 65 years. Arch Phys Med Rehabil 70:16, 1989.
24. Munnings F: Osteoporosis: What is the role of exercise? The Physician and Sportsmedicine 20(6):127, 1992.
25. Ettinger, B, et al: Contributions of vertebral deformities to chronic back pain and disability. J Bone Miner Res 7:449, 1992.

26. Ayalon, J, et al: Dynamic bone loading exercises for postmenopausal women: Effect on the density of the distal radius. Arch Phys Med Rehabil 68:280, 1987.
27. Nelson, ME, et al: Effects of high-intensity strength training on multiple risk factors for osteoporotic fractures. JAMA 272:1909, 1994.
28. Sinaki, M, and Mikkelsen, BA: Postmenopausal spinal osteoporosis: Flexion versus extension exercises. Arch Phys Med Rehabil 65:593, 1984.
29. Gold, DT: The clinical impact of vertebral fractures: Quality of life in women with osteoporosis. Bone 18:185S, 1996.
30. Guide to Physical Therapist Practice. Phys Ther 77:1163, 1997.
31. Jung, PI: Racial differences in hip fractures: A literature review. Issues on Aging 20(2):13, 1997.
32. Jabourian, AP, et al: Cognitive functions and fall-related fractures. Br J Psychiatry 165:122, 1994.
33. Gustafson, Y, et al: Acute confusional states in elderly patients treated for femoral neck fractures. J Am Geriatr Soc 36:525, 1988.
34. Jelicic, M, et al: Do psychosocial factors affect recovery from hip fracture in the elderly? A review of the literature. J Rehabil Sci 9(3):77, 1996.
35. Kisner, C, and Colby, LA: Therapeutic Exercise: Foundations and Techniques. 3rd ed. FA Davis, Philadelphia, PA, 1996.
36. Andrews, JR, et al: Elbow rehabilitation. In Brotzman, SB (ed): Clinical Orthopaedic Rehabilitation. Mosby, St Louis, MO, 1996.
37. Calandruccio, JH, et al: Rehabilitation of the hand and wrist. In Brotzman, SB (ed): Clinical Orthopaedic Rehabilitation. Mosby, St Louis, MO, 1996.
38. Knirk, JL, and Jupiter JB: Intra-articular fractures of the distal end of the radius in young adults. J Bone Joint Surg 63A:647, 1986.
39. Ryu, J, et al: Rheumatoid wrist reconstruction utilizing a fibrous nonunion and radiocarpal arthrodesis. J Hand Surg 10A:830, 1985.
40. Russell, TA, and Palmieri AK: Fractures of the pelvis, acetabulum, and lower extremity. In Brotzman, SB (ed): Clinical Orthopaedic Rehabilitation. Mosby, St Louis, MO, 1996.
41. Kellie, SE, and Brody, JA: Sex-specific and race-specific hip fractures. Am J Public Health 80:326, 1990.
42. Grisso, JA, et al: Risk factors for falls as a cause of hip fracture in women. N Engl J Med 324:1326, 1991.
43. Hinton, RY, and Smith, GS: The association of age, race, and sex, with the location of proximal femoral fractures in the elderly. J Bone Joint Surg 75A:752, 1993.
44. Salter, RB: Textbook of Disorders and Hip Injuries of the Musculoskeletal System. Williams & Wilkins, Baltimore, 1983.
45. Brotzman, SB, and Brasel, J: Foot and ankle rehabilitation. In Brotzman, SB (ed): Clinical Orthopaedic Rehabilitation. Mosby, St Louis, MO, 1996.
46. Lukert, BP: Vertebral compression fracture: How to manage pain, avoid disability. Geriatrics 49:22, 1994.
47. Zetterberg, C: Epidemiology of the lower extremity. In Nordin, M, et al: Musculoskeletal Disorders in the Workplace: Principles and Practice. Mosby, St Louis, MO, 1997.
48. Jobe, FW, et al: Rehabilitation of the shoulder. In Brotzman, SB (ed): Clinical Orthopaedic Rehabilitation. Mosby, St Louis, MO, 1996.
49. Cameron, HU, et al: Rehabilitation after total joint arthroplasty. In Brotzman, SB (ed): Clinical Orthopaedic Rehabilitation. Mosby, St Louis, MO, 1996.
50. Johnsson, R, et al: Physiotherapy after total hip replacement for primary arthrosis. Scand J Rehabil Med 20:43, 1988.
51. Angulo, DL, and Colwell, CW: Use of postoperative TENS and continuous passive motion following total knee replacement. J Ortho Sports Phys Ther 11:599, 1990.
52. Gose, JC: Continuous passive motion in the postoperative treatment of patients with total knee replacement: A retrospective study. Phys Ther 67:39, 1987.
53. Stralka, S: Reflex sympathetic dystrophy. In Brotzman, SB (ed): Clinical Orthopaedic Rehabilitation. Mosby, St Louis, MO, 1996.
54. Harrell, L, Massey, E: Hand weakness in the elderly. J Am Geriatr Soc 31:223, 1983.
55. White, EG, Mulley GP: Foot care for very elderly people: A community survey. Age Ageing 18(4):275, 1989.
56. Quarrier, NF, Wightman, AB: A ballet dancer with chronic hip pain due to a lesser trochanteric bony avulsion: The challenge of a differential diagnosis. J Orthop Sports Phys Ther 28:168, 1998.
57. Renstrom, AH: Tendon and muscle injuries in the groin area. Clin Sports Med 11:815, 1992.
58. Vogtle, LK, et al: An aquatic program for adults with cerebral palsy living in group homes. Physical Therapy Case Reports 1:250, 1998.
59. Danneskiold-Samsoe, B, et al: The effect of water exercise therapy given to patients with rheumatoid arthritis. Scand J Rehabil Med 19:31, 1987.

60. Bakker, C, et al: Cost effectiveness of group physical therapy compared to individualized therapy for ankylosing spondylitis: A randomized controlled trial. J Rheumatol 21:264, 1994.
61. Garvey, LA: Spinal cord injury and aquatics. Clinical Management 11(1):21, 1991.
62. Triggs, M: Orthopedic aquatic therapy. Clinical Management 11(1): 30, 1991.

 BIBLIOGRAPHY

Aisenbrey, JA: Exercise in the prevention and management of osteoporosis. Phys Ther 67:1100, 1987.

Andrews, JR, et al: Elbow rehabilitation. In Brotzman, SB (ed): Clinical Orthopaedic Rehabilitation. Mosby, St Louis, MO, 1996.

Angulo, DL, and Colwell, CW: Use of postoperative TENS and continuous passive motion following total knee replacement. J Ortho Sports Phys Ther 11:599, 1990.

Ayalon, J, et al: Dynamic bone loading exercises for postmenopausal women: Effect on the density of the distal radius. Arch Phys Med Rehabil 68:280, 1987.

Bakker, C, et al: Cost effectiveness of group physical therapy compared to individualized therapy for ankylosing spondylitis: A randomized controlled trial. J Rheumatol 21:264, 1994.

Brotzman, SB, and Brasel, J: Foot and ankle rehabilitation. In Brotzman, SB (ed): Clinical Orthopaedic Rehabilitation. Mosby, St Louis, MO, 1996.

Calandruccio, JH, et al: Rehabilitation of the hand and wrist. In Brotzman, SB (ed): Clinical Orthopaedic Rehabilitation. Mosby, St Louis, MO, 1996.

Cameron, HU, et al: Rehabilitation after total joint arthroplasty. In Brotzman, SB (ed): Clinical Orthopaedic Rehabilitation. Mosby, St Louis, MO, 1996.

Chandler, JM, et al: Is lower extremity strength gain associated with improvement in physical performance and disability in frail, community-dwelling elders? Arch Phys Med Rehabil 79:24, 1998.

Chow, R, et al: Effect of two randomised exercise programmes on bone mass of healthy postmenopausal women. BMJ 295:1441, 1987.

Danneskiold-Samsoe, B, et al: The effect of water exercise therapy given to patients with rheumatoid arthritis. Scand J Rehabil Med 19:31, 1987.

Engle, VF, et al: The experience of living-dying in a nursing home: self-reports of black and white older adults. J Am Geriatr Soc 46(9):1091, 1998. Available at [http://www.amgeriatrics.com/].

Ettinger, B, et al: Contributions of vertebral deformities to chronic back pain and disability. J Bone Miner Res 7:449, 1992.

Garvey, LA: Spinal cord injury and aquatics. Clinical Management 11(1):21, 1991.

Gold, DT: The clinical impact of vertebral fractures: Quality of life in women with osteoporosis. Bone 18:185S, 1996.

Gose, JC: Continuous passive motion in the postoperative treatment of patients with total knee replacement: a retrospective study. Phys Ther 67:39, 1987.

Grisso, JA, et al: Risk factors for falls as a cause of hip fracture in women. N Engl J Med 324:1326, 1991.

Guide to Physical Therapist Practice. Phys Ther 77:1163, 1997.

Gustafson, Y, et al: Acute confusional states in elderly patients treated for femoral neck fractures. J Am Geriatr Soc 36:525, 1988.

Harrell, L, and Massey, E: Hand weakness in the elderly. J Am Ger Soc 31:223, 1983.

Hinton, RY, and Smith, GS: The association of age, race, and sex, with the location of proximal femoral fractures in the elderly. J Bone and Joint Surg 75A:752, 1993.

Horak, FB, and Shumway-Cook, A: Clinical implications of posture control research. In Duncan, PW (ed): Balance: Proceedings of the APTA Forum. APTA, Washington, D.C., 1990.

Jabourian, AP, et al. Cognitive functions and fall-related fractures. Br J Psychiatry 165:122, 1994.

Jelicic, M, et al: Do psychosocial factors affect recovery from hip fracture in the elderly? A review of the literature. J Rehabil Sci 9(3):77, 1996.

Jobe, FW, et al: Rehabilitation of the shoulder. In Brotzman, SB (ed): Clinical Orthopaedic Rehabilitation. Mosby, St Louis, MO, 1996.

Johnsson, R, et al: Physiotherapy after total hip replacement for primary arthrosis. Scand J Rehabil Med 20:43, 1988.

Joseph, A, and Boult, C: Managed primary care of nursing home residents. J Am Geriatr Soc 46(9):1152, 1998. Available at [http://www.amgeriatrics.com/].

Jung, PI: Racial differences in hip fractures: A literature review. Issues On Aging 20(2):13, 1997.

Kellie, SE, and Brody, JA: Sex-specific and race-specific hip fractures. Am J Public Health 80:326, 1990.

Keshner, EA: Reflex, voluntary and mechanical processes in postural stabilization. In Duncan, PW (ed): Balance: Proceedings of the APTA Forum. APTA, Washington, D.C., 1990.

Kiely, DK, et al: Identifying nursing home residents at risk for falling. J Am Geriatr Soc 46(5):551, 1998. Available at [http://www.amgeriatrics.com/].

Kisner, C, and Colby, LA: Therapeutic Exercise: Foundations and Techniques, ed 3. FA Davis, Philadelphia, 1996.

Knirk, JL, and Jupiter JB: Intra-articular fractures of the distal end of the radius in young adults. J Bone Joint Surg 63A:647, 1986.

Koch, M, et al: An impairment and disability assessment and treatment protocol for community-living elderly persons. Phys Ther 74:286, 1994.

Leveille, SG, et al: Preventing disability and managing chronic illness in frail older adults: A randomized trial of a community-based partnership with primary care. J Am Geriatr Soc 46(10):1191, 1998. Available at [http://www.amgeriatrics.com/].

Lewis, CB, and Bottemley, JM: Geriatric Physical Therapy: A Clinical Approach. Appleton & Lange, Norwalk, CT, 1994.

Lukert, BP: Vertebral compression fracture: How to manage pain, avoid disability. Geriatrics 49:22, 1994.

Mion, LC, et al: Falls in the rehabilitation setting: Incidence and characteristics. Rehabilitation Nursing 14;17, 1989.

Munnings, F: Osteoporosis: what is the role of exercise? The Physician and Sportsmedicine 20(6):127, 1992.

Nashner, LM: Sensory, neuromuscular, and biomechanical contributions to human balance. In Duncan, PW (ed): Balance: Proceedings of the APTA Forum. APTA, Washington, D.C., 1990.

Nelson, ME, et al: Effects of high-intensity strength training on multiple risk factors for osteoporotic fractures. JAMA 272:1909, 1994.

Nevitt, MC, et al: Risk factors for injurious falls: A prospective study. J Gerontol 46:M164, 1991.

Nevitt, MC, and Cummings, SR: Type of fall and risk of hip and wrist fractures: The study of osteoporotic fractures. J Am Geriatr Soc 41:1126, 1993.

Patla, AE, et al: Identification of age-related changes in the balance-control system. In Duncan, PW (ed): Balance: Proceedings of the APTA Forum. APTA, Washington, D.C., 1990.

Quarrier, NF, and Wightman, AB: A ballet dancer with chronic hip pain due to a lesser trochanter bony avulsion: The challenge of a differential diagnosis. J Orthop Sports Phys Ther 28;168, 1998.

Renstrom, AH: Tendon and muscle injuries in the groin area. Clin Sports Med 11:815, 1992.

Russell, TA, and Palmieri AK: Fractures of the pelvis, acetabulum, and lower extremity. In Brotzman, SB (ed): Clinical Orthopaedic Rehabilitation. Mosby, St Louis, MO. 1996.

Ryu J, et al: Rheumatoid wrist reconstruction utilizing a fibrous nonunion and radiocarpal arthrodesis. J Hand Surg 10A:830, 1985.

Salter, RB: Textbook of Disorders and Injuries of the Musculoskeletal System. Williams & Wilkins, Baltimore, 1983.

Shumway-Cook, A, et al: The effect of multidimensional exercises on balance, mobility, and fall risk in the community-dwelling older adults. Phys Ther 77:46, 1997.

Sinaki, M, and Grubbs, NC: Back strengthening exercises: Quantitative evaluation of their efficacy for women aged 40 to 65 years. Arch Phys Med Rehabil 70;16, 1989.

Sinaki, M, and Mikkelsen, BA: Postmenopausal spinal osteoporosis: Flexion versus extension exercises. Arch Phys Med Rehabil 65:593, 1984.

Stralka, S: Reflex sympathetic dystrophy. In Brotzman, SB (ed): Clinical Orthopaedic Rehabilitation. Mosby, St. Louis, MO. 1996.

Tenetti, ME, et al: Risk factors for falls among elderly persons living in the community. N Engl J Med 319:1701, 1988.

Tresolini, CP, et al (eds): Working with patients to prevent, treat and manage osteoporosis: A curriculum guide for the health professions, ed 2. National Fund for Medical Education, San Francisco, CA, 1998.

Triggs, M: Orthopedic aquatic therapy. Clinical Management 11(1):30, 1991.

Vogtle, LK, et al: An aquatic program for adults with cerebral palsy living in group homes. Physical Therapy Case Reports 1:250, 1998.

White, EG, and Mulley GP: Foot care for very elderly people: a community survey. Age Ageing 18(4):275, 1989.

Winstein, CJ: Balance retraining: Does it transfer? In Duncan, PW (ed): Balance: Proceedings of the APTA Forum. APTA, Washington, D.C., 1990.

Woollacott, M: Postural control mechanisms in the young and old. In Duncan, PW (ed): Balance: Proceedings of the APTA Forum. APTA, Washington, D.C., 1990.

Zetterberg, C: Epidemiology of the lower extremity. In Nordin, M, et al (ed): Musculoskeletal Disorders in the Workplace: Principles and Practice. Mosby, St Louis, MO, 1997.

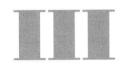

part **III**

CLINICAL APPLICATION OF ORTHOPEDIC CONDITIONS

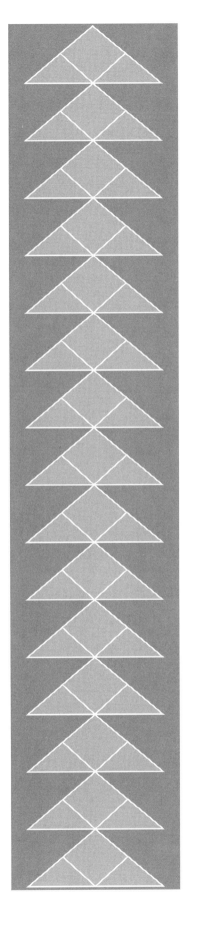

Introduction To Part III

Each subunit of Chapter 12 is a self-contained case study related to a chapter in the text. The respective text number is identified by the first number of the case study (e.g., 1–1 relates to materials presented in the first chapter of the text). Relevant clinical applications and role-playing exercises are structured within the case study to promote the acquisition and implementation of orthopedic skills presented in the text. The student should understand that all material needed to complete each case study may not be present in this textbook. To fully participate in the designed learning experience, the PTA student may have to access other educational resources, including professional journals, other relevant readings, the course instructor, and local professionals. Suggestions for case study preparation are made to ensure that the student is ready to participate in a selected exercise. The key to each case study is the critical analysis component, which promotes problem solving, creativity, and/or appropriate resource identification. If the student is having difficulty completing the respective case study, then he or she should refer to the recommended readings, organized by chapter, in Appendix B.

Chapter 13 provides the PTA student with brief orthopedic clinical scenarios that are divided into five functional categories

1. Handling skills
2. Interim assessment
3. Modalities
4. Modalities and exercise
5. Exercise

These tools can be used in a variety of ways, including repetitive practice, practical exams, and clinical simulations. The scenarios are designed to be broad in nature to allow for regional variations in implementation by physical therapy professionals.

As with the learning experience in Chapter 12, all of the resources needed to complete the practice scenarios are not included within the pages of this textbook. This is by instructional design to encourage the learner to become a critical consumer of the body of knowledge in the profession of physical therapy. Please do not grow discouraged and remember that the learning is in the doing,

Steven G. Lesh, MPA, PT, ATC
Assistant Professor of Physical Therapy
Arkansas State University

chapter **12**

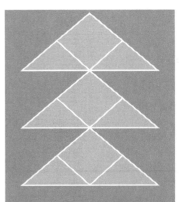

Case Studies

Outline

Text continues on page 468

OBJECTIVES

After completing this chapter, the PTA student will be able to:

1. Implement simulated orthopedic clinical skills presented in this text.
2. Critically discuss the implications of various clinical techniques.
3. Creatively solve problems relative to learned skills presented in this text.
4. Identify appropriate support resources necessary to solve problems.
   (**Note:** Specific learning objectives are identified within each case study.)

CASE STUDY 1–1   **ROLE OF THE PTA IN ORTHOPEDIC MANAGEMENT AND CLIENT COMPLIANCE**

Objectives
After completing the exercises in this case study, the PTA student will be able to:

1. Discuss the role of the PTA in orthopedic management, both under normal and unexpected conditions.
2. Critically discuss the implications of state laws governing the practice of the PTA.
3. Creatively investigate issues relative to client compliance.
4. Identify appropriate support resources necessary to solve problems related to this case.

Case
M.J. is a 15 y/o female basketball player and the plan of care has been delegated to you by the evaluating PT at the outpatient orthopedic clinic at which you are employed. Today is the first session that you will work with the client, and this is M.J.'s second visit to your clinic after her initial visit 2 days ago (the supervising PT completed the evaluation and developed the treatment plan at the first session). On reviewing M.J.'s chart you find the following significant information from the completed evaluation.

Hx: Client is s/p R ACL reconstruction 10 days after receiving a patellar tendon bone-to-bone graft. M.J. is anxious to return to competitive basketball as soon as possible.

O: Client is WBAT on R LE using two crutches and a hinged knee immobilizer that is locked into full extension. She is Ind with gait at this time. Circumferential measurements of the L LE compared to the R LE were as follows:

Location	R LE	L LE
Knee joint line	16 in.	13.5 in.
3 in. suprapatellar	17 in.	18 in.
3 in. infrapatellar	15 in.	14.5 in.

Suture line is anteriorly located on the R LE, 3 inches in length, originating at the inferior aspect of the patella moving distally. There is also a small incision ¼ inch in length over the superior aspect of the lateral femoral condyle. There is no drainage or odor noted from either incision, and the sutures are intact with mild scabbing noted.

A: Client is well motivated and is ready to begin rehabilitation.

P: ACL protocol as per Dr. Jones 3x/wk. Perform client education as appropriate. Initial session: evaluation, quad set instruction, and review of gait safety with client when using crutches.

Clinical Applications
This case study will examine the role of the PTA and client compliance.

Case Study Preparation
The supervising PT told M.J. that she would be following a specific protocol as per the orthopedic surgeon's orders, but the PT did not give the protocol to M.J. because she isn't yet ready to begin it. The PT discussed the protocol with her, but M.J. didn't remember much from the first day of therapy. M.J. would like you to provide her with some sources of education so she can learn more about her injury. To complete this case study, find the following items:

1. An educational pamphlet or a handout on knee injuries
2. An exercise protocol for ACL reconstructions (this may not be the specific protocol used by Dr. Jones, but try to find a complete protocol)
3. A resource on the World Wide Web for M.J. to review.

Role-Paying Exercise

1. As you introduce yourself to M.J., she begins to tell you about herself and the basketball injury that "blew" up her knee and her subsequent surgery. You ask her to describe how she is feeling and she responds as follows:

"I've been real tired, my knee really hurts and at times I get chills. I have been real frustrated, because those tightening exercises that guy told me to do are hard. Am I doing them right? When can I get this brace off and begin running?"

As the PTA treating this client how would you proceed? Discuss with your lab partner and instructor how you would begin M.J.'s treatment.

2. Have your lab partner become the client in this scenario. The lab partner is to become noncompliant with her exercise program because she is growing tired and frustrated with slow progress. She is ready to start playing basketball now and does not see the need for this exercise program any longer. Role-play to find out the reasons for her being noncompliant with the HEP and create solutions that would resolve the issues.

Critical Analysis

1. Investigate the physical therapy practice act in your state. Discuss with your lab partner and instructor when it is appropriate to modify the plan of treatment according to states laws. If your state still lacks legislation regarding the PTA, investigate one of the neighboring states.

CASE STUDY 2–1   **CONCEPTS OF PASSIVE RANGE OF MOTION, ACTIVE ASSISTIVE RANGE OF MOTION, ACTIVE RANGE OF MOTION, AND PROGRESSIVE RESISTIVE EXERCISE**

Objectives

After completing the exercises in this case study, the PTA student will be able to:

1. Implement simulated clinical skills of PROM, AAROM, AROM, and PRE.
2. Critically discuss the implications of various clinical orthopedic ROM and strengthening techniques.
3. Critically review professional literature related to ROM and strengthening exercises.
4. Identify appropriate support resources necessary to solve problems.

Case
September 19, 1999, 9:30 a.m.

> **S:** Client is a 37 y/o male s/p R RTC repair on 8/22/99 after sustaining a work-related injury. He presents today without an immobilizer and reports minimal discomfort in his neck, stating "my shoulder is fine." Client also reports that his doctor's visit yesterday went very well. New orders to "begin gentle PRE R Sh."
>
> **O: PROM:** R Sh supine—flex 135, abd 120, ER 35, IR 67, ext 35*
>   L Sh supine—flex 180, abd 180, ER 90, IR 80, ext 65*
>   **Visual inspection:** A well-healed scar appears superior to distal acromial arch. No drainage is noted. Soft tissue mobility is good superficially.
>   **MMT:** L shoulder: normal
>   R shoulder: flex poor+, abd poor+, ER poor+, IR fair–, ext fair–
> **A: Updated goals:**
>   **1.** Client to demonstrate R Sh increased strength by 1 muscle grade in 4 weeks.
>   **2.** Client able to lift R arm and hand to face to assist with simple grooming and ADLs.
>   **3.** Client to be Ind with home strengthening program.
> **P:** Begin PRE R Sh, continue PROM activities and progress to AAROM R Sh

*Ext measured supine passively by dangling arm from side of plinth.

Clinical Application

This was an actual note found in a client's chart and will serve as an appropriate learning tool for the PTA student to examine the concepts of PROM, AAROM, AROM, and PRE.

Case Study Preparation

1. Demonstrate appropriate technique in the application of the different ROM procedures including client positioning and appropriate hand placement.
2. Review and explain techniques for applying manual and mechanical resistance and be prepared to give examples under which circumstances each should be applied.
3. Discuss in small groups what types of "PRE" would be appropriate and which would be inappropriate for this client. Identify pros and cons for each mode of exercise selected.

Role-Playing Exercises

1. Perform PROM exercises on this client.
2. Progress the client to AAROM, as tolerated.
3. Having completed the first two ROM skills, assume the role of a PTA who has been told by the supervising PT to perform "PRE" on this client. Working with a lab partner, perform the selected mode(s) of exercise for your client. What types of responses would identify success or failure of the exercise program?
4. Assume that it is 4 weeks later and the client has been compliant with the prescribed program. The updated strength and functional goal has been achieved, and PROM is now within normal limits. Address question 3 under "Case Study Preparation" from this perspective.

Critical Analysis

1. Identify two different pieces of literature in a peer-reviewed professional journal that address an aspect presented in this case. Critically review the article and determine whether you can make clinical applications from information found in the literature review. Discuss this investigation with your instructor or a local professional.

CASE STUDY 2–2   APPLICATION OF MANUAL FORCE AND FUNCTIONAL USE OF STANDARDIZED ASSESSMENT FORMS

Objectives

After completing the exercises in this case study, the PTA student will be able to:

1. Implement simulated clinical skills relative to manual and mechanical resistance.
2. Critically discuss the implications of various clinical resistive exercise techniques.
3. Identify the clinical significance of Functional Independence Measure (FIM[SM]) forms or other standardized reporting forms.

Case

Mrs. Jones is a 54 y/o female s/p R hip Fx sustained in a MVA. After she was acutely stabilized in the ER, she underwent successful surgery receiving an ORIF of the R hip (intertrochanteric fracture). She now presents in the extended care facility in which you work. The supervising therapist has established a plan of treatment according to the FIM[SM] form ratings that are used in the facility. (FIM[SM] is a service mark of the Uniform Data System for Medical Rehabilitation, a division of U. B. Foundation Activities, Inc.). Plan of treatment includes:

1. Gait training with standard walker, score at admit (4)
2. Transfers from bed to chair and sit to stand, score at admit (5)
3. Bilateral LE strengthening—L LE with ankle weights, R LE with manual resistance
4. Client education specific to hip Fxs and rehabilitation protocols

Long-term goals include:

1. Independent gait using a standard walker (6) over level, smooth, and carpeted surfaces as well as uneven surfaces including ramps and curbs
2. Independent ability to climb stairs (6)
3. Independent transfers (7) to all surfaces including bed, chair, and bathtub bench

Clinical Applications

This case study will involve the application and clinical implications of manual force. A functional use of FIM^{SM} form scores and the clinical significance of standardized assessment forms will be investigated by the student.

Case Study Preparation

1. Obtain a FIM^{SM} form that is typically used in extended care facilities.
2. Review scoring system applied to FIM^{SM} assessment form.
3. Secure a 3-lb ankle weight.
4. Review techniques of manual resistance to the LEs.
5. Review lever systems and implications of increasing or decreasing the force arm.

Role-Playing Exercises

1. With your lab partner, apply treatment for LE strengthening as designed. Use a 3-lb ankle weight on one LE and manual resistance on the opposite extremity. Perform the following exercises:
   a. Supine SLRs
   b. Side-lying hip abduction
   c. Side-lying hip adduction
   d. Prone hip extension
   e. Seated large arc quads
   f. Prone hamstring curls
2. After the exercises are completed, form small groups to discuss the following:
   a. Does the quality of the resistance on each LE feel different to the "client"?
   b. Does the quality remain the same throughout the available ROM?
3. Quantify the exercises applied to the client's lower extremities.
4. Which exercised limb was under the more effective control of the therapist?
5. To effectively use the ankle weight, the client must be placed in antigravity positions. Are the same antigravity positions needed when applying manual resistance?
6. On the second day of treatment, the client is complaining of a soreness that "persisted most of the night in my right hip, but my left hip is fine." Discuss options for treatment at this point.

Critical Analysis

1. Investigate the three different classes of levers found in the human body. Which class best represents this scenario? Discuss how the resistance applied either manually or mechanically effects the working efforts of the muscle.
2. Discuss with your instructor or a local clinician the strengths and weaknesses of using FIM^{SM} instrument ratings. How does the use of this rating system improve consistency of documentation?

CASE STUDY 2–3   **ENERGY SYSTEMS IN THE HUMAN BODY, EXERCISE PARAMETERS, AND CLIENT PROGRESSION**

Objectives

After completing the exercises in this case study, the PTA student will be able to:

1. Implement simulated clinical skills related to aerobic exercise.
2. Critically discuss the clinical implications of the different energy systems in the human body.

3. Creatively solve problems relative to learned skills and applications presented in this text.
4. Identify appropriate conditions for client progression related to exercise parameters.

Case

M.W. is a 68 y/o female client with a history of osteoarthritis in her knees and ankles. She has remained active all of her life and does not want to let her current condition "slow" her down. Riding a stationary bike has been her primary source of exercise since her son purchased one for her 10 yrs ago. She tries to remain faithful to the exercise program, participating at least 3 times/wk exercising for 20 min each session. At times, she will ride once on the weekend.

M.W. entered the hospital at which you are employed for a TKR of her R knee. The surgery went well without complications, and the supervising PT has evaluated M.W. and placed her on your schedule. Plan of treatment includes the following:

1. CPM to R knee, 2x/day for 2 to 3 hours as tolerated
2. Cryotherapy to R knee, as tolerated for edema and pain management
3. Therapeutic exercise: QS, GS, SLR and AP
4. AAROM to R knee
5. Transfer training from side of bed
6. Gait training over level surfaces with standard walker

Clinical Applications

This case will compare the effectiveness of different energy systems in the human body, identify exercise parameters during exercise, and analyze circumstances in which a PTA may progress a client.

Case Study Preparation

To successfully complete this case study the student must:

1. Review the science of energy utilization in the human body and understand the clinical conditions that must be present for the respective energy system to be employed.
2. Review the terms related to the exercise prescription: *frequency, duration, intensity, repetition,* and *mode.*
3. Review legal and professional considerations specific to client progression and the role of the PTA.

Role-Playing Exercises

1. With your lab partner, perform the exercise program for this client. If you need help with any components of the program, check with your instructor or a local physical therapy professional. When performing the treatment session, the student playing the role of the client should perform the activities at an intensity level appropriate to that of a client who has just undergone a total knee replacement and is probably in pain. Allow frequent rest periods between each exercise component.
   a. After completing the treatment session, discuss with your partner which energy systems were used by this client during exercise. Was the student simulating the client fatigued in any way by performing the exercises? How can this client be challenged to promote return of strength and function?
   b. Implement the ideas presented to challenge this client in a second treatment session. Discuss with your lab partner which energy systems were involved and whether any fatigue occurred during the second session. How can this client be challenged to progress?
2. Have one partner assume the role of the supervising PT and have the student PTA report the progress of this client. Which suggestions for progression are indicated? Which changes or progressions appropriate to the established mode of exercises determined by the supervising PT in the plan of treatment can be made without first consulting the supervising PT?

3. The client has been discharged from the hospital and has returned for outpatient physical therapy. She has progressed steadily and is eager to return to her previous lifestyle and activity. She wants to resume riding her stationary bicycle to "keep up her health," but ROM in the R knee prevents intense exercise. The plan of treatment includes the following:

    a. Therapeutic exercise: QS, GS, PRE, SLRs with a limit of 3lbs., as per physician's orders

    b. Stationary bike for ROM to R knee

    c. Patellar and R knee joint mobilization

Have the lab partner ride the stationary bike for ROM purposes. This can be done by performing slow full rotations or performing ½ rotations forward and backward. Have the student PTA monitor the client's vital signs periodically during the exercise. Cycle for 15 minutes, then complete the rest of the exercise program. Discuss which energy system was used by this client. How can this client be challenged to improve her "good health"?

Critical Analysis

1. If a client is unable to aerobically exercise due to ROM limitations, should the cardiovascular benefits gained through aerobic exercise be deferred until the ROM limitations are resolved? Find current peer reviewed literature that would support or disprove your theory.

CASE STUDY 3–1	**RELIABILITY AND VALIDITY OF ORTHOPEDIC MEASUREMENT TOOLS**

Objectives

After completing the exercises in this chapter, the PTA student will be able to:

1. Properly implement the use of a hand dynamometer in simulated clinical simulations.

2. Critically discuss the implications of reliability and validity related to clinical orthopedic measurement tools.

Case

J.M. is a 47 y/o female factory worker. She c/o tingling and weakness in her R hand and reports that the symptoms have been gradually increasing over the last 2 months. The symptoms have now limited her ability to perform her routine job duties. She works at a local manufacturing plant in which she sits at an assembly line connecting small machine parts. The client is right-handed, but she uses both hands equally at work to perform her job. In the objective section of this client's initial assessment, you noticed that the grip strength was assessed at "max grip R hand 47 lb" and "max grip L hand 76 lb." Looking over the data from the initial evaluation, you noticed that an average of three gripping efforts for each hand (right-hand efforts were 76, 48, and 17; left-hand efforts were 81, 76, and 71) was measured on the third grip level from the base of the hand dynamometer to arrive at the "max grip" effort. You have been asked by the supervising therapist to measure this client's interim grip strength to assess the effectiveness to the therapy intervention program.

Clinical Application

This case study will examine the concepts of reliability and validity in measurement tools found in physical therapy.

Case Study Preparation

To complete this case study, the student must:

1. Obtain a hand dynamometer, such as a Jamar hand dynamometer, that has multiple grip size adjustments.

2. Review and explain the concept of validity and reliability.

3. Review and explain the concept of functional excursion.

Role-Playing Exercises

1. Repeat the original assessment on your lab partner: Squeeze the hand dynamometer set on the third level from the base three different times. Take the average of the three trials for the R hand and the average of three trials for the L hand.
2. From the data just collected, report your client's progress compared to the data from the intitial evaluation (assuming it has been 2 weeks since the initial evaluation).
3. Discuss the validity and reliability of this data set comparison (you need not discuss that the data are indeed from two differing individuals but assume this is actual data gathered from the same individual 2 weeks apart). What does the functional excursion of the gripping muscles (flexors) have to do with the setting level of the hand dynamometer?

Critical Analysis

1. Try the following method to assess hand grip strength using a hand dynamometer:
   a. Sit the client in a comfortable chair and face the client.
   b. Place the dynamometer in the client's R hand with the dial facing you and the grip width level set on the lowest or closest level to the base.
   c. Ask the client to squeeze, giving his or her best effort.
   d. Record data without revealing the score to the client.
   e. Repeat same effort in the L hand.
   f. Move dynamometer to the second level away from the dial and repeat steps b through e.
   g. Repeat on the third, fourth, and fifth levels of grip size.
   h. Document the recorded data on a graph, with the "X" axis being the grip levels 1 through 5 and the "Y" axis being the measure of strength either in kilograms or pounds. Make sure to always read the correct scale as most hand-held dynamometers will have both scales. The graphed data for the R and L hands should look something like the graph in Fig. 12–1.

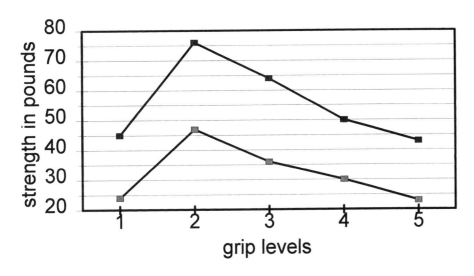

MJ Scenario A

simulated initial assessment data

FIG. 12–1

MJ Scenario B

simulated interim assessment (2 weeks)

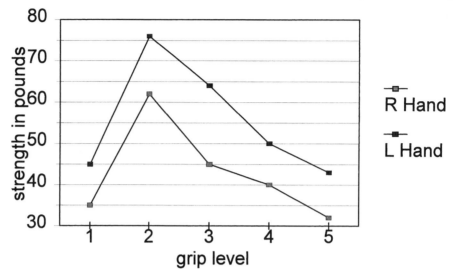

FIG. 12–2

MJ Scenario C

alternate initial assessment

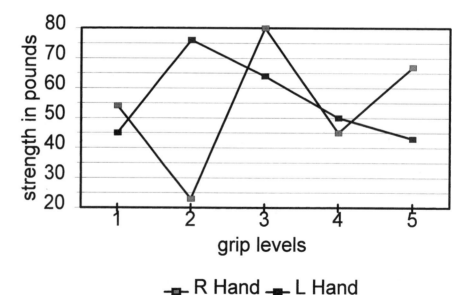

FIG. 12–3

2. Which aspects of reliability and validity in this graph can you discuss? Compare the results to M.J. Scenario B (Fig. 12–2), which was measured 2 weeks after a therapeutic exercise program was implemented. Discuss the elements of validity and reliability in comparing these two data sets, and compare these results to the data set in which the average of three trials was taken.

3. Examine the results graphed in Scenario C (Fig. 12–3) and discuss the reliability and validity of these data assuming that this was the initial assessment produced by M.J.

CASE STUDY 3–2   **ACTIVE INHIBITION TECHNIQUES TO IMPROVE RANGE OF MOTION AND FLEXIBILITY OF THE LOWER EXTREMITY**

Objectives

After completing the exercises in this case study, the PTA student will be able to:

1. Implement active inhibition techniques to improve ROM of the hamstring muscle.
2. Critically discuss the implications of various active inhibition techniques.
3. Critically evaluate the clinical and practical applications between manual and mechanical stretching techniques.

Case

E.L. is a 16 y/o female basketball player who has been complaining of "tightness" in her L hamstring limiting her ability to successfully compete on the basketball court. This athlete has had a history of muscular strains to her hamstring and most recently suffered a grade I hamstring strain during a practice session 4 weeks ago. At this time she has no significant pain in her posterior L thigh and an actively measured (AROM) SLR on the left reveals 60° of motion and on the right 95° of motion. The evaluation and plan of treatment completed by the supervising PT included the following:

1. Moist heat to L hamstring
2. Stretching to L hamstring using active inhibition techniques

Clinical Applications

The PTA will demonstrate understanding and appropriately use active inhibition techniques to improve ROM and flexibility of the LE.

Case Study Preparation

To successfully complete this case study, the student must:

1. Secure a standard goniometer.
2. Review and explain indications and contraindications for superficial moist heat.
3. Review correct measurement procedures to determine ROM of the hip and knee joint.
4. Review the different techniques of active inhibition found in the principles of PNF, which include HR, HRAM, CR, rhythmical rotation (RR), alternating isometrics (AI), and rhythmical stabilization (RS).
5. Review the following: motion occurring in anatomic planes of the LE, the function of the hamstring muscle working as a two-joint muscle, and combination motion that occurs in diagonal planes of the LE.

Role-Playing Exercises

1. With your lab partner, perform an interim assessment of AROM on this client comparing her SLR on the right versus the left. What role does the anatomic nature of the hamstring muscle group play in limiting hip flexion and knee extension simultaneously? Why? Does the position of the pelvis affect your measurement? Why?
2. Discuss with your lab partner the active inhibition techniques that would be appropriate for this client in promoting increased ROM of the L hamstring muscle. Which planes of motion would you use? Perform the techniques appropriately.

Critical Analysis

1. The application of therapeutic exercise in this scenario has used the principle of a short-duration stretch to a pathologically shortened tissue. Would a low-load, long-duration stretch be more effective in this scenario using some sort of mechanical device? Prepare a critical argument for or against the use of a low-load, long-duration mechanical device, supporting your decision with current professional literature.

CASE STUDY 3–3   VISUAL ASSESSMENT VERSUS GONIOMETRIC MEASUREMENT

Objectives

After completing the exercises in this case study, the PTA student will be able to:

1. Identify the clinical usefulness and limitations of visual estimations of joint ROM.
2. Critically discuss professional literature related to reliability and validity.

Case

D.B. is a 18 y/o male football player that has been rehabilitating an ACL grade I sprain in your clinic. The documented measurement of knee flexion taken by a student in the clinic does not appear to be accurate from your visual estimation.

Clinical Application

This case study will examine the concepts of reliability and validity as pertains to the measurement tools found in physical therapy.

Case Study Preparation

To complete this case study, the student must:

1. Obtain three different goniometers with various lengths of measuring arms or measurement dials (increments of measurement).
2. Review and relate the concept of validity and reliability.
3. Secure a chalkboard or dry erase board with writing utensils.

Role-Playing Exercises

1. On a chalk or dry erase board, make five different angles so that each leg of the angles are about 24 inches long. The figures should resemble those in Figure 12–4.

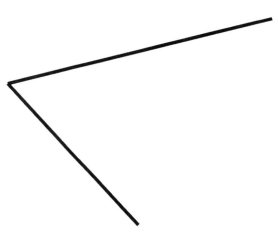

FIG. 12–4

	Visual Estimate	Goniometer A	Goniometer B	Goniometer C
Angle 1				
Angle 2				
Angle 3				
Angle 4				
Angle 5				

FIG. 12–5

2. On a piece of paper (without sharing information with your lab partner), perform the following:
   a. Have you and your lab partner visually estimate the measurement of each of the angles. Write the estimates down.
   b. Measure (both you and your lab partner independently) each of the angles with the various goniometers that you have secured. Document your results without collaborating the effort. The table that you are compiling should look something like Figure 12–5.
   c. Is there a difference between the goniometric measurements and the visual estimate?
   d. Is there a difference between the measurements obtained by the lab partners?
3. Repeat the same exercise with the following variation. Instead of drawing angles, place three dots on the board at least 24 inches apart, identifying one of the dots as the axis. The figures you draw should be similar to those in Figure 12–6.

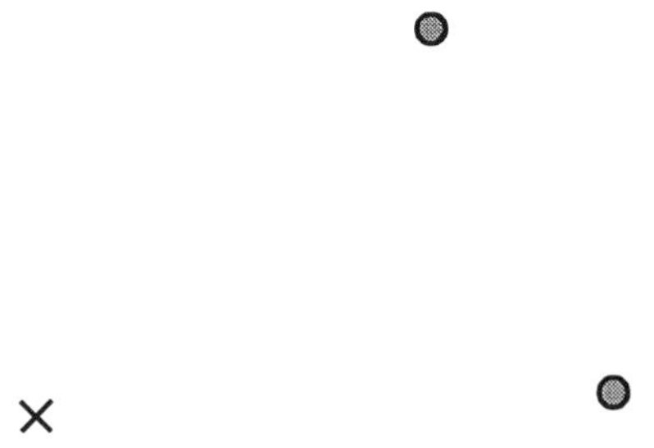

FIG. 12–6

Critical Analysis
1. Find the following research article (or similar peer-reviewed journal article) and develop a group discussion about the strengths and weaknesses of using visual estimations for ROM: Watkins, MA, et al: Reliability of goniometric measurements and visual estimates of knee range of motion obtained in a clinical setting. Phys Ther 71:90, 1991.

CASE STUDY 4–1   **MECHANICAL PLASTIC AND ELASTIC PROPERTIES AND BONY RESPONSE TO STRESS**

Objectives
After completing the exercises in this case, the PTA student will be able to:

1. Critically discuss the clinical implications related to the mechanical properties of plasticity and elasticity
2. Critically analyze current literature relative to the response of human tissue to exercise

Case

K.Y. is a 12 y/o female client with a congenitally acquired spinal cord injury at the segmental level of L2. She has been ambulatory all of her life using bilateral forearm crutches and bilateral KAFOs. She has no sensation or motor activity below the level of her lesion, is in good health, and has not had any other significant medical complications besides the normal childhood diseases. Recently, as she has been experiencing a growth period, she has found that ambulation is becoming difficult and tiring. The supervising PT in the rehabilitation hospital at which you are employed has ordered the client a manually adjustable, custom-fit wheelchair to assist with mobility. The PT has expressed concerns in the evaluation that this client may begin to experience orthopedic dysfunction as she makes the transition from being a full-time ambulator to being a full-time wheelchair user.

Clinical Applications

The clinical implications of the mechanical properties of elasticity and plasticity will be presented, and the response of selected human tissue to exercise will be identified.

Case Study Preparation

To successfully complete this case study, the student must:

1. Secure the following items: a plastic fork, therapeutic exercise putty with three different strengths, a pencil, a hammer, bilateral forearm crutches, wheelchair, and bilateral KAFOs or two straight-leg immobilizers.
2. Review the concepts of plasticity, elasticity, the stress-strain curve, and Wolff's law.

Role-Playing Exercises

1. For the first role-playing exercise, gather the plastic fork and the pencil.
   a. Gently bend the fork without causing it to break and release the stress. How far will the fork deform under the applied stress without breaking? What does this activity demonstrate? Does the fork bend any further or less if the deforming stress is applied very slowly? Repeat the same exercise with the pencil. Compare and contrast the results between the fork and the pencil.
   b. Repeat the bending of the fork, but hold the deforming stress without causing the fork to break. Examine the fork after various time intervals (10 seconds, 30 seconds and 60 seconds) under the deforming stress. Does the shape of the fork change? Does it always return to the original shape? What principle is being demonstrated? Repeat the same exercise with the pencil. Compare and contrast the results between the fork and the pencil.
   c. Gently bend the fork to the point at which the fork breaks. What does this activity demonstrate? Was there an effectively large plastic range of deformation noted?
   d. Grab both ends of the pencil and pull your fingers in opposite directions as hard as possible. What happens? What mechanical force is being applied to the pencil? Is the pencil able to easily withstand this force? What tissue in the body does this pencil represent?
2. For the second role-playing exercise, gather the three different exercise putties and the hammer.
   a. Mold each strength exercise putty into a ball of equivalent size. With the index finger of one hand, slowly push on the top of each newly formed ball. What happens? What is this principle demonstrating? Is there a different amount of force needed to deform each strength putty?
   b. Reform each putty ball. Apply the same "pulling" force to each putty ball as you did to the pencil in the previous exercise. What happens? What principle is being demonstrated? What is the nature of the force being applied?
   c. Reform each putty ball and place on a firm table. Discuss with your lab partner what would happen if you struck the putty with the hammer. After you have decided what should happen, then carefully strike each ball with the hammer. A great deal of force is not needed; simply use the momentum of the hammer to tap the top of each ball. What happened? What type of force was applied? Did you expect this? What principle was demonstrated?

3. K.Y., the client presented in this scenario, during 12 of ambulating on forearm crutches and bilateral forearm crutches, has provided external stress on her lower extremities. Demonstrate this type of gait pattern with your lab partner using bilateral forearm crutches and bilateral KAFOs (or two knee immobilizers). What benefits does K.Y. get from continuing to ambulate? What might happen to her if she becomes wheelchair bound? How is Wolff's law associated with this scenario?

Critical Analysis

1. Find two different current, peer-reviewed articles covering any aspect related to the response of the human skeletal system to exercise and stress. Topics that may contain pertinent information include: osteoporosis, development of children with spina bifida, effects of immobilized limbs, or human response to exercise. Critically analyze the professional works identifying topics related to the mechanical properties of the human tissue, the types of stresses placed on the tissue, and the responses of the selected tissue. Discuss with your instructor and fellow students the clinical implications of the knowledge that was gained from reading these researched investigations.

CASE STUDY 5–1 **CONTINUOUS PASSIVE MOTION AND LOW-LOAD STRETCHING**

Objectives

After completing the exercises in this case study, the PTA student will be able to:

1. Identify the appropriate healing conditions needed for an injured hand involving tendons and bone.
2. Compare and contrast the clinical implications of CPM and low-load dynamic stretching.
3. Critically discuss the implications of having a nonfunctional dominant hand as a result of an injury.

Case

C.H. is a 47 y/o factory worker who injured her L hand and elbow in an industrial accident 10 days ago. She sustained massive fractures to the radius, ulna, and proximal carpal bones as a large object fell onto her distal arm. She has undergone three orthopedic and reconstructive surgeries to stabilize and repair the damage from the crush injury. The surgeon, in her report to the PT, is concerned that because of the massive bony and soft-tissue injuries, this client is at great risk for loss of functional ROM in the forearm, wrist, hand, and digits. Her greatest concern is that the long finger tendons remain free from adhesion as the bony fractures heal. The surgeon asks the therapist for input in preventing potentially irreversible contractures of the tendons. After the client is surgically stabilized, the surgeon will allow gentle motion of all digits, but not at the wrist or forearm.

Clinical Applications

This case study is to be used to compare and contrast the clinical use of CPM and low-load dynamic stretching.

Case Study Preparation

To successfully complete this case study, the student must:

1. Review the healing process of tendons, ligaments, and bones including time frames for healing and prognosis for recovery.
2. Review the effects of immobilization on human tissue.
3. Review and explain the rationale behind the use of low-load stretching and continuous passive motion.
4. Review the anatomy of the forearm, hand, and wrist, examining the relationships of the long finger tendons to the forearm, wrist and digits.

5. Secure two 3 inches wide, single-length, elastic wraps and two flatboard splints about 14 inches long and 3 inches wide (a magazine folded in half will work nicely).

Role-Playing Exercises

1. Take one of the board splints and place it on the palmar surface of your lab partner's hand just proximal to the MCP joints. The splint (or magazine) should run from the MCP joints to just distal to the elbow. Use the 3-inch elastic wrap to secure the splint to the hand and forearm of your lab partner, making sure to leave the digits free to move. Now, take the second board splint and position it on the opposite arm of your lab partner in a similar fashion. Have your lab partner make a fist over the splint. Take the elastic wrap and secure the splint to the forearm and hand encompassing the fist so that the fingers are prevented from moving. When you are completed, this arm should resemble a club.
  - **a.** Compare and contrast the healing process of the bones, tendons, and muscular tissue for this client.
  - **b.** Describe the physiological effects on the joint capsule of the wrist.
  - **c.** Identify the role of collagen fibers in the healing process.
2. Have your lab partner describe the sensations that he or she is feeling as the wrist is immobilized. Working with this client, what can you do to lessen the effects of immobilization and promote healing and function?
3. It has now been 6 weeks after the injury, and the surgeon has removed the splint. The client has performed gentle AROM exercises to the digits as designed by her therapy team. The client describes some general stiffness in the digits, but there are no significant contractures present. The supervising therapist believes that the stiffness will soon resolve. However, there is markedly limited ROM of the wrist. Wrist flexion moves to 55°, and extension is slightly past the neutral position. What avenues of treatment are available for this client?

Critical Analysis

1. Discuss the clinical implications of the injury to the dominant hand of this client.

CASE STUDY 6–1   ATTITUDES TOWARD AGING

Objectives

After completing the exercises in this case study, the PTA student will be able to:

1. Interview a geriatric client.
2. Relate the clinical implications of aging.
3. Critically discuss professional literature related to the aging process.

Case

As you begin treatment on this 78 y/o male farmer, he begins a long discussion about what he did in his "younger years" and how this current ailment has "got him down." This client has been difficult to motivate in performing his exercises since sustaining a hip fracture in a fall at his home. Although you have a busy schedule, you patiently take the time to listen to the client describe his various life stories.

Clinical Applications

This case study will invite the student to examine his or her attitudes toward aging and develop clinical interviewing and critical listening skills.

Case Study Preparation

To successfully complete this case study, the student must:

1. Review the effects of normal aging.
2. Interview a geriatric client, either at a nursing home or in their home with appropriate permission. Ask the client to share stories about his or her life: the activities that the

client enjoys and events that were, or still are, special or memorable. This should be done as an individual assignment, not a collaborative effort by a group of students.

Role-Playing Exercises

1. Assume the role of the client that you interviewed. If the person used a walker, role-play the scenario as best possible. If the client was hard of hearing, role-play the scenario as best possible. In the role of your character, have your lab partner interview you as the geriatric client. When the interview has been completed, discuss with your partner how it felt to be a geriatric client.

2. Assume the role of the client presented in this scenario. Develop a "life story" to fit the character of this client. Have your lab partner interview you and try to increase your motivation to perform your exercise program.

3. Write your epitaph. When completed, place a date on your tombstone identifying how old you were when you died. Did you live a long, healthy life? Did you have a disabling condition? Did you die in a nursing home?

Critical Analysis

1. Discuss with your instructor the time concerns of listening to this client. Even though you have a busy schedule as a PTA, what are the implications of not taking time to listen or of quickly moving through the treatment session?

2. Identify two current peer-reviewed articles that discuss the effects of aging on humans. Form a roundtable discussion group to share what you have found related to concepts of aging. What implications does the published research have regarding the interactions of the PTA with the geriatric client?

CASE STUDY 7–1   PERIPHERAL JOINT MOBILIZATION AND REHABILITATION FUNCTIONAL EXPECTATIONS

Objectives

After completing the exercises in this case study, the PTA student will be able to:

1. Implement peripheral joint mobilization skills on a simulated surgically repaired shoulder.

2. Critically discuss the legal implications of peripheral joint mobilization techniques performed by the PTA.

3. Critically discuss rehabilitation implications of normal versus functional joint motion.

4. Identify and use appropriate support resources necessary to identify the clinical significance of current client medications.

Case

Hx: A 79 y/o white female client with a diagnosis of comminuted proximal R humerus Fx is now 1 week post-op after R shoulder total arthroplasty. Client fell as she was climbing steps at a local hardware store, landing on her R UE. She has been an Ind community ambulator before current onset of dysfunction, living with and caring for her husband who is legally blind. Medical history is unremarkable. Client is R hand dominant. Current medications are Darvocet-N and Phenergan. You will be treating the client at bedside in the extended care facility in which you are employed. The client is wearing an over-the-neck sling for her R UE and states that she has pain near her surgical incision.

Client goals: To return to Ind living with her husband as soon as possible. Her daughter will be able to assist until "she is on her feet [using her arm] again."

Plan of treatment: The supervising PT has included (1) gentle grade I and II joint oscillation mobilization techniques, (2) Codman's pendulum exercises, (3) PROM and AAROM to the R shoulder, and (4) gait training with a straight cane over level and uneven surfaces.

Clinical Applications

This case study will examine the clinical applications and implications of peripheral joint mobilization techniques performed by the PTA.

Case Study Preparation

1. Investigate the significance of this client's fall and injury to her R UE. What problems might this present for her in the future?
2. Look up in a drug handbook the current medications that this client is taking, and discuss the clinical importance of these medications.
3. Review peripheral joint mobilization techniques, indications, and contraindications.

Role-Playing Exercises

1. Demonstrate the rehabilitation techniques outlined in the plan of treatment on your lab partner. Which mobilization (directions) techniques are appropriate? How many oscillations of each technique are appropriate? How many repetitions of each AAROM, PROM, and Codman's pendulum exercises are appropriate? What other anatomic joints should you be concerned about?

Critical Analysis

1. Regarding joint mobilization for this client, why would this be a selected treatment modality? What are the legal issues of a PTA performing joint mobilization according to the practice act of your state?
2. What functional expectations do you have for this client? Is there a difference between normal and functional ROM? Is there a difference between normal and functional use expectations of the client?

CASE STUDY 7–2   CLINICAL IMPLICATIONS OF JOINT END-FEELS

Objectives

After completing the exercises in this chapter, the PTA student will be able to:

1. Differentiate between the three operational joint end-feels presented in this textbook.
2. Discuss possible human tissues that may be creating examiner end-feel.
3. Critique current literature related to peripheral joint mobilization.

Case

K.T. is a 21 y/o female who was injured in a MVA, suffering a TBI. She is currently comatose and has been admitted to the ICU for observation and treatment. The attending physician has ordered physical therapy 3×/day for cognitive stimulation, positioning, and the prevention of joint contractures. The supervising therapist has evaluated the client and implemented the following plan of treatment:

1. Family education regarding aspects of TBI relative to interaction and prognosis
2. Positioning schedule (turned every 2 hours from L side to back to R side)
3. Sensory stimulation
4. PROM ×4 extremities bid

You have been delegated to perform the PROM exercises for this client bid. The supervising therapist sees the client during the other session of the day, to promote sensory stimulation and ensure that positioning concerns for this client are addressed by nursing.

Clinical Applications

The student will compare and contrast the different types of normal and pathological end-feels.

Case Study Preparation
To successfully complete this case study the student must:

1. Review the operational examiner end-feels presented in Chapter 7.
2. Review the anatomy of the shoulder, elbow, wrist, hip, knee, and ankle paying close attention to the anatomical structures that cross each joint respectively. Identify the presence and function of any two-joint muscles that are present.

Role-Playing Exercises
1. Have your partner assume the role of the client in this case. The partner should be relaxed and will not interact during the scenario. Perform the PROM intervention ×4 extremities as designed in the plan of treatment with your eyes closed.
2. While performing PROM, pay particular attention to what you are perceiving at the end of ROM for the shoulder, elbow, wrist, hip, knee, and ankle. Describe the sensation to your partner or the instructor with each motion performed. To which category of end-feel does your perceived sensation of the end-feel belong?
3. Knowing the anatomy and kinesiology of each involved joint, discuss and analyze which tissues may be the limiting movement of the respective joints.

Critical Analysis
1. Identify two current research articles relating to the effectiveness of mobilization treatments. Form a roundtable discussion group and present what you have discovered. What implications do your findings have for your practice as a PTA?

CASE STUDY 8–1   **JUVENILE RHEUMATOID ARTHRITIS**

Objectives
After completing the exercises in this case study, the PTA student will be able to:

1. Implement a therapeutic program for a client with juvenile rheumatoid arthritis (JRA).
2. Discuss the clinical manifestation of JRA.
3. Identify appropriate community support resources necessary to solve problems for the client with JRA.

Case
A.D. is a 14 y/o female who has been complaining of swelling, pain, and stiffness in her hands, knees, and hips for about 2 months. She has been recently diagnosed with JRA. The pediatrician has referred A.D. and her mother to the outpatient physical therapy clinic at which you are employed. As the client enters the clinic, you note that she has a classic "arthritic" gait pattern. The client is taken into a treatment room for evaluation by the supervising PT.

Clinical Applications
This case study will investigate the management of a client with JRA.

Case Study Preparation
To successfully complete this case study, the student must:

1. Review the clinical manifestations of a client with JRA.
2. Review pathological gait deviations.
3. Secure the use of a paraffin bath and a lowboy whirlpool.

Role-Playing Exercises
1. What does a "classic" arthritic gait pattern look like? With your lab partner demonstrate several different types of gait patterns that may reflect how this client is ambulating. What are common characteristics to most arthritic gait patterns?
2. Once you have decided what this client's gait might look like, continue to imitate the gait pattern and leave the classroom, going to the cafeteria, main office, or just

outside. What does it feel like (either physically or psychologically) to simulate this gait pattern? What would it feel like to walk this way as a 14-year-old?

3. If you are feeling physical joint pain during the gait simulation, how would that same stress (applied to your healthy body) effect a client with JRA?

4. The supervising PT has completed her evaluation of this client and determines that a paraffin bath to the client's hands and a warm whirlpool might relieve some of the client's immediate symptoms. Perform this treatment accordingly.

5. In the whirlpool room during the treatment, the child's mother asks you the following question: "The other lady (supervising PT) mentioned something about (A.D.). Experiencing contractures in her hips? She said for (A.D.) to lay on her stomach for 20 minutes each day. What is a contracture and why does she have to lay on her stomach?" Answer the client accordingly.

Critical Analysis

1. Prepare a community resource notebook of support networks available for the client with JRA. Include in your notebook local, state, regional, national, and Internet-based resources available to support the needs of your client.

CASE STUDY 8–2   PEDIATRIC ELBOW FRACTURE AND DISLOCATION

Objectives

After completing the exercises in this case study, the PTA student will be able to:

1. Discuss appropriate elements of a plan of treatment related to the pediatric client with a fracture dislocation of the elbow.

2. Critically discuss the indications and contraindications of various treatment approaches and modalities for this condition.

Case

A pediatric client with a posterior dislocation and fracture of the elbow.

Clinical Applications

This case study will help the PTA student to critically understand the components of the prescribed plan of treatment for a posterior dislocation and fracture of the elbow.

Case Study Preparation

The PTA student must have a firm understanding of the concepts of etiology, mechanism of injury, tissue response to healing, applications of modalities, mobilization techniques, ROM exercises, strengthening exercises, and functional activities.

Role-Playing Exercises and Critical Analysis

Using a variety of professional literature, professional persons, and faculty mentors, describe the most appropriate management that this client will probably be receiving after the described accident. Divide up into six groups and investigate the following areas of probable treatment (**note:** All groups should work collaboratively to present a realistic plan of treatment for this client):

1. **Etiology and mechanism of injury:** This group will describe what the client looks like (demographics), how the injury happened, and what was the immediate medical care for the client?

2. **Modalities:** This group will investigate the appropriate use of modalities for this client. What is most likely to be used and why?

3. **ROM:** This group will investigate the proper use of ROM exercises for this client. When and why are theses exercises applied?

4. **Mobilization:** This group will describe the appropriate use of mobilization techniques for this client. Which techniques are used and why?

5. **Strengthening:** This group will describe and demonstrate the appropriate strengthening for this condition. How and why are the techniques applied?

6. Functional activities: This group will describe and demonstrate the appropriate functional retraining for the client after the injury. How and why are the techniques applied?

CASE STUDY 9–1   ACUTE LATERAL ANKLE SPRAIN

Objectives
After completing the exercises in this case study, the PTA student will be able to:

1. Implement a therapeutic program for an acute lateral ankle sprain.
2. Critically discuss the clinical implications of early aggressive motion versus immobilization in an acute ankle sprain.
3. Discuss the role of proprioception and kinesthesia in the rehabilitation of an acute ankle sprain and safe criteria for return to competition.

Case
N.W. is a 20 y/o female basketball player at the local college. The college is relatively small and has no full-time athletic training staff. When she injured her ankle in a game, she went to the ER for medical assistance. After taking x-rays and clearing the athlete of any fractures, the attending ER physician diagnosed N.W. with a grade II R lateral ankle sprain. She was given a pair of wooden axillary crutches (not properly fitted) and told to go to the PT in the morning. She was also told that she could put as much weight on her injured foot as she was comfortable with. N.W. arrives at the physical therapy clinic the next morning for assistance with her injury.

The supervising PT completed the evaluation and prescribed the following plan of treatment:

1. Cryotherapy to R ankle
2. Electrical stimulation for edema management and pain control
3. Gait training, WBAT R LE and properly fit crutches
4. AROM HEP to R ankle
5. Compression and elevation instruction

The athlete will attend daily sessions for the first week. The supervising PT will adjust the frequency upon re-evaluation of the injury in one week.

Clinical Applications
This case study will investigate the therapeutic intervention of an acute lateral ankle sprain and the role of proprioception and kinesthesia in the rehabilitation of an acute injury.

Case Study Preparation
To successfully complete this case study, the student must:

1. Design or obtain an ankle rehabilitation program.
2. Review the acute healing process and management of a ligamentous injury.
3. Secure an electrical stimulation machine, crutches, two 3-inch elastic wraps, and cryotherapy.

Role-Playing Exercises
1. Perform the plan of treatment on this client.

Critical Analysis
1. As this athlete heals and is encouraged to return to competition, critically discuss the role that proprioception and joint mechanoreceptors play in the ability of this athlete to compete successfully. What are the advantages and disadvantages of returning to play early? Find professional resources or literature to support or reject your position.

CASE STUDY 9–2   CHRONIC LATERAL EPICONDYLITIS

Objectives
After completing the exercises in this chapter, the PTA student will be able to:

1. Discuss appropriate elements of a plan of treatment related to the client with a chronic lateral epicondylitis.
2. Critically discuss the indications and contraindications of various treatment approaches and modalities for this condition.

Case
A client with a chronic lateral epicondylitis.

Clinical Applications
This case study will help the PTA student to critically understand the components of the prescribed plan of treatment to manage a client with a chronic lateral epicondylitis.

Case Study Preparation
The PTA student must have a firm understanding of the concepts of etiology, mechanism of injury, tissue response to healing, applications of modalities, mobilization techniques, ROM exercises, strengthening exercises, and functional activities.

Role-Playing Exercises and Critical Analysis
Using a variety of professional literature, professional persons, and faculty mentors, describe the most appropriate management that this client will probably be receiving for the described condition. Divide up into six groups and investigate the following areas of probable treatment (**note:** all groups should work collaboratively to present a realistic plan of treatment for this client):

1. **Etiology and mechanism of injury:** This group will describe what the client looks like (demographics), how the injury happened, and what the medical care was for the client?
2. **Modalities:** This group will investigate the appropriate use of modalities for this client. What is most likely to be used and why?
3. **ROM:** This group will investigate the proper use of ROM exercises for this client. When and why are these exercises applied?
4. **Mobilization:** This group will describe the appropriate use of mobilization techniques for this client. Which techniques are used and why?
5. **Strengthening:** This group will describe and demonstrate the appropriate strengthening for this condition. How and why are the techniques applied?
6. **Functional activities:** This group will describe and demonstrate the appropriate functional retraining for the client after the injury. How and why are the techniques applied?

CASE STUDY 10–1   WORK-RELATED CHRONIC LOWER BACK INJURY

Objectives
After completing the exercises in this case study, the PTA student will be able to:

1. Implement therapeutic program for a client with a chronic lower back injury.
2. Critically discuss the role that client education plays in a functional restoration program.
3. Critically discuss potential barriers to recovery for the chronically injured client.
4. Analyze worker's compensation benefits, guidelines, and restrictions relative to the rehabilitation of an injured worker.

Case
B.N. is a 38 y/o male factory worker who injured his back 12 weeks ago while lifting a box at work. He has had persistent pain in his lower back that he describes as "an

aching, sharp sensation." There are no radiating symptoms into either LE any longer, but he does complain of headaches on a regular basis. He has been in two different rehabilitation programs and has seen numerous physicians. He is currently being treated in the outpatient department at the hospital in which you are employed. Your facility does not have the equipment to be a work-hardening or work rehabilitation facility, but it does have a treadmill, stationary bike, basic passive modalities, and a number of small therapy tools, boxes, and wrist weights. While at work, this client must be able to successfully lift at least 10 lb frequently throughout the day from various levels. He must also tolerate standing on hard surfaces for extended periods of time, manipulating small objects, nuts, and bolts. The client attends physical therapy daily as part of his worker's compensation treatment guidelines. The facility receives a flat reimbursement for the client's 4-hour daily sessions. The supervising PT has evaluated this client and has established the following plan of treatment:

1. Aerobic exercise to reverse deconditioning
2. Cryotherapy for pain control
3. Work-simulated activities including lifting, standing, and manipulating objects
4. Client education emphasizing physical work readiness and fitness maintenance

Clinical Applications

This case study will investigate the issues relative to the management of a client with a chronic low back injury, including treatment, barriers to recovery, and worker's compensation guidelines.

Case Study Preparation

To successfully complete this case study, the student must:

1. Review the treatment implications for a client with a chronic low back injury.
2. Secure or design a functional restoration program for a client with chronic low back pain.
3. Secure cryotherapy, small ankle weights, stationary bike, treadmill, nuts, bolts, exercise putty, and magazines.

Role-Playing Exercises

1. Implement the plan of treatment on your lab partner and document the session accordingly. Why does this plan of treatment de-emphasize passive modalities?
2. Plan a client education session for a group of injured workers. What aspects of education are necessary in promoting the safe return to work?
3. Plan a client education session for a group of noninjured workers. How is this session different from the session for an injured group of workers?

Critical Analysis

1. Discuss with your lab partner the potential barriers to recovery for this client. How can these barriers be identified, overcome, or managed?
2. Investigate the regulations related to workman's compensation in your state. What are the guidelines for rehabilitation, rights of the worker, and conditions for return to work?

CASE STUDY 10–2   **ACTIVITY MODIFICATION FOR THE INJURED WORKER BY THE REHABILITATION TEAM**

Objectives

After completing the exercises in this case study, the PTA student will be able to:

1. Implement simulated clinical skills related to activity modification.
2. Critically discuss the clinical implications of job modification and returning the client to work.

3. Identify appropriate support resources necessary to solve problems associated with this case.

Case

M.M. is 46 y/o female factory worker who arrives at your clinic with complaints of pain and discomfort in her R shoulder. She explains to the evaluating PT that she must repeatedly use her arm to reach into an overhead bin to retrieve a part and place the part onto the machine that is slowly passing by on the assembly line. The supervising PT has indicated that the client has an impingement syndrome from repeated stress at work. The management of the condition consisted of rest, iontophoresis with dexamethasone, and rotator cuff strengthening. After 2 weeks, the symptoms in the arm were significantly better, and the client became anxious to return to her job. The supervising PT directs you to construct a functional restoration program to prepare this client to safely return to her job duties.

Clinical Applications

Modification of the activities performed by a client at work is sometimes necessary to prevent the recurrence of symptoms. The student will investigate how to creatively modify activities for clients to safely return to work.

Case Study Preparation

To successfully complete this case study, the student must:

1. Review and describe the mechanism of injury of repetitive stress injuries.
2. Relate the biomechanics of the shoulder girdle.
3. Design a functional restorative exercise program for the UE.

Role-Playing Exercises

1. Assume the role of the PTA in this case. Design exercises that will functionally retrain the client and prepare her both physically and mentally for a safe return to work.
2. Design an educational packet for the client to follow for the prevention of similar symptoms in the future.
3. Design, discuss, and implement strategies for the client to modify her work environment to lessen the risk of reinjury.

Critical Analysis

1. Find two current pieces of literature related to repetitive stress syndromes in the workplace. Critically analyze the articles identifying educational concepts and job modification techniques used to prevent the return of symptoms associated with repetitive stress disorders.

CASE STUDY 11–1   REHABILITATION AND PROGRESSION OF THE CLIENT WITH A FRACTURED PATELLA

Objectives

After completing the exercises in this case study, the PTA student will be able to:

1. Implement clinical application skills of gait training, gait analysis, functional electrical stimulation, and knee rehabilitation protocols.
2. Critically discuss the implications of written evaluation components necessary for effective treatment.
3. Critically discuss appropriate exercise protocols for the knee.
4. Discuss client progression with supervising physical therapist.

Case

Hx: A 66 y/o female client with a diagnosis of R patella Fx was referred to the outpatient clinic at which you are employed after receiving inpatient physical therapy services following surgical fixation of the fractured patella. She is now 6 weeks postoperative status. Onset of present disability occurred when the client stepped up onto a curb and "lost her balance," landing on the anterior surface of her R knee. She is now an Ind ambulator, using a rolling walker and wearing a straight-leg immobilizer on R LE. She ambulates over level surfaces and small curbs, short distances in the community. She lives alone in an accessible retirement community environment and has the ability to ride a shuttle bus to and from her scheduled appointments or for shopping. She must be able to climb the two steps into the bus because it does not have a wheelchair lift. She will have physical assistance from the bus driver if needed. Relevant medical history includes stable angina, osteoporosis, and peptic ulcer disease. Medications being taken include Cardizam, Tums, Pepcid, Fosamax, Xanax, and Darvocet-N.

Evaluation

The documented evaluation was markedly brief and in a narrative handwritten format. You were able to distinguish the following important aspects related to the client's status:

1. There was marked R knee pain with flexion.
2. R quad strength was poor.
3. R knee flexion was 30° (measured with a standard goniometer).
4. Knee ext was passively 0°.
5. Active terminal extension R knee was −15° (demonstrated by an extensor lag during SLR of −15°).
6. All other ROM was WFL.
7. The supervising therapist had written a gait evaluation that consisted of "WB status WBAT w/RW and immobilizer R LE Ind short functional community distances. No significant deviations. Stairs NT."

Plan of Treatment

1. E-stim (FES) to R quads
2. Gait training, progressing as tolerated to include steps
3. Ther ex protocol for R quad strengthening
4. No aggressive ROM exercises of R knee, as per physician's orders.

Clinical Applications

This case study will examine knee rehabilitation for a geriatric client and the role of the PTA in progressing the client.

Case Study Preparation

To successfully complete this case study, the student must:

1. Secure a straight-leg immobilizer and a rolling walker.
2. Obtain an exercise protocol for quadriceps femoris strengthening.
3. Review the clinical use of a functional electrical stimulation unit, including indications and contraindications for electrical stimulation.
4. Review gait patterns and gait deviations.

Role-Playing Exercises

1. Gait train your lab partner over level and uneven surfaces, demonstrating the gait pattern that this client is probably using.
2. Perform a gait assessment on your partner. Do you feel that there are "no significant deviations"?
3. Perform E-stim (FES) to the R quads as well as the therapeutic exercise protocol for R quad strengthening. Does the client's difficulty with terminal knee extension on the right change your protocol?
4. Given the ROM limitation orders by the physician, do you feel that this will limit your ability to rehabilitate this client's R knee?

Critical Analysis

1. You received a phone call from the physician today. He has just seen the client and informed you that he was pleased with the bone healing (patella) and to "push motion

of the R knee." Document the phone order appropriately, and discuss your recommendations with the supervising PT. You have been the only therapist who has seen this client over the past 2 weeks.

CASE STUDY 11–2   **CONTINUOUS PASSIVE MOTION AFTER TOTAL KNEE REPLACEMENT AND THE PRACTICAL APPLICATION OF COMPRESSION GARMENTS**

Objectives

After completing the exercises in this case study, the PTA student will be able to:

1. Implement simulated clinical skills for the CPM machine and compression garments.
2. Critically discuss the rationale for the use of compression garments and CPM after a total knee replacement.
3. Identify and use appropriate support resources necessary to identify the clinical significance of current client medications.

Case

Upon arrival to work at the Jonesboro Medical Center, you see a new client's name on your schedule. The supervising PT completed the evaluation late in the evening the previous night and you are now to implement the plan of treatment. The physician's orders on the chart simply stated, "Order PT, WBAT R LE." The PT evaluation was as follows:

S: Hx: Client is a 56 y/o black female w/Dx of osteoarthritis and s/p R TKA post-op 2 days. PMH include a L TKA 6 months ago. Medications: Feldene, Coumadin, Tylox. Client's social Hx includes living at home independently with husband who is in good health. Client appears well motivated to perform her rehabilitation.

O: Incision on R knee is dressed with sterile 4 × 4 gauze pads and large cotton wrap under full leg-length compressive stockings. Examination of the R knee on removal of dressing reveals a 10-inch longitudinal incision held securely with staples and a post-op drain located laterally superior to the knee joint line. No drainage or odor is noted, but knee appears moderately swollen and is warm to the touch around the incision.

   AROM: R Knee (E/F) –5° to 45° with moderate pain
            L Knee (E/F) 0° to 95° with no pain
   PROM: R Knee (E/F) –5° to 82° with moderate pain
            L Knee (E/F) 0° to 95°
   MMT: R quads—trace, client has significant difficulty contracting quadriceps muscle
            L quads—good–, client is able to lock L knee
            R hamstrings—fair–
            L hamstrings—good
   Sensation: R LE is intact to light touch and pain; L LE was not tested.
   Functional assessment: WB status is WBAT.
   Gait: Contact guard assist using standard walker over level surfaces 300 ft. Stairs were not tested.
   Transfers: Sit to stand from hospital bed is Ind. Minimum assistance for stand to sit in chair.
   Bed mobility: Rolling and come to sit are Ind.

A: Client appears well motivated and eager to go home.
   STG (1 wk):
       1. R knee AROM to be 0° to 85° to facilitate Ind transfers and gait.
       2. R knee quads to be fair– to facilitate Ind transfers and gait.

LTG (2 weeks):
1. Client to be Ind with gait using appropriate assistive device over level surfaces.
2. Client to be Ind with all functional transfers.
3. Client to be Ind with HEP.

P: Client to be seen bid in hospital teaching QSs, SLRs, AROM R LE, heel slides, APs, gait training, transfer training, and instructions for use of CPM.

Clinical Application
This case study will examine the efficacy of CPM after a total knee replacement, including the practical application of compression garments and CPM machines.

Case Study Preparation
1. Secure the following supplies and equipment: full leg-length compressive stocking, several 4 × 4 gauze pads, cotton wrapping, and access to a knee CPM machine.
2. Identify the role of the medications that this client is taking.
3. Identify and review the rationale for wearing full leg-length compressive stockings.

Role-Playing Exercises
1. On your lab partner, attempt to place a full length compressive stocking over a mock surgical dressing of several 4 × 4s and a full cotton wrap.
2. Apply a CPM to your partner's knee and adjust properly. Go through the recommended procedures for setting your machine, and establish a treatment session that would be applicable for the case study client.

Critical Analysis
1. Discuss with your instructor the role that the CPM plays in the rehabilitation of this client.
2. Find three current articles in the professional literature on the effectiveness of CPM after a TKR surgery. Form a roundtable discussion group and analyze these with peers.

CASE STUDY 11–3   MANAGEMENT OF THE CLIENT IN THE HOME SETTING

Objectives
After completing the exercises in this case study, the PTA student will be able to:

1. Discuss the unique requirements of managing a client in the home setting.
2. Identify the appropriate communication chain and supervision requirements for the PTA working in a home health environment.
3. Creatively incorporate therapeutic exercises to effectively manage the client in the home health setting.
4. Relate appropriate emergency procedures for managing unforeseen situations in the home health setting.

Case
N.G. is a 78 y/o female that you are treating in her home.

Clinical Applications
The student will investigate the unique nature of managing a client in the home health setting.

Case Study Preparation
To successfully complete this case study, the student must:

1. Review and identify rules and regulations related to the PTA treating clients in the home health environment.

Role-Playing Exercises

1. With your lab partner, determine the impairments and functional limitations that your client presents with.
2. Using nothing but common household items, develop an exercise program for N.G. to follow to help improve her functional status.
3. Repeat this exercise with a new set of impairments and functional limitations.

Critical Analysis

1. Critically discuss the supervision requirements and the regulations imposed on the PTA working in the home health setting.
2. Critically discuss and make appropriate recommendations in an emergency situation related to managing the client in the home setting: You are walking N.G. in her home and she suddenly falls to the floor and is in pain.

CASE STUDY 11–4   FALLING AND BALANCE

Objectives

After completing the exercises in this case study, the PTA student will be able to:

1. Discuss and demonstrate the mechanisms and strategies for maintaining balance.
2. Critically discuss risk factors related to falling.
3. Develop guidelines for a fall prevention program.

Case

K.R. is an 87 y/o female nursing home resident who is being treated after she sustained a fractured hip in a fall in her room. The nursing supervisor has mandated that the rehabilitation team develop a fall prevention program in the facility because there have been too many falls and fall-related injuries to the residents.

Clinical Applications

This case will present a critical inquiry into the need for and development of fall prevention programs.

Case Study Preparation

To successfully complete this case study, the student must:

1. Investigate and demonstrate the various balancing strategies used to maintain upright balance.
2. Review the risk factors related to falling.

Role-Playing Exercises

1. With your lab partner, demonstrate the various balance mechanisms and strategies used by clients to prevent a fall (fixed support—ankle synergy and hip synergy, change in support—stepping and grasping).
   a. Which strategies are used for small challenges to stability?
   b. Which strategies are used for greater challenges to stability?
2. Try to elicit the mechanisms in your lab partner with their eyes open and with their eyes closed. Is there a difference?

Critical Analysis

1. Either using the identified risk factors related to falls presented in Chapter 11, or use an outside source, critically discuss why each factor is on the list.
2. Using at least three different sources of professional literature, develop a fall prevention program for this nursing home resident. Key elements that should be included are presented in Chapter 11.

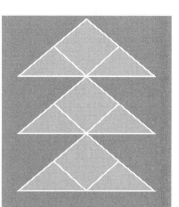

chapter 13

Practice Scenarios

ORTHOPEDIC CLIENT HANDLING SKILLS

CLIENT HANDLING SKILLS SCENARIO 1

Items Needed to Complete Scenario

> Gait Belt

This orthopedic client is s/p TKR on the right. The supervising PT has instructed you to assist this client out of bed and into the wheelchair. She has a history of severe RA and has significant difficulty performing weight-bearing activities, including transferring from the side of bed. Discuss strategies for assisting this client safely out of bed and into the wheelchair. Perform the most appropriate transfer and document accordingly.

CLIENT HANDLING SKILLS SCENARIO 2

Items Needed to Complete Scenario

> Gait Belt

This orthopedic client is s/p THR on the left. The supervising PT has instructed you to assist this client out of bed and into the wheelchair. The client is very motivated to begin her rehabilitation and reports having very little discomfort in her L hip. Discuss strategies for assisting this client safely out of bed and into the wheelchair. Perform the most appropriate transfer and document accordingly.

CLIENT HANDLING SKILLS SCENARIO 3

Items Needed to Complete Scenario

> Sliding Board
> Gait Belt

This 54 y/o female client is a Bil AK amputee who must be taught independent transfers from bed to wheelchair. Instruct her in the most appropriate sliding board transfers and document accordingly.

CLIENT HANDLING SKILLS SCENARIO 4

Items Needed to Complete Scenario

> Gait Belt

This 28 y/o male client with complete C5 quadriplegia has entered your rehabilitation hospital after recent surgery to correct LE contractures of both ankles. The surgery consisted of a heel cord-lengthening procedure to assist with his mobility during transfers. You are to begin therapeutic exercises with this client and must safely transfer him to the mat in your gym. Discuss strategies for safely transferring this client to the exercise mat. Perform the most appropriate transfer and document accordingly.

CLIENT HANDLING SKILLS SCENARIO 5

Items Needed to Complete Scenario

> An Assistant

You are an employee at a nursing home who is called by the supervising nurse to assist in placing a client back in bed. It appears that the client had fallen to the floor as she was trying to get out of bed. The supervising nurse has cleared the client after a physical exam and asks for your suggestions on the most appropriate way to lift the client from the floor back into the bed. Give recommendations and assist this client in returning to bed, with the help of the supervising nurse.

CLIENT HANDLING SKILLS SCENARIO 6

Items Needed to Complete Scenario

> Bed Sheet
> Two Assistants
> Reclining Wheelchair

This client is a 16 y/o male who has undergone surgical spinal fixation for a recent spinal fracture. The client arrives for a therapy session in a solid CTLSO body jacket (turtle shell–type with cervical collar). To take him to the therapy gym, you must assist him out of bed and into a fully reclined wheelchair. He is unable to tolerate any position but supine at this time. The supervising PT has recommended that you perform a bed sheet transfer, safely moving the client from the bed to the reclined wheelchair. Perform this transfer and document accordingly.

CLIENT HANDLING SKILLS SCENARIO 7

Items Needed to Complete Scenario

> Mechanical Lift
> Wheelchair

This client is completely dependent for all transfers. He is too large to lift safely. You must use the mechanical lift to safely perform this maneuver. Perform the mechanical lift transfer from hospital bed to wheelchair. Ensure that the client is comfortable in the wheelchair because he may be up in the wheelchair for an undetermined length of time. Document this activity accordingly.

CLIENT HANDLING SKILLS SCENARIO 8

Items Needed to Complete Scenario

> Axillary Crutches
> Ankle ROM HEP
> Gait Belt

This client has been evaluated by a PT in your outpatient facility with a diagnosis of acute grade II R ankle sprain. Client c/o pain with weight bearing. Signs include moderate swelling anteriorly and laterally in the R ankle, as well as significant pain to palpation over sinus tarsi region and inferior to the lateral malleolus. ROM is significantly limited because of pain. X-rays have ruled out fracture. You are instructed to (1) fit the client with crutches, (2) teach gait (TTWB) on level and uneven surfaces, and (3) teach the client AROM exercises for the R ankle. Document your session accordingly.

CLIENT HANDLING SKILLS SCENARIO 9

Items Needed to Complete Scenario

> Standard Walker
> Gait Belt

This 75 y/o male client is 24 hours postop status, R THR surgery. The supervising PT has evaluated the client in the a.m., and for the p.m. therapy session, you are instructed to perform gait training for short distances over level surfaces from side of bed. The client's weight-bearing status is TTWB on the right for balance only. The PT documented that during the a.m. session, the client was a bit dizzy when sitting at the side of bed, needing moderate assistance to transfer from sit to stand. The client reports to you that he is eager to begin walking. Perform the gait training session.

CLIENT HANDLING SKILLS SCENARIO 10

Items Needed to Complete Scenario

> Gait Belt

Your client is a 65 y/o female with a history of severe RA. She has undergone a recent TKR on her L knee and is having difficulty getting out of bed. She feels much better if she just stays in bed and keeps a pillow propped under her surgical knee. Work with this client on moving from supine to sit and from sit to stand at the side of bed. Discuss with her the potential danger and problems that may occur from her positioning of the knee in bed. Demonstrate beginning isometric quadriceps exercises and AAROM for the L knee.

CLIENT HANDLING SKILLS SCENARIO 11

Items Needed to Complete Scenario

> Gait Belt
> Axillary Crutches
> Steps and Ramps

This 24 y/o male basketball player recently suffered a grade II ankle sprain. After being evaluated by the supervising PT, the POT calls for (1) fitting of axillary crutches, (2) gait training over level surfaces (WBAT), and (3) gait training over uneven surfaces and stairs. Document your session accordingly.

CLIENT HANDLING SKILLS SCENARIO 12

Items Needed to Complete Scenario

> Gait Belt
> Parallel Bars
> Two Long-Leg Immobilizers (or Actual KAFOs)

Your client is a 16 y/o female with a complete L1 level lesion due to SCI. She has been tremendously motivated to walk and has shown good progress during her rehabilitative stay. She is now to begin gait skills using the parallel bars and Bil KAFOs (simulated with knee immobilizers). Instruct this client in (1) sit to stand from wheelchair into parallel bars, (2) balance activities in the parallel bars when standing erect, and (3) a swing-to gait pattern in the parallel bars. Document your session accordingly.

CLIENT HANDLING SKILLS SCENARIO 13

Items Needed to Complete Scenario

> Gait Belt
> Standard Walker
> Two Long-Leg Immobilizers (or Actual KAFOs)

The client in Client Handling Skills Scenario 12, who you have been working with regularly, has improved as expected with her gait and balance skills inside the parallel bars. She is now ready to be progressed to outside of the parallel bars using a standard walker. When the client is up in the parallel bars, progress her out the end of the bars to the walker. Continue gait training over level surfaces using a swing-to gait pattern. Document your session accordingly.

CLIENT HANDLING SKILLS SCENARIO 14

Items Needed to Complete Scenario

> Gait Belt
> Forearm Crutches
> Floor Mat
> Two Long-Leg Immobilizers (or Actual KAFOs)

The same client in Orthopedic Client Handling Skills Scenarios 12 and 13 continues to progress accordingly. She is pleased with her ability to ambulate but reports that the walker is slowing her down. Progress this client to using Bil forearm crutches with a swing-through gait pattern. Also, begin working on falling skills to ensure her safety as a potential community ambulator. Document your session accordingly.

CLIENT HANDLING SKILLS SCENARIO 15

Items Needed to Complete Scenario

> Gait Belt
> Standard Walker
> Wheelchair

Your client is a 87 y/o male who has been hospitalized for several weeks with a diagnosis of pneumonia. He c/o inability to walk because of LE weakness. The supervising PT has upgraded his POT to include gait training (no weight-bearing limitations) from the side of the bed. Perform a gait training session with this client. Keep in mind that he is weak and may need frequent rests.

CLIENT HANDLING SKILLS SCENARIO 16

Items Needed to Complete Scenario

> Gait Belt
> Wheelchair
> Bedside Commode

Your client is a 58 y/o female who has suffered a compound fracture of the R ankle. She is non–weight bearing on the affected side and is wearing a plaster cast AK immobilizing the foot, ankle, and knee. You are to teach her how to transfer effectively from the wheelchair to the bed and bedside commode. Document your session accordingly.

CLIENT HANDLING SKILLS SCENARIO 17

Items Needed to Complete Scenario

Gait Belt

You have been selected by the chief PT of the department to give inservice training on lifting to a new class of nurses' aides. You have 20 minutes to cover the concepts of body mechanics, lifting, and safe transferring of clients. Prepare and present your inservice training complete with handouts.

CLIENT HANDLING SKILLS SCENARIO 18

Items Needed to Complete Scenario

Gait Belt

You have been selected by the department's chief PT to give inservice training on transferring clients to the newly hired staff. You are to effectively cover (1) dependent pivot transfer, (2) dependent sliding board transfer, and (3) two-man lift.

CLIENT HANDLING SKILLS SCENARIO 19

Items Needed to Complete Scenario

Bed Sheet
Tilt Table
Hospital Gurney

This client has been in LE orthopaedic traction for 4 weeks and has been in the supine position since that time. The supervising PT has given you instructions to transfer the client out of bed. She is at risk for orthostatic hypotension. The POT includes a progressive sitting program with the goal of sitting upright in a wheelchair for 15 minutes. Perform an appropriate transfer to the tilt table from a hospital gurney and then an appropriate treatment session on the tilt table. Document your session accordingly.

CLIENT HANDLING SKILLS SCENARIO 20

Items Needed to Complete Scenario

Axillary Crutches

This 14 y/o male client comes to your outpatient clinic after a recent same-day arthroscopic procedure to his R knee. The supervising therapist has asked you to fit the client with a pair of axillary crutches and instruct him in a PWB (25%) gait pattern. Instruct the client (1) how to safely ambulate over level surfaces and (2) how to ascend and descend steps using the crutches. Document your session accordingly.

CLIENT HANDLING SKILLS SCENARIO 21

Items Needed to Complete Scenario

Tilt Table
Hospital Gurney
Bed Sheets
Stethoscope
Blood Pressure Cuff

This client has been in orthopedic traction after sustaining multiple LE fractures in a MVA 6 weeks ago. The physician has ordered to begin progressive weight bearing on the injured LEs. The supervising PT is greatly concerned over the ability of the client to tolerate an upright posture needed for weight bearing because of the length of time the client has been supine. The decision has been made to use a tilt table to begin weight bearing and work on orthostatic hypotension problems. Perform an appropriate transfer onto the tilt table, and then perform a treatment session gradually progressing the client as tol. Document your session accordingly.

CLIENT HANDLING SKILLS SCENARIO 22

Items Needed to Complete Scenario

> Tilt Table
> Hospital Gurney
> Bed Sheets
> Stethoscope
> Blood Pressure Cuff

This 28 y/o client with SCI has recently undergone cervical spinal fixation and arrives for treatment in a halo device. The client has not been out of the supine position since the onset of his injury. The supervising PT has instructed you to begin working with the client to increase sitting tolerance. The means to accomplish this goal is the use of a tilt table. Perform an appropriate transfer onto the tilt table, and then perform a treatment session gradually progressing the client as tol. Document your session accordingly.

CLIENT HANDLING SKILLS SCENARIO 23

Items Needed to Complete Scenario

> Tilt Table
> Hospital Gurney
> Bed Sheets
> Stethoscope
> Blood Pressure Cuff
> Reclining Wheelchair
> Standard Walker

This 75 y/o female client has recently undergone a THA revision for the third time. She has a history of dislocating her R hip. The physician has ordered gait training but wants to avoid any significant hip flexion or adduction. After discussing this difficult scenario with the supervising PT, the decision was made to initiate gait training with this client from an upright position using a tilt table to avoid excessive hip motion during the transition from sitting to standing. Perform an appropriate transfer onto the tilt table from a gurney. Perform a treatment session moving the client from supine to standing, followed by gait training using a standard walker from the standing position. Return the client to a supine position after the gait training session is complete. Discuss any contraindications and the method for assisting the client quickly to a supine position in an emergency situation. Document your session accordingly.

CLIENT HANDLING SKILLS SCENARIO 24

Items Needed to Complete Scenario

> Standard Walker
> Gait Belt

This 78 y/o client who resides in a nursing home has recently returned from the hospital with a surgically repaired hip fracture. The orders from the surgeon call for 50% weight bearing. The supervising PT has completed the evaluation and delegated his treatment to you for gait training and balance skills. Perform the gait training session, and document your results accordingly.

 # ORTHOPEDIC INTERIM ASSESSMENT

INTERIM ASSESSMENT SCENARIO 1

Items Needed to Complete Scenario

    Standard Goniometer

After treating this client with L supraspinatus tendinitis, you are to perform an interim assessment of ROM and muscle testing. The client is still mildly tender to palpation over the belly of the muscle. His subjective symptoms of pain with abduction are less, and he is now able to sleep all night without waking up because of pain. Document your results accordingly.

INTERIM ASSESSMENT SCENARIO 2

Items Needed to Complete Scenario

    Standard Goniometer

After treating this client for an acute grade II lateral ankle sprain on the right, you are to perform an interim assessment of ROM and muscle testing. The client is moderately tender over the lateral inferior portion of the lateral malleolus. The client reports that he exercises "sometimes." Mild edema persists in the sinus tarsi region, and he ambulates with a single crutch. Perform an interim assessment, and document your results accordingly.

INTERIM ASSESSMENT SCENARIO 3

Items Needed to Complete Scenario

    Standard Goniometer

After treating this client for chronic "tennis elbow" on the left, you are to perform an interim assessment of ROM and muscle testing. The client is mildly tender over the lateral aspect of the forearm and, in particular, has "an aching in her elbow" when she arises in the morning. The client is anxious to return to playing tennis and has asked you when this will be possible. Document the interim assessment accordingly. What instruction regarding protection of the injury would you give her? When can she return to play, and how do you determine this?

INTERIM ASSESSMENT SCENARIO 4

Items Needed to Complete Scenario

    Standard Goniometer
    Hand Dynamometer
    Pinch Dynamometer

After treating this client for a carpal tunnel release on the R wrist, you are to perform an interim assessment for ROM, grip, and pinch strength. Document your results accordingly. Was your test valid and reliable? How would you make this determination?

INTERIM ASSESSMENT SCENARIO 5

Items Needed to Complete Scenario

Standard Goniometer

After treating this 18 y/o client s/p ORIF of the L femur, you are to perform an interim assessment of ROM and muscle testing of the hip and knee. The client is 6 weeks postop status and feels that she is progressing steadily. She has no c/o pain or irritation. The scar is healed and mobile. Document your results accordingly.

INTERIM ASSESSMENT SCENARIO 6

Items Needed to Complete Scenario

Cervical Goniometer

Your client is recovering from a cervical soft-tissue injury suffered in a MVA 2 months ago. There exists a minimal loss of ROM in all cervical planes. Perform an interim assessment on this client's cervical ROM, and document your results accordingly.

INTERIM ASSESSMENT SCENARIO 7

Items Needed to Complete Scenario

Standard Goniometer

Your client is a 28 y/o male who suffered a fracture of his R distal radius and ulna in an industrial accident. During your treatment progression of moist heat, AROM exercises, and gentle mobilization techniques to the wrist and forearm, you note increased flexibility and movement. Perform an interim assessment for AROM of the L forearm and wrist, and document your results accordingly.

INTERIM ASSESSMENT SCENARIO 8

Items Needed to Complete Scenario

Stethoscope
Blood Pressure Cuff
Standard Goniometer

This 47 y/o client with a history of hypertension has been treated in your facility after a rotator cuff repair of the L shoulder. Perform an interim assessment of her vital signs and PROM measurements for her L shoulder. Document the objective data in an appropriate progress note.

INTERIM ASSESSMENT SCENARIO 9

Items Needed to Complete Scenario

Knowledge of Manual Muscle Testing

The same client as in Interim Assessment Scenario 8 is in need of an interim assessment of manual muscle testing for the shoulder. Perform an appropriate interim assessment, and document your results appropriately.

INTERIM ASSESSMENT SCENARIO 10

Items Needed to Complete Scenario

Knowledge of Manual Muscle Testing

The client you have been treating sustained a distal R humeral fracture 8 weeks ago. Your treatment has included the use of moist heat, ROM exercises, and strengthening exercises. Perform an interim assessment of manual muscle testing for the elbow. Document your results accordingly.

INTERIM ASSESSMENT SCENARIO 11

Items Needed to Complete Scenario

Knowledge of Manual Muscle Testing
Hand Dynamometer

The client you have been treating was injured in a MVA 6 weeks ago, sustaining multiple trauma to the upper extremities and trunk. In the accident she "injured her L hand some how" but sustained no fractures. The treatment has consisted of electrical stimulation for pain control as well as ROM and strengthening exercises to the L UE. Perform an interim assessment of manual muscle testing for the wrist and functional grip strength test of the hand. Document your results accordingly.

INTERIM ASSESSMENT SCENARIO 12

Items Needed to Complete Scenario

Knowledge of Manual Muscle Testing

The client you have been treating has been receiving ultrasound and moist heat for greater trochanteric bursitis on the left. Perform an interim assessment of manual muscle testing for the hip. Document your results accordingly.

INTERIM ASSESSMENT SCENARIO 13

Items Needed to Complete Scenario

Knowledge of Manual Muscle Testing

This 16 y/o female track athlete injured her R knee in a fall over a hurdle. The diagnosis was a patellar contusion. She has been treated for 2 weeks receiving stretching, ice, and electrical stimulation for pain. Perform an interim assessment of manual muscle testing for the knee. Document your results accordingly.

INTERIM ASSESSMENT SCENARIO 14

Items Needed to Complete Scenario

Knowledge of Manual Muscle Testing

Your client is recovering 6 weeks after a grade II lateral ankle sprain that was sustained as she stepped into a hole at a local park. Perform an interim assessment of manual muscle testing for the ankle. Document your results accordingly.

INTERIM ASSESSMENT SCENARIO 15

Items Needed to Complete Scenario

Standard Goniometer
Tape Measure

This 21 y/o male football player has been receiving physical therapy under your care for 4 weeks. His original injury was a grade III ACL tear with meniscal involvement on the right, and he is now recovering 5 weeks after reconstructive surgery to repair the torn ligament and removal of the injured meniscus (partial menisectomy). Treatment has included AROM exercises, closed-chain exercises (WBAT), electric stimulation to R quadiceps for muscle re-education and cryotherapy for edema and pain management. You are to perform an interim assessment of R knee AROM and PROM, followed by circumferential measurements of the R thigh, calf, and knee joint. Document your results accordingly.

INTERIM ASSESSMENT SCENARIO 16

Items Needed to Complete Scenario

Standard Goniometer
Tape Measure

This 76 y/o female client has been seen in her home for the last 3 weeks after returning from an extended care facility. She received reconstructive surgery to her L shoulder resulting in a total shoulder arthroplasty. Surgery was performed as a result of a humeral fracture sustained due to a fall that occurred while she was watering her plants outdoors. She c/o moderate pain in her L shoulder and hand, and there has been persistent edema in her L UE and hand. The surgical incision is healed with no drainage or open areas noted. Perform an interim assessment of PROM to the L UE and circumferential measurements using your tape measure. Document your results accordingly. Discuss your results with your supervising therapist. What concerns are there for this client? Are there other methods for measuring UE or hand edema that may be effective?

INTERIM ASSESSMENT SCENARIO 17

Items Needed to Complete Scenario

Knowledge of Manual Muscle Testing for Cervical Region

This client is close to achieving her established therapy goals after sustaining a muscular strain (grade I) to her neck extensor muscles in an MVA. Perform an interim assessment of cervical muscle strength to report back to the supervising PT. Document your results accordingly.

INTERIM ASSESSMENT SCENARIO 18

Items Needed to Complete Scenario

Tape Measure

This 84 y/o client is home from an extended care facility where she was undergoing rehabilitation after a fractured L ankle. On your regular home health visit, she c/o swelling in her affected leg distally. Perform circumferential measurements to the L ankle and lower leg and report to the supervising PT. What instructions would you give this client? What is your rationale for giving these instructions?

INTERIM ASSESSMENT SCENARIO 19

Items Needed to Complete Scenario

Tape Measure

This 58 y/o client has been receiving kidney dialysis 2×/wk over the last 6 months. The client has recently been experiencing significant swelling and pain in the L elbow of the area where the dialysis machine tubes are attached. The client has an indwelling venous portal for easy venous access, and the surgeon is concerned about the excessive swelling. The surgeon referred the client to physical therapy for assessment and treatment of the edema. The supervising PT has implemented a treatment program of intermittent compression pump and elevation to help with edema control. After treating this client, perform a circumferential measurement to report to the supervising PT regarding progress.

 # ORTHOPEDIC MODALITIES

MODALITIES SCENARIO 1

Items Needed to Complete Scenario

TENS Unit

After evaluation by the supervising PT, you are to instruct a patient on the home use of a TENS unit for a chronic cervical dysfunction. The patient has already been instructed and issued a written HEP for cervical ROM ex and is awaiting your instructions.

MODALITIES SCENARIO 2

Items Needed to Complete Scenario

Lumbar Traction Unit
Hot Packs
Massage Lotion

This 34 y/o male client has subacute back dysfunction. The treatment protocol prescribed by the supervising PT calls for lumbar traction with moist heat followed by lumbar massage. Perform treatment, and document your session accordingly.

MODALITIES SCENARIO 3

Items Needed to Complete Scenario

TENS Unit

The supervising PT has instructed you to apply a TENS unit to an outpatient who has been complaining of L lateral hip pain and needs to control pain when she is working. What precautions and protocols for use would you suggest to this client?

MODALITIES SCENARIO 4

Items Needed to Complete Scenario

> Electrical Stimulation Unit
> Cryotherapy

This client has already been evaluated by a PT in your outpatient facility and has a diagnosis of acute grade II R ankle sprain. Symptoms include client's complaints of pain with weight bearing. Signs include moderate swelling anteriorly and laterally in the R ankle as well as significant pain to palpation over sinus tarsi region and inferior to the lateral malleolus. ROM is significantly limited because of pain. X-rays have ruled out fracture. The POT includes E-stim and ice to the R ankle for pain control and decrease of swelling. Perform treatment appropriately, and document your session accordingly.

MODALITIES SCENARIO 5

Items Needed to Complete Scenario

> Moist Heat
> IFC

This client has been evaluated by a PT in your facility. You notice the diagnosis is as follows: chronic lumbar strain to paraspinal muscles bilaterally L3-S1. Symptoms include client complaints of dull ache in lower back that "doesn't ever go away." Signs are negative for visual deformity in the lumbar region, but the client is tender to palpation over the spinous processes of L3 and L4. Visually inspect and palpate the area to be treated. POT includes (1) MHP, (2) IFC, and (3) soft-tissue massage. Document your session accordingly.

MODALITIES SCENARIO 6

Items Needed to Complete Scenario

> Ultrasound Machine

This client has been evaluated by a PT in your outpatient facility. The diagnosis for this client is a supraspinatus tendinitis of the L UE. The client c/o tenderness in his L shoulder when he abducts his L arm and is point tender to your palpation along the superior aspect of the head of the humerus as you passively extend the client's shoulder. The client notes that this discomfort has persisted for about 2 weeks, and he is unsure why the pain began. The POT calls for an US to the insertion of the supraspinatus tendon. Perform the treatment with appropriate parameters, and document your session accordingly.

MODALITIES SCENARIO 7

Items Needed to Complete Scenario

> Iontophoresis Machine

The diagnosis for this client is R "tennis elbow." The supervising PT designs the POT to include iontophoresis with dexamethasone to R lateral epicondyle. Perform the treatment, and document your session accordingly.

MODALITIES SCENARIO 8

Items Needed to Complete Scenario

Ice Cup

This 15 y/o female soccer player has a history of infrapatellar irritation and most recently has been diagnosed with Osgood-Schlatter disease. The supervising therapist has instructed you to teach the client how to use an ice massage at home to control pain and irritation. Perform the treatment, and document the session accordingly.

MODALITIES SCENARIO 9

Items Needed to Complete Scenario

Ice Pack
CPM Machine

This 57 y/o male client is recovering 1 week after L TKR surgery and has just arrived at home. After the first home health visit by the evaluating PT 2 days ago, you have arrived to follow the established POT, which includes (1) CPM of 2 hours' duration, 3×/day progressing ROM as tol, (2) ice for pain and edema control, (3) quad sets, (4) ROM exercises, (5) patellar mobilization, and (6) progress to PRE when tolerated. Ensure that the CPM machine is properly fit to the client's L knee, and apply the cryotherapy appropriately. Document the session accordingly.

MODALITIES SCENARIO 10

Items Needed to Complete Scenario

Whirlpool Extremity Tank
Elastic Wrapping

This 18 y/o football player has an acutely sprained L ankle (grade II). The supervising PT wants to aggressively treat the ankle as the athlete is anxious to return to play as soon as possible. The chief problems include moderate edema and stiffness. The treatment for this client includes (1) cool whirlpool to promote ROM and reduce swelling, (2) ROM exercises in the tank, and (3) elastic wrap to ankle when client is not in tank. Perform the treatment as outlined, and document the session accordingly.

MODALITIES SCENARIO 11

Items Needed to Complete Scenario

Whirlpool, Lowboy or Full-body

The physician has referred this client who experiences chronic back pain to your facility for whirlpool treatment. The supervising PT, finding no contraindications to the order, has implemented the POT of whirlpool to the lumbar spine. The client reports that the "water massage" makes him feel better. Perform the treatment as outlined, and document the session accordingly.

MODALITIES SCENARIO 12

Items Needed to Complete Scenario

Ultrasound Unit

The supervising PT has delegated a new client to you for implementation of the established POT. The client's diagnosis is greater trochanteric bursitis of the L hip. The client reports significant aching in her L lateral leg that radiates down into her L knee. The POT includes US to the L hip. Perform this aspect of the POT, and document the session accordingly.

 # ORTHOPEDIC MODALITIES AND EXERCISE

MODALITIES AND EXERCISE SCENARIO 1

Items Needed to Complete Scenario

> Intermittent Compression Pump
> Wall Pulley And/or Cane

A 51 y/o female s/p L radical mastectomy arrives for physical therapy with marked edema in her L UE. The evaluation is completed, and you are to document circumference measurements and begin an intermittent compression therapy program to assist with edema reduction. Pay close attention to length of treatment and instructions to the patient. She is very anxious about her condition. Also instruct her on self-ROM exercises at home.

MODALITIES AND EXERCISE SCENARIO 2

Items Needed to Complete Scenario

> Paraffin Bath
> Various Gripping Devices

This 59 y/o male client fell with a resultant fracture to the second and third proximal phalanxes of the R hand. The fractures are now well healed (6 weeks postinjury), but the client is having trouble with flexion of the MCP of the second and third digits of his dominant R hand. The treatment protocol is for paraffin bath followed by Binnell's tendon gliding exercises, various gripping exercises, and mobilization to the MCP of the second and third digits. Perform the prescribed treatment, and document the session accordingly.

MODALITIES AND EXERCISE SCENARIO 3

Items Needed to Complete Scenario

> Standard Walker
> Knee CPM
> FES Unit

This 63 y/o female client is having difficulty contracting her R quadriceps muscle as she is s/p TKR 1 week ago. You have been treating her using CPM, quad sets (which she is having difficulty performing), hamstring stretching, gait training with a walker (WBAT), and transfer training. She can go home from the hospital when her quadriceps become functional. Her incision is healing well, with no signs of infection. Set the client up in a CPM device for R knee, and make a suggestion for improvement to the supervising PT.

MODALITIES AND EXERCISE SCENARIO 4

Items Needed to Complete Scenario

> Short-wave Diathermy
> Straight Cane

This client has been evaluated by a PT in your outpatient facility. The client was found to have chronic greater trochanteric bursitis on the R hip. The POT includes SWD to R hip and fitting the client with a straight cane. Perform the treatment (be sure to check for any precautions or contraindications) and gait-train the client over level and uneven surfaces. Document your session accordingly.

MODALITIES AND EXERCISE SCENARIO 5

Items Needed to Complete Scenario

    US and E-Stim Combination
    Moist Heat
    Wall Pulley

This client has been evaluated by the supervising PT in your facility. The diagnosis is documented as a subacute strain (grade I) of the L supraspinatus muscle. Symptoms include c/o pain over the belly of the muscle and at the muscular insertion. Client also reports pain when she lifts her arm overhead. Signs are negative for visual deformity, and AROM of the L shoulder is flex 0° to 110°, abd 0° to 75°, and ER 0° to 45°, with all other motions WNL. Perform the POT of (1) moist heat, (2) US and E-Stim combination, and (3) AAROM using wall pulley. Document your session accordingly.

MODALITIES AND EXERCISE SCENARIO 6

Items Needed to Complete Scenario

    Cryotherapy
    E-Stim or IFC unit

This client has been evaluated by the supervising PT in your outpatient facility. The diagnosis is acute pain secondary to chondromalacia patellae of the R knee. Symptoms include client's complaints of anterior knee pain when sitting for prolonged periods of time or when climbing stairs. Signs are positive for crepitus posterior to the patella with movement. ROM is full. The POT includes (1) cryotherapy, (2) E-Stim for pain control, (3) quad sets (pain free), (4) SLR and hip adduction, PRE 1-lb weight cuff distally around ankle ×2 sets of 20 reps. Document your session accordingly.

MODALITIES AND EXERCISE SCENARIO 7

Items Needed to Complete Scenario

    US Machine
    Resistive Tubing or Weight Cuffs.

The diagnosis for this client is R "tennis elbow." The supervising PT designs the POT to include (1) US, (2) R common wrist extensor stretching, (3) PRE to R wrist extensors, and (4) ice after exercise. Perform the treatment session, and document your session accordingly.

MODALITIES AND EXERCISE SCENARIO 8

Items Needed to Complete Scenario

    Whirlpool Extremity Tank
    Therapeutic Putty
    Knowledge of Joint Mobilization Techniques

This client has been treated for a crush injury to the R hand that was sustained in a fall from a ladder. The fractures in the hand are healed, but the client is still having ROM and strength deficits in all digits. She has difficulty making a fist and has generally no strength in her grip. The supervising PT has identified the treatment to include

(1) whirlpool for ROM exercise, (2) mobilization to the MCP and PIP joints of digits 2 through 4, and (3) gripping exercises to R hand. Perform the treatment as indicated, and document your session accordingly.

MODALITIES AND EXERCISE SCENARIO 9

Items Needed to Complete Scenario

> Bucket Large Enough for an Ankle and Foot
> Ice
> Ankle ROM Exercise Handout
> Elastic Wrap

This college baseball player has been referred to your clinic from an orthopedic surgeon for an acute ankle sprain (grade I) on the right. Because of an insurance visit limitation, the client has one visit to physical therapy. The supervising PT has evaluated the client and established a treatment program of home icing, AROM, compression and gait as tol. The supervising PT has asked you to instruct the client in (1) the use of an ice bucket at home to do ROM exercises in the bucket, (2) compression and elevation of ankle, (3) home ankle ROM program, and (4) gait WBAT. Perform the treatment session, and document your session accordingly.

 # ORTHOPEDIC EXERCISE

EXERCISE SCENARIO 1

Items Needed to Complete Scenario

> HEP for ACL Rehabilitation

This 16 y/o female basketball player is s/p ACL reconstruction (2 weeks) on her R knee. This is her second visit for physical therapy, and the supervising PT wants you to instruct her in a rehab program as she is limited to one more visit because of managed care limitations. She must perform her exercise program independently. She has fair–quadriceps at this time, has difficulty performing an SLR, and uses a protective immobilizer and one crutch for gait assistance. Demonstrate her HEP and have her perform a return demonstration. Be sure to include a discussion about signs of infection and progression of the exercise program. Issue the client a written HEP.

EXERCISE SCENARIO 2

Items Needed to Complete Scenario

> HEP for THR

This client is 6 weeks s/p THR on the left. The client does not complain of pain and is using a standard walker for ambulating. Gait deviations include a lateral trunk lurch as he brings his body weight over his L LE during stance phase to help stabilize the pelvis. Review THR precautions with the client and ensure that his exercises are adequate. Give the client written instructions. Tell your supervising PT what you think may be causing the lateral trunk lurch.

EXERCISE SCENARIO 3

Items Needed to Complete Scenario

> HEP for Ankle
> LE Proprioception Exercise

After evaluation by the supervising PT, you are to instruct this 16 y/o male basketball player in an ankle rehabilitation program. He is s/p (4 weeks) grade II lateral ankle sprain, with no pain or swelling. ROM is not limited at this time, but his balance "just doesn't feel right, yet." He is notably weak in ankle PF and eversion. Issue the client a written HEP, and document your treatment.

EXERCISE SCENARIO 4

Items Needed to Complete Scenario

> HEP for Grip Strengthening
> Gripping Items

This 35 y/o female client is 4 weeks s/p CTR on the right. The supervising PT has ordered client instruction in soft-tissue self-mobilization techniques to the surgical release region. The scar appears well healed, with no gapping or drainage present, but significant soft-tissue limitations are noted. Instruct the client in gripping and coordination exercises that she may perform at home.

EXERCISE SCENARIO 5

Items Needed to Complete Scenario

> Balance and Proprioceptive Exercises for LE

This client is 6 months s/p R ACL reconstruction. You are to instruct the client in four advanced balancing and proprioceptive exercises that the client can perform at home. He is anxious to return to playing basketball in the fall.

EXERCISE SCENARIO 6

Items Needed to Complete Scenario

> None

The client is a 73 y/o male client who has been hospitalized in the ICU of your hospital after a fall at home. He has suffered an injury to his head and a fracture to his R hip. Currently the client is unconscious and generally non responsive. The R LE is kept in skeletal traction fixating the hip fracture until the orthopedic surgeon is able to repair the fracture. The supervising PT in your department feels that this client is at risk for developing loss of ROM in the L LE and Bil UE. The established POT includes PROM exercises to Bil UE and L LE. Perform the treatment, and document your session accordingly.

EXERCISE SCENARIO 7

Items Needed to Complete Scenario

> Gait Belt
> Standard Walker
> Wheelchair
> CPM Machine

This client is a 54 y/o female s/p 1 week R TKR. The physician's orders instruct that the client is to be PWB on the R LE to 50 lbs. The physical therapy POT includes (1) gait training with standard walker over level surfaces, (2) AROM to R knee, (3) quad sets, (4) ankle pumps, (5) patellar mobilization, (6) CPM bid for 2-hour duration. Perform the treatment, and document your session appropriately.

EXERCISE SCENARIO 8

Items Needed to Complete Scenario

> A Partner
> Knowledge of PNF Stretching Techniques

This 20 y/o male basketball player has been experiencing L hamstring problems all season. The supervising PT has seen the client intermittently during the season as reinjury to the hamstring muscle occurs. Under the current plan, the supervising PT has written orders for active inhibition stretching techniques for the hamstring muscle, including CR, HR, and HRAM to help improve flexibility. Perform a treatment session that includes these stretching techniques. Explain the neurophysiological basis for each therapeutic intervention. If reinjury continues, what instructions would you give the athlete? What factors lead to this determination?

EXERCISE SCENARIO 9

Items Needed to Complete Scenario

> Straight Cane
> Over-the-door Pulleys

The supervising PT has asked you to instruct a client in three different ways to perform self-ROM to the shoulder for a home program. Instruct her in the appropriate parameters of the HEP.

EXERCISE SCENARIO 10

Items Needed to Complete Scenario

> Ankle Weight

Your client describes that when the ankle weight is placed around her thigh when performing an SLR that it is significantly easier to perform than if the weight is around the ankle. Describe the mechanical principles behind this process, and describe their clinical relevance.

EXERCISE SCENARIO 11

Items Needed to Complete Scenario

> Elastic Tubing or Band
> Shoulder Home Program

This client has been treated in your facility for impingement syndrome of the R shoulder. The supervising PT feels that he is ready for a home program of PRE for the R shoulder. Instruct the client in a home program of PRE using elastic tubing or band. Document the parameters of the home program.

EXERCISE SCENARIO 12

Items Needed to Complete Scenario

> Elastic Tubing or Weight
> Elbow Home Program

You have been treating a client who sustained a proximal radial fracture in a skiing accident. After conferring with the supervising PT, you feel that the client is ready to progress to strengthening exercises. Design and implement a strengthening program for the client to use at home including elbow and forearm motions. Document your session accordingly.

EXERCISE SCENARIO 13

Items Needed to Complete Scenario

> Elastic Tubing or Weight
> Resistive Putty
> Wrist and Hand Home Program

Your client has sustained a massive crush injury to his L hand in an industrial accident. After discussing his progress with the supervising PT, the client's POT has been upgraded to include PRE for the L wrist and hand. Design a strengthening program for the client to use at home, and instruct the client in the program. Ensure that the program addresses the functional needs of the client. Document your session accordingly.

EXERCISE SCENARIO 14

Items Needed to Complete Scenario

> Resistive Tubing or Weights
> Hip Home Program

This client is recovering from a greater trochanteric bursitis of the L hip. The supervising PT wants you to instruct the client in PREs for the L hip. Design a program for the client to use at home, and instruct the client in the program. Document your session accordingly.

EXERCISE SCENARIO 15

Items Needed to Complete Scenario

> Resistive Tubing or Weights
> Knee Home Program

This 14 y/o hockey player is recovering from tendinitis to his L patellar tendon. The supervising PT wants you to instruct him in a home program of PRE for the L knee. Design a program for the client to use at home, and instruct the client in the program. Document your session accordingly.

EXERCISE SCENARIO 16

Items Needed to Complete Scenario

> Resistive Tubing or Weights
> Ankle Home Program

Your instructor in PTA school twisted her ankle as she was climbing off of a mat after closing a window. The physician cleared her injury of any fracture, diagnosing the injury as a grade I lateral ankle sprain, and instructed her "to keep off the ankle until it was feeling better." After the acute injury has resolved, the instructor has asked you to demonstrate your knowledge of a home program by instructing her in PRE for the R ankle. Design an appropriate program for the instructor to use at home if it were prescribed by the supervising therapist.

EXERCISE SCENARIO 17

Items Needed to Complete Scenario

Variety of Tools Such as a Straight Cane, Wall, Balance Board, or Slide Board
Scapular Stabilization Program

This 14 y/o female athlete has been having scapular and shoulder pain on the R side. The supervising PT has identified the problem as poor scapular stabilization strength. The supervising PT has instructed you to design and instruct this client in scapular stabilization exercises. Document your session accordingly.

EXERCISE SCENARIO 18

Items Needed to Complete Scenario

Closed-Chain Exercise Program for LE

Your client is an 18 y/o male athlete with an ACL reconstruction on his R knee. He has progressed through his program well and has had no complications in his rehabilitation. The supervising PT has instructed you to begin-closed chain exercises for the LE with this client. Construct a closed-chain Ex program, and instruct the client in the program. Document your session accordingly.

EXERCISE SCENARIO 19

Items Needed to Complete Scenario

William's Flexion Ex Program

The supervising PT has assigned you a client that has subacute low back injury. The diagnosis from the physician is "facet syndrome," with orders to instruct the client in "William's Flexion Ex as tol." The supervising PT agrees with the diagnosis and wants you to instruct this client in a William's flexion Ex protocol. Document your session accordingly.

EXERCISE SCENARIO 20

Items Needed to Complete Scenario

McKenzie Extension Program

The supervising PT has assigned you a client that has a subacute low back injury. The diagnosis from the physician is "bulging disk," with orders to instruct in "Extension exercises as tol." The client has localized lumbar discomfort and pain that radiates into the posterior thigh on the left. The supervising PT agrees with the diagnosis, and wants you to instruct this client in a McKenzie extension Ex protocol. Document your session accordingly.

EXERCISE SCENARIO 21

Items Needed to Complete Scenario

Lumbar Stabilization Program

This client, who works in a local manufacturing plant, has persistent lumbar dysfunction. The supervising PT has instructed you to teach the client in a dynamic lumbar stabilization program to protect his back while he is at work. Document your session accordingly.

EXERCISE SCENARIO 22

Items Needed to Complete Scenario

Cervical Posture Handout

This 38 y/o secretary has been complaining of headaches, eye strain, and a "tired" feeling in the back of her neck. The supervising therapist has evaluated her and established that the problem is postural in nature. The POT is to include (1) postural retraining and (2) cervical isometric exercises. Provide the client with a postural education handout covering the principles of proper posture when sitting at a workstation, and instruct her in cervical isometric exercises. Document your session accordingly.

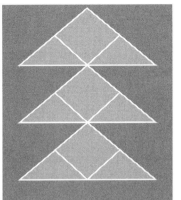

Abbreviations List

The following list contains common abbreviations used by orthopedic physical therapy professionals for documentation purposes. It should not be considered complete nor comprehensive. Before using abbreviations when documenting client status or progression, ensure that their use follows established policy and procedure for the facility. Be aware that there are inherent dangers to documenting with abbreviations, including miscommunication of appropriate information.

↑	increase	c̄	with
↓	decrease	CC	chief complaint
//	parallel	CGA	contact guard assist
abd	abduction	c/o	complains of
add	adduction	CPM	continuous passive motion
ACL	anterior cruciate ligament	CR	contract-relax
ADL	activity of daily living	CTLSO	cervical-thoracic-lumbar-sacral orthosis
AE	above elbow		
AFO	ankle-foot orthosis		
AI	alternating isometrics	CTR	carpal tunnel release
		d/c	discharged or discontinued
AK	above knee		
amb	ambulation	DF	dorsiflexion
AP	anterior-posterior or ankle pump	DJD	degenerative joint disease
AROM	active range of motion	DOB	date of birth
		Dx	diagnosis
AAROM	active assistive range of motion	ER	emergency room or external rotation
as tol	as tolerated	E-Stim	electrical stimulation
Ⓑ or Bil	bilateral	ex	exercise
BE	below elbow	ext or /	extension
bid	twice a day	F	female or fair muscle strength grade
BK	below knee		
BP	blood pressure	FES	functional electrical stimulation
bpm	beats per minute		

flex or √	flexion	**NT**	not tested
FWB	full weight bearing	**NWB**	non–weight bearing
Fx	fracture	**OOB**	out of bed
G	Good muscle strength grade	**OP**	outpatient
GS	gluteal set	**ORIF**	open reduction and internal fixation
Gt	gait or gait training	**OT**	occupational therapy
HOB	head of bed	**p̄**	after
HEP	home exercise plan (program)	**P**	poor muscle strength grade
HNP	herniated nucleus pulposus	**PCL**	posterior cruciate ligament
HP	hot pack	**PF**	plantar flexion
HR	hold-relax	**PIP**	proximal interphalangeal
HRAM	hold-relax active movement	**PMH**	pertinent medical history
Hx	history		
Ⓘ or Ind	Independent	**PNF**	proprioceptive neuromuscular facilitation
ICU	intensive care unit		
IEP	individual education program	**postop**	postoperative
IFC	interferential current	**POT**	plan of treatment
IR	internal rotation	**PRE**	progressive resistive exercises
JRA	juvenile rheumatoid arthritis	**prn**	as needed
Jt	joint	**PROM**	passive range of motion
KAFO	knee-ankle-foot orthosis	**pt**	patient
L	left	**PT**	physical therapy or physical therapist
LBP	low back pain		
LCL	lateral collateral ligament (fibular)	**PTA**	physical therapist assistant
LE	lower extremity	**PWB**	partial weight bearing
LOB	loss of balance		
LTG	long-term goal	**qid**	four times a day
M	male	**QS**	quad set
max	maximal or maximum	**R**	right
MCL	medial collateral ligament (tibial)	**RA**	rheumatoid arthritis
		RD	radial deviation
MCP	metacarpophalangeal	**reps**	repetitions
MHP	moist hot pack	**r/o**	rule out
min	minimal or minimum	**ROM**	range of motion
MMT	manual muscle test	**RR**	rhythmical rotation
mob	mobilization or mobility	**RS**	rhythmical stabilization
mod	moderate or modified	**RTC**	rotator cuff
		RW	rolling walker
MVA	motor vehicle accident	**Rx**	treatment
		SBA	standby assist
N	normal muscle strength grade	**SCI**	spinal cord injury
		Sh	shoulder
N/A	not applicable	**SLR**	straight-leg raise

SOB	short of breath or side of bed	**TKR**	total knee replacement
s/p	status post	**TMJ**	temporomandibular joint
STG	short-term goal		
sup	superior or supervised	**TTWB**	touch toe weight bearing
SWD	short-wave diathermy	**Tx**	traction
		tx	treatment
T	trace muscle strength grade	**UE**	upper extremity
		UD	ulnar deviation
TBI	traumatic brain injury	**US**	ultrasound
TDWB	touch down weight bearing	**WB**	weight bearing
		WBAT	weight bearing as tolerated
TENS	transcutaneous electrical nerve stimulation	**wc or w/c**	wheelchair
		WFL	within functional limits
THA	total hip arthroplasty		
Ther Ex	therapeutic exercise	**WNL**	within normal limits
THR	total hip replacement	**×1**	one person, one time
		×2	two persons, two times
tid	three times a day		
TKA	total knee arthroplasty	**y/o**	year(s) old
TKE	terminal knee extension		

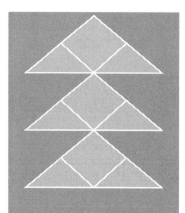

appendix B

Recommended Readings

PART I GENERAL ORTHOPEDIC PRINCIPLES

CHAPTER 1   ROLE OF THE PHYSICAL THERAPIST ASSISTANT IN ORTHOPEDICS

Gahimer, JE, and Domholdt, E: Amount of patient education in physical therapy practice and perceived effects. Phys Ther 76:1089, 1996.

Guide for Conduct of the Affiliate Member. APTA Core Documents. PT Magazine of Physical Therapy 6(1):81, 1998.

Robinson, AJ, et al: Physical therapists' perception of the roles of the physical therapist assistant. Phys Ther 74:571, 1994.

Schunk, C, et al: PTA practice: In reality. Clinical Management 12(6):88, 1992.

Sluijs, EM, et al: Correlates of exercise compliance in physical therapy. Phys Ther 73:771, 1993.

CHAPTER 2   EXERCISE PRINCIPLES

Bandy, WD, et al: Adaptations of skeletal muscle to resistance training. J Orthop Sports Phys Ther 12:248, 1990.

Binder-Macleod, SA: Introduction: Skeletal muscle. Phys Ther 73:829, 1993.

Clamann, HP: Motor unit recruitment and the gradation of muscle force. Phys Ther 73:830, 1993.

Davies, GJ, et al: Assessment of strength. In Malone, TR et al (eds): Orthopedic and Sports Physical Therapy, ed 3. Mosby, St Louis, MO, 1997.

Dean, E: Physiology and therapeutic implications of negative work: A review. Phys Ther 68:233, 1988.

Fitzgerald, GK, et al: Exercise-induced muscle soreness after concentric and eccentric isokinetic contractions. Phys Ther 71:505, 1991.

Hopp, JF: Effects of age and resistance training on skeletal muscle: A review. Phys Ther 73:361, 1993.

Kisner, C, and Colby, LA: Therapeutic Exercise: Foundations and Techniques, ed 3. FA Davis, Philadelphia, 1996.

Lippert, L: Clinical Kinesiology for the Physical Therapist Assistant, ed 2. FA Davis, Philadelphia. 1994.

Lieber, RL, and Bodine-Fowler, SC: Skeletal muscle mechanics: Implications for rehabilitation. Phys Ther 73:844, 1993.

Norkin, CC, and Levangie, PK: Joint Structure and Function: A Comprehensive Analysis, ed 2. FA Davis, Philadelphia, 1992.

Prentice, WE: Rehabilitation Techniques in Sports Medicine, ed 2. Mosby, St Louis, MO, 1994.

Salter, RB: Textbook of Disorders and Injuries of the Musculoskeletal System, ed 2. Williams & Wilkins, Baltimore, 1983.

Sanders, B: Exercise and rehabilitation concepts. In Malone, TR (eds): Orthopedic and Sports Physical Therapy, ed 3. Mosby, St Louis, MO, 1997.

CHAPTER 3   RANGE OF MOTION

Bandy, WD, et al: The effect of time and frequency of static stretching on flexibility of the hamstring muscles. Phys Ther 77:1090, 1997.

Clark, S, et al: Effects of ipsilateral anterior thigh soft tissue stretching on passive unilateral straight-leg raise. J Orthop Sports Phys Ther 29:4, 1999.

Gajdosik, RL: Effects of static stretching on maximal length and resistance to passive stretch on short hamstring muscles. J Orthop Sports Phys Ther 14:250, 1991.

Gogia, PP, et al: Reliability and validity of goniometric measurements at the knee. Phys Ther 67:192, 1987.

James, B, and Parker, AW: Active and passive mobility of lower limb joints in elderly men and women. Am J Phys Med. 68:162, 1989.

Johnson, J, and Silverberg, R: Serial casting of the lower extremity to correct contractures during the acute phase of burn care. Phys Ther 75:262, 1995.

Kisner, C, and Colby, LA: Therapeutic Exercise: Foundations and Techniques, ed 3. FA Davis, Philadelphia, 1996.

Knott, M, and Voss, D: Proprioceptive Neuromuscular Facilitation: Patterns and Techniques. Harper & Row, New York, 1968.

Light, KE, et al: Low-load prolonged stretch vs. high-load brief stretch in treating knee contractures. Phys Ther 64:330, 1984.

Lippert, L: Clinical Kinesiology for the Physical Therapist Assistant, ed 2. FA Davis, Philadelphia, 1994.

McClure, PW, et al: The use of splints in the treatment of joint stiffness: Biological rationale and an algorithm for making clinical decisions. Phys Ther 74:1101, 1994.

Moore, MA, and Kukulka, CG: Depression of Hoffmann reflexes following voluntary contraction and implications for proprioceptive neuromuscular facilitation therapy. Phys Ther 71:321, 1991.

Norkin, CC, and White, DJ: Measurement of Joint Motion: A Guide to Goniometry, ed 2. FA Davis, Philadelphia, 1995.

Phillips, WE, and Audet, M: Use of serial casting in the management of knee joint contractures in an adolescent with cerebral palsy. Phys Ther 70:521, 1990.

Prentice, WE: Rehabilitation Techniques in Sports Medicine, ed 2. Mosby, St Louis, MO, 1994.

Rheault, W, et al: Intertester reliability and concurrent validity of fluid based and universal goniometers for active knee flexion. Phys Ther 68:1676, 1988.

Riddle, DL, et al: Goniometric reliability in a clinical setting: Shoulder measurements. Phys Ther 67:68, 1987.

Roach, KE, and Miles, TP: Normal hip and knee active range of motion: The relationship to age: Phys Ther 71:656; 1991.

Rothstein, JM, et al: Goniometric reliability in a clinical setting: Elbow and knee measurements. Phys Ther 63:1611, 1983.

Salter, RB, et al: Clinical application of basic research on continuous passive motion for disorders and injuries of synovial joints. J Orthop Res 1:324, 1984.

Salter, RB: Textbook of Disorders and Injuries of the Musculoskeletal System, ed 2. Williams & Wilkins, Baltimore, 1983.

Watkins, MA, et al: Reliability of goniometric measurements and visual estimates of knee range of motion obtained in a clinical setting. Phys Ther 71:90, 1991.

CHAPTER 4 MECHANICAL PROPERTIES OF THE HUMAN BODY

Lippert, L: Clinical Kinesiology for the Physical Therapist Assistant, ed 2. FA Davis, Philadelphia. 1994.

Kisner, C, and Colby, LA: Therapeutic Exercise: Foundations and Techniques, ed 3. FA Davis, Philadelphia, 1996.

Riegger-Krugh, C: Bone. In Malone, TR, et al (eds): Orthopedic and Sports Physical Therapy, ed 3. Mosby, St Louis, MO, 1997.

Salter, RB: Textbook of Disorders and Injuries of the Musculoskeletal System, ed 2. Williams & Wilkins, Baltimore, 1983.

CHAPTER 5 TISSUE RESPONSE TO HEALING

Basso, DM, and Knapp, L: Comparison of two continuous passive motion protocols for patients with total knee implants. Phys Ther 67:360, 1987.

Cailliet, R: Knee Pain and Disability. FA Davis, Philadelphia, 1972.

Covey, MH, et al: Efficacy of continuous passive motion devices with hand burns. J Burns Care Rehabil 9(4):397, 1988.

Cummings, GS, and Tillman, LJ: Remodeling of dense connective tissue in normal adult tissues. In

Currier, DP, and Nelson, RM (eds): Dynamics of Human Biologic Tissues. FA Davis, Philadelphia, 1992.

Davis, D: Continuous passive motion for total knee arthroplasty. Phys Ther 64:709, 1984.

deAndrade, JR, et al: Joint distension and reflex muscle inhibition in the knee. J Bone Joint Surg [Am] 47:313, 1965.

Enneking, WF, and Horowitz, H: The intra-articular effects of immobilization on the human knee. J Bone Joint Surg 54A:973, 1972.

Fredericks, CM, and Saladin, LK: Pathophysiology of the Motor System: Principles and Clinical Presentations. FA Davis, Philadelphia, 1996.

Gose, JC: Continuous passive motion in the postoperative treatment of patients with total knee replacement: A retrospective study. Phys Ther 67:39, 1987.

Hardy, MA: The biology of scar formation. Phys Ther 69:1014, 1989.

Keene, JS, and Malone, TR: Ligament and muscle-tendon unit injuries. In Malone, TR, et al (eds): Orthopedic and Sports Physical Therapy, ed 3. Mosby, St Louis, MO, 1997.

Kisner, C, and Colby, LA: Therapeutic Exercise: Foundations and Techniques, ed 3. FA Davis, Philadelphia, 1996.

Lippert, L: Clinical Kinesiology for the Physical Therapist Assistant, ed 2. FA Davis, Philadelphia, 1994.

MacKay-Lyons, M: Low-load, prolonged stretch in treatment of elbow flexion contractures secondary to head trauma: A case report. Phys Ther 69:292, 1989.

McCarthy, MR, et al: The clinical use of continuous passive motion in physical therapy. J Orthop Sports Phys Ther 15:132, 1992.

Norkin, CC, and Levangie, PK: Joint Structure and Function: A Comprehensive Analysis, ed 2. FA Davis, Philadelphia, 1992.

Noyes, FR: The functional properties of knee ligament and alterations induced by immobilization: A correlative biomechanical and histological study in primates. Clin Orthop 123:210, 1977.

Noyes, FR, and Mangine, RE: Early knee motion after open and arthroscopic anterior cruciate ligament reconstruction. Am J Sports Med 15:149, 1987.

Salter, RB: Textbook of Disorders and Injuries of the Musculoskeletal System, ed 2. Williams & Wilkins, Baltimore, 1983.

Spencer, JD, et al: Knee joint effusion and quadriceps reflex inhibition in man. Arch Phys Med Rehabil 65:171, 1984.

Stap, LJ, and Woodfin, PM: Continuous passive motion in the treatment of knee flexion contractures: A case report. Phys Ther 66:1720, 1986.

Stillwell, DM, et al: Atrophy of quadriceps muscle due to immobilization of the lower extremity. Arch Phys Med Rehabil 48:289, 1967.

Vaughan, VG: Effects of upper limb immobilization on isometric muscle strength, movement time, and triphasic electromyographic characteristics. Phys Ther 69:119, 1989.

CHAPTER 6   NORMAL AGING

Aisenbrey, JA: Exercise in the prevention and management of osteoporosis. Phys Ther 67:1100, 1987.

Brown, M: Resistance exercise effects on aging skeletal muscles in rats. Phys Ther 69:46, 1989.

Di Fabio, RP, and Emasithi A: Aging and the mechanisms underlying head and postural control during voluntary motion. Phys Ther 77:458, 1997.

Hopp, JF: Effects of age and resistance training on skeletal muscle: A review. Phys Ther 73:361, 1993.

Hollander, LL: Normal aging. In Logigian, MK (ed): Adult Rehabilitation: A Team Approach for Therapists. Little, Brown & Co, Boston, 1982.

Jackson, O: Brain function, aging, and dementia. In Umphred, DA (ed). Neurological Rehabilitation, ed 3. Mosby, St Louis, MO, 1995.

Kisner C, and Colby, LA: Therapeutic Exercise: Foundations and Techniques, ed 3. FA Davis, Philadelphia, 1996.

Lewis, CB: Aging: The Health Care Challenge. FA Davis, Philadelphia, 1985.

Lewis, CB, and Bottemley, JM: Geriatric Physical Therapy: A Clinical Approach. Appleton & Lange, Norwalk, CT, 1994.

Lewthwaite, R: Motivational considerations in physical activity involvement. Phys Ther 70:808, 1990.

Light, KE: Information processing for motor performance in aging adults. Phys Ther 70:820, 1990.

Salter, RB: Textbook of Disorders and Injuries of the Musculoskeletal System. Williams & Wilkins, Baltimore, 1983.

Schmitz, TJ: Sensory assessment. In O'Sullivan, SB, and Schmitz, TJ (eds): Physical Rehabilitation: Assessment and Treatment, ed 3. FA Davis, 1994.

Shumway-Cook, A, et al: Predicting the probability for falls in community-dwelling older adults. Phys Ther 77:812, 1997.

Thompson, LV: Effects of age and training on skeletal muscle physiology and performance. Phys Ther 74:77, 1994.

Van Sant, F: Life-span development in functional tasks. Phys Ther 70:788, 1990.

Woollacott, MJ, and Shumway-Cook A: Changes in posture control across the life span: A systems approach. Phys Ther 70:799, 1990.

CHAPTER 7   CONCEPTS OF MOBILIZATION

Farrell, JP, and Jensen, GM: Manual therapy: A critical assessment of role in the profession of physical therapy. Phys Ther 72:843, 1992.

Di Fabio, RP: Efficacy of manual therapy. Phys Ther 72:853, 1992.

Hoppenfeld, S: Physical Examination of the Spine and Extremities. Appleton-Century-Crofts, Norwalk, CT, 1976.

Kessler, RM, and Hertling, D: Management of Common Musculoskeletal Disorders: Physical Therapy Principles and Methods, ed 3. Lippincott, Philadelphia, PA, 1996.

Kisner, C, and Colby, LA: Therapeutic Exercise: Foundations and Techniques, ed 3. FA Davis, Philadelphia, PA, pp 183–233, 1996.

Riddle, DL: Measurements of accessory motion: critical issues and related concepts. Phys Ther 72:865, 1992.

PART II MANAGEMENT OF ORTHOPEDIC CONDITIONS

CHAPTER 8   PEDIATRIC CLIENTS

Behrens, BJ, and Michlovitz, SL: Physical Agents: Theory and Practice for the Physical Therapist Assistant. FA Davis, Philadelphia, 1996.

Brotzman, SB (ed): Clinical Orthopaedic Rehabilitation. Mosby, St Louis, MO, 1996.

Guide to Physical Therapist Practice. Phys Ther 77:1163, 1997.

Kessler, RM, and Hertling, D: Management of Common Musculoskeletal Disorders: Physical Therapy Principles and Methods, ed 3. Lippincott, Philadelphia, 1996.

Kisner, C, and Colby, LA: Therapeutic Exercise: Foundations and Techniques, ed 3. FA Davis, Philadelphia, 1996.

Malone, TR, et al (eds): Orthopedic and Sports Physical Therapy, ed 3. Mosby, St Louis, MO, 1997.

Pediatric Orthopedics, pt I. Phys Ther 71:875, 1991.

Pediatric Orthopedics, pt II. Phys Ther 72:1, 1992.

Rothstein, et al: The Rehabilitation Specialist's Handbook, ed 2. FA Davis, Philadelphia, 1998.

Staheli, LT: Pediatric Orthopaedic Secrets. Hanley & Belfus, Philadelphia, 1997.

CHAPTER 9   INJURIES FROM AN ACTIVE LIFESTYLE

ACL surgery and rehabilitation (special section). J Orthop Sports Phys Ther 15:256, 1992.

Behrens, BJ, and Michlovitz, SL: Physical Agents: Theory and Practice for the Physical Therapist Assistant. FA Davis, Philadelphia, 1996.

Brotzman, SB (ed): Clinical Orthopaedic Rehabilitation. Mosby, St Louis, MO, 1996.

Calliet, R: Foot and Ankle Pain, ed 2. FA Davis, Philadelphia, 1983.

Guide to Physical Therapist Practice. Phys Ther 77:1163, 1997.

Kessler, RM, and Hertling, D: Management of Common Musculoskeletal Disorders: Physical Therapy Principles and Methods, ed 3. Lippincott, Philadelphia, 1996.

Kisner, C, and Colby, LA: Therapeutic Exercise: Foundations and Techniques, ed 3. FA Davis, Philadelphia, 1996.

Malone, TR, et al (eds): Orthopedic and Sports Physical Therapy, ed 3. Mosby, St Louis, MO, 1997.

Outcomes Effectiveness of Physical Therapy: An Annotated Bibliography. American Physical Therapy Association, Alexandria, VA, 1994.

Prentice, WE: Rehabilitation Techniques in Sports Medicine, ed 2. Mosby, St Louis, MO, 1994.

Rothstein, JM, et al: The Rehabilitation Specialist's Handbook, ed 2. FA Davis, Philadelphia, 1998.

CHAPTER 10   REPETITIVE STRESS OR WORK-RELATED INJURIES

Behrens, BJ, and Michlovitz, SL: Physical Agents: Theory and Practice for the Physical Therapist Assistant. FA Davis, Philadelphia, 1996.

Brotzman, SB (ed): Clinical Orthopaedic Rehabilitation. Mosby, St Louis, MO, 1996.

Calliet, R: Low Back Pain Syndrome, ed 3. FA Davis, Philadelphia, 1981.

Calliet, R: Neck and Arm Pain, ed 2. FA Davis, Philadelphia, 1981.

Guide to Physical Therapist Practice. Phys Ther 77:1163, 1997.

Kessler, RM, and Hertling, D: Management of Common Musculoskeletal Disorders: Physical Therapy Principles and Methods, ed 3. Lippincott, Philadelphia, 1996.

Kisner, C, and Colby, LA: Therapeutic Exercise: Foundations and Techniques, ed 3. FA Davis, Philadelphia, 1996.

Malone, TR, et al (eds): Orthopedic and Sports Physical Therapy, ed 3. Mosby, St Louis, MO, 1997.

Nordin, M, et al: Musculoskeletal Disorders in the Workplace. Mosby, St Louis, 1997.

Outcomes Effectiveness of Physical Therapy: An Annotated Bibliography. American Physical Therapy Association, Alexandria, VA, 1994.

Rothstein, JM, et al: The Rehabilitation Specialist's Handbook, ed 2. FA Davis, Philadelphia, 1998.

CHAPTER 11   GERIATRIC POPULATION

Behrens, BJ, and Michlovitz, SL: Physical Agents: Theory and Practice for the Physical Therapist Assistant. FA Davis, Philadelphia, 1996.

Brotzman, SB (ed): Clinical Orthopaedic Rehabilitation. Mosby, St Louis, MO, 1996.

Calliet, R: Hand Pain and Impairment, ed 3. FA Davis, Philadelphia, 1982.

Guide to Physical Therapist Practice. Phys Ther 77:1163, 1997.

Kessler, RM, and Hertling, D: Management of Common Musculoskeletal Disorders: Physical Therapy Principles and Methods, ed 3. Lippincott, Philadelphia, 1996.

Kisner, C, and Colby, LA: Therapeutic Exercise: Foundations and Techniques, ed 3. FA Davis, Philadelphia, 1996.

Lewis, CB: Aging: the Health Care Challenge. FA Davis, Philadelphia, 1985.

Lewis, CB, and Bottemley, JM: Geriatric Physical Therapy: A Clinical Approach. Appleton & Lange, Norwalk, CT, 1994.

May, BJ: Home Health and Rehabilitation: Concepts of Care. FA Davis, Philadelphia, 1993.

Malone, TR, et al (eds): Orthopedic and Sports Physical Therapy, ed 3. Mosby, St Louis, MO, 1997.

Outcomes Effectiveness of Physical Therapy: An Annotated Bibliography. American Physical Therapy Association, Alexandria, VA, 1994.

Rothstein, JM, et al: The Rehabilitation Specialist's Handbook, ed 2. FA Davis, Philadelphia, 1998.

INDEX

Italic numbers indicate figures; italic *t* indicates tables.